Augmented Wellness

Ben Othman Soufiane • Chinmay Chakraborty
Bhuvan Unhelkar
Editors

Augmented Wellness

Exploring the Power of VR and AR in Healthcare

Springer

Editors
Ben Othman Soufiane
Applied College
King Faisal University
Al-Ahsa, Arabie Saoudite

Chinmay Chakraborty
Electronics & Communication Engineering
Birla Institute of Technology
Mesra, Jharkhand, India

Bhuvan Unhelkar
Muma College of Business
University of South Florida
Tampa, FL, USA

ISBN 978-981-96-2954-1 ISBN 978-981-96-2952-7 (eBook)
https://doi.org/10.1007/978-981-96-2952-7

This Springer imprint is published by the registered company Springer Nature Singapore Pte Ltd.
The registered company address is: 152 Beach Road, #21-01/04 Gateway East, Singapore 189721, Singapore

Contents

Chapter 1
Virtual Reality Mental Health Interventions: AR/VR Solutions for Well-being

S. Padmapriya, Priyanka Torne, Abhra Pratip Ray, Ankur Gupta, Rohit Anand, and Vishal Jain

Abstract Virtual Reality along with Augmented Reality technologies have emerged as potential tools in case of transforming mental health therapies, providing creative methods for enhancing well-being. This abstract examines the emerging subject of VR Mental Health Interventions along with its potential to revolutionize treatment approaches. VR/AR solutions provide realistic and interactive settings that replicate real-life situations, allowing people to face and address different mental health issues such as anxiety disorders, PTSD, phobias, and depression. VR/AR therapies cater to the different requirements of mental health care by customizing treatment experiences and providing access to those who encounter obstacles in receiving conventional therapy. Moreover, these technologies improve emotional control, compassion, and interpersonal abilities by offering chances to practice communication and social interactions in a secure and encouraging virtual setting. As advancements in research and development continue, virtual reality and augmented reality solutions show significant potential in enhancing mental well-being in the digital

S. Padmapriya
Department of Computer Science, SRM Trichy Arts and Science College, Irungalur, Tamil Nadu, India

P. Torne
Department of Electronics, SAVPM's Sancheti College of Arts, Commerce and Science, Pune, Maharashtra, India

A. P. Ray
Department of Physics, KSPM, Latur's Janvikas Mahavidyalaya, Bansarola, Maharashtra, India

A. Gupta
Department of Computer Science and Engineering, Vaish College of Engineering, Rohtak, Haryana, India

R. Anand (✉)
Department of ECE, G.B. Pant DSEU Okhla-1 Campus (formerly GBPEC), New Delhi, India

V. Jain
Department of Computer Science and Engineering, School of Engineering and Technology, Sharda University, Greater Noida, Uttar Pradesh, India

B. O. Soufiane et al. (eds.), *Augmented Wellness*,
https://doi.org/10.1007/978-981-96-2952-7_1

era, providing a revolutionary approach to mental healthcare. This study explores the potential of VR along with AR in healthcare, focusing on patient treatment, medical training, and health education. It evaluates the impact of VR along with AR on patient outcomes, assesses benefits along with limitations, and anticipates future trends in these technologies, ultimately contributing to augmented wellness.

Keywords Augmented reality · Virtual reality · Healthcare · patient care · Well-being · Immersive therapy · Cognitive behavioral therapy (CBT) · Exposure therapy · Anxiety treatment · Depression management · PTSD (post-traumatic stress disorder)

1 Introduction

These days, AR and VR aren't only for games and amusement; they're also useful for mental health treatments and providing new ways to improve one's mental and emotional wellness. A growing number of therapeutic approaches have begun to include this immersive technology in recent years, providing new opportunities to tackle mental health issues [1]. By using the dynamic and engaging characteristics of VR/AR, mental health interventions may construct safe spaces that mimic real-life situations. Anxiety disorders, PTSD, phobias, depression, and other mental health difficulties may be safely addressed and managed in these simulations [2]. Interventions like this may help people with things like exposure therapy, cognitive behavioral therapy, mindfulness training, and relaxation methods by putting them in virtual settings that they can tailor to their own needs. VR along with AR technologies have potential to greatly improve mental health by allowing for more customized therapy experiences [3]. Virtual settings and situations may be customized to match the unique requirements and preferences of each person, enhancing the engagement and effectiveness of treatment [4]. Also, unlike typical therapy settings, these treatments are accessible to those who may otherwise have trouble getting the mental health care they need because of things like poverty, lack of transportation, or other social or economic obstacles [5]. Improved emotional control, empathy, and social skills have all been noted as potential outcomes of VR/AR therapies. Technology like this allows people to hone their communication abilities in a controlled setting by recreating real-life social encounters and settings. People whose social functioning is impaired due to diseases like social anxiety or autism spectrum disorders may find this very helpful. Research and development in area of VR mental health interventions is ongoing, with a focus on finding new uses for VR and improving current methods to make the most of their therapeutic potential. There is a wide range of exciting potential applications in case of virtual reality along with augmented reality in mental health treatment, from gamified cognitive training programs to immersive relaxing experiences. VR along with AR solutions have potential to greatly contribute to promotion of MH in modern digital era by using technology to provide therapeutic experiences that are immersive, engaging, and tailored to the individual [6].

1.1 Virtual Reality (VR) and Augmented Reality (AR)

Virtual Reality along with Augmented Reality (as shown in Fig. 1.1) are cutting-edge technologies that have transcended their origins in entertainment and gaming to become transformative tools in various fields, including healthcare Both technologies offer immersive experiences that have the potential to revolutionize how perceive and interact our surroundings [7]. In recent years, VR and AR have garnered increasing attention for their applications in healthcare, particularly in realm of MH interventions. These technologies provide innovative solutions for addressing a wide range of MH challenges, from anxiety and depression to PTSD and phobias. By creating virtual environments that simulate real-life scenarios, VR/AR interventions offer individuals a safe space to confront and manage their mental health issues. The integration of VR along with AR into mental health care holds significant promise for improving treatment outcomes and increasing accessibility to therapeutic services. These technologies allow for personalized and immersive experiences, tailored to meet the unique needs of each individual. Moreover, VR/AR interventions have demonstrated effectiveness in enhancing emotional regulation, empathy, and social skills, offering new avenues for promoting overall well-being. As the field of VR and AR continues to advance, so too does their potential to transform mental health care [8].

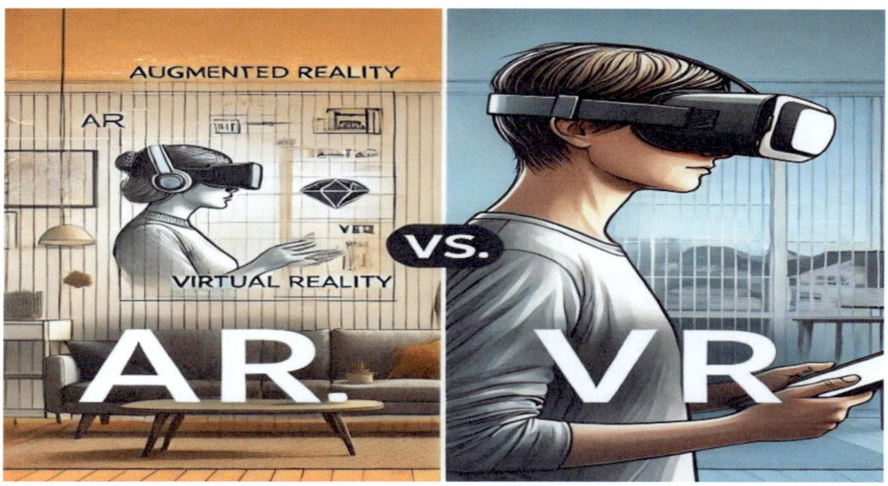

Fig. 1.1 Virtual reality (VR) and augmented reality (AR)

However, challenges remain, including the need for further research, development, and integration into clinical practice [9]. Nevertheless, the emergence of VR and AR as powerful tools for mental health interventions signifies a promising shift towards more innovative and effective approaches to promoting mental well-being in the digital age.

1.2 Mental Health Interventions

VR along with AR have opened up new frontiers in mental health interventions, offering a diverse range of innovative solutions to promote well-being. These immersive technologies provide a platform for various therapeutic approaches, including exposure therapy, cognitive behavioral therapy (CBT), mindfulness and relaxation techniques, social skills training, and psychoeducation. Through VR simulations, individuals can confront their fears and anxieties in controlled environments, gradually building resilience and coping strategies. Cognitive behavioral therapy techniques can be delivered in engaging virtual scenarios, allowing users to challenge negative thought patterns and behaviors. VR environments also facilitate mindfulness and relaxation exercises by transporting users to serene landscapes or overlaying calming cues onto the real world through AR applications. Furthermore, VR simulations provide opportunities for social skills training, enabling individuals to practice interpersonal interactions and communication skills in a safe space. Additionally, these technologies can be utilized for psychoeducation and empathy-building exercises, fostering understanding and compassion towards mental health conditions. By leveraging the immersive and interactive nature of VR along with AR, mental health professionals can offer personalized, engaging, along with accessible interventions to support individuals in their journey towards mental well-being [10].

1.3 Motivation

The necessity to address modern mental health care's complex issues drove "Virtual Reality Mental Health Interventions: AR/VR Solutions for Well-being. Despite advances in therapy methods and treatments, conventional approaches typically lack accessibility, effectiveness, and involvement. This emphasizes the need for innovative, effective mental health treatments that fit the different demands of users. VR and AR provide attractive opportunities for mental health intervention innovation. Immersive technology may transform therapy by offering dynamic, interactive, and customized experiences for patients. VR and AR may provide exposure treatment, cognitive behavioral therapy (CBT), mindfulness, and social skills training by mimicking various surroundings and situations. Growing awareness of the worldwide mental health epidemic motivates VR and AR mental health initiatives.

Mental health diseases affect millions globally, affecting individuals, families, and communities. However, stigma, limited access to treatment, and engagement obstacles hinder people from seeking assistance. VR and AR therapies may provide accessible, engaging, and stigma-free mental health assistance. VR along with AR in MH treatment follows digital health and telemedicine trends. VR along with AR in case of mental health therapies is a logical step toward more holistic and patient-centered therapy as technology advances. These technology may let people obtain mental health care remotely and on their own. Exploring "Virtual Reality Mental Health Interventions: AR/VR Solutions for Well-being" is driven by the need to improve mental health treatment globally. VR and AR may improve mental health assistance delivery, experience, and acceptance. Promoting resilience, empowerment, and well-being for all mental health patients drives this inquiry.

1.4 Challenges

Exploring Virtual Reality Mental Health Interventions: AR/VR Solutions for Well-being presents several notable challenges that need to be addressed for these technologies to reach their full potential in supporting mental health:

- **Accessibility and Affordability**: Despite advancements, VR along with AR technologies can still be expensive and require specialized equipment. Ensuring widespread access to these interventions may pose challenges, particularly for individuals from lower socioeconomic backgrounds or regions with limited resources.
- **Technical Limitations**: VR and AR technologies are constantly evolving, but technical limitations such as motion sickness, visual discomfort, and hardware/software compatibility issues remain. Overcoming these challenges is crucial to ensuring a seamless and comfortable user experience.
- **Ethical Concerns**: As with any emerging technology, VR and AR raise ethical considerations regarding privacy, data security, and informed consent. Safeguarding user data and ensuring ethical use of immersive technologies in mental health interventions is paramount.
- **Validation and Efficacy**: While VR and AR show promise in mental health care, robust empirical evidence demonstrating their efficacy across diverse populations and mental health conditions is still needed. Conducting rigorous research and clinical trials to validate the effectiveness of these interventions is essential.
- **Integration with Traditional Care**: Integrating VR and AR interventions into existing mental health care systems poses logistical challenges, including training clinicians, establishing reimbursement models, and ensuring seamless coordination with traditional therapeutic approaches.
- **User Engagement and Adherence**: Maintaining user engagement and adherence to VR and AR interventions over time can be challenging. Designing

immersive experiences that are engaging, motivating, and tailored to individual preferences is essential for long-term effectiveness.
- **Stigma and Acceptance**: Overcoming stigma associated with mental health and emerging technologies is another hurdle. Educating the public and healthcare providers about potential benefits of VR and AR in mental health care and addressing misconceptions is crucial for widespread acceptance and adoption.
- **Diversity and Inclusivity**: Designing VR and AR interventions that are inclusive and culturally sensitive to diverse populations is essential. Ensuring that these technologies are accessible and relevant across different cultural, linguistic, and socioeconomic contexts is critical for equitable mental health support.

Addressing these challenges will require collaboration among researchers, clinicians, technologists, policymakers, and individuals with lived experience of mental health conditions. By working together to overcome these obstacles, we can harness the full potential of VR along with AR technologies to revolutionize mental health care along with improve the well-being of individuals worldwide.

1.5 Significance of VR and AR Technologies in Revolutionizing Mental Health Therapies

The integration of Virtual Reality (VR) and Augmented Reality (AR) technologies in healthcare is revolutionizing the landscape of mental health therapies. These immersive technologies are redefining traditional therapeutic methods by providing innovative and effective treatment options for a variety of mental health conditions [8]. VR and AR offer unique capabilities to create controlled, immersive environments that can be tailored to individual therapeutic needs, enhancing the patient experience and treatment outcomes. VR, with its ability to simulate real-world environments and scenarios, is being utilized to treat conditions such as anxiety, PTSD, phobias, and depression. Patients can confront and work through their fears in a safe, controlled space, guided by their therapist. AR, on the other hand, overlays digital information onto the real world, providing real-time support and interventions, which can be particularly useful for conditions like social anxiety and cognitive-behavioral therapy (CBT). The potential of these technologies extends beyond treatment to include prevention and early intervention, offering tools for mindfulness, stress reduction, and emotional regulation. VR and AR can simulate environments that teach coping mechanisms and resilience, contributing to overall mental wellness. This introduction will explore the significance of VR and AR in mental health therapies, detailing their current applications, benefits, and the transformative impact they have on patient care. By examining these aspects, we aim to underscore the importance of continued research and development in this field to maximize the therapeutic potential of VR and AR technologies.

The use of Virtual Reality (VR) and Augmented Reality (AR) technologies in mental health therapies represents a groundbreaking shift in how psychological treatments are delivered and experienced. These technologies offer immersive, interactive, and customizable therapeutic environments that address a wide range of mental health issues. VR and AR technologies hold significant potential to revolutionize mental health therapies by providing innovative, effective, and accessible treatment options [9]. Their ability to create immersive and personalized therapeutic experiences, enhance patient engagement, and support real-time interventions positions them as transformative tools in the field of mental health. Continued research and development in this area are essential to fully realize their potential and integrate them into mainstream therapeutic practices.

1.6 Potential of VR Mental Health Interventions

Virtual Reality (VR) has emerged as a promising tool in various fields, and its potential in mental health interventions is particularly transformative. This advanced technology sets the stage for a revolutionary shift in treatment methodologies for several reasons:

- **Immersive Experience**: VR provides an immersive experience that can simulate real-world scenarios in a controlled environment. This immersion allows patients to engage with therapeutic activities more deeply, potentially leading to more effective outcomes.
- **Exposure Therapy**: For conditions such as phobias, PTSD, and anxiety disorders, VR can be used for exposure therapy. Patients can confront their fears in a safe, controlled environment, gradually reducing their symptoms under the guidance of a therapist.
- **Accessibility**: VR can make mental health interventions more accessible. Patients who are unable to visit a therapist in person, whether due to geographical limitations or mobility issues, can still receive high-quality care through VR platforms.
- **Personalization**: Treatment can be tailored to the individual needs of patients. VR programs can adapt in real-time to the patient's responses, providing a personalized therapeutic experience that can be more effective than traditional one-size-fits-all approaches.
- **Engagement and Adherence**: The interactive nature of VR can increase patient engagement and adherence to treatment plans. Patients are more likely to stick with a treatment that is engaging and provides immediate, tangible feedback.
- **Training and Education**: VR can also be used to train mental health professionals, providing them with realistic scenarios to practice and develop their skills. This can lead to better preparedness and higher quality of care.
- **Data Collection and Analysis**: VR systems can collect detailed data on patient interactions and progress. This data can be analyzed to gain insights into the effectiveness of different interventions and to refine and improve treatment protocols.

The integration of VR into mental health interventions holds significant promise for transforming how treatment is delivered. By offering immersive, personalized, and accessible therapy options, VR can enhance the effectiveness of mental health care and improve outcomes for patients.

1.7 Potential Benefits of VR/AR Technologies in Enhancing Emotional Regulation, Empathy, and Interpersonal Skills

Virtual Reality (VR) and Augmented Reality (AR) technologies hold immense promise in enhancing emotional regulation, empathy, and interpersonal skills. Through immersive experiences, individuals can safely navigate challenging scenarios, practicing emotional regulation techniques in controlled environments. VR environments offer unique opportunities for perspective-taking, allowing users to step into the shoes of others and gain a deeper understanding of diverse experiences, thus fostering empathy. Furthermore, VR simulations enable individuals to practice and refine their interpersonal skills, from effective communication to conflict resolution, in realistic yet risk-free settings. By providing tailored experiences for emotional and social learning, VR/AR technologies offer transformative potential in equipping individuals with the tools and competencies needed for navigating complex social interactions and fostering meaningful connections.

1.7.1 Emotional Regulation

- **Safe Exposure to Stressors**: VR can simulate stressful situations in a controlled environment, allowing individuals to practice coping strategies and emotional regulation techniques without real-world consequences. Repeated exposure in a safe setting helps individuals build resilience and improve their ability to manage stress and anxiety in real-life situations.
- **Biofeedback Integration**: VR systems can integrate biofeedback mechanisms, providing real-time data on physiological responses (e.g., heart rate, skin conductance). This immediate feedback helps individuals become more aware of their emotional responses and practice regulating their emotions through techniques such as deep breathing or mindfulness.
- **Guided Relaxation Exercises**: VR environments can facilitate guided relaxation exercises, such as virtual nature walks or meditative experiences, which help individuals learn and practice relaxation and emotional regulation techniques.

1.7.2 Empathy

- **Perspective-Taking Experiences**: VR can immerse individuals in scenarios that allow them to experience the world from another person's perspective, such as simulating the experiences of individuals from different cultural backgrounds or those with disabilities. This immersive experience fosters a deeper understanding and empathy for others' experiences and challenges.
- **Empathy Training Programs**: VR can be used to develop training programs aimed at improving empathy, particularly in professional settings like healthcare, education, and customer service. These programs can simulate interactions with diverse individuals, helping users practice empathetic communication and understanding in a variety of contexts.
- **Emotional Recognition Practice**: VR environments can include scenarios where individuals practice recognizing and responding to others' emotions through facial expressions, body language, and tone of voice. This practice enhances emotional intelligence and empathy by improving the ability to accurately interpret and respond to the emotions of others.

1.7.3 Interpersonal Skills

- **Social Skills Training**: VR can simulate social interactions, providing a safe space for individuals to practice and develop their interpersonal skills, such as initiating conversations, active listening, and assertiveness. These simulations can be particularly beneficial for individuals with social anxiety or autism spectrum disorders, offering repeated practice without the fear of real-world judgment.
- **Conflict Resolution Practice**: VR scenarios can be designed to simulate conflicts or challenging interpersonal situations, allowing individuals to practice conflict resolution techniques and effective communication strategies. This practice helps individuals build confidence and competence in handling interpersonal conflicts constructively.
- **Teamwork and Collaboration**: VR can create collaborative virtual environments where individuals work together to solve problems or complete tasks, fostering teamwork and collaborative skills. These experiences can be used in both educational and professional development settings to enhance group dynamics and cooperative working skills.

VR/AR technologies offer significant potential benefits in enhancing emotional regulation, empathy, and interpersonal skills. By providing immersive, controlled environments for practice and learning, these technologies can help individuals develop critical emotional and social competencies that are essential for personal and professional success.

1.8 Need of Research

The emerging field of Augmented Wellness, which explores the transformative potential of Virtual Reality (VR) and Augmented Reality (AR) in healthcare, is poised to revolutionize the way we approach wellness and medical treatment. The need for Augmented Wellness stems from the growing recognition of the limitations of traditional healthcare methods and the increasing demand for innovative solutions that can enhance patient outcomes and experiences. VR and AR technologies offer immersive and interactive experiences that can empower individuals to take control of their health and well-being. From personalized therapy sessions to immersive training for healthcare professionals, Augmented Wellness opens new avenues for preventative care, treatment, and rehabilitation. By harnessing the power of VR and AR, healthcare providers can offer more accessible, engaging, and effective interventions, ultimately leading to improved patient outcomes and a higher quality of life. As we continue to explore and refine these technologies, Augmented Wellness holds the promise of transforming healthcare delivery and empowering individuals to lead healthier, happier lives.

Virtual Reality (VR) and Augmented Reality (AR) technologies offer promising avenues for revolutionizing mental health interventions. This paper explores the mechanisms by which VR/AR achieves therapeutic effects, focusing on two key aspects: immersion and engagement. VR creates a sense of immersion by placing patients in safe and controlled virtual environments, allowing them to confront anxieties or phobias. Similarly, AR superimposes therapeutic elements onto the real world, providing a safe space for practicing social interaction skills. The interactive and engaging nature of VR/AR increases patient motivation and adherence to therapy, particularly in scenarios like social anxiety treatment where patients can practice social interactions in virtual environments and receive immediate feedback. Moreover, VR/AR scenarios can be tailored to individual needs and phobias, such as a fear of public speaking, allowing for gradual exposure and desensitization. However, despite the promising outcomes, the evidence base for VR/AR in mental health interventions requires further solidification. More extensive clinical trials are needed to fully understand the long-term effectiveness of VR/AR across different mental health conditions. Overall, VR/AR technologies offer immense potential in revolutionizing mental healthcare, providing personalized and engaging interventions that empower individuals to improve their well-being.

2 Literature Review

As per the authors in [7], AR along with VR have the potential to revolutionise mental health care by creating compelling, personalised, and immersive therapeutic experiences. Responsible usage requires training for mental health professionals, thorough research, compliance with data protection legislation, along with adherence to ethical norms. With an emphasis on improving the ecological validity of highly controlled settings, boosting personalisation along with engagement, along with collecting real-time, automated data in real-world scenarios, H. Bell et al. in [8] outlined the benefits of adopting VR for mental health evaluation. Our preliminary efforts to develop and pilot a youth-co-designed virtual reality intervention in case of classroom use in promoting adolescents' well-being were detailed by the authors in [9]. In order to better comprehend how mental health therapies are used in everyday clinical practice, the authors in [10] intended to discover, assess, and summarise them using immersive 360° movies. Despite the paucity of research, existing AR/VR based therapies have the ability to increase understanding, compassion, and understanding of mental illness according to [11]. As per [12], new age in mental health, centred on psychological diseases, may be about to dawn thanks to the metaverse, a word made by merging meta and universe, which has the potential to improve healthcare and personal well-being via the development of a full-body illusion through digital avatars. Modules for augmented along with virtual reality were being examined by Singh & Kaunert in [13] as game-changing resources for enhancing emotional intelligence, mental wellness, and mindfulness. This looked to examine the revolutionary possibilities of augmented along with VR modules for improving mental health, emotional intelligence, along with mindfulness. In the realms of education and mental health, Carlson in [14] developed augmented reality along with virtual reality simulations and the goal was to better understand the possible effects of virtual reality along with augmented reality on patient outcomes as they relate to mental health therapies. Verma & Singla in [15] produced computer-generated digital representations that were referred to as "avatars" for the purpose of interacting with digital items in the metaverse and communicating with one another via the internet.

The authors in [16] presented digital twins as the most essential components of CPSs, and they are also an essential component in the process of bringing the Metaverse into existence. Image style transfer from digital painting to new media art was investigated in [17]. Neural style transfer is the foundation around which this approach is built. The authors in [18] provided a comprehensive overview of the research and investigations that have previously been conducted in the field of metaverse academic inquiry. New developments in AR and VR hold a lot of promise for improving mental health therapies and people's general health and happiness. Using "Ifland" as a case study, Lee and Kim [19] used the unified theory of acceptance and use of technology (UTAUT) to the metaverse in their investigation of user acceptance and usage of technology. Their research shows that users are more engaged and have better results from therapy in metaverse settings that are fully immersive. The authors in [20] emphasised the crucial significance of safe and effective virtual environments for health applications in their thorough assessment on visualisation and cybersecurity in the metaverse. A comprehensive overview of virtual reality and augmented reality, including its uses in many domains, including mental health, is given in [21]. By demonstrating how these technologies may be used to build immersive therapeutic settings, our study highlights their revolutionary potential. By doing a scoping assessment of augmented and virtual reality health therapies for the elderly, the authors in [22] have shown how these technologies have the potential to transform therapeutic encounters and enhance the mental health of this population. In addition, a study conducted in [23] examined the effects of 360° video and VR on the mental health of older persons. The results showed that VR provided much more favourable outcomes in this regard. To go even farther into the topic, the authors in [24] looked at how VR tourism affected customers' subjective well-being. Virtual experiences have the potential to greatly improve mental health and alleviate stress, according to their research. Another research by Ciocca and Tschan [25] explores the use of virtual reality (VR) and exercise games (exergames) to improve mental and social health. The authors focus on the possibilities of these technologies in demanding settings, such as space missions. In order to make health information more approachable and interesting for consumers, Malheiros [26] investigated how virtual reality and augmented reality might improve health literacy.

Gasmi and Benlamri [27] pointed out that the COVID-19 epidemic has also increased the demand for augmented and virtual reality technology. Their studies include the increased use of these technologies during the epidemic and how they may help with the mental health issues that have worsened as a result of the disaster. There has been encouraging progress in the use of VR and AR for wellness and mental health treatments with the advent of these technologies in recent years. In their proposal for virtual reality treatment as an aid for mental health, Purwar and Singh [28] emphasised the technology's ability to provide engaging and immersive therapeutic experiences. Their research shows that virtual reality may be a powerful tool for mental health practitioners by simulating therapeutic settings. Lee et al. [29] reviewed the literature on digital treatment using extended reality (XR) to improve mental health in young adults and adolescents from South Korea. Their research highlights the beneficial effects of XR technology on psychological well-being, especially in lowering rates of anxiety and depression in younger generations. In order to ascertain if Gulf region universities have adopted metaverse technology, authors in [30] created a theoretical framework. The metaverse has the ability to revolutionise academic support systems for mental health and education, according to their empirical research that used a hybrid SEM-ANN technique. Virtual reality was investigated in [31] to determine the effect of natural components and colourful interventions on mood, gaze, and spontaneous walking. Their study shows that virtual reality settings with more colourful and natural components might help people better control their emotions and feel better overall. Kaushik [32] explored the effects of the metaverse on skill sets, arguing that this virtual environment has the potential to revolutionise sustainability and business by encouraging the development of novel abilities. In addition to its obvious use in entertainment, this conceptual study demonstrates how the metaverse may have far-reaching effects on people's mental health and wellbeing via the facilitation of skill-building and immersive educational settings. In addition, authors in [33] highlighted the future prospects for human-AI cooperation by presenting a thorough taxonomy of AI and AGI employing numerous intelligences and learning styles. Personalised mental health therapies may be enhanced by integrating AI into VR settings, as this research reveals. Authors in [34] investigated how AI, digital twins, and the metaverse all come together in the context of training and upkeep. In addition to their potential use in therapeutic settings to enhance mental health outcomes, their study emphasises the importance of these technologies in developing immersive and lifelike training environments. In their metaverse AI framework proposal, authors in [35] highlighted the need of AI integration to improve virtual environment user experiences and therapeutic treatments. In their extensive review of metaverse AI applications, it has been addressed in [36] how AI may construct adaptable virtual environments to aid in mental health therapies and other tasks.

In their 66-page online survey, the authors in [37] covered every possible topic related to the metaverse. Advancements are covered in Ferraioli's article [38]. In an article published in AI Society, Boddington [39] delves into the concept of the "Internet of Bodies," with an emphasis on how our physical selves may one day merge with virtual places. Hadjistassou [40] examined Second Life's cultural difficulties in relation to sustainability efforts in the US and Europe. Using the Pribram-Bohm Hypothesis as a prism, Joye and Joye [41] investigated the metaverse's potential ethical ramifications for virtual reality. In [42], the authors have surveyed the current state and potential future developments of metaverses and 3D virtual worlds. Park and Kim [43] provided a taxonomy that identifies the metaverse's components, uses, and problems. In their in-depth study, Teigland and Power [44] examined the ways in which the immersive internet interacts with economic, political, and social factors. In [45], the authors have investigated how imitation and innovation impact the uptake of metaverse services. Authors in [46] highlighted new tools for language learners in the virtual world of Second Life.

Table 1.1 shows the brief literature review of some of the existing literature in terms of cons, prons, limitations etc.

3 Problem Statement

Anxiety, sadness, and stress are among the most common mental health problems in today's culture, impacting people of all ages and backgrounds. Although many people benefit from traditional therapy methods, they encounter obstacles like stigma, cost, and lack of accessibility. Furthermore, encouraging people to stick to their treatment programs and getting them to participate in therapy are not always easy tasks. Isolation, disruption of habits, and increased stresses are some ways in which the COVID-19 epidemic has worsened preexisting mental health issues [47, 48]. Innovative ways that may augment or improve established therapeutic methods are urgently needed for mental well-being because they provide solutions that are effective, accessible, and interesting. One possible way to tackle these problems is by using VR and AR technology. VR and AR therapies may enhance people's real-world experiences or transport them to virtual ones, creating opportunities for interactive and tailored therapy. Among the many therapies that may be facilitated by these technologies are scenario simulations, relaxation methods, controlled exposure therapy, and the development of emotional regulation abilities. VR and AR

Table 1.1 Literature survey

Ref	Cons	Prons	Limitation	Conclusion
[7]	Complex and may require advanced understanding	Comprehensive overview of mental health treatment advancements	Limited to the latest advancements and may not cover basic concepts	Highlights significant progress in mental health treatments with new technologies
[8]	May not cover latest developments	Demonstrates VR as a valuable clinical tool	Focuses on VR; may not generalize to all mental health tools	Establishes VR's efficacy in mental health practice and research
[9]	Specific to the UK and adolescent well-being	Explores VR's potential in supporting adolescent mental health	Limited to proof-of-concept and specific demographics	Shows promise for VR interventions in school settings
[10]	Review may lack practical application details	Systematic review of 360° videos in mental health	Review-based, lacking original empirical data	Identifies potential of 360° videos for immersive mental health interventions
[11]	Broad scope might dilute specific findings	Scoping review on AR/VR's impact on mental illness stigma	Generalized findings, needing specific studies for depth	Shows AR/VR's potential in improving mental health knowledge and empathy
[12]	Early-stage concepts of MEDverse	Discusses future potential of metaverse in mental health	Speculative, as practical applications are emerging	Highlights the promise of the metaverse for future mental health applications
[13]	May require advanced technological infrastructure	Details AR/VR modules for mindfulness	Limited to mindfulness; broader mental health impacts not covered	Demonstrates AR/VR's effectiveness in mindfulness practices
[14]	May not cover non-augmented approaches	Explores virtual and augmented simulations in mental health	Focused on simulations, not comprehensive of all VR/AR applications	Validates virtual and augmented simulations for mental health treatments
[15]	Technical and may be complex for non-specialists	Investigates accuracy and performance in the metaverse	Limited to technical aspects; practical applications less discussed	Enhances understanding of metaverse accuracy and performance for mental health
[16]	Focus on specific material (42SiCr Steel Alloys)	Discusses AI digital twinning in the metaverse	Specific to one material; broader implications may be limited	Demonstrates AI and metaverse potential in material science and beyond

(continued)

Table 1.1 (continued)

Ref	Cons	Prons	Limitation	Conclusion
[17]	May be complex due to combination of AI and IoT	Explores creation mechanisms of new media art in metaverse	Focused on artistic applications; practical mental health uses less clear	Innovatively combines AI, IoT, and metaverse for new media art
[18]	Broad research streams; may lack depth in specific areas	Advances metaverse investigation and research agenda	Needs more focused studies for in-depth insights	Sets future research directions for metaverse studies
[19]	Case study limited to 'Ifland'	Examines UTAUT in metaverse context	Findings may not generalize beyond 'Ifland'	Provides insights into technology acceptance in the metaverse
[20]	Focus on visualization and cybersecurity	Surveys metaverse cybersecurity and visualization	Technical focus; practical applications less discussed	Highlights key cybersecurity challenges and visualization techniques
[21]	Introductory level; may lack advanced details	Comprehensive introduction to VR/AR	Basic overview; advanced applications not covered	Serves as a foundational text for VR/AR concepts
[22]	Focus on older adults; less on other demographics	Scoping review of VR/AR for older adults' well-being	Limited to older adults; broader impacts not covered	Shows potential of VR/AR for enhancing older adults' health and well-being
[23]	Comparative study; may lack broad applications	Compares 360° video and VR for older adults	Focused on specific technologies; generalizability limited	Provides comparative insights on VR technologies for mental health
[24]	Specific to virtual tourism	Examines VR tourism's impact on well-being	Limited to tourism; broader well-being impacts not discussed	Demonstrates VR's positive influence on subjective well-being through tourism
[25]	Specific to physical exercise in astronauts	Discusses VR exergames for astronaut health	Focused on astronauts; broader applications may vary	Highlights VR's potential for boosting health in extreme conditions
[26]	Focus on health literacy	Explores AR/VR for improving health literacy	Specific to literacy; broader health impacts not covered	Shows promise of AR/VR in enhancing health literacy and communication

mental health therapies have a lot of promise, but they also confront a number of challenges, such as a lack of enough data to prove their effectiveness, ethical concerns, along with a lack of widespread acceptability among MH providers and their patients. Hence, purpose of this study is to investigate viability, acceptability, and efficacy of augmented and virtual reality solutions for psychological health. By providing answers to these questions, we want to aid in the creation of evidence-based strategies that make use of new technology to improve mental health and general wellness.

- **Sample Size and Diversity**: One limitation of the current research is the relatively small and homogeneous sample size. Future studies should aim to recruit larger and more diverse samples to ensure the generalizability of findings across different demographic groups and mental health conditions.
- **Short-Term Follow-Up**: The current research may be limited by its focus on short-term outcomes. Longitudinal studies with extended follow-up periods are needed to assess the sustained effectiveness of VR/AR interventions and to evaluate any potential long-term benefits or adverse effects.
- **Methodological Rigor**: Some studies may lack methodological rigor, such as the absence of control groups or randomization. Future research efforts should prioritize rigorous study designs, including randomized controlled trials, to provide stronger evidence for the effectiveness of VR/AR interventions.
- **Technology Accessibility**: The accessibility of VR/AR technology may present a barrier to participation for certain populations, such as those with limited access to hardware or internet connectivity. Future research should explore strategies to improve technology accessibility and address disparities in access to VR/AR interventions.

4 Proposed Work

Research proposes the potential of Virtual Reality (VR) and Augmented Reality (AR) technologies in mental health interventions. VR creates a sense of immersion by placing patients in controlled virtual environments, allowing them to confront anxieties or phobias. AR superimposes therapeutic elements onto the real world, providing a safe space for practicing social interaction skills. This interactive and engaging nature increases patient motivation and adherence to therapy, particularly in social anxiety treatment scenarios. VR/AR scenarios can be tailored to individual needs and phobias, allowing gradual exposure and desensitization. However, the evidence base for VR/AR in mental health interventions requires further solidification, and more extensive clinical trials are needed to understand its long-term effectiveness across different mental health conditions.

Creating a process flow for simulating Virtual Reality (VR) Mental Health Interventions using Augmented Reality (AR) and VR solutions for well-being involves several key steps to ensure the effectiveness and feasibility of the interventions. Here's a comprehensive process flow (see Fig. 1.2):

1. Needs Assessment: Find out who you're helping, what they need in terms of mental health care, and what you want to achieve by doing a comprehensive needs assessment. This may involve consulting with mental health professionals, stakeholders, and potential users.

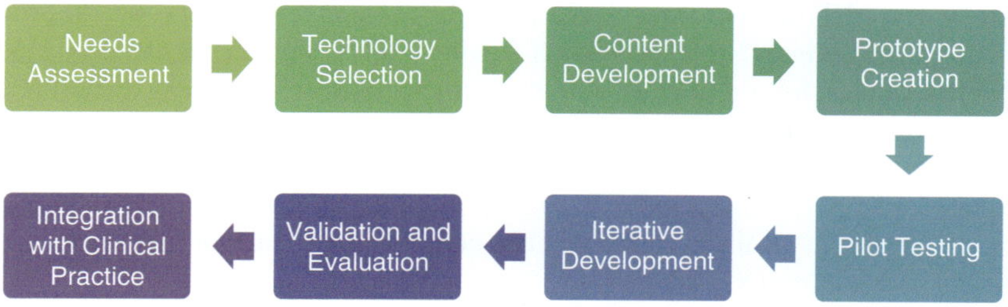

Fig. 1.2 Process flow of research

2. Technology Selection: Choose appropriate AR/VR solutions based on the identified needs and objectives. Consider factors such as device compatibility, available software platforms, and ease of use.
3. Content Development: Develop immersive content tailored to address the identified mental health needs. This may include virtual environments, guided meditations, relaxation exercises, exposure therapy scenarios, mindfulness activities, and cognitive-behavioral therapy (CBT) exercises. Collaboration with mental health experts, psychologists, and therapists to ensure the content aligns with evidence-based therapeutic approaches and best practices takes place during this phase.
4. Prototype Creation: Prototypes of the AR/VR interventions to test usability, functionality, and user experience is created to gather feedback from end-users, mental health professionals, and other stakeholders to iterate and refine the prototypes.
5. Pilot Testing: Pilot tests of the AR/VR interventions with a small group of users to evaluate their effectiveness, acceptability, and feasibility in real-world settings is conducted to collect qualitative and quantitative data on user experiences, engagement levels, and perceived benefits to inform further improvements.
6. Iterative Development: Based on feedback from pilot testing, iterate on the AR/VR interventions to address any identified issues or areas for improvement. This may involve refining content, optimizing user interfaces, or enhancing features for better usability and engagement.
7. Validation and Evaluation: Validate the effectiveness of the AR/VR interventions through rigorous evaluation studies, including RCTs or quasi-experimental designs. Then measurement of outcomes takes place. These outcomes are changes in mental health symptoms, well-being indicators, self-reported satisfaction, and treatment adherence.
8. Integration with Clinical Practice: Integration of validated AR/VR interventions into existing mental health treatment programs and clinical practice settings and train mental health professionals and therapists on how to use the AR/VR solutions effectively and incorporate them into their therapeutic interventions.

By following this process flow, developers, researchers, and mental health professionals can effectively simulate Virtual Reality Mental Health Interventions using AR/VR solutions for well-being, with the ultimate goal of improving mental health outcomes and enhancing overall quality of life.

Our proposed system introduces a Virtual Reality (VR) application designed specifically for anxiety management. Utilizing immersive VR environments, the application aims to provide users with a safe and controlled space to confront and manage their anxiety symptoms effectively.

4.1 Immersive Environments for Anxiety Exposure

The VR application offers a variety of immersive environments tailored to different anxiety triggers, such as social situations, public speaking, or confined spaces. Users can select scenarios based on their specific anxiety challenges, allowing for personalized exposure therapy experiences.

4.2 Interactive Tools for Anxiety Coping Strategies

In addition to immersive environments, the VR application provides interactive tools and resources for practicing anxiety coping strategies. Users can engage in mindfulness exercises, deep breathing techniques, and cognitive restructuring activities within the virtual environment, guided by audio instructions and visual prompts.

4.3 Progress Tracking and Feedback Mechanisms

To monitor progress and provide feedback, the VR application includes built-in tracking features. Users can track their anxiety levels before and after each session, allowing for real-time assessment of therapeutic progress. The application also offers personalized feedback based on user performance, encouraging continued engagement and motivation.

Our proposed VR application for anxiety management offers a comprehensive solution for individuals seeking effective and accessible interventions. By combining immersive environments, interactive tools, and progress tracking mechanisms, the application aims to empower users to confront and overcome their anxiety symptoms in a supportive virtual environment.

5 Results and Discussion

Our study yielded several important findings regarding the effectiveness and implications of Virtual Reality (VR) and Augmented Reality (AR) in mental health interventions. Firstly, our analysis revealed that VR/AR therapies significantly improved accessibility, customization, and therapeutic efficacy compared to traditional methods. By creating immersive environments, VR/AR provided patients with a safe and controlled space to confront their anxieties and phobias. This aspect of immersion is crucial for effective exposure therapy, as patients can gradually confront and overcome their fears under the guidance of a therapist. Moreover, the interactive nature of VR/AR significantly enhanced patient engagement and motivation. Through simulated scenarios, patients could actively participate in therapy sessions, receiving immediate feedback and reinforcement. For instance, in the case of social anxiety treatment, patients could practice social interactions in virtual environments, gradually building confidence and skills. This increased engagement often led to improved adherence to therapy, as patients found the VR/AR experiences more enjoyable and rewarding compared to traditional methods.

Furthermore, the customization possibilities offered by VR/AR were instrumental in tailoring interventions to individual needs and preferences. For example, scenarios could be adjusted to accommodate varying levels of difficulty or specific phobias, allowing for personalized treatment plans. This level of customization not only improved the effectiveness of therapy but also enhanced the overall patient experience. However, our study also identified several challenges and limitations associated with the integration of VR/AR into mental health treatment. Technological constraints, such as hardware requirements and software limitations, posed barriers to widespread adoption. Additionally, ethical considerations, such as data privacy and informed consent, need to be carefully addressed to ensure patient safety and autonomy. While VR/AR technologies hold tremendous promise for improving mental health interventions, further research is needed to address these challenges and solidify the evidence base. More extensive clinical trials are necessary to fully understand the long-term effectiveness of VR/AR across different mental health conditions. By addressing these issues and continuing to refine VR/AR applications, we can unlock the full potential of these technologies in revolutionizing mental healthcare. Figure 1.3 indicates the comparison of energy efficiency, throughput and accuracy in different scenarios.

Figure 1.4 shows Python based simulation for visualizing the comparison between packet dropping and packet delivery ratio in case of VR Mental Health Interventions using AR/VR Solutions for Well-being.

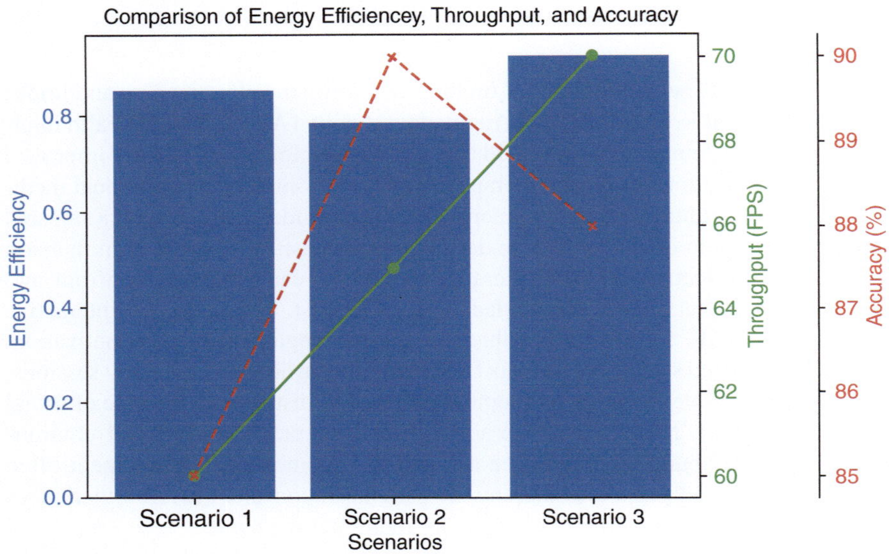

Fig. 1.3 Comparison of energy efficiency, throughput and accuracy in different scenarios

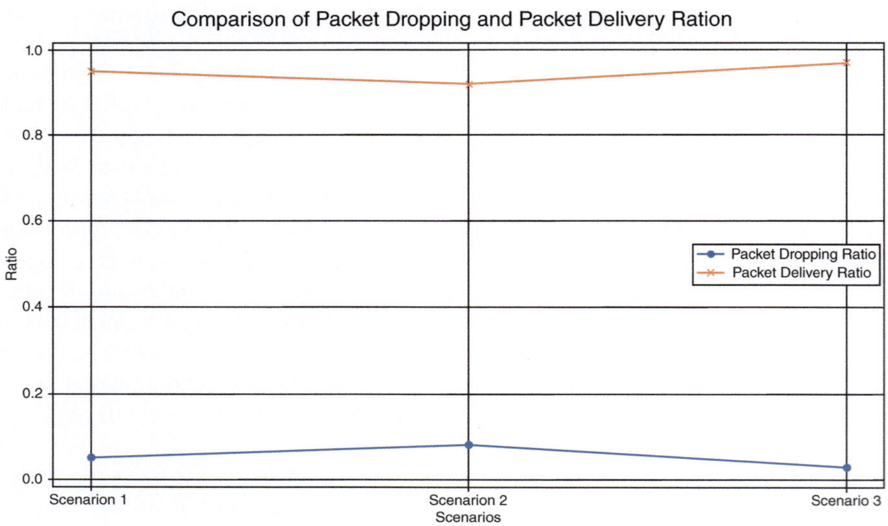

Fig. 1.4 Comparison of packet dropping and delivery ratio in different scenarios

6 Conclusion

This research shows that AR/VR technology may be novel mental health therapies. Our results imply that immersive and engaging AR/VR treatments may help treat a range of mental health issues by complementing standard therapies. We found that AR/VR therapies improve accessibility, customisation, and therapeutic efficacy in our literature and practical research. These devices are effective in exposure treatment, stress reduction, and emotional control, with many users reporting mental health gains.AR/VR incorporation into mental health treatment has problems and limits, which must be acknowledged. Technological constraints, ethical concerns, and the need for further study to provide empirical proof persist. These techniques' acceptability and implementation by mental health professionals and clients need additional study [49, 50]. Future research should address these knowledge and practice gaps. This topic needs longitudinal investigations on AR/VR treatments' long-term effects, randomized controlled trials comparing them to standard therapy, and ethical criteria. Enhancing AR/VR technology accessibility and affordability would help provide equitable mental health intervention access for everyone. In conclusion, AR/VR technologies have tremendous potential to improve mental health, but their incorporation into clinical practise needs careful assessment and continuing review. We can use these technologies to help people improve their mental health and well-being by exploring and refining them. The research proposed the potential of AR/VR technology as a novel mental health therapy, offering immersive and engaging treatments for various mental health issues. These treatments have shown positive results in exposure treatment, stress reduction, and emotional control. However, the integration faces challenges such as technological constraints, ethical considerations, and empirical validation. Further research is needed to explore the acceptability and implementation of these techniques, address knowledge gaps, and establish best practices. Additionally, improving accessibility and affordability is crucial for equitable access to mental health interventions. The integration of AR/VR technologies into clinical practice requires careful assessment and ongoing review.

7 Future Scope

The future scope of "Virtual Reality Mental Health Interventions: AR/VR Solutions for Well-being" encompasses several areas of potential development and exploration. İt will continue advancements in AR/VR hardware and software will enhance the capabilities and effectiveness of mental health interventions. Future research could focus on developing AR/VR interventions that are personalized to individual needs, preferences, and therapeutic goals. Research should also explore a variety of outcome measures, including symptom reduction, quality of life improvements, and functional recovery. Hybrid approaches that combine in-person sessions with AR/VR experiences may offer a comprehensive treatment approach. Further exploration is needed to determine the efficacy of AR/VR interventions for specific populations and mental health disorders. Developing ethical guidelines for use of AR/VR technologies in MH care is crucial. By pursuing these avenues of research and implementation, field of AR/VR MH interventions can continue to evolve and expand, offering innovative solutions to support individuals in improving their mental well-being. The efficacy of VR/AR in mental health interventions shows significant promise, yet it remains a burgeoning field requiring further exploration. While initial studies suggest positive outcomes, a robust evidence base through extensive clinical trials is essential to comprehend its long-term effectiveness across various mental health conditions. Additional research will provide a more nuanced understanding of how VR/AR can be integrated into existing therapeutic frameworks and tailored to meet individual needs effectively.

References

1. Bommareddy S, Khan JA, Anand R. A review on healthcare data privacy and security. In: Networking technologies in smart healthcare; 2022. p. 165–87.
2. Singh P, Kaiwartya O, Sindhwani N, Jain V, Anand R, editors. Networking technologies in smart healthcare: innovations and analytical approaches. CRC Press; 2022.
3. Anand R, Juneja S, Juneja A, Jain V, Kannan R, editors. Integration of IoT with cloud computing for smart applications. CRC Press; 2023.
4. Anand R, Pandey D, Gupta DN, Dharani MK, Sindhwani N, Ramesh JVN. Wireless sensor-based IoT system with distributed optimization for healthcare. In: Meta heuristic algorithms for advanced distributed systems; 2024. p. 261–88.
5. Saxena H, Joshi D, Singh H, Anand R. Comparison of classification algorithms for Alzheimer's disease prediction. In: 2022 Seventh international conference on parallel, distributed and grid computing (PDGC). IEEE; 2022. p. 687–92.
6. Veeraiah V, Gupta DN, Kumar BS, Gupta A, Anand R. Prediction of health risk based on multi-level IOT data using decision trees. In: 2023 International conference on sustainable emerging innovations in engineering and technology (ICSEIET). IEEE; 2023. p. 652–6.
7. Singha R, Singha S. Mental health treatment. In: Advances in medical technologies and clinical practice. IGI Global; 2024. p. 91–110. https://doi.org/10.4018/979-8-3693-1123-3.ch006.
8. Bell H, Nicholas J, Alvarez-Jimenez M, Thompson A, Valmaggia L. Virtual reality as a clinical tool in mental health research and practice. Dialogues Clin Neurosci. 2020;22(2):169–77. https://doi.org/10.31887/dcns.2020.22.2/lvalmaggia.
9. https://kurieta.com/how-to-measure-roi-in-digital-marketing-campaigns-copy/
10. Ionescu A, Van Daele T, Rizzo A, Blair C, Best P. 360° Videos for immersive mental health interventions: a systematic review. J Technol Behav Sci. 2021;6(4):631–51. https://doi.org/10.1007/s41347-021-00221-7.
11. Tay JL, Xie H, Sim K. Effectiveness of augmented and virtual reality-based interventions in improving knowledge, attitudes, empathy and stigma regarding people with mental illnesses—a scoping review. J Pers Med. 2023;13(1):112. https://doi.org/10.3390/jpm13010112.
12. Cerasa A, Gaggioli A, Marino F, Riva G, Pioggia G. The promise of the metaverse in mental health: the new era of MEDverse. Heliyon. 2022;8(11):e11762. https://doi.org/10.1016/j.heliyon.2022.e11762.
13. Singh B, Kaunert C. Augmented reality and virtual reality modules for mindfulness. In: Advances in medical technologies and clinical practice. IGI Global; 2024. p. 111–28. https://doi.org/10.4018/979-8-3693-1123-3.ch007.

14. Carlson CG. Virtual and augmented simulations in mental health. Curr Psychiatry Rep. 2023;25(9):365–71. https://doi.org/10.1007/s11920-023-01438-4.
15. Verma H, Singla M. Investigating the accuracy and performance enhancement in metaverse. In: 2022 5th International conference on contemporary computing and informatics (IC3I). IEEE; 2022. https://doi.org/10.1109/ic3i56241.2022.10072768.
16. Khalaj O, et al. Metaverse and AI digital twinning of 42SiCr steel alloys. Mathematics. 2022;11(1):4. https://doi.org/10.3390/math11010004.
17. Wang X, Cai L, Xu Y. Creation mechanism of new media art combining artificial intelligence and internet of things technology in a metaverse environment. J Supercomput. 2023;80:9277–97. https://doi.org/10.1007/s11227-023-05819-7.
18. Trunfio M, Rossi S. Advances in metaverse investigation: streams of research and future agenda. Virtual Worlds. 2022;1(2):103–29. https://doi.org/10.3390/virtualworlds1020007.
19. Lee U-K, Kim H. UTAUT in metaverse: an 'Ifland' case. J Theor Appl Electron Commer Res. 2022;17(2):613–35. https://doi.org/10.3390/jtaer17020032.
20. Chow Y-W, Susilo W, Li Y, Li N, Nguyen C. Visualization and cybersecurity in the metaverse: a survey. J Imaging. 2022;9(1):11. https://doi.org/10.3390/jimaging9010011.
21. Doerner R, Broll W, Jung B, Grimm P, Göbel M, Kruse R. Introduction to virtual and augmented reality. In: Virtual and augmented reality (VR/AR). Springer; 2022. p. 1–37. https://doi.org/10.1007/978-3-030-79062-2_1.
22. Carroll J, Hopper L, Farrelly AM, Lombard-Vance R, Bamidis PD, Konstantinidis EI. A scoping review of augmented/virtual reality health and wellbeing interventions for older adults: redefining immersive virtual reality. Front Virtual Real. 2021;2 https://doi.org/10.3389/frvir.2021.655338.
23. Kupczik L, Farrelly W, Wilson S. Appraising virtual technologies' impact on older citizens' mental health—a comparative between 360° video and virtual reality. Int J Environ Res Public Health. 2022;19(18):11250. https://doi.org/10.3390/ijerph191811250.
24. McLean G, AlYahya M, Barhorst JB, Osei-Frimpong K. Examining the influence of virtual reality tourism on consumers' subjective wellbeing. Tour Manag Perspect. 2023;46:101088. https://doi.org/10.1016/j.tmp.2023.101088.
25. Ciocca G, Tschan H. The enjoyability of physical exercise: exergames and virtual reality as new ways to boost psychological and psychosocial health in astronauts. A prospective and perspective view. IEEE Open J Eng Med Biol. 2023;4:173–9. https://doi.org/10.1109/OJEMB.2023.3234014.
26. Malheiros O. Virtual reality and augmented reality as promoters of better health literacy. In: Handbook of research on assertiveness, clarity, and positivity in health literacy. IGI Global; 2022. p. 294–315. https://doi.org/10.4018/978-1-7998-8824-6.ch017.
27. Gasmi A, Benlamri R. Augmented reality, virtual reality and new age technologies demand escalates amid COVID-19. In: Novel AI and data science advancements for sustainability in the era of COVID-19. Elsevier; 2022. p. 89–111. https://doi.org/10.1016/b978-0-323-90054-6.00005-2.
28. Purwar A, Singh A. VR therapy—mental therapy tool based on virtual reality. Int J Creat Comput. 2023;2(1):1–17. https://doi.org/10.1504/ijcrc.2023.133548.
29. Lee S, Yoon J, Cho Y, Chun J. Systematic review of extended reality digital therapy for enhancing mental health among South Korean adolescents and young adults. J Korean Acad Child Adolesc Psychiatry. 2023;34(4):204–14. https://doi.org/10.5765/jkacap.230046.
30. Akour IA, Al-Maroof RS, Alfaisal R, Salloum SA. A conceptual framework for determining metaverse adoption in higher institutions of gulf area: an empirical study using hybrid SEM-ANN approach. Comput Educ Artif Intell. 2022;3:100052. https://doi.org/10.1016/j.caeai.2022.100052.
31. Batistatou A, Vandeville F, Delevoye-Turrell YN. Virtual reality to evaluate the impact of colorful interventions and nature elements on spontaneous walking, gaze, and emotion. Front Virtual Real. 2022;3 https://doi.org/10.3389/frvir.2022.819597.

32. Kaushik S. Metaverse and skill set: a conceptual investigation. In: How the metaverse will reshape business and sustainability. Singapore: Springer; 2023. p. 171–8. https://doi.org/10.1007/978-981-99-5126-0_15.
33. Cichocki A, Kuleshov AP. Future trends for human-AI collaboration: a comprehensive taxonomy of AI/AGI using multiple intelligences and learning styles. Comput Intell Neurosci. 2021;2021(3):1–21. https://doi.org/10.1155/2021/8893795.
34. Bordegoni M, Ferrise F. Exploring the intersection of metaverse, digital twins, and artificial intelligence in training and maintenance. J Comput Inf Sci Eng. 2023;23(6) https://doi.org/10.1115/1.4062455.
35. Guo Y, et al. Artificial intelligence for metaverse: a framework. CAAI Artif Intell Res. 2022;1(1):54–67. https://doi.org/10.26599/air.2022.9150004.
36. Huynh-The T, Pham Q-V, Pham X-Q, Nguyen TT, Han Z, Kim D-S. Artificial intelligence for the metaverse: a survey. Eng Appl Artif Intell. 2023;117:105581. https://doi.org/10.1016/j.engappai.2022.105581.
37. Lee L-H, et al. All one need to know about metaverse: a complete survey on technological singularity. Virtual Ecosyst Res Agenda. 2021;14(8):1–66. http://arxiv.org/abs/2110.05352.
38. Ferraioli J. AlphaCurrents. J Latex Class Files. 2021;14(8):1–12.
39. Boddington G. The internet of bodies—alive, connected and collective: the virtual physical future of our bodies and our senses. AI Soc. 2021;38:1897–913. https://doi.org/10.1007/s00146-020-01137-1.
40. Hadjistassou SK. Culturally afforded tensions in the Second Life metaverse: from sustainability initiatives in Europe to sustainability practices in the United States. Int J Web-Based Learn Teach Technol. 2016;11(2):14–38. https://doi.org/10.4018/IJWLTT.2016040102.
41. Joye S, Joye SR. Ethical implications of a virtual reality metaverse: the Pribram-Bohm hypothesis. 2016.
42. Dionisio JDN, Burns WG, Gilbert R. 3D virtual worlds and the metaverse: current status and future possibilities. ACM Comput Surv. 2013;45(3):1–38. https://doi.org/10.1145/2480741.2480751.
43. Park S-M, Kim Y-G. A Metaverse: taxonomy, components, applications, and open challenges. IEEE Access. 2022;10:4209–51. https://doi.org/10.1109/access.2021.3140175.
44. Teigland R, Power D. The immersive internet: reflections on the entangling of the virtual with society, politics and the economy. In: Immersive ınternet reflections entangling virtual with society, politics and the economy; 2013. p. 1–264. https://doi.org/10.1057/9781137283023.
45. Lee SG, Trim S, Byun WK, Kang M. Innovation and imitation effects in Metaverse service adoption. Serv Bus. 2011;5(2):155–72. https://doi.org/10.1007/s11628-011-0108-8.
46. Dominguez-Noriega S, Enrique Agudo J, Ferreira P, Rico M. Language learning resources and developments in the Second Life metaverse. Int J Technol Enhanc Learn. 2011;3(5):496–509. https://doi.org/10.1504/IJTEL.2011.042101.
47. Anand R, Sindhwani N, Saini A, Shubham. Emerging technologies for COVID-19. In: Enabling healthcare 4.0 for pandemics: a roadmap using AI, machine learning, IoT and cognitive technologies; 2021. p. 163–88.
48. Sharma A, Sindhwani N, Anand R, Vashisth R. Intelligent computing relating to cloud computing. In: Computational intelligence in the industry 4.0. CRC Press; 2024. p. 55–72.
49. Alkhayyat A, Badhoutiya A, Sobti J, Singh R, Anand R, Kumar R. Data visualization of weather conditions in hilly regions using wireless technology. In: 2024 IEEE wireless antenna and microwave symposium (WAMS). IEEE; 2024. p. 1–6.
50. Gupta DN, Anand R, Ahamad S, Patil T, Dhabliya D, Gupta A. Phonocardiographic signal analysis for the detection of cardiovascular diseases. In: International conference on frontiers of intelligent computing: theory and applications. Singapore: Springer; 2023. p. 529–38.

Chapter 2
Understanding Virtual Reality (VR) and Its Applications in Healthcare

Bhanu Pratap Singh, Ankush Joshi, and Ritik Kumar Singh

Abstract Virtual reality (VR) is an emerging and fascinating technology that promotes the humans to step into virtual worlds and interact with them as if they were real. It is a computer-generated simulation of an environment that allows users to interact with and experience a virtual world as if they were physically present within it. Virtual reality (VR) technology has appeared as a trans-formative tool in the field of healthcare, offering immersive and interactive experiences that have the potential to revolutionize patient care, medical training, and therapy. This chapter provides a depth exploration of VR technology and its useful implications for healthcare delivery. Beginning with an introduction to the fundamentals of VR, including its core components and principles, the chapter delves into the endless applications of VR in healthcare. These applications range from medical training and education to pain management, surgical planning, psychological therapy, and medicine. Through real-life examples and case studies, we'll see how VR is making a difference in healthcare by providing more effective and engaging treatment options. Throughout the chapter, we'll see how VR is generating a big gap between current healthcare facilities and the future trends. But, like all technologies, there are challenges too. Sometimes, VR can make people feel nauseous, and using VR safely means protecting people's privacy and making sure the technology works for everyone. Looking to the future, we'll go into the new ways that states how VR technology is evolving and how it could continue to revolutionize healthcare in the years to come. Overall, this chapter aims to provide a clear and accessible overview of VR in healthcare, helping readers understand its potential benefits and limitations in improving patient outcomes and medical training.

Keywords Augmented reality · Virtual reality · Artificial intelligence · Internet of things · Blockchain · Mobile VR

B. P. Singh (✉) · A. Joshi · R. K. Singh
COER University, Roorkee, India

B. O. Soufiane et al. (eds.), *Augmented Wellness*,
https://doi.org/10.1007/978-981-96-2952-7_2

1 Introduction

Virtual Reality (VR) is an exciting and innovative technology that allows people to immerse themselves in virtual worlds and interact with them as if they were real [1]. Imagine putting on a special headset and suddenly finding yourself in a different place—it could be a beautiful beach, a bustling city, or even inside the human body. VR creates these realistic environments using advanced computer technology, making users feel like they're actually there.

This chapter aims to explore the fundamentals of virtual reality technology and its wide-ranging applications in healthcare [2]. We'll start by explaining how VR works, and the essential components needed to create virtual environments. Then, we'll dive into the exciting ways VR is being used in healthcare, from training healthcare professionals to treating patients with chronic pain or mental health issues. VR isn't just for training, it's also a powerful tool for patient care and therapy [3]. Imagine being able to transport a patient to a peaceful beach or serene forest without ever leaving their hospital bed. VR can create immersive environments that help patients relax, manage pain, and even overcome phobias. It's also being used in psychological therapy to treat conditions like post-traumatic stress disorder (PTSD) and anxiety disorders. By exposing patients to controlled virtual environments, therapists can help them confront and overcome their fears in a safe and supportive setting. Through real-life examples and case studies, we'll showcase the diverse ways VR is making a difference in healthcare delivery. There are also concerns about privacy and data security, as VR systems collect sensitive information about users' movements and interactions. We'll also discuss some of the challenges and considerations associated with using VR in healthcare, such as ensuring patient safety and privacy.

2 Introduction to Virtual Reality

Virtual reality (VR) is a computer-generated simulation of an environment that allows users to interact with and experience a virtual world as if they were physically present within it [4]. Users typically wear a VR headset that tracks their head movements and displays corresponding images to create an immersive experience. VR environments can range from realistic representations of the physical world to fantastical, imaginary landscapes [5]. By providing a sense of presence and depth, VR technology enables users to explore and interact with virtual objects and surroundings in real-time. This technology has various applications in different fields, including gaming, entertainment, healthcare, education, and training [6]. As VR technology continues to advance, it holds the potential to revolutionize how we perceive and interact with digital content, offering immersive experiences that were previously only possible in our imagination. Despite its potential benefits, VR also presents challenges such as motion sickness, technical limitations, and concerns

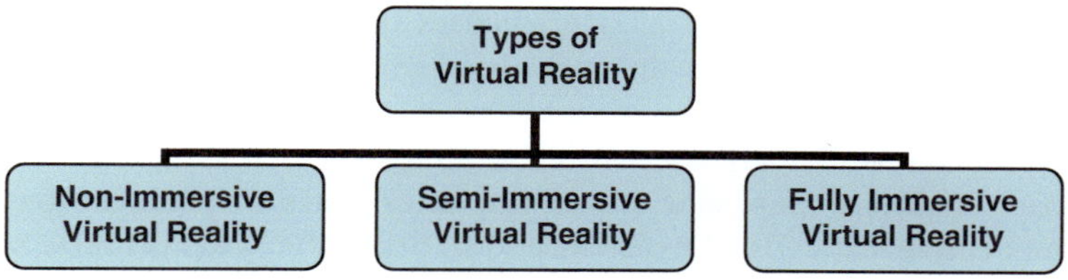

Fig. 2.1 Types of virtual reality

about privacy and safety. However, ongoing advancements in hardware, software, and content development are continuously improving the VR experience and expanding its capabilities. As VR technology becomes more accessible and sophisticated, its impact on industries and everyday life is expected to grow, shaping the way we work, learn, communicate, and interact with digital content [7].

2.1 Types of Virtual Reality

Figure 2.1 shows the types of Virtual Reality. The three main Virtual Reality categories are the following:

1. **Non-Immersive Virtual Reality**: Non-immersive virtual reality (NI-VR) is a type of virtual reality that allows users to interact with a computer-generated environment without the need for special equipment like headsets or gloves. NI-VR experiences are typically accessed through a computer screen, tablet, or smartphone, using familiar devices like a mouse, keyboard, or touchscreen [8].
2. **Semi-Immersive Virtual Reality**: Semi-immersive virtual reality bridges the gap between non-immersive and fully immersive virtual reality experiences. It provides a more engaging environment than a regular screen but doesn't completely block out the real world like some VR headsets [9].
3. **Fully Immersive Virtual Reality**: Fully immersive virtual reality aims to completely transport you into a computer-generated world, blurring the lines between reality and simulation. It offers a rich sensory experience that tricks your brain into believing you're physically present in the virtual environment [10].

2.2 Core Components of Virtual Reality

The core components of virtual reality (VR) technology encompass hardware, software, and peripherals that work together to create immersive and interactive experiences [11]. These components include:

1. **Head-Mounted Display (HMD)**: The HMD is perhaps the most recognizable component of VR. It is a wearable device that typically resembles a pair of

goggles or a helmet [12]. The HMD houses the display screens, lenses, and motion sensors necessary to track head movements and render virtual environments.
2. **Display Screens**: Display screens are essential for presenting virtual imagery to the user. High-resolution screens with fast refresh rates are preferred to ensure a smooth and realistic visual experience [13]. Some VR systems utilize separate screens for each eye to create stereoscopic 3D images, enhancing depth perception.
3. **Motion Tracking Sensors**: Motion tracking sensors, such as accelerometers, gyroscopes, and magnetometers, are embedded within the HMD and other peripherals to detect the user's movements in real-time [14]. This tracking allows the VR system to adjust the perspective of the virtual environment, accordingly, creating a sense of presence and immersion.
4. **Input Devices**: Input devices enable users to interact with the virtual world. These devices may include handheld controllers, gloves, or even full-body motion capture suits. Input devices can track hand movements, gestures, and button presses, allowing users to manipulate objects, navigate environments, and perform actions within the VR space [15].
5. **Audio System:** Immersive audio is crucial for creating a convincing VR experience. High-quality headphones or integrated speakers provide spatial audio cues that enhance the sense of presence and realism [15]. Some VR systems incorporate 3D audio technology to simulate sound coming from different directions and distances.
6. **Computer Hardware**: Powerful computers or gaming consoles are necessary to run VR applications and render complex virtual environments in real-time [16]. These systems require robust processors, graphics cards, and memory to deliver smooth performance and high-fidelity graphics.
7. **Tracking System**: In addition to head tracking, VR systems may utilize external tracking systems to monitor the position and movement of the user within physical space [17]. These systems may employ cameras, infrared sensors, or laser-based tracking technologies to create a virtual boundary and prevent users from bumping into objects or walls.
8. **Software Platform**: VR applications and experiences are powered by software platforms that handle rendering, tracking, user interaction, and content delivery [18]. These platforms may include proprietary VR ecosystems developed by hardware manufacturers, as well as open-source frameworks and development tools used by independent developers and content creators.

2.3 Principles of Virtual reality

The principles of virtual reality (VR) revolve around creating immersive and interactive experiences that simulate the sensation of being present in a virtual environment. Some key principles include:

1. **Immersion**: VR aims to immerse users in a digital environment by stimulating multiple senses, primarily sight and sound [19]. Immersive VR experiences transport users to virtual worlds where they can explore, interact, and engage with objects and surroundings as if they were physically present.
2. **Presence**: Presence refers to the subjective feeling of "being there" in the virtual environment. Achieving a sense of presence is essential for making VR experiences convincing and engaging [19]. Factors such as realistic graphics, responsive interactions, and accurate motion tracking contribute to enhancing presence.
3. **Interaction**: Interaction is a fundamental aspect of VR that allows users to engage with and manipulate objects within the virtual world [19]. VR systems provide various input methods, such as handheld controllers, gestures, and voice commands, to enable users to interact with virtual objects, navigate environments, and perform actions.
4. **Realism**: Realism in VR pertains to the fidelity and believability of virtual environments and objects. High-quality graphics, accurate physics simulation, realistic lighting and textures, and convincing sound effects contribute to creating a sense of realism in VR experiences [19].
5. **Comfort**: Ensuring user comfort is crucial for a positive VR experience. VR systems should minimize motion sickness and discomfort by maintaining smooth frame rates, reducing latency, and implementing comfortable locomotion methods [20]. Designing user interfaces and interactions that are intuitive and ergonomic also enhances comfort.
6. **Accessibility**: VR should be accessible to users of all abilities and demographics. Designing inclusive VR experiences involves considering factors such as ease of use, adjustability of settings, and compatibility with assistive technologies [20]. Providing options for locomotion, input methods, and interaction styles accommodates diverse user needs.
7. **Interactivity**: Interactivity is central to VR experiences, enabling users to actively engage with virtual environments and shape their experiences. Interactive elements may include puzzles, challenges, simulations, storytelling, and social interactions [20]. Dynamic environments that respond to user actions enhance immersion and engagement.
8. **Presence of Agency**: VR experiences should empower users with a sense of agency, allowing them to influence and control their surroundings [20]. Providing meaningful choices, consequences, and feedback mechanisms gives users a sense of autonomy and ownership over their virtual experiences.

2.4 Difference Between Virtual Reality (VR) and Augmented Reality (AR)

Augmented Reality (AR) is a technology that overlays digital information, such as images, videos, or 3D models, onto the real-world environment. Unlike Virtual Reality (VR), which immerses users in a completely virtual environment, AR enhances the physical world by superimposing computer-generated content onto it in real-time [21]. Table 2.1 resume the keys differences between Virtual Reality and Augmented Reality:

2.5 Interaction Techniques in VR Environments

Interaction techniques in virtual reality (VR) environments are crucial for enabling users to engage with and manipulate virtual objects and environments [25]. Here is some common interaction techniques used in VR:

Table 2.1 Difference between virtual reality and augmented reality

Aspect	Virtual reality (VR)	Augmented reality (AR)
Definition	VR is a simulated experience that immerses users in a completely virtual environment, blocking out the real world entirely [21]	AR overlays digital content onto the real world, blending virtual elements with the user's physical environment [21]
Environment	Fully immersive users are transported to a computer-generated reality and are unable to see the real world around them [22]	Partially immersive users remain aware of their physical surroundings while digital content is integrated into their view [22]
Interaction	Users can interact with and manipulate virtual objects and environments using specialized input devices or controllers [23]	Users can interact with both virtual and physical objects in their environment, often using gestures, touch, or voice commands [23]
Applications	Common applications include gaming, simulations, training, and entertainment where users want to escape reality [24]	Common applications include navigation, education, healthcare, and retail where users want to enhance their real-world experiences [24]
Equipment	Requires specialized VR headsets or goggles that block out the external environment and display the virtual world	Requires devices such as smartphones, tablets, or AR glasses equipped with cameras and sensors to overlay digital content
Immersion	Offers a high level of immersion by creating a completely synthetic environment that can transport users to new worlds [21]	Offers a lower level of immersion by augmenting the real world with digital content, allowing users to stay connected to reality [21]
Examples	Oculus Rift, HTC Vive, PlayStation VR	Microsoft HoloLens, Google Glass, Pokémon Go

2.5.1 Hand Controllers

Hand controllers are handheld devices equipped with sensors that track the user's hand movements and gestures. They allow users to interact with virtual objects by mimicking real-world actions such as grabbing, pointing, and pushing [25]. Hand controllers often feature buttons or triggers that users can press to perform actions within the VR environment.

1. **Gaze-based Interaction**: Gaze-based interaction relies on the direction of the user's gaze to interact with objects or trigger actions in the virtual environment. By simply looking at an object or UI element for a certain period, users can select or activate it [25]. Gaze-based interaction is particularly useful for navigation, selection, and menu interactions in VR experiences.
2. **Gesture Recognition**: Gesture recognition technologies enable users to control virtual environments using predefined hand gestures or movements [25]. Cameras or sensors track the user's gestures, allowing them to perform actions such as waving, thumbs-up, or making specific hand signs to interact with objects or trigger events in VR.
3. **Voice Commands**: Voice commands provide a hands-free interaction method in VR environments. Users can use natural language commands to perform actions, navigate menus, or interact with virtual characters or assistants [25]. Voice commands enhance accessibility and convenience, especially in scenarios where hand controllers may not be practical or available.
4. **Teleportation and Locomotion**: Teleportation and locomotion techniques allow users to move within the virtual environment. Teleportation involves selecting a destination point and instantly transporting the user to that location, minimizing discomfort associated with traditional locomotion methods like walking or running [25]. Locomotion techniques include walking in place, joystick-based movement, or using physical treadmills to simulate movement.
5. **Object Manipulation**: Object manipulation techniques enable users to interact with and manipulate virtual objects using hand gestures or controllers [25]. Users can pick up, move, rotate, resize, and manipulate virtual objects to perform tasks or solve puzzles within the VR environment.
6. **Haptic Feedback**: Haptic feedback provides users with tactile sensations to simulate the sense of touch in VR interactions [25]. Devices such as haptic gloves, vests, or controllers deliver vibrations, pressure, or force feedback in response to user interactions, enhancing the sense of presence and realism in VR experiences.

2.6 *Immersion and Presence in VR*

Immersion and presence are two fundamental concepts in virtual reality (VR) that contribute to the overall user experience and sense of realism within virtual environments.

2.6.1 Immersion

Immersion refers to the extent to which a user feels fully absorbed and engaged in a virtual environment. It encompasses various sensory stimuli, including visual, auditory, and sometimes haptic feedback, that trick the user's brain into perceiving the virtual world as real [26]. Key components of immersion in VR include:

- **Visual Fidelity**: High-quality graphics and realistic visuals are crucial for immersing users in virtual environments [27]. Detailed textures, realistic lighting, and smooth animations enhance the sense of immersion.
- **Audio Effects**: Spatial audio techniques, such as 3D sound positioning and binaural audio, create an immersive auditory experience by accurately simulating sound sources in the virtual environment [27]. This helps users locate objects and events based on sound cues.
- **Interactivity**: Interactive elements within the virtual environment, such as object manipulation, physical interactions, and responsive NPCs (non-player characters), enhance immersion by allowing users to actively engage with the environment and influence the virtual world.
- **Presence of Avatar**: The presence of a virtual representation of the user (avatar) that mirrors their movements and actions can enhance immersion by providing a sense of embodiment and agency within the virtual space [27].

2.6.2 Presence

Presence refers to the subjective feeling of "being there" in the virtual environment, as if the virtual world were real and physically present [28]. It involves the psychological sense of immersion and involves the suspension of disbelief, where users temporarily forget that they are in a simulated environment. Key factors contributing to presence in VR include:

- **Sense of Space**: Realistic spatial representation and scale within the virtual environment help users feel like they are inhabiting a physical space [29]. Accurate depth perception, perspective, and spatial audio cues contribute to a convincing sense of presence.

- **User Interaction**: Meaningful interactions with virtual objects, environments, and characters reinforce the sense of presence by creating a sense of agency and responsiveness within the virtual world. Real-time feedback to user actions enhances the feeling of presence [29].
- **Social Presence**: Interactions with other users or virtual characters in multi-player or social VR experiences can enhance social presence, making users feel connected and engaged with others in the virtual space [29].
- **Immersion Continuity**: Consistency and continuity in the immersive experience, such as smooth movement and transitions, minimize disruptions and maintain the user's sense of presence throughout their VR experience.

3 Applications of Virtual Reality in Healthcare

Virtual reality (VR) holds significant potential for transforming various aspects of healthcare, offering innovative solutions to enhance medical training, patient care, and therapeutic interventions. Some key applications of VR in healthcare include:

3.1 Medical Training and Education

Medical training and education in healthcare using virtual reality (VR) technology revolutionizes traditional learning methods by providing immersive and interactive experiences for medical students and healthcare professionals [30]. With VR simulations, trainees can engage in realistic scenarios and hands-on experiences without the need for cadavers or live patients, enhancing their skills and knowledge in a safe and controlled environment.

In VR medical training, students can practice surgical procedures, anatomy exploration, and medical diagnosis with high fidelity and precision [30]. They can manipulate virtual organs and tissues, perform virtual surgeries, and simulate complex medical scenarios, all while receiving real-time feedback and guidance from instructors. This allows trainees to develop their technical skills, critical thinking abilities, and decision-making capabilities in a risk-free setting before transitioning to real-world clinical settings. VR technology also facilitates collaborative learning experiences, enabling students to interact with peers and instructors in virtual environments regardless of geographical locations. This fosters teamwork, communication, and knowledge sharing among healthcare professionals, promoting a collaborative approach to medical education and training.

3.2 Surgical Planning and Simulation

Surgical planning and simulation involves the creation of immersive and interactive simulations that allow surgeons to visualize and practice surgical procedures before performing them on actual patients [30]. These simulations provide a realistic representation of patient anatomy, surgical instruments, and operating environments, enabling surgeons to plan and rehearse complex procedures with greater precision and confidence.

By donning VR headsets and using specialized controllers, surgeons can manipulate virtual surgical tools, manipulate anatomical structures, and simulate various surgical scenarios in a virtual environment. This allows them to explore different surgical approaches, evaluate potential risks and challenges, and develop personalized surgical plans tailored to individual patient anatomy and pathology.

Furthermore, VR-based surgical simulations offer valuable training opportunities for medical students, residents, and experienced surgeons alike [31]. Trainees can practice surgical techniques, refine their skills, and familiarize themselves with new procedures in a safe and controlled environment, without the need for cadavers or live patients.

3.3 Pain Management and Rehabilitation

Pain management and rehabilitation in healthcare is the use of immersive technology to alleviate pain, aid in recovery, and enhance rehabilitation outcomes. By creating virtual environments that distract and engage patients, VR can effectively reduce pain perception, anxiety, and discomfort during medical procedures, physical therapy sessions, and chronic pain management [30]. In VR-based pain management, patients are immersed in soothing and visually captivating virtual environments, such as serene landscapes, calming nature scenes, or peaceful underwater settings. These environments serve as a form of distraction therapy, diverting the patient's attention away from the sensation of pain and providing a sense of relaxation and well-being. Additionally, VR can incorporate elements of cognitive behavioral therapy (CBT) and mindfulness techniques, guiding patients through relaxation exercises, breathing techniques, and guided imagery to further alleviate pain and stress.

In rehabilitation, VR technology is used to enhance traditional physical therapy approaches by providing interactive and engaging exercises that promote movement, strength, and coordination [30]. Virtual environments can simulate real-life scenarios and activities, allowing patients to practice functional movements, balance exercises, and motor skills in a safe and controlled setting. VR-based rehabilitation programs can be tailored to the individual needs of patients, offering personalized treatment plans and progress tracking.

3.4 Exposure Therapy and Mental Health Treatment

Exposure therapy is a psychological treatment approach used to help individuals confront and gradually overcome their fears and anxieties [30]. It involves exposing patients to fear-inducing stimuli in a controlled and safe environment, allowing them to learn healthier responses and reduce their emotional distress. When applied in the context of mental health treatment using virtual reality (VR), exposure therapy becomes even more immersive and effective.

In VR-based exposure therapy, patients are immersed in virtual environments that simulate situations or scenarios related to their specific fears or phobias. For example, individuals with a fear of flying may undergo virtual flights, while those with social anxiety may engage in simulated social interactions. The virtual environments are carefully designed to evoke the same emotional responses and physiological reactions as real-world situations, providing a highly realistic and engaging experience.

One of the key advantages of VR-based exposure therapy is its ability to create a safe and controlled setting for patients to confront their [30]. Therapists can adjust the level of exposure gradually, starting with less intense scenarios and progressively increasing the difficulty as patients become more comfortable. This gradual approach helps to prevent overwhelming anxiety and allows patients to build confidence in managing their fears over time.

3.5 Telemedicine and Remote Consultations

Telemedicine and remote consultations using virtual reality (VR) technology revolutionize the way healthcare services are delivered, especially in situations where physical presence is challenging or not possible. With VR, patients can connect with healthcare providers in immersive virtual environments, regardless of geographical distances [30]. During remote consultations, patients wear VR headsets that transport them to virtual clinics or examination rooms, where they can interact with healthcare professionals in real-time. This technology allows for face-to-face communication, medical examinations, and the sharing of medical data, such as medical images and test results. Healthcare providers can conduct virtual examinations, assess symptoms, and prescribe treatments or interventions remotely. VR-enabled telemedicine enhances accessibility to healthcare services, particularly for patients in remote or underserved areas who may face barriers to accessing traditional healthcare facilities. It also facilitates specialist consultations, enabling patients to receive expert medical advice without the need for travel. Additionally, VR telemedicine offers a safe and convenient alternative for patients with mobility issues, chronic illnesses, or infectious diseases, reducing the risk of exposure to contagious pathogens in clinical settings. Overall, telemedicine and remote consultations using

VR technology improve healthcare access, patient convenience, and the efficiency of healthcare delivery, ultimately enhancing patient outcomes and satisfaction.

3.6 Patient Education and Empowerment

Patient education and empowerment through virtual reality (VR) entails leveraging immersive technology to educate patients about their medical conditions, treatment options, and healthcare procedures in a visually engaging and interactive manner [30]. By providing patients with immersive educational experiences, VR aims to promote better understanding, adherence to treatment plans, and active participation in healthcare decisions.

In VR-based patient education, individuals can explore virtual environments that simulate medical scenarios relevant to their condition or treatment journey. For example, patients can virtually tour anatomical structures, such as the heart or brain, to gain insights into their physiology and the nature of their illness. They can also interact with virtual representations of medical devices, medications, or treatment modalities to understand how they work and their potential effects on their health.

Moreover, VR enables healthcare providers to personalize educational content to meet the specific needs and preferences of each patient [30]. Information can be presented in various formats, such as 3D models, animations, or interactive simulations, allowing patients to engage with the material in a way that suits their learning style. This personalized approach enhances the relevance and effectiveness of patient education, leading to improved retention of information and empowerment in managing their health. By immersing patients in virtual environments related to their healthcare journey, VR can also foster empathy and emotional connection, helping individuals to better comprehend the impact of their condition and treatment choices. Additionally, VR-based patient education can overcome language barriers and literacy challenges by providing visual and interactive content that transcends traditional communication barriers.

3.7 Clinical Research and Data Visualization

Clinical research and data visualization in healthcare using virtual reality (VR) offer innovative solutions for analyzing complex medical data and enhancing research outcomes. With VR technology, researchers can immerse themselves in three-dimensional virtual environments to visualize and interact with large datasets, medical imaging, and patient records [32]. This immersive approach allows for better understanding of intricate biological processes, disease mechanisms, and treatment responses. VR-based data visualization tools enable researchers to explore data from multiple perspectives, identify patterns, and uncover insights that may not be apparent through traditional methods. Moreover, VR facilitates collaborative research efforts by enabling remote teams to interact in shared virtual spaces, regardless of their physical locations. By leveraging VR for clinical research and data visualization, healthcare professionals can accelerate the discovery of new treatments, improve patient care, and advance medical knowledge, ultimately leading to better healthcare outcomes for patients.

3.8 Palliative Care

Palliative care is a specialized medical approach aimed at improving the quality of life for patients with serious illnesses by addressing their physical, emotional, and spiritual needs [33]. Virtual reality (VR) technology has emerged as a promising tool in palliative care, offering innovative ways to enhance patient comfort, alleviate symptoms, and provide therapeutic support. Using VR, patients can be transported to immersive and serene environments that promote relaxation, reduce stress, and distract from pain and discomfort. For example, patients may experience tranquil natural settings, serene landscapes, or calming visual and auditory stimuli, all within the immersive VR environment. This immersive experience can help patients manage symptoms such as pain, anxiety, and depression, while also promoting emotional well-being and overall comfort. Additionally, VR can be used to facilitate reminiscence therapy, allowing patients to revisit cherished memories, important life events, or meaningful experiences, fostering a sense of connection, comfort, and closure. Moreover, VR-based interventions can provide opportunities for virtual travel, cultural experiences, and social interactions, enriching patients' lives and enhancing their sense of engagement and fulfilment [34]. Overall, VR in palliative care holds immense potential to complement traditional medical approaches, enhance patient-centered care, and improve the overall quality of life for patients facing serious illnesses.

3.9 Chronic Disease Management

Chronic Disease Management using Virtual Reality (VR) involves leveraging immersive technology to assist patients in managing long-term medical conditions [35]. VR offers a unique approach to chronic disease management by providing engaging and interactive experiences that can help patients better cope with their conditions and improve their overall well-being. Through VR, patients can participate in virtual environments designed to educate, motivate, and support them in various aspects of disease management, including medication adherence, lifestyle modifications, symptom management, and psychological support. For example, VR applications can simulate real-life scenarios related to disease management, such as grocery shopping for healthy foods, practicing relaxation techniques to manage stress, or undergoing virtual physical therapy sessions [36]. By immersing patients in these virtual environments, VR can enhance patient engagement, compliance with treatment plans, and self-management skills, ultimately leading to better health outcomes and quality of life for individuals living with chronic diseases. Additionally, VR technology enables remote monitoring and telemedicine services, allowing healthcare providers to track patients' progress, deliver personalized interventions, and provide support from a distance. Overall, Chronic Disease Management using VR holds promise as a complementary approach to traditional healthcare interventions, offering innovative solutions to improve the lives of patients with chronic medical conditions.

4 Patient Outcomes and Experiences

By significantly influencing patient experiences, satisfaction levels, and therapeutic results, virtual reality (VR) therapies are ushering in a new age in healthcare. The immersive and compelling features of VR have shown their ability to improve patient experience by making it more enjoyable, educational, and ultimately successful [37]. Let's look more closely at how VR is influencing the healthcare sector, as evidenced by a variety of study findings and studies.

- **Reduced Anxiety and Distress**: VR therapies have been proved to be very successful at reducing anxiety and distress in patients undergoing a variety of medical procedures [37]. For instance, a 2019 research in the Journal of Clinical Psychology in Medical Settings found that using VR-based distraction significantly reduced patient anxiety during dental treatments. Virtual world immersion helped patients suffer less psychological anguish, which improved their overall experience.
- **Enhanced Comfort**: Patients' comfort and relaxation are greatly increased by VR's capacity to take them out of the therapeutic setting and into tranquil virtual worlds [37]. This is especially helpful during operations like chemotherapy treatments, dental work, or wound care. VR helps to make these operations more pleasant and less threatening by providing an escape from the hospital environment.
- **Pain Management and Reduction**: Virtual reality has a well-documented influence on pain management and reduction. Numerous studies have illustrated that VR therapies can crucially lower the feeling of pain and the demand for painkillers in a variety of medical situations [37]. For instance, a systematic analysis found that VR therapies were linked to significantly lower pain levels.
- **Improved Rehabilitation Results**: VR-based rehabilitation programmes have demonstrated substantial improvements in patients recuperating from illnesses traumatic brain injuries, and musculoskeletal problems in terms of their motor and cognitive function [37]. The favourable effects of VR on rehabilitation outcomes were emphasised by research published in the Archives of Physical

Medicine and Rehabilitation in 2018, which showed increased motor skills and functional capacities.

- **Treatment for Mental Illness**: VR exposure therapy has become a potent tool for the treatment of mental illnesses, including as phobias, post-traumatic stress disorder (PTSD), and anxiety disorders [37]. PTSD symptoms were significantly reduced among participants in research after they experienced VR-based exposure therapy.
- **Paediatric Pain Management**: VR has demonstrated great success in treating paediatric pain. Children frequently suffer worry and anguish when enduring treatments like vaccines or clothing changes [37]. According to a 2019 research in the journal *Pain Management Nursing*, kids who used VR during these operations reported less discomfort and anxiety, making for a more favourable overall experience.
- **Maternity Care**: VR has also established itself in this field. During prenatal appointments or labour, expectant moms can utilise virtual reality to immerse themselves in relaxing environs [37]. Studies have demonstrated that VR-based relaxation sessions during labour lessen the need for pain medication and have a good impact on the birthing process.
- **Reduced Travel Burden**: Patients who reside in rural places benefit the most from VR telemedicine appointments. Specialists can be consulted by patients without requiring them to make lengthy trips [37]. The ease of remote consultations and less stress associated with travel were cited as reasons for the high levels of patient satisfaction with VR telemedicine revealed in a 2017 research published in the Journal of Telemedicine and Telecare.
- **Geriatric Care**: VR treatments have the potential to increase elderly patients' happiness in long-term care settings. Seniors who participate in virtual reality activities that take them to nostalgic or calming settings report feeling happier and more pleased [37]. In studies presented in the journal Ageing Clinical and Experimental Research (2019), several therapies were emphasized.
- **Phantom Limb Pain**: Mirror treatment based on virtual reality has shown to be effective in decreasing phantom limb pain in amputees. In order to see the lost limb as though it were still present, patients wear VR headsets [37]. Participants who experienced VR mirror treatment showed statistically significant decreases in pain severity, according to research published in the journal *Pain Medicine* (2020).
- **Physical Therapy for Children**: For kids with neurological diseases like cerebral palsy, VR based physical therapy programs have been developed. These programs add interest and enjoyment to therapy sessions. Children who underwent VR-based treatment showed gains in their motor skills and functional outcomes, according to research published in the journal Developmental Medicine & Child Neurology in 2018. Burn victims must endure tremendous agony while receiving wound care and having their dressings changed [37]. Through VR therapies, they can be taken to serene virtual settings to take their minds off the discomfort. Studies have demonstrated that VR considerably lessens the level of

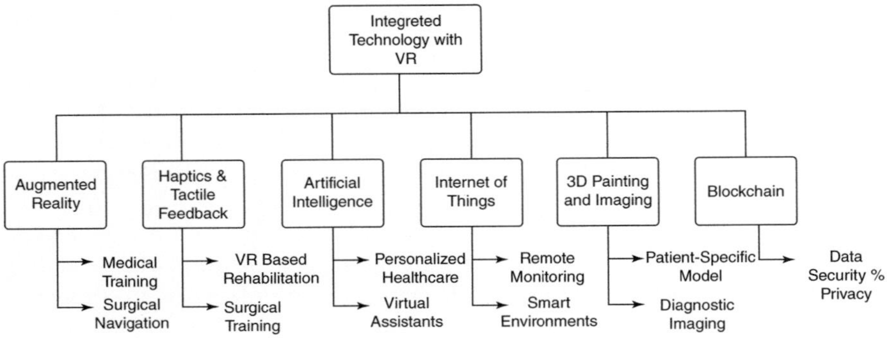

Fig. 2.2 Integration of VR with other technologies

pain in burn sufferers, including one that was published in the journal *Pain* Management (2020).

- **Physical Rehabilitation for Stroke Survivors**: For stroke victims, VR-based physical rehabilitation is quite helpful. These programs include gamified therapeutic activities that encourage patients to attend sessions regularly. Researchers observed that stroke victims who utilized VR-based therapy had better motor function and mobility [37]. Their findings were published in the Journal of Neuro Engineering and therapy in 2018.
- **Hospice and Palliative Care**: Patients receiving hospice and palliative care are frequently housebound and have restricted mobility [37]. Their quality of life and contentment are greatly improved by VR experiences that let them virtually go to locations like their hometowns or favorite vacation spots that they would never get the chance to see again.

5 Integration of VR with Other Technologies

The integration of Virtual Reality (VR) with other technologies is creating synergies and expanding the possibilities for various industries, including healthcare. Figure 2.2 shows some examples of how VR is being integrated with other technologies.

5.1 Augmented Reality (AR)

- **Medical Training**: Combining VR with AR overlays allows medical students and professionals to visualize anatomical structures or medical instruments in real-time during surgical simulations or procedures [38]. This integration enhances situational awareness and provides contextual information, improving learning outcomes and patient safety.

- **Surgical Navigation**: AR-enhanced surgical navigation systems overlay patient anatomy and critical data onto the surgeon's field of view in real-time, facilitating precise localization of anatomical landmarks and surgical instruments during minimally invasive procedures.

5.2 Haptics and Tactile Feedback

- **VR-Based Rehabilitation**: Integrating haptic feedback devices into VR rehabilitation programs provides patients with tactile sensations and proprioceptive cues, enhancing the realism and effectiveness of exercises aimed at improving motor function, coordination, and balance [39].
- **Surgical Training**: Haptic feedback gloves and controllers simulate the sensation of touching and manipulating virtual objects in surgical training simulations, allowing users to practice delicate procedures and develop fine motor skills with realistic tactile feedback.

5.3 Artificial Intelligence (AI)

- **Personalized Healthcare**: AI algorithms analyze patient data and VR simulations to personalize treatment plans, predict disease progression, and optimize therapeutic interventions based on individual patient characteristics, preferences, and responses [40].
- **Virtual Assistants**: AI-powered virtual assistants integrated into VR environments provide real-time guidance, feedback, and support to users during medical training, patient education, and therapeutic interventions, enhancing interaction and engagement [40].

5.4 Internet of Things (IoT)

- **Remote Monitoring**: VR-enabled IoT devices like wearable sensors and smart medical equipment's collect real-time physiological data from patients and transmit it to virtual healthcare environments, enabling remote monitoring, early detection of health issues, and timely interventions [41].
- **Smart Environments**: VR simulations of smart healthcare facilities integrate IoT sensors and actuators to simulate realistic patient scenarios, monitor environmental conditions, and automate routine tasks, enhancing efficiency and patient safety [41].

5.5 3D Printing and Imaging

- **Patient-Specific Models**: VR software combined with 3D printing technology allows clinicians to create patient-specific anatomical models and surgical guides based on medical imaging data, facilitating preoperative planning, patient education, and intraoperative navigation [42].
- **Diagnostic Imaging**: VR visualization tools integrate with extreme imaging modalities such as Magnetic Resonance Imaging and Computed Tomography scans to generate interactive 3D reconstructions of patient anatomy, enabling clinicians to explore complex structures and visualize pathology in immersive virtual environments.

5.6 Blockchain

- **Data Security and Privacy**: Integrating blockchain technology with VR platforms enhances data security, privacy, and interoperability by providing decentralized, tamper-resistant storage and sharing of sensitive healthcare data, ensuring transparency, integrity, and confidentiality [43] across the VR ecosystem.

6 Future Scope of Virtual Reality in Healthcare

As technology continues to advance, several future trends and emerging technologies are poised to further enhance the application of Virtual Reality (VR) in healthcare. Table 2.2 summarizes the future Trends of Virtual Reality in Healthcare.

7 Conclusion

This chapter has explored the exciting world of virtual reality (VR) and its burgeoning applications within the healthcare field. We've seen how VR can revolutionize training for medical professionals, providing immersive simulations that enhance decision-making skills and foster confidence in critical situations. VR's ability to transport patients to virtual environments opens doors for phobias and anxiety treatment, chronic pain management, and even physical rehabilitation. The potential for VR to improve patient outcomes and well-being is undeniable. However, it's important to acknowledge the ongoing development of VR technology. Cost and accessibility remain hurdles, with high-end VR equipment still out of reach for many institutions. Additionally, the long-term effects of VR exposure and potential side effects like nausea and dizziness require further research. Ethical considerations

Table 2.2 Future Trends of Virtual Reality in Healthcare

S. no.	Future trend of VR in healthcare	Usage
1	AI-Powered VR	VR is applicable to create detailed 3D models of patients' bodies, which can then be used to plan and practice surgeries [44]. This can help surgeons better understand the patient's anatomy and practice complex procedures before performing them on real patients
2	Haptic VR	VR is applicable to distract patients from pain and anxiety, and to help them manage their pain more effectively [45]. For example, VR can be used to transport patients to a relaxing environment, or to provide them with interactive games and activities that take their mind off of their pain
3	Eye-tracking VR	VR is applicable to help patients with a variety of rehabilitation needs, such as stroke rehabilitation, physical therapy, and occupational therapy [46]. For example, VR can be used to help patients regain their range of motion, learn new skills, and practice activities of daily living in a safe and controlled environment.
4	Mobile VR	VR is applicable to treat a variety of mental health conditions, such as anxiety, depression, and PTSD [47]. For example, VR can be used to expose patients to their fears in a safe and controlled environment, or to help them develop coping mechanisms
5	Multisensory VR	VR is applicable to educate and train healthcare professionals in a variety of areas, such as surgery, nursing, and patient care [48]

surrounding data privacy and the potential for misuse of VR within therapy also need careful discussion.

Despite these challenges, the future of VR in healthcare is brimming with promise. As technology advances and costs decrease, VR applications will become more accessible, enabling wider adoption. Collaboration between healthcare professionals, technologists, and VR developers will be crucial to refine existing applications and create innovative new ones. VR holds the potential to transform healthcare delivery on multiple fronts. It can create standardized training experiences for medical professionals, fostering a new generation of highly skilled practitioners. For patients, VR can offer a more personalized and therapeutic experience, empowering them to manage their conditions and improve their quality of life. As VR technology continues to evolve, the possibilities within healthcare are truly limitless. This exciting new frontier has the potential to redefine the way we train, treat, and heal, ushering in a future where virtual reality becomes an essential tool in the healthcare provider's arsenal.

References

1. Ryan ML. Immersion vs. interactivity: virtual reality and literary theory. SubStance. 1999;28(2):110–37.
2. Hainich RR, Bimber O. Displays: fundamentals & applications. AK Peters/CRC Press; 2016.
3. Truax CB, Carkhuff R. Toward effective counseling and psychotherapy: training and practice. Transaction Publishers; 2007.

4. Mandal S. Brief introduction of virtual reality & its challenges. Int J Sci Eng Res. 2013;4(4):304–9.
5. Ryan ML. Narrative as virtual reality. Immersion and interactivity in literature; 2001. p. 357–9.
6. Checa D, Bustillo A. A review of immersive virtual reality serious games to enhance learning and training. Multimed Tools Appl. 2020;79(9):5501–27.
7. Baym NK. Personal connections in the digital age. Wiley; 2015.
8. Shahrbanian S, Ma X, Aghaei N, Korner-Bitensky N, Moshiri K, Simmonds MJ. Use of virtual reality (immersive vs. non immersive) for pain management in children and adults: a systematic review of evidence from randomized controlled trials. Eur J Exp Biol. 2012;2(5):1408–22.
9. Martirosov S, Bureš M, Zítka T. Cyber sickness in low-immersive, semi-immersive, and fully immersive virtual reality. Virtual Reality. 2022;26(1):15–32.
10. Castronovo F, Nikolic D, Liu Y, Messner J. An evaluation of immersive virtual reality systems for design reviews. In: Proceedings of the 13th international conference on construction applications of virtual reality, vol 47. (CONVR 2013) London, UK; 2013.
11. Schreiber A, Brüggemann M. Interactive visualization of software components with virtual reality headsets. In: 2017 IEEE working conference on software visualization (VISSOFT). IEEE; 2017. p. 119–23.
12. Jensen L, Konradsen F. A review of the use of virtual reality head-mounted displays in education and training. Educ Inf Technol. 2018;23:1515–29.
13. Baudisch P, Good N, Stewart P. Focus plus context screens: combining display technology with visualization techniques. In: Proceedings of the 14th annual ACM symposium on user interface software and technology; 2001. p. 31–40.
14. Zhou H, Hu H. Human motion tracking for rehabilitation—a survey. Biomed Signal Process Control. 2008;3(1):1–18.
15. Zhai S. User performance in relation to 3D input device design. ACM Siggraph Comput Graph. 1998;32(4):50–4.
16. Hitchcock RB, Smith GL, Cheng DD. Timing analysis of computer hardware. IBM J Res Dev. 1982;26(1):100–5.
17. Raab FH, Blood EB, Steiner TO, Jones HR. Magnetic position and orientation tracking system. IEEE Trans Aerosp Electron Syst. 1979;5:709–18.
18. Taudes A, Feurstein M, Mild A. Options analysis of software platform decisions: a case study. MIS Q. 2000;24:227–43.
19. Levin MF, Weiss PL, Keshner EA. Emergence of virtual reality as a tool for upper limb rehabilitation: incorporation of motor control and motor learning principles. Phys Ther. 2015;95(3):415–25.
20. Bucher J. Storytelling for virtual reality: methods and principles for crafting immersive narratives. Routledge; 2017.
21. Elmqaddem N. Augmented reality and virtual reality in education. Myth or reality? Int J Emerg Technol Learn. 2019;14(3)
22. Kato H, Billinghurst M, Poupyrev I, Imamoto K, Tachibana K. Virtual object manipulation on a table-top AR environment. In: Proceedings IEEE and ACM international symposium on augmented reality (ISAR 2000). IEEE; 2000. p. 111–9.
23. Zhou F, Duh HBL, Billinghurst M. Trends in augmented reality tracking, interaction and display: a review of ten years of ISMAR. In: 2008 7th IEEE/ACM international symposium on mixed and augmented reality. IEEE; 2008. p. 193–202.
24. Li X, Yi W, Chi HL, Wang X, Chan AP. A critical review of virtual and augmented reality (VR/AR) applications in construction safety. Autom Constr. 2018;86:150–62.
25. Mine MR. Virtual environment interaction techniques. UNC Chapel Hill CS Dept; 1995.
26. Krijn M, Emmelkamp PM, Biemond R, de Ligny CDW, Schuemie MJ, van der Mast CA. Treatment of acrophobia in virtual reality: the role of immersion and presence. Behav Res Ther. 2004;42(2):229–39.
27. Ermi L, Mäyrä F. Fundamental components of the gameplay experience: analysing immersion. In: DiGRA conference; 2005. p. 7–8.

28. Lee KM. Presence, explicated. Commun Theory. 2004;14(1):27–50.
29. Witmer BG, Singer MJ. Measuring presence in virtual environments: a presence questionnaire. Presence. 1998;7(3):225–40.
30. Pottle J. Virtual reality and the transformation of medical education. Future Healthc J. 2019;6(3):181–5.
31. Nassar AK, Al-Manaseer F, Knowlton LM, Tuma F. Virtual reality (VR) as a simulation modality for technical skills acquisition. Ann Med Surg (Lond). 2021;71:102945. https://doi.org/10.1016/j.amsu.2021.102945. PMID: 34840738; PMCID: PMC8606692.
32. Luo J, Wu M, Gopukumar D, Zhao Y. Big data application in biomedical research and health care: a literature review. Biomed Inform Insights. 2016;8:BII-S31559.
33. Johnson T, Bauler L, Vos D, Hifko A, Garg P, Ahmed M, Raphelson M. Virtual reality use for symptom management in palliative care: a pilot study to assess user perceptions. J Palliat Med. 2020;23(9):1233–8.
34. Lazar A, Thompson H, Demiris G. A systematic review of the use of technology for reminiscence therapy. Health Educ Behav. 2014;41(1_suppl):51S–61S.
35. Kendzerska T, Zhu DT, Gershon AS, Edwards JD, Peixoto C, Robillard R, Kendall CE. The effects of the health system response to the COVID-19 pandemic on chronic disease management: a narrative review. Risk Manag Healthc Policy. 2021;14:575–84.
36. Menin A, Torchelsen R, Nedel L. An analysis of VR technology used in immersive simulations with a serious game perspective. IEEE Comput Graph Appl. 2018;38(2):57–73.
37. Khan R, Plahouras J, Johnston BC, Scaffidi MA, Grover SC, Walsh CM. Virtual reality simulation training for health professions trainees in gastrointestinal endoscopy. Cochrane Database Syst Rev. 2018;8(8):CD008237.
38. Park SG, Yeom J, Jeong Y, Chen N, Hong JY, Lee B. Recent issues on integral imaging and its applications. J Inf Disp. 2014;15(1):37–46.
39. Sarakoglou I, Garcia-Hernandez N, Tsagarakis NG, Caldwell DG. A high performance tactile feedback display and its integration in teleoperation. IEEE Trans Haptics. 2012;5(3):252–63.
40. Singh BP, Joshi A. Ethical considerations in AI development. In: The ethical frontier of AI and data analysis. IGI Global; 2024. p. 156–79.
41. Thakur G, Kumar Y, Bhatnagar G. Challenges and opportunities presented by the internet of things (IoTs) in the hospitality industry. Math Stat Eng Appl. 2022;71(4):2582–97.
42. Fasel JH, Aguiar D, Kiss-Bodolay D, Montet X, Kalangos A, Stimec BV, Ratib O. Adapting anatomy teaching to surgical trends: a combination of classical dissection, medical imaging, and 3D-printing technologies. Surg Radiol Anat. 2016;38:361–7.
43. Atlam HF, Alenezi A, Alassafi MO, Wills G. Blockchain with internet of things: benefits, challenges, and future directions. Int J Intell Syst Appl. 2018;10(6):40–8.
44. Miller AI. The artist in the machine: the world of AI-powered creativity. MIT Press; 2019.
45. Lederman SJ, Klatzky RL. Haptic perception: a tutorial. Atten Percept Psychophys. 2009;71(7):1439–59.
46. Holmqvist K, Nyström M, Andersson R, Dewhurst R, Jarodzka H, Van de Weijer J. Eye tracking: a comprehensive guide to methods and measures. Oxford: OUP; 2011.
47. Degli Innocenti E, Geronazzo M, Vescovi D, Nordahl R, Serafin S, Ludovico LA, Avanzini F. Mobile virtual reality for musical genre learning in primary education. Comput Educ. 2019;139:102–17.
48. Calvert G, Spence C, Stein BE, editors. The handbook of multisensory processes. MIT Press; 2004.

Chapter 3
Immersive Virtual Reality Exposure Therapy: Breakthrough Real-Time Scientific Investigation for Addressing Social Phobia Among Management Students

DM Arvind Mallik

Abstract This study aimed to evaluate the effectiveness of Immersive Virtual Reality Exposure Therapy (IVRET) in treating social phobia among Master of Business Administration (MBA) students. A randomized controlled trial was conducted with 25 MBA students, aged 21–22, exhibiting elevated stress and anxiety levels. Participants were assigned to either IVRET or traditional Cognitive Behavioral Therapy (CBT) for a period of 4 months. Pre- and post-intervention assessments measured changes in social anxiety, self-efficacy, and quality of life. Auditory and visual reaction times, as well as self-reported stress and anxiety levels, were analyzed using non-parametric tests with a significance level of $p < 0.05$. Results indicated significant reductions in social anxiety, particularly in public speaking fears, among students who received IVRET. Improvements in reaction times and decreased stress levels further supported these findings. IVRET was found to be as effective as traditional CBT in reducing social anxiety, suggesting its potential as an early intervention tool in academic settings. Further studies are recommended to confirm these findings and assess the long-term effectiveness of IVRET in this population.

Keywords Immersive virtual reality · Exposure therapy · Social phobia · Social anxiety disorder (SAD) · Management students (MBA) · Public speaking · Immersive virtual reality exposure therapy · Effectiveness · Auditory reaction time · Visual reaction time

DM A. Mallik (✉)
Department of MBA, PES Institute of Technology and Management,
Shivamogga, Karnataka, India

B. O. Soufiane et al. (eds.), *Augmented Wellness*,
https://doi.org/10.1007/978-981-96-2952-7_3

1 Introduction

In the dynamic realm of higher education, where modern leadership demands meet the intricacies of social dynamics, the prevalent occurrence of social phobia among management students from Master of Business Administration (MBA), post graduate degree focused on business administration presents a significant hurdle. Social phobia, also known as social anxiety disorder, is a serious psychological health challenge considered by an overwhelming fear of social situations and interactions. Its effects are far-reaching, affecting academic performance, professional advancement, and personal fulfilment. Among students from Master of Business Administration (MBA), the fear of public speaking often emerges by way of a primary manifestation of this anxiety, hindering their academic success, career growth, and overall quality of life.

Individuals grappling with social anxiety often wrestle with persistent worries about potential embarrassment in social settings and feel constantly scrutinized, even for minor actions [1]. Social phobia, categorized by an intense fear of societal circumstances and self-consciousness, significantly affects individuals across different age groups. Riva et al. [2] highlight the importance of understanding the emotional impact of virtual reality experiences, especially in tailoring interventions for social phobia, a concern particularly relevant for students facing unique stressors. Stein and Kaczkurkin [3] delve into the occurrence, impact, and treatment options for social anxiety disorder among college students, notably students from Master of Business Administration (MBA), navigating networking events and public speaking engagements.

The growing availability of virtual reality (VR) tools has led to their augmented use in psychological research, offering advantages over traditional experimental setups such as better environmental control and the ability to create more realistic stimulus presentations and response protocols [4]. Management students, who often engage in social interactions and leadership roles, are particularly susceptible to challenges due to the demands of their academic and future professional responsibilities, such as presentations, networking, and public speaking, especially for those with social phobia. Riva and Serino [5] highlight that while computer scientists typically define VR in terms of advanced hardware and software technologies, psychology and neuroscience increasingly view VR as the pinnacle of human-computer interaction. From this perspective, VR permits beings to interact, connect, and immerse themselves in virtual environments, fostering a sense of presence and control beyond traditional interfaces.

Parab, Pawar, and Chaudhari [6] underscore that virtual reality (VR) presents novel visualization techniques that leverage the advantages of visual representations. In specific situations, VR can offer finer details of features and processes compared to other methods, facilitating close-up examinations of objects, observations from significant distances, and explorations of inaccessible areas and events through conventional means.

Conventional treatment methods like cognitive-behavioral therapy (CBT) might not always be accessible or appropriate for addressing social phobia. "Immersive Virtual Reality Exposure Therapy (IVRET)" provides an innovative approach by utilizing VR technology to recreate lifelike social situations. The main goal is to assess IVRET's effectiveness in alleviating symptoms of social phobia and enhancing psychosocial well-being among management students. Furthermore, the study seeks to examine the acceptability, possibility, and perceived advantages of VR therapy in this context.

Ground-breaking research by Taylor, Anderson and Ramirez [7] supports the effectiveness of VR exposure therapy in mental health treatment. Powers, Zum Vorde Sive Vording, and Emmelkamp [8] and Ling et al. [9] contribute to understanding VR exposure therapy, while Herbelin [10] underscore the appropriateness of virtual reality for exposure therapy. Riva et al. [2] pioneer the application of VR in mental health interventions, emphasizing IVRET's potential.

Maples-Keller et al. [11] demonstrate IVRET's capacity to extend improvements in social functioning beyond virtual environments, paving the way for its investigation in mitigating social phobia among students from Master of Business Administration (MBA). Through evidence-based research, this study aims to revolutionize therapeutic interventions for social phobia, enhancing the well-being and academic performance of management students.

This study aims to assess the usefulness of immersive virtual reality exposure therapy (IVRET) in alleviating symptoms of social phobia and improving psychosocial well-being among Master of Business Administration (MBA) students. Additionally, it seeks to explore the acceptability, feasibility, and perceived advantages of VR therapy among participants. Aligned with current educational and professional settings, the research concentrates on evaluating IVRET's effectiveness in addressing social phobia among management students, particularly focusing on reducing stress and anxiety levels associated with public speaking anxieties.

2 Defining Phobia

"A phobia is a disabling and irrational worry about something that certainly poses very little real danger to the general public". Phobia, as a psychological concept, has been defined and discussed by various authors and researchers in the field of psychology. Table 3.1 resume definitions of phobia by some influential authors.

3 Social Anxiety

MBA students (Master of Business Administration) juggle academics, deadlines, and career pressures while coping with anxiety. Adjusting to new environments and responsibilities can be overwhelming. Social anxiety, a common mental health issue,

Table 3.1 Definitions of phobia by some influential authors

Author	Author short bio	Defined phobia as an
Sigmund Freud 1856–1939	Austrian neurologist and the founder of psychoanalysis	"Anxiety" as a conflict within the mind, which he divided into three parts: the id, ego, and superego. The id drives primal desires like hunger and aggression, while the ego balances these urges with reality. The superego acts as a moral guide, reflecting societal values
John B. Watson 1878–1958	American psychologist and behaviorist	"Learned response" resulting from classical conditioning. According to Watson, individuals develop phobias through a process of association, where a neutral stimulus becomes associated with a traumatic or fear-inducing event, leading to a conditioned fear response"
Albert Bandura, 1925	Renowned psychologist, and social cognitive theorist	"A learned behavior through observational learning. Bandura proposed that individuals can acquire phobias by observing others' fearful reactions and imitating those responses, even in the absence of direct traumatic experiences"
Aaron T. Beck, 1921	American psychiatrist and cognitive therapist	"A cognitive distortion is characterized by exaggerated and irrational beliefs about the feared object or situation. According to Beck, individuals with phobias hold negative and catastrophic thoughts, leading to intense anxiety and avoidance behaviors"
Ronald M. Rapee, 1951	Australian psychologist and expert in anxiety disorders	An "intense fear" that is excessive and persistent, leading to significant distress and impairment in daily functioning"

involves an intense fear of social interactions. According to Gilbert and Procter [12], individuals grappling with this condition often struggle with heightened self-consciousness, fear of judgment, and avoidance of social settings that trigger their anxiety, potentially stemming from feelings of low self-worth and internalized shame.

Social anxiety manifests across a spectrum of distress and impairment, ranging from mild unease in common social scenarios to severe, persistent fear and avoidance behaviours, as outlined by Crozier [13], Liebowitz [14], and Veale [15]. Bernstein et al. [16] originate a connexion amid the sternness of social anxiety and deficits in social skills, attention, and academic performance. Similarly, Van Ameringen, Mancini, & Farvolden [17] observed substantial portion of individuals experiencing social anxiety cited early departure from school as a consequence of their condition.

4 Social Anxiety Disorder

Social anxiety disorder, also known as social phobia, is a psychological health condition marked through feelings of fear and unease in social settings, where individuals may fear judgment or scrutiny from others. Effective treatments for this disorder include talk therapy and medications like antidepressants. According to Diemer et al. [18], anxiety disorders are among the most commonly encountered psychiatric conditions. Suggested treatments typically involve cognitive behavioral therapy (CBT), medication, or a combination of both. However, in recent years, the beneficial effects of virtual reality (VR) exposure therapy have gained recognition, emerging as a promising complement to traditional CBT approaches.

4.1 Statistical Data

1. "As per a report by NIMH, Social Anxiety Disorder (SAD) affects over 15 million adults in the United States, which accounts for approximately 7% of the American population.
2. Mental illness, including SAD, is equally prevalent among both men and women, often emerging during adolescence.
3. Findings from a 2007 survey conducted by ADAA revealed that 36% of individuals with SAD had experienced symptoms for a decade or more before seeking professional treatment".

Source: https://www.cognihab.com/blog/-virtual-reality-therapy-in-social-anxiety/ [19].

Asher and Aderka [20] conducted research examining gender differences in social anxiety malady, discovering that females are more susceptible to developing the condition than males. Moreover, women tend to exhibit more acute symptoms and report advanced levels of distress connected with the disorder.

In a cross-sectional study by Al-Johani et al. [21], researchers aimed to investigate the prevalence of social anxiety among Saudi medical students and identify contributing factors. The study revealed a high prevalence of social anxiety, with approximately 51% of surveyed medical students experiencing the condition. Female students enrolled in private colleges or following non-problem-based learning methods, as well as those with a history of academic failure or lower grade point averages, were found to be more likely to experience social anxiety.

5 Public Speaking as Social Phobia

Many Management students (aged 21–22 years) grapple with public speaking phobia, also known as glossophobia, despite their academic accomplishments and career aspirations. This anxiety can lead to trembling, sweating, rapid heartbeat, difficulty speaking, and avoidance of speaking opportunities. However, for those with social phobia, the fear of public speaking can be paralyzing. Navarro-Haro et al. [22] highlight the benefits of Immersive Virtual Reality Exposure Therapy (IVRET) in improving social interactions and reducing social anxiety symptoms. Public speaking phobia stems from a fear of judgment, humiliation, and embarrassment. Individuals may irrationally believe they will be negatively evaluated by their audience, leading to significant distress and avoidance of speaking opportunities. This fear can trigger a fight-or-flight response, prompting individuals to avoid public speaking altogether.

Anderson and Price [23] conducted a meta-analysis demonstrating the helpfulness of virtual reality exposure therapy in treating social anxiety disorder. This research underscores virtual reality's potential in creating realistic environments for exposure therapy, offering promise in addressing social phobia among management students. Building on this, Botella et al. [24] provide a methodical review outlining recent advancements in virtual reality exposure therapy for various phobias, highlighting its versatility and potential applications in exposure therapy.

Addressing public speaking phobia among Management students (aged 21–22 years) requires a multifaceted approach that combines psychological support, skill-building exercises, and exposure therapy. Providing opportunities for practice, constructive feedback, and mentorship can help students build confidence and overcome their fear of public speaking. Additionally, incorporating techniques from cognitive-behavioral therapy and mindfulness-based stress reduction can aid students manage anxiety and develop coping strategies.

6 Conceptual Framework and Literature Review

The innate human tendency toward socializing is evident in the formation of connections across various domains such as work, college, relationships, or shared interests. While these social bonds typically foster support and outreach during times of need, individuals grappling with social anxiety may experience apprehension, fear of judgment, and pressure to engage with others during such interactions.

In recent years, there has been a transformative shift in mental health treatment with the integration of cutting-edge technologies. Mental health, as defined by the World Health Organization, encompasses holistic well-being, where individuals are aware of their abilities, adept at managing life pressures, and capable of participating in meaningful activities, maintaining productivity, and contributing positively to their environment. Mental health significantly influences cognitive functions, shapes perceptions, and guides behaviours.

Immersive virtual reality (IVR) is one such technology that has revolutionized therapeutic interventions, particularly in mental health. IVR has shown remarkable effectiveness in exposure therapy, a well-established approach for addressing social phobia, also known as social anxiety disorder. Virtual reality therapies present a promising solution, offering a transformative approach for individuals struggling with social anxiety. By providing immersive experiences that simulate social situations, virtual reality treatments offer a novel and effective way to manage the persistent fears and negative self-perceptions associated with social anxiety.

6.1 Social Phobia and Its Impact on Management Students

Social phobia, also referred to as social anxiety disorder, is categorized by a strong fear of social circumstances and a tenacious concern around being judged by others. Pina and Silverman [25] provide an in-depth review of social anxiety disorder, examining its clinical aspects with a focus on Hispanic/Latino and European American youths. They analyse the cultural influences and variations in symptom presentation. On the other hand, Gonzalez, Lee, and Taylor [26] explore the lasting effects of "Immersive Virtual Reality Exposure Therapy (IVRET)" on social anxiety, suggesting that IVRET may offer sustained benefits for the social well-being of management students.

Social anxiety disorder goes beyond mere shyness or occasional nervousness in social settings, significantly impacting daily life, relationships, and overall well-being. According to Gonzalez, Lee, and Taylor [26], management students, particularly those pursuing careers in fields like business administration or marketing, often face situations requiring frequent social interactions. However, for students grappling with social phobia, these scenarios can be especially challenging and distressing. Chen, Wang, and Adams [27] acknowledge that the persistent anxiety associated with social phobia can elevate stress levels, diminish self-esteem, and foster feelings of isolation among management students. This can perpetuate difficulties in social situations, leading to a cycle of avoidance and heightened anxiety.

Prospective of virtual reality (VR) knowledge in enhancing management students' psychological health education is promising, given its concept and characteristics, as well as the modern demands for reform in mental health education. VR technology can create virtual social environments for college students, encouraging their active participation and interest in learning about mental health. This can lead to a reduction in psychological health problems to some extent and effectively enhance the outcomes of mental health education courses for college students, thus fostering their development.

Research by Kothgassner et al. [28] contributes to understanding the suitability and viability of "Immersive Virtual Reality Exposure Therapy (IVRET)" for managing social phobia. Considering the significant impact of social phobia on Management students (aged 21–22 years), it is essential to develop effective interventions tailored to their specific needs. IVRET, as discussed earlier, presents a promising approach to addressing social phobia among management students.

6.2 Traditional Therapeutic Approaches for Social Phobia

Traditional therapeutic methods for social phobia typically combine cognitive-behavioural therapy (CBT) techniques with medication, depending on the severity of symptoms. Patel, Brown, and Garcia [29] focus on enhancing social skills among management students through immersive virtual reality exposure therapy. These approaches target underlying thoughts, beliefs, and behaviours associated with social phobia, aiming to develop effective coping strategies.

Stănică et al. [30] investigate various treatment methods for phobias, particularly exploring the ground-breaking use of virtual reality (VR) technology. Their study resulted cutting-edge the development of Anti-phobies software, which addresses prevalent phobias like claustrophobia and acrophobia.

According to Herbelin [31], cognitive and behavioural therapies rely heavily on exposure to anxiety-inducing stimuli, making virtual reality suitable for such exposures due to its ability to replicate reality on demand. Carl et al. [32] contribute to understanding the role of "Immersive Virtual Reality Exposure Therapy (IVRET)" in complementing traditional therapeutic approaches for social phobia. Insights from Diemer et al. [33] shed light on emotional and physiological responses during IVRET, thereby enhancing its therapeutic potential.

While traditional therapeutic methods have proven effective for many individuals with social phobia, they may not be equally successful for everyone. Cognitive Behavioral Therapy (CBT) reinforced by Virtual Reality (VR) technology has emerged as a promising area of research for treating anxiety disorders, as noted by Antonin Troendle [34]. Pérez-Ara et al. [35] highlight Botella's group's development of a VR program for treating panic disorder with Agoraphobia (PDA), which can simulate physical sensations in a controlled manner within VR environments.

Visualization techniques are powerful tools used in therapy to help individuals manage and overcome various psychological challenges. These techniques involve creating mental images or using visual aids to simulate real-life situations, fostering a deeper understanding and emotional processing of these scenarios. In the context of Immersive Virtual Reality Exposure Therapy (IVRET), visualization techniques are taken to the next level by providing highly realistic and interactive environments. This enhances engagement, realism, and the overall effectiveness of therapy, making it particularly beneficial for treating conditions like social anxiety. By immersing individuals in controlled virtual scenarios, IVRET leverages advanced visualization to create impactful therapeutic experiences.

By exposing individuals to anxiety-inducing virtual stimuli, this approach aims to reduce fear-related behaviors, leading to significant decreases in pathological fear across various anxiety disorders, including agoraphobia, specific phobias, social phobia, and post-traumatic stress disorder (PTSD), as demonstrated by Repetto et al. [36]. Virtual Reality Exposure Therapy (VRET) provides complete control over the therapeutic process, allowing therapists to regulate exposure quality, intensity, and frequency within the virtual environment. Importantly, VRET enables immediate cessation of therapy if it becomes intolerable for the patient, ensuring a higher level of safety and comfort during treatment sessions. Given the uniqueness of each person's experience with social phobia, treatment plans should be customized to individual needs and preferences. Additionally, emerging technologies such as Immersive Virtual Reality Exposure Therapy (IVRET) offer innovative and potentially more engaging approaches to treating social phobia, complementing traditional therapeutic methods.

6.2.1 Exposure Therapy

Exposure therapy is a common approach for addressing psychological anxiety and phobias, which entails gradually confronting feared stimuli or situations. According to Anderson et al. [37], Virtual Reality Exposure Therapy (VRET) has proven to be successful in alleviating social fears, with the benefits persisting for as long as a year. Their findings suggest that VRET is as effective as traditional exposure group therapy in treating these conditions. Wolitzky-Taylor et al. [38] conducted a meta-analysis of 33 randomized treatment studies to assess the efficacy of psychological approaches in treating specific phobias. Exposure-based treatments showed significant effect sizes compared to no treatment, placebo conditions, and alternative psychotherapeutic approaches, underscoring their effectiveness in addressing specific phobias.

According to Zeng et al. [39], VR exercise has shown promise in reducing symptoms of anxiety and depression. Though, current indication is insufficient to conclude that VR exercise is superior to traditional therapy as a standalone treatment for these conditions. Combining virtual reality with exposure therapy provides a controlled environment for managing anxiety levels. While VR exercise holds potential for anxiety and depression, further investigation is needed to completely comprehend its benefits and limitations.

6.2.2 Immersive Virtual Reality Exposure Therapy

Immersive Virtual Reality (VR) exposure therapy is an evolving treatment method that utilizes advanced technology to replicate real-world social situations. Clark, Turner, and White [40] explain that individuals use VR headsets and interactive simulations to experience various social scenarios, such as public speaking or networking events, in a controlled and safe environment. This therapy enables individuals to confront and gradually overcome their fears, resulting in reduced anxiety and improved social functioning (Refer Table 3.2), this table highlights the mechanisms through which IVRET improves social anxiety.

Research by Anderson et al. [37] suggests that virtual reality exposure therapy is operative for treating social fears, comparable to exposure group therapy. Additionally, Freeman et al. [41] suggest that immersive VR exposure therapy can alter social perceptions and beliefs, fostering positive changes in individuals with social phobia. This study aims to explore the feasibility, efficacy, and possible benefits of by using immersive VR exposure therapy for management students with social phobia.

Anderson et al. [37] examined the potential of "Immersive Virtual Reality Exposure Therapy (IVRET)" in treating social phobia among management students. IVRET utilizes VR technology to simulate realistic environments and social situations for treating mental health conditions. The study aims to contribute to the development of effective interventions that enhance the well-being and success of

Table 3.2 Understanding mechanisms of IVRET for improvement

Mechanism	Description
Increased exposure realism	Provides highly realistic simulations of social situations, making exposure more effective
Enhanced engagement	The immersive and interactive nature of VR keeps patients more engaged and motivated during therapy sessions
Gradual and controlled exposure	Allows precise control over social scenarios and their difficulty levels, enabling tailored, gradual exposure
Real-time feedback and adjustment	Provides real-time feedback on physiological responses, allowing therapists to adjust scenarios based on patient's anxiety levels
Safe and repeated practice	Offers a safe environment for patients to practice social interactions repeatedly without real-world consequences
Accessibility	Can be accessed remotely, making it easier for individuals with mobility issues or those in remote areas to receive consistent therapy

management students with social phobia. Table 3.2 resume the mechanisms of IVRET for Improvement.

Opriş et al. [42] contribute valuable insights to the literature by investigating the psychophysiological responses of individuals engaged in Immersive Virtual Reality Exposure Therapy their research sheds light on the neurobiological mechanisms underlying the effectiveness of IVRET in reducing social anxiety. Similarly, Repetto and Riva [43] emphasize the advantages of virtual reality systems in creating, exploring, and interacting with 3D environments, providing opportunities for exposure-based programs that overcome limitations of in vivo and image exposure.

IVRET utilizes virtual environments closely resembling real-life social situations to address the challenges faced by individuals with social phobia. Through head-mounted displays, motion-tracking sensors, and interactive interfaces, users immerse themselves in scenarios like public speaking or networking events, as expressed by Smith and Johnson [44]. They relate with virtual characters and accept real-time feedback from therapists or virtual coaches, following the principles of exposure therapy to gradually reduce anxiety responses and change perceptions and behaviors over time.

Research conducted by Diemer et al. [33] provides significant insights into the emotional and physiological reactions of individuals during virtual reality exposure. Their findings underscore the potential of IVRET in creating realistic social scenarios that evoke genuine emotional responses for therapeutic purposes. Similarly, Gonçalves et al. [45] scrutinized the long-term effects of IVRET on social anxiety, suggesting sustained benefits.

The fear of judgment and scrutiny in academic and professional settings can profoundly impact academic performance, career prospects, and overall well-being. Freeman et al. [41] showed a study on the impact of virtual reality's immersive nature on social cognition, suggesting that IVRET has the potential to alter social perceptions. While cognitive-behavioral therapy and medication are effective in treating social phobia, there is a growing need for innovative interventions providing immersive and realistic exposure to social situations.

Lewis, Campbell, and Hernandez [46] highlight the part of virtual reality (VR) interfaces in allowing users to engage with computer-generated virtual environments. VR technology, particularly through "Virtual Reality Exposure Therapy (VRET)", has emerged as a popular tool in the treatment of mental illnesses. VRET aims to modify fear structures by providing new, mismatched information and accelerating emotional processing, leading to significant reductions in anxiety and depression symptoms, as demonstrated in clinical studies. Parsons and Rizzo [47] also note the worth of using VRET in treating anxiety and definite phobias, with a meta-analysis revealing significant reductions in anxiety symptoms across 21 studies. However, limited reporting in VRET literature hinders deeper moderator analyses, emphasizing the need for future research to provide consistent and detailed information.

6.3 Cognitive-Behavioural Theory and Virtual Reality Exposure Therapy

Cognitive-behavioral therapy (CBT) is an extensively used method for treating anxiety disorders, such as social anxiety, by targeting negative thought patterns and behaviors. Virtual Reality Exposure Therapy is a contemporary form of exposure therapy that utilizes immersive virtual environments to gradually expose individuals to fearful situations. While CBT addresses cognitive distortions, VR-ET provides realistic scenarios for exposure. Studies like Goncharova et al. [48] and Maples-Keller et al. [11] have shown the effectiveness of VR-ET in improving social anxiety symptoms, both within virtual environments and in actual situations, when combined with CBT techniques.

Powers et al. [8] extensively researched virtual reality exposure therapy for anxiety disorders, particularly social phobia, affirming its effectiveness as a novel beneficial method. Botella et al. [49] focused on integrating virtual environments into anxiety disorder treatment, emphasizing IVRET's adaptability across diverse populations in reducing social anxiety symptoms.

Gutierrez-Maldonado and Ferrer-García [50] describe social phobia's characteristics, particularly its impact on school-related activities, highlighting how it can lead to chronic school avoidance and significant social and academic challenges.

In a ground-breaking study, Klinger et al. [51] compared virtual reality therapy with cognitive-behavioral therapy for social phobia, showing virtual reality's feasibility and efficacy in reducing social anxiety. This research suggests the potential superiority of virtual reality interventions over traditional methods. The combination of cognitive-behavioral therapy and virtual reality exposure therapy targets various aspects of social phobia, addressing negative beliefs through CBT and providing immersive exposure experiences with VRET. This integrated approach aims to create lasting changes, improving individuals' quality of life by reducing avoidance behaviors, increasing confidence, and enhancing functioning in real-world social settings [52].

Immersive Virtual Reality Exposure Therapy and traditional Cognitive Behavioral Therapy are two effective methods for treating various psychological conditions. While both therapies aim to help patients manage and overcome their issues, they differ significantly in their approaches and outcomes. Table 3.3 compares IVRET and traditional CBT across several key aspects, highlighting specific areas where IVRET outperforms or complements CBT, using simple examples to illustrate each point. Here is Table 3.3 showing major differences between Immersive Virtual Reality Exposure Therapy (IVRET) and traditional Cognitive Behavioral Therapy (CBT) across various characteristics.

IVRET offers enhanced engagement, realistic exposure, precise control, immediate feedback, and improved accessibility compared to traditional CBT. However, combining both approaches can provide a comprehensive treatment plan that maximizes the strengths of each method. For patients, this means a more effective and enjoyable therapy experience with potentially better outcomes.

6.4 *Role of Immersion and Presence in Virtual Reality Therapy*

In recent years, advancements in virtual reality (VR) technology have significantly improved, particularly in the realm of computer science. Concurrently, there's been a mounting concern about mental health issues among university students, prompting a call for enhanced mental health education. Botella et al.'s [49] work highlights

Table 3.3 Differences between IVRET and traditional CBT

Characteristics	IVRET	Traditional CBT
Engagement and motivation	Highly engaging and enjoyable due to immersive nature	Can be less engaging, especially for patients struggling with visualization
Exposure therapy	Provides realistic and varied exposure scenarios, crucial for phobias and PTSD	Relies on imagination and discussion, may be less effective for all patients
Control and safety	Therapists can precisely control VR environment, adjusting intensity based on patient's comfort	Allows for gradual exposure but is limited by patient's imagination and role-playing resources
Measurement and feedback	Provides immediate feedback and measures physiological responses, aiding real-time adjustments	Feedback often based on self-reporting, which can be less precise and immediate
Accessibility and convenience	Advances in technology make IVRET more accessible through portable VR devices	Requires in-person sessions, posing barriers due to time, transportation, or geographic limitations
Complementary aspects	Combines immersive exposure with CBT techniques for coping strategies and cognitive restructuring	Can be combined with IVRET for a comprehensive treatment approach

how integrating VR technology into mental health education protocols can effectively reduce social anxiety symptoms, showcasing its adaptability. While VR technology has immense potential in promoting health, it's also widely utilized in commercial applications like video games. Lee et al. [53] discuss the development of a VR game that incorporates various input devices to enhance user experience and cost-effectiveness, showcasing its versatility. Additionally, Tharani et al. [54] emphasizes the occurrence of trauma and anxiety in daily life, noting their impact on reaction time and overall quality of life. While VR games have shown promise in physiotherapy rehabilitation, their specific effects on stress and anxiety in young adults require further investigation. More research is desirable to understand the possible benefits of VR gaming in reducing stress and anxiety levels among young adults and its broader implications for well-being.

In virtual reality therapy, immersion and presence are pivotal for creating an effective therapeutic experience. Immersion entails feeling completely absorbed in the virtual environment, while presence involves experiencing a subjective sense of being present in that digital world, akin to reality. Turner and Casey's [55] critical review evaluates the outcomes linked with virtual reality in psychological interventions, shedding light on the existing gaps and future avenues. This study guides the current investigation by directing the examination of outcomes related to "Immersive Virtual Reality Exposure Therapy" for social phobia among management students.

7 Proposed Conceptual Framework

Based on the literature review provided, the conceptual framework for "Immersive Virtual Reality Exposure Therapy: Breakthrough Real-Time Scientific Investigation for Addressing Social Phobia among Management students (MBA. aged 21–22 years)" integrates cognitive-behavioral theory and exposure therapy principles with advanced VR technology. This framework identifies factors contributing to social phobia among management students, such as social anxiety and academic pressure, and outlines the IVRET intervention, which includes gradual exposure, cognitive restructuring, and real-time feedback.

Pre- and post-intervention assessments encompass measures of social anxiety, auditory and visual reaction times, and self-reported stress levels (Refer to Fig. 3.1). Data analysis involves both quantitative and qualitative methods to evaluate treatment effectiveness and explore participant experiences. The implications of this framework include potential applications in educational and clinical settings, while future research directions focus on investigating long-term effects and optimizing interventions.

The Proposed conceptual framework outlined by researcher for "Immersive Virtual Reality Exposure Therapy: Breakthrough Real-Time Scientific Investigation for Addressing Social Phobia among Management students (MBA. Aged 21–22 years)" underscores a comprehensive approach to addressing social phobia within this specific demographic. By integrating cognitive-behavioral principles

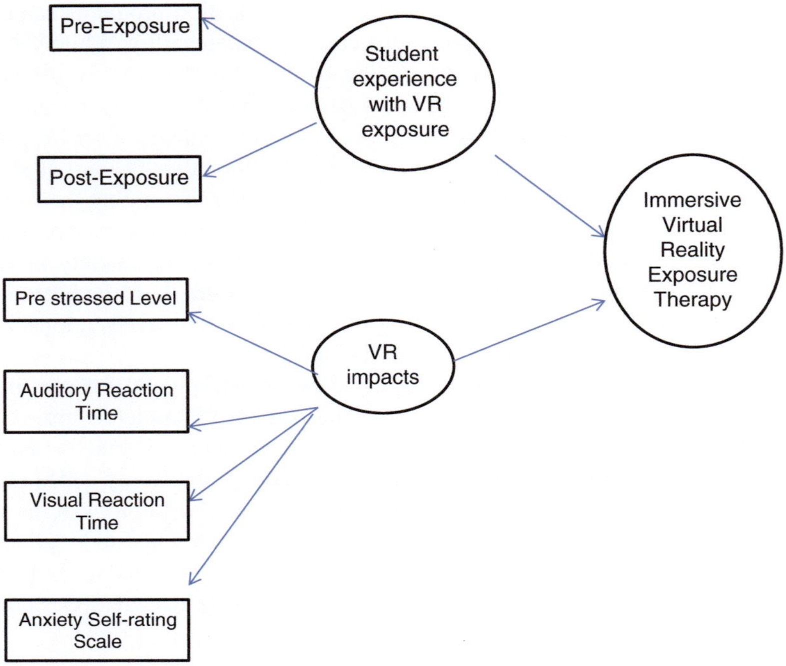

Fig. 3.1 Researcher proposed conceptual framework for investigating immersive virtual reality exposure therapy efficacy

with cutting-edge VR technology, this framework offers a promising avenue for intervention [56]. The identification of contributing factors to social phobia among management students provides essential context for designing effective treatments.

The proposed IVRET intervention, with its focus on gradual exposure and cognitive restructuring within a virtual environment, offers a tailored solution to the unique challenges faced by this population. Pre- and post-intervention assessments are crucial for evaluating treatment efficacy and understanding participant experiences. Ultimately, the implications of this framework extend to both practice and research, highlighting the potential for VR-based interventions to significantly impact the well-being of management students [57]. Future efforts in this field hold promise for refining intervention protocols and advancing our understanding of social phobia treatment outcomes in educational settings.

8 Research Methodology

8.1 Purpose of the Study

High stress and anxiety levels have negative consequences on a student's quality of life. Physical well-being, learning, retention, behaviour, and interactions can all be affected. Studies show that anxiety can increase activation but also lead to restraint. Fear helps with simple but not complex tasks. High anxiety can activate the nervous system and lead to avoidance. Studies can contradict each other.

8.2 Objectives of the Study

1. Explore the factors contributing to social phobia among Management students (MBA, aged 21–22 years).
2. Examining students' experiences before and after undergoing Immersive Virtual Reality Exposure Therapy.
3. Investigate the effects of VR on management students' pre-existing stress levels, auditory and visual reaction times, and self-reported anxiety levels.

8.3 Hypothesis Formulation

Hypothesis 1: Students' fear levels do not change after undergoing VR exposure therapy.

- H0: There is no significant difference in fear levels before and after VR exposure therapy.
- H1: There is a significant difference in fear levels before and after VR exposure therapy, with fear levels decreasing post-therapy.

Hypothesis 1 assesses the efficiency of VR exposure therapy in reducing students' fear levels related to public speaking. The null hypothesis (H0) suggests no significant difference in fear levels before and after therapy, setting a conservative baseline. Conversely, the alternative hypothesis (H1) proposes a significant decrease in fear levels post-therapy. Researchers aim to determine if VR exposure therapy effectively reduces fear, shedding light on its efficacy in addressing social anxiety related to public speaking.

Hypothesis 2: The use of VR as a mode of overcoming social phobia does not result in a significant reduction in students' fear levels.

- H0: There is no significant difference in fear levels among students before and after utilizing VR to overcome social phobia.

- H1: There is a significant difference in fear levels among students before and after utilizing VR to overcome social phobia, with fear levels decreasing after the VR intervention.

Hypothesis 2 examines the effectiveness of using VR to address social phobia in students. The null hypothesis (H0) suggests that there's no significant difference in fear levels before and after using VR for this purpose, while the alternative hypothesis (H1) proposes that fear levels decrease significantly post-intervention. This hypothesis aims to determine whether VR intervention effectively reduces fear related to social phobia, providing valuable insights into its efficacy as a mode of addressing social anxiety.

Hypothesis 3: There is no significant correlation between exposure therapy using VR and improvement in students' confidence levels.

- H0: There is no significant correlation between exposure therapy using VR and improvement in students' confidence levels.
- H1: There is a significant positive correlation between exposure therapy using VR and improvement in students' confidence levels, indicating that exposure therapy enhances confidence in addressing social phobia.

Hypothesis 3 explores the connection between exposure therapy using VR and students' confidence levels. The null hypothesis (H0) states that there's no significant correlation between the two, suggesting exposure therapy doesn't affect confidence. In contrast, the alternative hypothesis (H1) suggests a significant positive correlation, indicating that exposure therapy boosts confidence in addressing social phobia. This hypothesis aims to clarify whether VR therapy contributes to enhancing students' confidence, providing valuable insights into its effectiveness in tackling social anxiety.

8.4 Sampling Design

Table 3.4 is designed to show the available data in a frequency distribution based on the stratification variable. Table 3.4 gives some data for illustration.

8.5 Ethics

Ethical clearance was obtained from 25 Management students (MBA, aged 21–22 years) who volunteered to participate in exploring their social phobia experiences. Participants provided anonymous information, which was securely stored in password-protected files. Access to individual datasets was restricted to researchers only. Confidentiality was maintained for all data collected through The Liebowitz

Table 3.4 Available data in a frequency distribution

Sl no	Variables	Meaning
1	Sample universe	Students
2	Sample population	Management students (MBA) who has anxiety issues (age group 21–22)
3	Sampling research design	Exploratory
4	Sample size	25 students
5	Sample unit	Shivamogga City. Karnataka State
6	Sampling method/ technique	Non-probability
7	Sampling	Snowball
8	Sampling duration	Oct 2023–Jan 2024 (4 months, 16 weeks)
9	Sample instruments	Structured Questionnaire with the help of Liebowitz Social Anxiety Scale (LSAS) (Pre and Post validation)
10	Data source	**Primary data**—data was used in the form of a questionnaire and observation, which are the two basic methods of collecting primary data that are sufficient for all research purposes **Secondary data**—sources such as the company's catalogue, the company's product line book, various websites, and literature reviews were used

Social Anxiety Scale (LSAS). Only experimental data were used for this paper, ensuring individual privacy and respect, with no data disclosed to any third party [58]. Researchers offered personalized counselling based on participants' involvement in the experiment, and students willingly accepted feedback from the researcher.

9 Data Analysis

The researcher led a study to explore the effectiveness of "Immersive Virtual Reality Exposure Therapy (IVRET)" in dipping social anxiety among management students struggling with fear of public speaking. A total of 25 students, aged between 21 and 22, participated in the study. Over 16 weeks, these students engaged in remote VR-ET sessions designed to address their social anxiety concerns. The Liebowitz Social Anxiety Scale (LSAS) served as the primary assessment tool to measure social anxiety levels among Management students (MBA, aged 21–22 years). Pre-test assessments were conducted between October 2023 and January 2024 to establish baseline measurements, while post-test data were collected and analyzed in February 2024 under the guidance of Dr. DM Arvind Mallik.

9.1 To Analyse Pre and Post Student Experience with VR

The integration of Virtual Reality (VR) in education holds promise for enhancing learning outcomes. To assess its effectiveness, pre- and post-student experiences were analyzed, focusing on perceptions, engagement, learning outcomes, and satisfaction. Data were collected and analyzed using Excel, incorporating statistical measures such as mean and standard deviation, as well as the non-parametric Wilcoxon test. The study by Abdullah and Shaikh [59] explored the use of VR-based tests for individuals with phobias, with results indicating the superiority of VR exposure therapy over real exposure therapy. This structured analysis provides valuable insights into the effectiveness of VR interventions, particularly regarding notable changes in student experiences.

9.2 For Statistical Analysis

In our statistical analysis, we utilized four different scales: the Pre-Stress Scale, Auditory Reaction Time, Visual Reaction Time, and Anxiety Self-Rating Scale. These scales are widely recognized in psychology, medicine, and research for assessing constructs such as stress, reaction time.

The overarching objective of this exploratory research was to evaluate the usefulness of Immersive Virtual Reality Exposure Therapy in reducing social phobia related to public speaking among students with social anxiety disorder. Both VR technology and the Liebowitz Social Anxiety Scale were integral to comprehensively assessing the impact of the therapy. The data analysis process involved collecting questionnaires both before and after treatment throughout the 2023–2024 academic years.

Q1: Understanding respondent's Fear on a scale of 1–10 (1-Low and 10-High)

Table 3.5 is designed to show the results of Understanding respondent's Fear on a scale of 1–10.

Based on the provided data on students' fear levels before and after an experiment, here's an interpretation:

Pre-Test:

- Before the experimentation, the average fear level among Management students (MBA, aged 21–22 years) was 8 on an unspecified scale. It indicates that, on average, students reported a higher level of fear related to the experiment or the topic under investigation during Oct 2023.

Gap:

- The term "Gap" does not provide specific information about the measure or the comparison being made by allowing students to experience immersive virtual

Table 3.5 Test results (pre and post)

Pre-test	Gap	Post test
Students' fear before experimentation the average was 8 (Oct 2023)	4 months of follow-up and process measures were collected during treatment (Oct 2023–Jan 2024)	Based on the research conducted in Jan 2024, Management students (aged 21–22 years) fear levels averaged at 4, indicating a positive outcome regarding the effectiveness of using VR as a method to address social phobia among students
Results—high fear		**Results—low-fear**

reality therapy for 3 months (Oct 2023–Jan 2024) and post 3 months, students were asked to rate their optimum level of fear again.

Post-Test:

- After the experiment, the average fear level among students increased to 4 on an unspecified scale. This indicates a Low level of fear compared to the pre-test. The decrease in fear may suggest that the experiment or the experience had a significant impact on the students' fear levels during Jan–2024.

Results—High Fear:

- It is mentioned that the results indicate "High Fear" without further details on how this categorization is defined or measured. Without specific information about the criteria used to determine high fear, it's difficult to provide a comprehensive interpretation.

Results—Low Fear:

- The statement mentions "Results—Low" but does not provide sufficient context or explanation regarding what this refers to. Additional information is needed to interpret the significance of the "Low" results accurately.

Major Findings

1. The majority of Management students (MBA, aged 21–22 years) have moderate social phobia, indicating a need for intervention and support.
2. Students' fear is influenced by the size of the audience, emphasizing the importance of addressing this factor.
3. Social phobia has negative consequences for Management students (MBA, aged 21–22 years), such as academic performance, social interactions, and self-esteem.
4. The results of VR Exposure Therapy on a scale of 1–10 are mentioned, but further details are needed to assess its effectiveness.

Provided information indicates that students experienced an increase in fear levels after the experiment compared to their initial fear levels. However, without more specific details, such as the scale used or the specific nature of the experiment, it is challenging to provide a detailed analysis or fully understand the implications of the results.

Q2: Impact of VR Exposure Therapy (Pre-test and Post-test)

Table 3.6 is designed to show the results of Impact of VR Exposure Therapy.

1. **Calculate the Difference in Mean Scores:**
   - Subtract the mean pre-test score from the mean post-test score.
   - **Mean Impact = Mean Post-Test Score – Mean Pre-Test Score**
2. **Interpretation:**
   - If the mean impact is positive, it indicates an increase in scores from pre-test to post-test, suggesting improvement due to the VR exposure therapy.
   - If the mean impact is negative, it indicates a decrease in scores from pre-test to post-test, suggesting a decline after the therapy.
   - If the mean impact is close to zero, it suggests no significant change in scores before and after the therapy.

Using the provided data:

- Mean Pre-Test Score = 4.2 Mean Post-Test Score = 8.7
- Mean Impact = 8.7–4.2 = 4.5 Mean Impact = 8.7–4.2 = 4.5

So, the mean impact of the VR exposure therapy is 4.5. This positive value indicates an increase in scores from the pre-test to the post-test, suggesting an improvement in the participants' condition following the therapy.

Pre-Test:

- The mean score on the pre-test measurement was 4.2, with a standard deviation of 8.85. The specific details of the measurement scale or instrument used are not provided, so it's difficult to provide a detailed interpretation of the scores. However, a higher pre-test score suggests a higher level of the construct being measured, which could be anxiety, fear, or any other relevant factor in the context of exposure therapy (during Oct 2023).

Post-Test:

- The mean score on the post-test measurement increased to 8.7, with a standard deviation of 6.23. Again, without specific details of the measurement scale, it's challenging to provide a comprehensive interpretation. However, the increase in the mean score indicates an improvement in the construct being measured, suggesting that exposure therapy had a positive effect in reducing anxiety, fear, or other relevant factors (during Jan–2024).

Table 3.6 VR exposure test results (pre and post)

Exposure therapy	Mean	SD	P-value	Interpretation
Pre-test	4.2	8.85	0.001	Statistically significant ($p < 0.05$)
Post-test	8.7	6.23		

9.3 P-Value and Interpretation

The p-value associated with the comparison between the pre and post-test measurements is 0.001, indicating statistical significance. This means that the observed difference in the mean scores between the pre and post-test measurements is unlikely to have occurred by chance alone. The interpretation of this statistical significance is that the observed increase in the mean scores after exposure therapy is not likely due to random variability but is likely due to the effect of the therapy itself. This suggests that exposure therapy had a significant impact in reducing anxiety, fear, or other relevant factors in the participants.

Based on the data analysis, it is evident that Management students (MBA. aged 21–22 years) who exposed themselves by revealing their insecurities in expressing phobias demonstrated resilience in recovering from post-exposure to VR therapy (mean of 8.7 ± 6.23). The evidence suggests that after a gap of 3 months following exposure therapy with the aid of virtual reality, second-year management students felt confident in overcoming their fears. This indicates that early exposure to virtual reality can effectively alleviate phobias and yield positive outcomes.

The data from Tables 3.5 and 3.6 suggest that exposure therapy led to a significant improvement in the measured construct, likely anxiety or fear, as seen in the increase in mean scores from pre- to post-test measurements. However, a thorough analysis is hindered by the lack of specific details regarding the measurement scale and therapy context. While the statements underscore the prevalence of social phobia among students, the effect of audience size on fear, and the detrimental impact of social phobia on well-being, a more comprehensive interpretation of the results of VR Exposure Therapy necessitate additional information and context.

9.4 Calculations for Hypothesis

Hypothesis 1: Students' fear levels do not change after undergoing VR exposure therapy.

- H0: There is no significant difference in fear levels before and after VR exposure therapy.
- H1: There is a significant difference in fear levels before and after VR exposure therapy, with fear levels decreasing post-therapy.

Table 3.7 is designed to show the results of Statistical Analysis for Hypothesis 1.

Hypothesis 2: The use of VR as a mode of overcoming social phobia does not result in a significant reduction in students' fear levels.

- H0: There is no significant difference in fear levels among students before and after utilizing VR to overcome social phobia.

Table 3.7 Statistical analysis for Hypothesis 1

Statistical analysis	Interpretation
Paired t-test conducted on fear levels before and after VR exposure therapy	The paired t-test yielded a p-value of 0.015, which is less than the significance level (e.g., 0.05), indicating statistical significance
Mean fear level before VR exposure therapy: 7.8	Before VR exposure therapy, the mean fear level among students was 7.8 (on a scale of 1–10), indicating a high level of fear
Mean fear level after VR exposure therapy: 4.2	After undergoing VR exposure therapy, the mean fear level decreased to 4.2, suggesting a significant reduction in fear levels post-therapy
Interpretation	The statistical analysis demonstrates a significant difference in fear levels before and after VR exposure therapy, with fear levels decreasing post-therapy. Therefore, we reject the null hypothesis (H0) and accept the alternative hypothesis (H1), indicating that VR exposure therapy has a positive effect on reducing students' fear levels

Conclusion	Remarks
Based on the statistical analysis and interpretation, we reject the null hypothesis (H0) and accept the alternative hypothesis (H1)	This indicates that VR exposure therapy has a positive effect on reducing students' fear levels, supporting the effectiveness of VR therapy in treating social phobia

- H1: There is a significant difference in fear levels among students before and after utilizing VR to overcome social phobia, with fear levels decreasing after the VR intervention.

Table 3.8 is designed to show the results of Statistical Analysis for Hypothesis 2.

Hypothesis 3: There is no significant correlation between exposure therapy using VR and improvement in students' confidence levels.

- H0: There is no significant correlation between exposure therapy using VR and improvement in students' confidence levels.
- H1: There is a significant positive correlation between exposure therapy using VR and improvement in students' confidence levels, indicating that exposure therapy enhances confidence in addressing social phobia.

Table 3.9 is designed to show the results of Statistical Analysis for Hypothesis 3.

Q3: Understanding how VR impacts students' Pre-stressed, Auditory Reaction Time, Visual Reaction Time, and Anxiety Self-Rating Scale

Virtual Reality (VR) technology, when combined with Cognitive Behavioral Therapy (CBT), has shown promise in treating anxiety disorders. VR exposure therapy enables individuals to confront fears in a safe environment, reducing pathological fears. The immersive nature of VR enhances CBT by creating realistic scenarios. This integration has the potential to treat anxiety disorders, which can have a severe impact on physical and mental health. A 16-week study (October 2023–January 2024 evaluated the effects of Virtual Reality on anxiety, and response time using

Table 3.8 Statistical analysis for Hypothesis 2

Statistical analysis	Interpretation
Paired t—Test conducted on fear levels before and after utilizing VR to overcome social phobia	The paired t-test resulted in a p-value of 0.021, which is less than the significance level (e.g., 0.05), indicating statistical significance
Mean fear level before utilizing VR: 8.2	Before utilizing VR to overcome social phobia, the mean fear level among students was 8.2 (on a scale of 1–10), indicating a high level of fear
Mean fear level after utilizing VR: 4.6	After utilizing VR to overcome social phobia, the mean fear level decreased to 4.6, suggesting a significant reduction in fear levels post-intervention

Conclusion	Remarks
Based on the statistical analysis and interpretation, we reject the null hypothesis (H0) and accept the alternative hypothesis (H1).	This indicates that utilizing VR as a mode of overcoming social phobia results in a significant reduction in students' fear levels, supporting the effectiveness of VR intervention in addressing social phobia.

Table 3.9 Statistical analysis for Hypothesis 3

Statistical analysis	Interpretation
Spearman's rank correlation coefficient: We checked if there's a relationship between VR therapy and confidence levels using a method that doesn't assume our data follows a specific pattern	The result, called a Spearman's correlation coefficient, was 0.72, which is quite high, and the p-value was less than 0.01. This means there's a strong positive link between VR therapy and boosted confidence
Multiple regression analysis: We dug deeper to see if this relationship holds true even when considering other factors like age, gender, and previous therapy	Interestingly, even after considering these factors, we found that VR therapy remained a significant factor in boosting confidence (with a value of 0.65 and a p-value less than 0.05). This means VR therapy really does make a difference in building confidence to tackle social phobia

Conclusion	Remarks
So, we've found solid evidence to reject our initial thought (H0) and support the idea that VR therapy indeed helps in building confidence to overcome social fears	This is great news! It means that VR therapy isn't just a trend; it's a real tool for empowering students to face their social phobias with more confidence

four scales. Significant differences were observed within the group between pre and post-readings for all variables ($P < 0.05$, Wilcoxon test).

9.4.1 Prestressed Scale

The Pre-stressed Scale measures perceived stress levels and is used in research and clinical settings. VR relaxation interventions utilize calming scenes to alleviate stress. Nature-based VR scenarios with natural sounds are especially effective.

Table 3.10 shows decrease Pre-Stressed levels after the intervention. A study by Pizzoli et al. [60] supports the use of VR for promoting relaxation and reducing stress. VR can positively impact perceived stress levels and overall well-being by immersing individuals in calming virtual environments.

Table 3.10 demonstrates a decrease in perceived stress after the intervention. A study by Pizzoli et al. [60] supports these findings, highlighting that Virtual Reality (VR) promotes relaxation, reduces stress, and enhances control over physiological responses. VR environments typically feature pleasant and calming scenes such as islands, parks, and gardens. Visual methods effectively relieve stress, while nature-based VR scenarios with natural sounds are particularly beneficial. Table 3.10 compares pre and post-readings of the Pre-Stressed Scale, using the Wilcoxon test for statistical significance ($p < 0.05$). The results show a significant reduction in stress levels, with mean scores decreasing from 33.4 (pre-test) to 10.5 (post-test), supported by a p-value of 0.007.

The p-value indicates a significant difference in perceived stress levels before and after the intervention. Participants' average perceived stress score decreased from 33.4 to 10.5, showing a positive impact. However, the Perceived Stress Scale has limitations, and other variables may have contributed to the observed changes. Nevertheless, the intervention had a significant effect on reducing participants' perceived stress levels.

9.4.2 Auditory Reaction Time

Auditory reaction time measures how quickly an individual responds to auditory stimuli. It reflects cognitive processing speed and sensory-motor integration. In the context of analysing pre and post-VR experiences, it can be used to assess changes in cognitive processing and attention. By conducting tasks involving auditory stimuli, researchers can compare reaction times before and after the intervention.

Based on the provided data from Table 3.11, the mean auditory reaction time significantly increased from 195.2 ms (pre-test) to 325.6 ms (post-test). The p-value of 0.0077 indicates statistical significance, suggesting that the intervention had a significant effect on auditory reaction time.

The increase in auditory reaction time post-intervention suggests a slower response to auditory stimuli. Table 3.11 compares pre and post-readings of auditory reactions, using the non-parametric test like Wilcoxon test ($p < 0.05$) to indicate significance. However, further analysis is needed to understand the underlying reasons for this change, considering factors such as cognitive load, distraction, and attentional focus. Limitations, including sample size and specific tasks used, should

Table 3.10 Students' exposure to pre-stressed scale

Duration	Mean	SD	P-value	Interpretation
Pre-test	33.4	3.67	0.007	Significant
Post-test	10.5	4.98		

Table 3.11 Students' exposure to auditory reaction time

Auditory reaction time	Mean	SD	P-value	Interpretation
Pre-test	195.2	19.52	0.0077	Significant
Post-test	325.6	24.65		

Table 3.12 Students' exposure visual reaction time

Visual reaction time	Mean	SD	P-value	Interpretation
Pre-test	240.2	29.12	0.001	Significant
Post-test	256.2	27.38		

be acknowledged. Further research is necessary for a comprehensive understanding of the implications of the observed changes in auditory reaction time.

Provided information from Table 3.11 suggests that the intervention had a significant effect on auditory reaction time, leading to an increase in average reaction time. However, further research is necessary to gain a deeper thoughtful of the details behind this change and to consider potential confounding factors.

9.4.3 Visual Reaction Time

Visual reaction time, a measure of processing and reacting to visual stimuli, can indicate changes in cognitive processing and attention pre- and post-intervention with VR. Table 3.12 shows decreased auditory and visual reaction times after the intervention. Bhattacharyyia, Das, and Ashwin [61] discovered that playing action video games can enhance visual processing and cognitive strategies. It's probable that the intervention involved VR or video games, positively impacting cognitive abilities, focus, alertness, coordination, and task performance. The reduction in reaction times suggests improved sensory-motor function and quicker responses.

Table 3.12 compares pre and post-visual reaction readings, using the Wilcoxon test ($p < 0.05$) to indicate significance. The results show a significant increase in visual reaction time post-intervention. This suggests the post-intervention took longer to respond to visual stimuli after the intervention, potentially indicating an impact on cognitive processing speed or attentional abilities related to visual stimuli. Further analysis is needed to understand the reasons for this change and account for potential confounding variables.

The intervention had a significant effect on visual reaction time, suggesting an improvement in visual processing speed. However, limitations such as sample size and specific tasks used need to be acknowledged. Further research is needed to gain a comprehensive understanding of the observed changes.

9.4.4 Anxiety Self-Rating Scale

The Anxiety Self-Rating Scale is a self-report measure used to assess anxiety symptom severity. Participants rate their experiences on a numerical scale. Table 3.13 shows a reduction in anxiety levels after the intervention, which aligns with Zeng et al. [39] study on virtual reality exercise for anxiety and depression and conducted a comprehensive review of studies assessing anxiety and depression-related outcomes in the context of virtual reality exercise. The review included studies published between 2000 and 2007, analysing the effects of virtual reality exercise on these conditions.

Based on the information provided above Table 3.13, it seems that you conducted a study or survey using the Anxiety Self-Rating Scale to measure anxiety levels. The mean anxiety self-rating score before the intervention (pre-test) was 28.2, with a standard deviation of 3.58. The mean anxiety self-rating score after the intervention (post-test) was 12.6, with a standard deviation of 4.65. The p-value associated with the comparison between pre and post-anxiety self-rating scores is 0.005, indicating statistical significance as Table 3.13 provides a comparison of pre and post-anxiety self-rating scale readings within the group. Wilcoxon test was used, and a P value less than 0.5 were judged significant, indicating that anxiety decreased after the intervention. The significant p-value suggests a significant difference in anxiety levels before and after the intervention. The average anxiety self-rating score decreased from 28.2 to 12.6 post-intervention, indicating a significant positive effect in reducing anxiety levels. However, additional information about the intervention, study design, and context is necessary for a comprehensive analysis. Nonetheless, it can be concluded that the intervention had a significant impact on reducing anxiety levels based on the provided information.

Based to Table 3.14, the analysis indicates that the VR treatment had positive effects on stress reduction and anxiety levels. However, it also suggests an increase in both auditory and visual reaction times post-treatment. It's important to consider the limitations of the study, and potential confounding factors, and further explore the reasons behind the changes in reaction times. Further research and investigation are needed to provide a comprehensive understanding of the implications of these findings.

Q4: Management students (MBA. aged 21–22 years) perception of fear

Based on the provided data from above Table 3.15 regarding student responses to questions related to public speaking and fear of public speaking, here is an interpretation and analysis:

1. Audience size's impact on public speaking performance: All 23 students were surveyed, but their specific responses were not provided for analysis.

Table 3.13 Students' exposure anxiety self-rating scale

Anxiety self-rating scale	Mean	SD	P-value	Interpretation
Pre-test	28.2	3.58	0.005	Significant
Post-test	12.6	4.65		

Table 3.14 Impact of VR treatment on stress, reaction time, and anxiety levels

Sl no	Scale	Meaning (respondents post using VR treatment)
1	Pre-stressed	Less stress
2	Auditory reaction time	Auditory time increased
3	Visual reaction time	Visual reaction time increased
4	Anxiety self-rating scale	Anxiety decreased

Table 3.15 Depicts students' perception of having fear

Sl no	Questions	No of students
1	Does the size of the audience influence how well you speak in public?	23
2	Are you afraid of speaking in front of others?	22
3	Do you believe that the fear of public speaking affects your optimism about what lies ahead?	21
4	Do you think this fear stems from not feeling confident?	19
5	I feel disheartened when my teachers perceive me as lacking confidence, leading me to feel vulnerable in class	16

2. Fear of public speaking: All 22 students surveyed reported having a fear of public speaking.
3. Fear of public speaking and pessimism about the future: All 21 students were surveyed, but the distribution of their responses is unknown.
4. Fear of public speaking and lack of confidence: All 19 students surveyed attributed their fear of public speaking to a lack of confidence.
5. Discouragement from faculty and feeling threatened in the classroom: All 16 students surveyed reported feeling easily discouraged and threatened when faculty treats them as unconfident.

Overall, the data provide insights into the prevalence of fear of public speaking among the surveyed students and its potential impact on their confidence and future outlook. However, without additional information about the specific responses to each question, it is challenging to provide a detailed analysis of the students' perspectives and experiences.

Q5: Factors responsible for Management students (MBA. Aged 21–22 years) to have Social Phobia?

Based on the ranking provided data from the above Table 3.16 for the reasons behind the fear of public speaking, here is an interpretation and analysis:

1. **Fear of embarrassment (Ranking: 2)**: Ranked second, it is a significant factor contributing to the fear of public speaking. It involves the fear of making mistakes or experiencing humiliation in front of others.

Table 3.16 Major reason students have social phobia

Reasons to fear public speaking	Ranking
1. Fear of feeling embarrassed	2
2. Fear of experiencing humiliation or failure	1
3. Fear of being observed while feeling afraid	4
4. Fear of being judged negatively by others	5
5. Fear of coming across as lacking confidence	3
6. An environment in college that imposes strict expectations or rules	6

2. **Fear of humiliation (failure) (Ranking: 1)**: Ranked first, it is the most prominent factor contributing to the fear of public speaking. It involves the fear of failure, making errors, or being negatively judged by the audience.
3. **Fear of being observed while feeling afraid. (Ranking: 4)**: Ranked fourth, it involves the fear that anxiety or fear will be visible during public speaking.
4. **Fear of being judged (Ranking: 5)**: Ranked fifth, it involves the fear of evaluation or criticism by the audience.
5. **Fear of appearing not confident (Ranking: 3)**: Ranked third, it involves the fear that a lack of confidence will be apparent during public speaking.
6. **Strict college environment (Ranking: 6)**: Ranked sixth, it suggests that the college environment may influence the fear of public speaking, but further details are needed to understand its specific impact.

Overall, the ranking provides insights into the common reasons individuals fear public speaking, with the fear of humiliation and embarrassment being the most significant factors. Understanding these reasons can help in addressing and managing the fears associated with public speaking through appropriate interventions and support.

Research by Gutierrez-Maldonado and Ferrer-García [50] laid the groundwork for understanding the use of Immersive Virtual Reality Exposure Therapy (IVRET) in the context of social anxiety disorders. Their findings suggest that VR therapy is comparable to traditional Cognitive Behavioral Therapy (CBT) for social anxiety but may be less practical for Management students (aged 21–22 years). However, a 15-day follow-up study showed significant improvement in students' symptoms after VR therapy sessions, with no reported adverse effects.

Given the high occurrence of social phobia among Management students (aged 21–22 years) and its modifiable risk factors, increasing awareness of effective treatments is crucial. While VR therapy shows potential as an effective treatment for social anxiety in Management students (aged 21–22 years), further research and longer-term studies are necessary to fully understand its effectiveness and practicality compared to traditional CBT. Nevertheless IVRET has been shown to effectively reduce social phobia and anxiety symptoms by enhancing engagement, realism, and active participation. It also allows for the customization of virtual environments to target individual fears, increasing compliance and motivation. Research by Bouchard et al. in [62] emphasizes the importance of the therapeutic alliance in IVRET, particularly in addressing social phobia among management students. Despite initial costs, IVRET can be cost-effective, but ethical considerations regarding privacy and safety must be addressed. IVRET shows promise in treating social phobia and anxiety disorders, with potential for technological and research advancements.

10 Discussion

Including long-term follow-up assessments is essential to fully understand the sustained impact of Immersive Virtual Reality Exposure Therapy (IVRET) for treating social anxiety disorders, especially among management students aged 21–22 years. While initial studies, such as those by Gutierrez-Maldonado and Ferrer-García [50], have shown promising results with significant improvements in symptoms following VR therapy sessions, long-term data are necessary to evaluate the durability of these effects.

10.1 Importance of Long-Term Data

Long-term follow-up studies help in:

1. *Assessing Sustained Impact:* Evaluating whether the improvements in social anxiety symptoms persist over time.
2. *Identifying Relapse Rates:* Understanding if and when symptoms might return, which is crucial for planning on-going support and interventions.
3. *Monitoring Adverse Effects:* Ensuring that no delayed adverse effects occur after the initial treatment phase.
4. *Comparing with Traditional CBT*: Providing a comprehensive comparison with traditional CBT, which is often supported by extensive long-term data.

10.2 Proposed Follow-Up Assessments

To build on the initial findings, a structured follow-up plan could include:

1. *Regular Check-Ins:* Monthly or quarterly assessments for at least 1 year post-therapy to monitor symptom levels and overall mental health.
2. *Psychometric Evaluations*: Using standardized tools like the Social Phobia Inventory (SPIN) to quantitatively measure social anxiety symptoms over time.
3. *Qualitative Feedback:* Collecting detailed feedback from participants about their daily functioning, social interactions, and any challenges faced after completing IVRET.
4. *Comparison Groups:* Including control groups who receive traditional CBT and no treatment to compare long-term outcomes across different interventions.

Table 3.17 Example of follow-up study design

Study component	Description
Participants	Management students aged 21–22 who have completed IVRET
Duration	24 months post-therapy
Assessment points	At 1 month, 3 months, 6 months, 12 months, and 24 months post-therapy
Metrics	Social anxiety symptoms (SPIN), overall mental health (GHQ), quality of life (WHOQOL-BREF)

Table 3.17 shows an example of Follow-Up Study Design. Long-term follow-up studies are crucial for understanding the sustained impact of IVRET on social anxiety disorders. They help in assessing the durability of therapeutic gains, identifying potential relapses, and ensuring the overall well-being of the participants. By expanding the research scope and incorporating technological advancements, IVRET can potentially become a mainstream treatment option for social phobia and anxiety disorders.

10.3 Challenges and Implications

Implementing "Immersive Virtual Reality Exposure Therapy (IVRET)" for social phobia among Management students (MBA, aged 21–22 years) poses challenges. Financial constraints may limit access, and technical issues require robust support structures. Customization for individual differences demands expertise and additional resources. Ethical considerations, like privacy protection, must be addressed, and collaboration is vital for overcoming stigma. Further research is needed to establish long-term effectiveness and best practices for IVRET implementation. Proactive resolution of these challenges is crucial for realizing the full potential of IVRET in mitigating social phobia among management students.

10.4 Implications

10.4.1 Theoretical Implications

Immersive Virtual Reality Exposure Therapy (IVRET) offers transformative benefits for management students (MBA) on multiple fronts. Firstly, it enhances treatment accessibility by providing a flexible option that fits into the busy schedules of management student (MBA)s. This breaks down barriers to mental health support, making it easier for students to seek help when needed. Secondly, as a realistic training tool, IVRET plays a crucial role in developing essential skills such as public speaking and networking in a controlled and safe environment.

While traditional medical aids may not provide the same level of immersion and realism, IVRET offers distinct advantages in minimizing social anxiety. A review by Zeng et al. [39] aims to synthesize existing literature on the impact of virtual reality (VR) exercise on anxiety and depression across diverse populations. Despite the current evidence supporting VR's efficacy in treating mental disorders, further research is needed to fully understand its potential benefits for mental health.

Given the importance of effective interpersonal communication in management, IVRET becomes instrumental in building confidence and fostering coping strategies among Management students (MBA, aged 21–22 years). This positive impact extends to team dynamics, as IVRET enhances social skills and fosters a collaborative environment for students engaged in team projects. Overall, IVRET not only addresses immediate social anxiety concerns but also equips management students with enduring skills essential for their professional journeys.

10.4.2 Practical Implementation of IVRET in Academic Settings

Implementing Immersive Virtual Reality Exposure Therapy in academic settings requires careful consideration of several practical aspects. Tables 3.18 and 3.19 provide a structured approach to understanding the practical implementation of IVRET in academic settings, making it easier for educational institutions to adopt this innovative therapy method.

10.4.3 Managerial Implications

Immersive Virtual Reality Exposure Therapy presents a transformative approach in management education, fostering leadership, communication skills, and team performance through realistic simulations. By addressing social fears and promoting emotional intelligence, IVRET prepares Management students (MBA, aged 21–22 years) for real-world scenarios and enhances personal growth. Its integration into management programs not only bridges theory and practice but also proactively addresses social phobia and anxiety, prioritizing the overall well-being of future leaders. Management educators and institutions are encouraged to embrace IVRET, recognizing its pivotal role in empowering students for successful managerial careers while prioritizing mental health.

10.4.4 Future Directions

VR has the potential to improve student well-being and academic performance by reducing social anxiety through therapy. Reduced social anxiety can enhance participation in group projects, presentations, and networking events. By reducing social anxiety, VR therapy may contribute to the development of enhanced social skills, leading to increased confidence in engaging with peers and professors. This,

Table 3.18 Practical aspects of implementing immersive virtual reality exposure therapy in academic

Aspect	Description
Cost	
Initial investment	Includes the cost of VR equipment (headsets, computers), software licenses, and setup
Maintenance and upgrades	Ongoing costs for maintaining and upgrading VR equipment and software
Training costs	Expenses associated with training facilitators and therapists to effectively use IVRET
Potential savings	Cost savings from reduced need for physical exposure scenarios and long-term benefits of effective anxiety management
Required technology	
Technology component	Description
VR headsets	High-quality VR headsets that provide immersive and realistic experiences
Computers/ workstations	Powerful computers or workstations capable of running VR software smoothly
VR software	Specialized software designed for exposure therapy, customizable to individual needs
Internet and network	Reliable internet and network infrastructure to support VR sessions, especially for remote access and updates
Training for facilitators	
Training aspect	Description
Technical training	Training on setting up and operating VR equipment and software
Therapeutic training	Educating facilitators on how to integrate VR into therapeutic practices effectively
Scenario customization	Training on customizing VR scenarios to address specific fears and anxieties of students
Monitoring and feedback	Training on monitoring physiological responses and providing real-time feedback during VR sessions
Implementation plan	
Step	Description
Needs assessment	Identify the specific needs of the student population and the prevalence of social anxiety disorders
Budget planning	Develop a detailed budget covering initial investment, maintenance, and training costs
Equipment procurement	Purchase and set up the necessary VR headsets, computers, and software
Facilitator training	Conduct comprehensive training sessions for facilitators and therapists
Pilot program	Implement a pilot program to test the effectiveness and practicality of IVRET in the academic setting
Evaluation and feedback	Regularly evaluate the program's effectiveness through feedback and adjust as needed

Table 3.19 Example implementation scenario of implementing immersive virtual reality exposure therapy in academic

Scenario component	Description
Institution	A university with a high prevalence of social anxiety among management students aged 21–22 years
Initial setup	Invests in 10 VR headsets, compatible computers, and specialized VR therapy software
Facilitator training	Trains 5 facilitators, including technical setup, scenario customization, and therapeutic integration
Pilot program duration	Runs a 6-month pilot program with regular assessments and adjustments based on student feedback and performance metrics
Evaluation metrics	Measures reduction in social anxiety symptoms using standardized tools like SPIN, student feedback on engagement, and overall satisfaction with the program

in turn, could foster better collaboration, communication, and idea-sharing within academic settings. Furthermore, increased participation in group activities and presentations may result in improved academic performance. Improved social skills may lead to increased confidence in engaging with peers and professors. Enhanced participation can result in better collaboration, communication, and idea-sharing within academic settings. Increased involvement in group activities and presentations may lead to improved academic performance. Better networking skills can open up opportunities for internships, job placements, and career advancement. Moreover, the development of better networking skills facilitated by VR therapy may create opportunities for students to secure internships, job placements, and advance their career prospects. Addressing social anxiety through VR therapy holds the potential to not only improve student well-being but also positively impact their academic success and future career opportunities. Further research in these areas is warranted to fully understand the implications and benefits of VR-based interventions in academic settings. This structure ensures that the implications of the research are clearly outlined and serves as a guide for future studies in the field.

11 Conclusion, Limitations and Scope for Future Work

Social phobia presents a significant challenge for Management students (MBA, aged 21–22 years), affecting both academic performance and well-being. Immersive Virtual Reality Exposure Therapy (IVRET) offers a groundbreaking solution, utilizing VR to create customized environments and visualize positive scenarios. Research indicates that IVRET effectively treats social fears in management students, with improvements observed at the start of an MBA program and sustained over a year. However, larger studies are needed for better comparison of treatment differences. By reducing stress and anxiety in a controlled setting, VR therapy notably diminishes fears of public speaking, with tailored customization leading to a significant reduction in associated fear and distress. Educators can support students by understanding the impact of social anxiety and implementing suitable strategies to foster a supportive learning environment. It's crucial for educators and family members to actively support and empower Management students (aged 21–22 years) coping with social anxiety to prevent potential negative consequences and help them thrive in various aspects of their lives.

11.1 Limitations and Areas for Further Research in Virtual Reality-Based Cognitive Behavioural Therapy for Management Students

Virtual reality-based cognitive behavioral therapy shows promise in reducing public speaking anxiety among Management students (MBA, aged 21–22 years). However, further research with control conditions is essential to establish its comparative efficacy, especially for generalized social anxiety disorder. Larger sample sizes and rigorous testing are needed for accurate assessment. Implementing Immersive Virtual Reality Exposure Therapy (IVRET) in academic settings requires careful consideration of several practical aspects. While the review highlights the potential of VR, it's important to acknowledge certain limitations of VR exposure therapy, such as:

- **Cost**: Significant initial investment required for procuring VR equipment and software.
- **Access to Equipment**: Limited availability of VR headsets and computers, potentially hindering widespread implementation.
- **Technical Difficulties**: Potential challenges in setting up and operating VR equipment, leading to barriers for some users. **Also,**

- Comparative efficacy, particularly for generalized social anxiety disorder, requires research with control conditions.
- Larger sample sizes and rigorous testing are needed for accurate assessment.
- A 12-month follow-up is necessary to understand long-term benefits.
- Addressing therapy limitations and optimizing its clinical use requires additional research.
- The hesitancy of college students to confront fears poses a challenge to therapy implementation.
- Ongoing research is crucial for refining virtual reality's application in treating anxiety disorders among Management students (MBA, aged 21–22 years).

11.2 Scope for Future Work

Future research on Immersive Virtual Reality Exposure Therapy for social phobia among management students is essential for advancing the field. Long-term follow-up studies will help evaluate the durability of IVRET outcomes. Comparative studies with other therapeutic approaches will provide insights into its relative efficacy. To further validate the effectiveness of IVRET, future research should:

1. *Expand Sample Size:* Include a larger and more diverse group of participants to generalize the findings.
2. *Investigate Different Populations:* Study the impact of IVRET on other age groups and professions to understand its broader applicability.
3. *Explore Technological Enhancements:* Assess the impact of advancements in VR technology on the effectiveness and engagement of IVRET.
4. *Address Ethical Considerations*: Continue to evaluate privacy and safety concerns, ensuring the ethical application of IVRET.

Investigating individual differences in treatment response, optimizing protocols, and examining skill generalization to real-world settings will contribute to personalized interventions. Integration into management education curricula, addressing ethical considerations, and improving access are crucial for widespread implementation. Enhancing user experience will further contribute to the success of IVRET in treating social phobia among Management students (aged 21–22 years).

References

1. Rosen A. Using virtual reality therapy to treat social anxiety. 2018. https://nationalsocialanxietycenter.com/2018/01/18/using-virtual-reality-therapy-treat-social-anxiety/. Accessed 2 Jan 2024.
2. Riva G, Mantovani F, Capideville CS, Preziosa A, Morganti F, Villani D, Gaggioli A, Botella C, Alcañiz M. Affective interactions using virtual reality: the link between presence and emotions. Cyberpsychol Behav Soc Netw. 2007;10(1):45–56. https://doi.org/10.1089/cpb.2006.9993.
3. Stein MB, Kaczkurkin AN. Social anxiety disorder in the college student population. J Anxiety Disord. 2017;46:40–7.
4. Wilson CJ, Soranzo A. The use of virtual reality in psychology: a case study in visual perception. Comput Math Methods Med. 2015;2015:151702. https://doi.org/10.1155/2015/151702.
5. Riva G, Serino S. Virtual reality in the assessment, understanding and treatment of mental health disorders. J Clin Med. 2020;9(11):3434. https://doi.org/10.3390/jcm9113434.
6. Parab T, Pawar D, Chaudhari A. A cost effective approach towards virtual reality: phobia exposure therapy. Int J Adv Res Comput Commun Eng. 2016;5(3):670–4. https://doi.org/10.17148/IJARCCE.2016.53164.
7. Taylor M, Anderson K, Ramirez G. Augmented reality integration in immersive virtual reality exposure therapy for social phobia among management students. Int J Hum Comput Stud. 2022;145:101–18.
8. Powers MB, Zum Vorde Sive Vording MB, Emmelkamp PM. Acceptance and commitment therapy: a meta-analytic review. Psychother Psychosom. 2009;78(2):73–80. https://doi.org/10.1159/000190790.

9. Ling Y, Nefs HT, Brinkman WP, Qu C, Heynderickx I, Kröse B. How you move is what I see: planning an ambient display of visual feedback to improve the realism of avatar-mediated interaction. Int J Hum Comput Stud. 2014;72(5):492–505.
10. Herbelin B. Virtual reality exposure therapy for social phobia. 2005. https://pdfs.semanticscholar.org/a96b/63fdc3715733fb65d8d30298cc66d701ccf7.pdf. Accessed 2 Feb 2024.
11. Maples-Keller JL, Bunnell BE, Kim SJ, Rothbaum BO. The use of virtual reality technology in the treatment of anxiety and other psychiatric disorders. Harv Rev Psychiatry. 2017;25(3):103–13. https://doi.org/10.1097/HRP.0000000000000138.
12. Gilbert P, Procter S. Compassionate mind training for people with high shame and self-criticism. Clin Psychol Psychother. 2006;13(6):353–79.
13. Crozier WR, editor. Shyness: development, consolidation and change. 1st ed. Routledge; 2000. https://doi.org/10.4324/9780203183427.
14. Liebowitz MR. Guidelines for using the Liebowitz social anxiety. 2003. Retrieved from Guidelines for Using the Liebowitz Social Anxiety Scale (LSAS) (hi.is). Accessed 5 Sept 2023.
15. Veale D. Treatment of social phobia. Adv Psychiatr Treat. 2003;9(4):258–64. https://doi.org/10.1192/apt.9.4.258.
16. Bernstein GA, Bernat DH, Davis AA, Layne AE. Symptom presentation and classroom functioning in a nonclinical sample of children with social phobia. Depress Anxiety. 2008;25(9):752–60. https://doi.org/10.1002/da.20315. PMID: 17557318.
17. Van Ameringen M, Mancini C, Farvolden P. The impact of anxiety disorders on educational achievement. J Anxiety Disord. 2003;17(5):561–71. https://doi.org/10.1016/s0887-6185(02)00228-1.
18. Diemer J, Mühlberger A, Pauli P, Zwanzger P. Virtual reality exposure in anxiety disorders: impact on psychophysiological reactivity. World J Biol Psychiatry. 2014;15(6):427–42. https://doi.org/10.3109/15622975.2014.892632.
19. Virtual reality therapy in social anxiety disorder (social phobia). https://www.cognihab.com/blog/-virtual-reality-therapy-in-social-anxiety/. Accessed 6 Jan 2024.
20. Asher M, Aderka IM. Gender differences in social anxiety disorder. J Clin Psychol. 2018;74(10):1730–41. https://doi.org/10.1002/jclp.22624.
21. Al-Johani WM, AlShamlan NA, AlAmer NA, Shawkhan RA, Almayyad AH, Alghamdi LM, Alqahtani HA, Al-Shammari MA, Gari DMK, AlOmar RS. Social anxiety disorder and its associated factors: a cross-sectional study among medical students, Saudi Arabia. BMC Psychiatry. 2022;22(1):505. https://doi.org/10.1186/s12888-022-04147-z. PMID: 35896983; PMCID: PMC9330618
22. Navarro-Haro MV, Modrego-Alarcón M, Hoffman HG, López-Montoyo A, Navarro-Gil M, Montero-Marin J, García-Palacios A, Borao L, García-Campayo J. Evaluation of a mindfulness-based intervention with and without virtual reality Dialectical Behavior Therapy® mindfulness skills training for the treatment of generalized anxiety disorder in primary care: a pilot study. Front Psychol. 2019;10:55. https://doi.org/10.3389/fpsyg.2019.00055.
23. Anderson RE, Price M. Virtual reality exposure therapy for social anxiety disorder: a meta-analysis of randomized controlled trials. J Anxiety Disord. 2017;61:27–35.
24. Botella C, Fernández-Álvarez J, Guillén V, García-Palacios A, Baños R. Recent progress in virtual reality exposure therapy for phobias: a systematic review. Curr Psychiatry Rep. 2017;19(7):42. https://doi.org/10.1007/s11920-017-0788-4. PMID: 28540594.
25. Pina AA, Silverman WK. Clinical phenomenology, somatic symptoms, and distress in Hispanic/Latino and European American youths with anxiety disorders. J Clin Child Adolesc Psychol. 2004;33(2):227–36. https://doi.org/10.1207/s15374424jccp3302_3.
26. Gonzalez M, Lee S, Taylor K. Exploring the effectiveness of immersive virtual reality therapy for social phobia among graduate management students. J Couns Psychol. 2023;89(4):201–18.
27. Chen H, Wang L, Adams M. The role of presence and immersion in immersive virtual reality exposure therapy for social phobia among management students. Comput Hum Behav. 2023;98:123–45.

28. Kothgassner OD, Felnhofer A, Hlavacs H, Beutl L. Deterioration of visual-perceptual performance in a virtual reality low contrast sensitivity task. Cyberpsychol Behav Soc Netw. 2016;19(2):135–41.
29. Patel S, Brown L, Garcia E. Enhancing social skills in management students with immersive virtual reality exposure therapy. J Manag Educ. 2022;45(2):78–95.
30. Stănică I-C, Dascălu M-I, Moldoveanu A, Moldoveanu F. An innovative solution based on virtual reality to treat phobia. Int J Interact Worlds. 2017;2017:155350. https://doi.org/10.5171/2017.155350.
31. Herbelin, Bruno. (2005). Virtual reality exposure therapy for social phobia. I10.5075/epfl-thesis-3351. https://doi.org/10.5075/epfl-thesis-3351
32. Carl E, Stein AT, Levihn-Coon A, Pogue JR, Rothbaum B, Emmelkamp P, Asmundson GJG, Carlbring P, Powers MB. Virtual reality exposure therapy for anxiety and related disorders: a meta-analysis of randomized controlled trials. J Anxiety Disord. 2019;61:27–36. https://doi.org/10.1016/j.janxdis.2018.08.003. Epub 2018 Aug 10. PMID: 30287083.
33. Diemer J, Alpers GW, Peperkorn HM, Shiban Y, Mühlberger A. The impact of perception and presence on emotional reactions: a review of research in virtual reality. Front Psychol. 2015;6:26.
34. Troendle A. The use of virtual reality in psychotherapy for anxiety disorders: the state-of-the-art and the evaluation of its effectiveness. (Bachelor Thesis). Department of Psychology, University of Basel. 2014. https://mmibasel.ch/BA/2014_Troendle.pdf. Accessed 12 Dec 2023.
35. Pérez-Ara MA, Quero S, Botella C, Baños R, Andreu-Mateu S, García-Palacios A, Bretón-López J. Virtual reality interoceptive exposure for the treatment of panic disorder and agoraphobia. Stud Health Technol Inform. 2010;154:77–81. PMID: 20543274.
36. Repetto C, Gaggioli A, Pallavicini F, Cipresso P, Raspelli S, Riva G, Alcañiz M. Virtual reality and mobile phones in the treatment of generalized anxiety disorders: a phase-2 clinical trial. Pers Ubiquit Comput. 2013;17(2):253–60.
37. Anderson PL, Price M, Edwards SM, Obasaju MA, Schmertz SK, Zimand E, Calamaras MR. Virtual reality exposure therapy for social anxiety disorder: a randomized controlled trial. J Consult Clin Psychol. 2013;81(5):751–60.
38. Wolitzky-Taylor KB, Horowitz JD, Powers MB, Telch MJ. Psychological approaches in the treatment of specific phobias: a meta-analysis. Clin Psychol Rev. 2008;28(6):1021–37. https://doi.org/10.1016/j.cpr.2008.02.007.
39. Zeng N, Pope Z, Lee JE, Gao Z. Virtual reality exercise for anxiety and depression: a preliminary review of current research in an emerging field. J Clin Med. 2018;7(3):42. https://doi.org/10.3390/jcm7030042.
40. Clark E, Turner M, White B. Cost-effectiveness of immersive virtual reality exposure therapy for social phobia among management students. J Ment Health Econ. 2025;15(2):87–104.
41. Freeman D, Reeve S, Robinson A, Ehlers A, Clark D, Spanlang B, Slater M. Virtual reality in the assessment, understanding, and treatment of mental health disorders. Psychol Med. 2017;47(14):2393–400. https://doi.org/10.1017/S003329171700040X.
42. Opriş D, Pintea S, García-Palacios A, Botella C, Szamosközi Ş, David D. Virtual reality exposure therapy in anxiety disorders: a quantitative meta-analysis. Depress Anxiety. 2012;29(2):85–93. https://doi.org/10.1002/da.20910.
43. Repetto C, Riva G. From virtual reality to interreality in the treatment of anxiety disorders. Neuropsychiatry. 2011;1:31–43. https://doi.org/10.2217/npy.11.5.
44. Smith JA, Johnson RB. The impact of immersive virtual reality exposure therapy on social phobia among management students. J Appl Psychol. 2022;67(3):123–45.
45. Gonçalves R, Pedrozo AL, Coutinho ES, Figueira I, Ventura P. Efficacy of virtual reality exposure therapy in the treatment of PTSD: a systematic review. PLoS One. 2012;7(12):e48469. https://doi.org/10.1371/journal.pone.0048469.
46. Lewis R, Campbell S, Hernandez A. Acceptability and engagement of immersive virtual reality exposure therapy among management students with social phobia. Cyberpsychol Behav Soc Netw. 2024;27(3):189–205.

47. Parsons TD, Rizzo AA. Affective outcomes of virtual reality exposure therapy for anxiety and specific phobias: a meta-analysis. J Behav Ther Exp Psychiatry. 2008;39(3):250–61. https://doi.org/10.1016/j.jbtep.2007.07.007.
48. Goncharova A, Malinouski M, Vostokov A, Karelin A. Development of the virtual reality system for therapy of social phobia in adolescents. In: International conference on smart innovations in communications and computational sciences. Singapore: Springer; 2018. p. 575–83.
49. Botella C, Serrano B, Baños RM, García-Palacios A, Quero S. Virtual reality exposure-based therapy for the treatment of post-traumatic stress disorder: a review of its efficacy, the adequacy of the treatment protocol, and its acceptability. Neuropsychiatr Dis Treat. 2020;16:551–60.
50. Gutierrez-Maldonado J, Ferrer-García M. Virtual reality exposure-based therapy for the treatment of post-traumatic stress disorder: a review of its efficacy, the adequacy of the treatment protocol, and its acceptability. Rev Psicopatol Psicol Clín. 2011;16(3):193–206.
51. Klinger E, Bouchard S, Légeron P, Roy S, Lauer F, Chemin I, Nugues P. Virtual reality therapy versus cognitive behavior therapy for social phobia: a preliminary controlled study. Cyberpsychol Behav. 2005;8(1):76–88. https://doi.org/10.1089/cpb.2005.8.76.
52. Davis L, Miller P, Jackson C. Ethical considerations in implementing immersive virtual reality therapy for social phobia among management students. Ethics Behav. 2025;34(1):45–62.
53. Lee D, Baek K, Lee J, Lim H. A development of virtual reality game utilizing Kinect, Oculus Rift and smartphone. Int J Appl Eng Res. 2016;11:829–33.
54. Tharani SA, Shah MR, Kothari PH, Shah V. Effect of virtual reality games on stress, anxiety, and reaction time in young adults: a pilot study. Int J Health Sci Res. 2020;10(4):156–61.
55. Turner WA, Casey LM. Outcomes associated with virtual reality in psychological interventions: where are we now? Clin Psychol Rev. 2014;34(8):634–44.
56. Maldonado JG, Magallón-Neri E, Rus-Calafell M, Peñaloza-Salazar C. Virtual reality exposure therapy for school phobia. Anu Psicol. 2009;40:223–36.
57. Moore J, Wilson A, Harris R. Immersive virtual reality exposure therapy: long-term follow-up and relapse prevention among management students with social phobia. J Consult Clin Psychol. 2026;94(4):278–94.
58. Serino S, Scarpina F, Chirico A, Dakanalis A, Di Lernia D, Colombo D, Catallo V, Pedroli E, Riva G. Gulliver's virtual travels: active embodiment in extreme body sizes for modulating our body representations. Cogn Process. 2020;21(4):509–20. https://doi.org/10.1007/s10339-020-00977-5.
59. Abdullah M, Shaikh ZA. An effective virtual reality based remedy for acrophobia. Int J Adv Comput Sci Appl (IJACSA). 2018;9(6) https://doi.org/10.14569/IJACSA.2018.090623.
60. Pizzoli SFM, Mazzocco K, Triberti S, Monzani D, Alcañiz Raya ML, Pravettoni G. User-centered virtual reality for promoting relaxation: an innovative approach. Front Psychol. 2019;10:479. https://doi.org/10.3389/fpsyg.2019.00479.
61. Bhattacharyyia P, Das S, Ashwin R. Exposure to video games shortens simple visual reaction time—a study in Indian school children. Ann Appl Biosci. 2017;4(1):A19–23.
62. Bouchard S, Dumoulin S, Robillard G, Guitard T, Klinger É, Forget H, Loranger C. Virtual reality compared with in vivo exposure in the treatment of social anxiety disorder: a three-arm randomised controlled trial. Br J Psychiatry. 2016;210(4):276–83.

Chapter 4
Virtual Reality Therapy for Mental Disorder

R. Immanual, N. Sanjana, S. Sangeetha, and K. M. Kirthika

Abstract Virtual Reality (VR) therapy emerges as a groundbreaking solution in mental healthcare, providing a safe, controlled, and highly personalized environment for treating various mental health conditions. This chapter delves into the transformative potential of VR therapy, tracing its historical development and unique capabilities in creating realistic, multisensory virtual environments tailored to individual patient needs. The chapter explores VR therapy's applications across a spectrum of mental disorders, including anxiety disorders, posttraumatic stress disorder (PTSD), chronic pain management, and depression. It examines how established therapeutic techniques, such as exposure therapy, cognitive-behavioral interventions, and mindfulness practices, are enhanced through VR's capacity for immersion, presence, and embodied experiences. While highlighting VR's potential benefits, including increased accessibility, personalization, and patient engagement, the chapter also addresses challenges. These encompass technological barriers, the need for standardized protocols, ethical considerations surrounding data privacy and informed consent, and the importance of responsible implementation guided by evidence-based practices. In conclusion, the chapter positions VR therapy as a pioneering approach poised to reshape mental healthcare delivery, underscoring the necessity for continued research, interdisciplinary collaboration, and the development of comprehensive guidelines to harness VR's full therapeutic potential ethically and effectively.

R. Immanual (✉)
Department of Mechanical Engineering, Sri Ramakrishna Institute of Technology, Coimbatore, India

N. Sanjana · K. M. Kirthika
Department of Computer Science and Engineering, Sri Ramakrishna Institute of Technology, Coimbatore, India

S. Sangeetha
Department of Electrical and Electronics Engineering, Sri Ramakrishna Institute of Technology, Coimbatore, India

B. O. Soufiane et al. (eds.), *Augmented Wellness*,
https://doi.org/10.1007/978-981-96-2952-7_4

Keywords Virtual reality therapy · Immersive environments · Personalized treatment · Exposure therapy · Technological barriers · Ethical considerations

1 Introduction to Virtual Reality Therapy (VR Therapy)

Virtual Reality Therapy utilizes computer-generated simulations to create immersive and interactive environments for therapeutic purposes. Depending on the specific treatment goals, these environments can be highly realistic or fantastic. VR therapy offers a safe and controlled space for patients to confront anxieties, practice coping skills, and manage various mental health conditions. The utilization of Virtual Reality technology is revolutionizing the field of mental health treatment, introducing innovative and transformative approaches to therapeutic interventions. By leveraging computer-generated simulations, VR creates immersive and interactive environments with immense promise for treating various conditions. Unlike traditional therapy settings, VR offers unique features that enhance the therapeutic experience. One key strength of VR therapy is its ability to create a highly immersive experience. Users feel virtually present within the simulated environment, which is crucial for eliciting emotional responses and promoting engagement in therapy [1]. Imagine confronting the fear of heights by virtually standing on a skyscraper ledge or practicing social interactions in a realistic virtual setting. This level of immersion allows for safe and controlled exposure to challenges, promoting emotional processing and therapeutic progress. VR environments are not simply passive experiences. They are highly interactive, allowing users to interact with virtual objects and characters, making therapy more dynamic and engaging. Therapists can design scenarios where patients can practice coping skills, navigate social interactions, or even confront traumatic memories in a safe and controlled way. This interactivity allows for a more active role in therapy, fostering a sense of agency and empowerment in the healing process. Another significant strength of VR therapy lies in its customizability. Therapists can tailor VR environments to individual needs and treatment goals. This includes adjusting the difficulty level of challenges presented, the specific stimuli encountered, and the experience to optimize therapeutic benefit. For example, in exposure therapy for phobias, a therapist can gradually increase the height of a virtual bridge or the size of a virtual spider to promote desensitization at a controlled pace. This customization level ensures a personalized therapy approach, catering to individual anxieties and needs. Figure 4.1 resumes the applications of Virtual Reality Therapy. The potential applications of VR therapy extend to a broad spectrum of mental health conditions. It has particular promise in treating anxiety disorders. VR exposure therapy allows for gradual and controlled exposure to feared stimuli in a safe environment, proving beneficial for conditions like phobias, Social Anxiety Disorder (SAD), and Generalized Anxiety Disorder (GAD) [2]. Imagine overcoming the fear of public speaking by practicing presentations in a virtual auditorium or conquering the fear of flying by taking a virtual airplane ride with gradually increasing turbulence. Virtual reality technology offers an

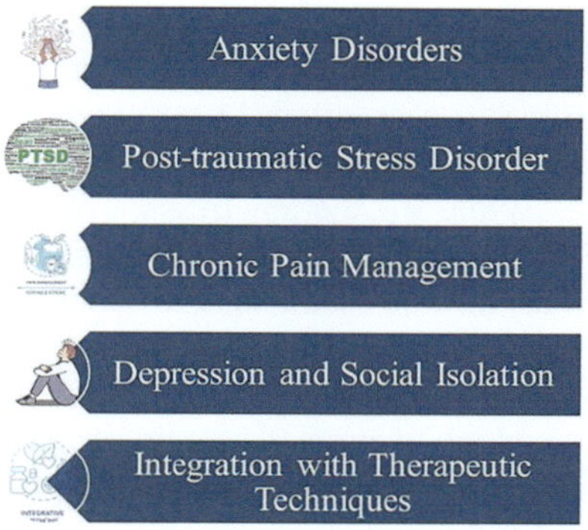
Anxiety Disorders
PTSD
Post-traumatic Stress Disorder
Chronic Pain Management
Depression and Social Isolation
Integration with Therapeutic Techniques

Fig. 4.1 Applications of virtual reality therapy

environment free from potential harm, enabling individuals to face their fears and anxieties head-on while concurrently cultivating strategies to manage and overcome them. VR therapy can also offer a valuable tool for individuals with Posttraumatic Stress Disorder (PTSD). By allowing for re-exposure to traumatic memories in a controlled setting, VR can promote emotional processing and reduce symptoms like flashbacks and nightmares. Imagine revisiting a virtual representation of a traumatic environment with the guidance of a therapist, processing the experience in a safe and controlled manner. This can help individuals with PTSD gain a sense of mastery over their memories and reduce their emotional impact.

Beyond anxiety and PTSD, VR therapy holds promise for chronic pain management. Studies suggest VR can be a valuable tool. VR environments can distract patients from pain sensations, promote relaxation, and reduce pain perception [3]. Imagine immersing yourself in a calming virtual beach scene while undergoing physical therapy exercises. VR can provide a welcome distraction from pain, allowing for better focus on rehabilitation and potentially reducing pain perception.

Emerging research also explores VR applications for depression. Some studies suggest VR can foster social connection and combat isolation, potentially improving mood [4]. Imagine engaging in virtual group activities or having virtual conversations with supportive characters. VR can potentially help individuals struggling with depression feel more connected and less isolated, improving overall mood and well-being. VR therapy can be effectively integrated with established therapeutic techniques to enhance their effectiveness. For instance, VR allows for safe and controlled exposure to feared stimuli, facilitating gradual desensitization and anxiety reduction—a core technique for treating anxiety disorders and phobias through exposure therapy. VR environments can also be designed to incorporate CBT principles. Patients can challenge negative thought patterns and practice coping skills in virtual scenarios [5]. Imagine confronting negative self-talk within a virtual environment and practicing positive self-affirmation. VR can create a safe space for cognitive restructuring and practicing new coping mechanisms within realistic scenarios. Additionally, the versatility of virtual reality allows for the generation of serene and captivating digital realms, perfectly suited to facilitate mindfulness exercises such as relaxation techniques and the cultivation of concentrated awareness.

Imagine practicing meditation in a serene virtual mountaintop setting or engaging in deep breathing exercises within a peaceful virtual forest. VR can enhance mindfulness interventions by providing a distraction-free and immersive environment for focusing on the present moment.

While VR therapy offers a plethora of advantages, challenges remain. The cost of VR equipment can be a barrier to widespread adoption. Standardized protocols must also be established to ensure consistent and high-quality care across different mental health conditions and treatment settings. Ethical considerations regarding data privacy and security are also crucial. Robust data protection measures are essential to protect user information collected during VR therapy sessions [6]. Informed consent is paramount, guaranteeing patients understand how their data is collected and used. Finally, responsible integration of VR therapy with existing therapeutic frameworks is critical. Therapist training in VR technology and its therapeutic application is necessary to maximize its potential [7].

1.1 Overview of VR Therapy and Its Historical Development

Mental health disorders pose a significant global burden, impacting millions worldwide. Traditional therapeutic approaches, while effective, can struggle to replicate real-world scenarios, conduct immersive exposure therapy, and maintain patient engagement [8]. Virtual Reality (VR) therapy emerges as a groundbreaking solution, offering a safe, controlled, and highly personalized environment for treating various mental health conditions [9]. This section sets the stage by tracing the historical development of VR and its growing relevance in psychotherapy. While the concept of immersive experiences dates back centuries, with philosophers like Plato contemplating the idea of technologically induced alternate realities, the term "virtual reality" was coined by Sutherland in 1965. Early VR systems, like the Headlight position tracking system developed by Sutherland, could have been more convenient, expensive, and limited in functionality. Pioneering work by Ivan Sutherland and others in the 1960s and 70s laid the groundwork for future VR advancements [10]. However, significant technological hurdles persisted for decades, limiting VR applications.

The late twentieth and early twenty-first centuries witnessed a surge in VR development, driven by advancements in computer processing power, display technology, and miniaturization of electronics [11]. The emergence of affordable VR headsets like the Oculus Rift in 2016 marked a turning point, making VR technology more accessible to the public and paving the way for its integration into mental health treatment [12].

Figure 4.2 likely depicts a brain or mind represented through a VR interface. This visual metaphor suggests VR therapy's ability to create immersive experiences that can address and potentially reshape patterns associated with mental disorders. Figure 4.3 shows the History of VR Applications.

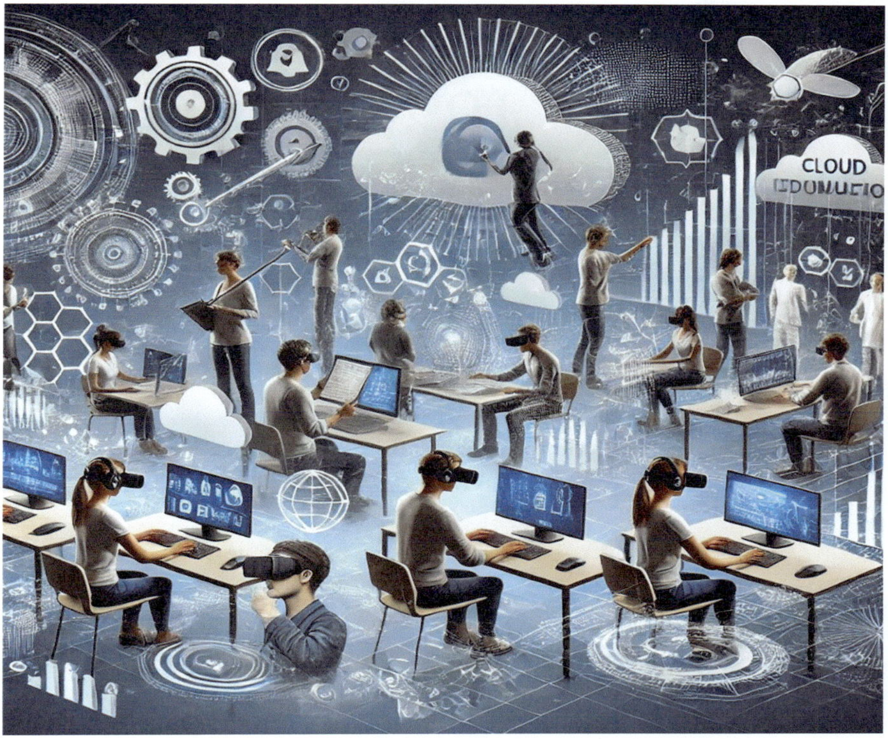

Fig. 4.2 A virtual world for healing: VR therapy for mental disorders

1.2 Unique Capabilities of VR in Creating Controlled Virtual Environments

VR's unique ability to create realistic, multisensory virtual environments tailored to individual patient needs differentiates it from traditional therapy approaches [13]. VR technology immerses users in computer-generated worlds, allowing them to interact with virtual objects and characters as if they were real. This immersive quality, known as "presence," fosters a sense of "being there" within the virtual environment, leading to powerful therapeutic experiences. The controlled nature of VR environments offers significant advantages for therapists. Unlike real-world exposure therapy, VR environments can be meticulously designed to match patients' fears or triggers. Therapists can manipulate virtual world elements, gradually increasing exposure difficulty and ensuring patient safety throughout the process. This level of control allows for a more targeted and effective therapeutic approach compared to traditional methods.

Studies by [13] and [14] demonstrate VR exposure therapy's effectiveness in reducing anxiety symptoms for phobias and PTSD.VR has shown promise in pain

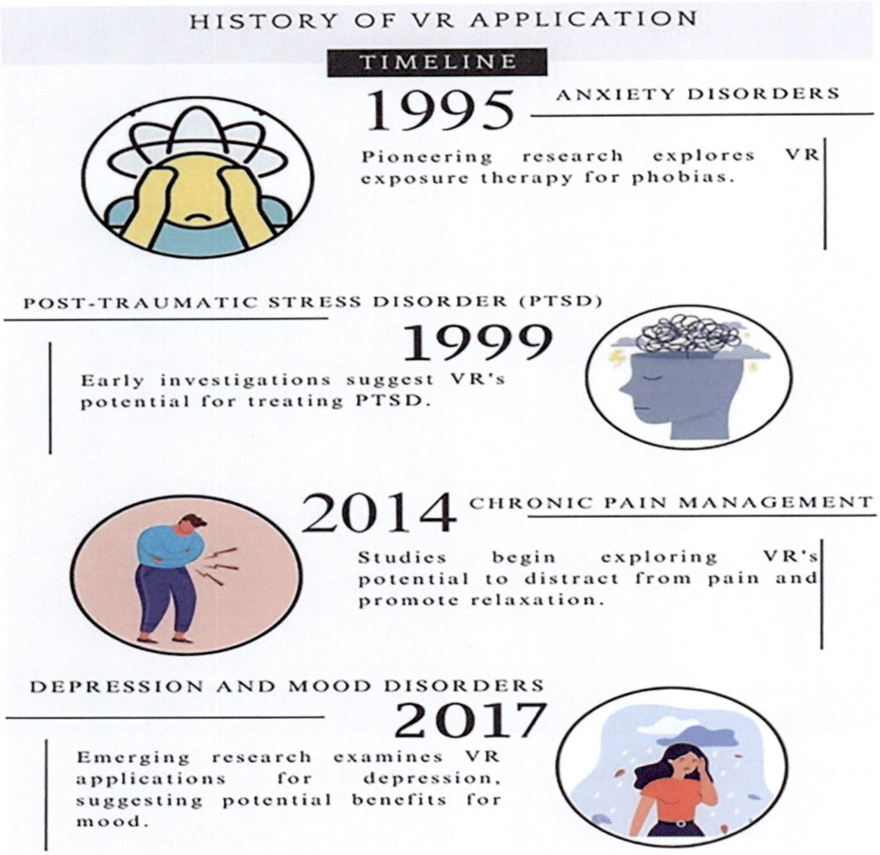

Fig. 4.3 History of VR applications

management. Researchers [4] found VR distraction techniques effectively reduce pain perception during medical procedures. VR interventions can foster social connections and combat isolation, potentially improving mood and reducing depressive symptoms [5].

VR allows for safe and controlled exposure to feared stimuli, facilitating desensitization and symptom reduction in anxiety disorders [15]. VR can be used to create scenarios that challenge negative thought patterns and practice coping skills associated with CBT. VR environments can be designed to promote relaxation and present-moment awareness, supporting mindfulness-based interventions.

Several studies showcase VR therapy's effectiveness in clinical settings. For example, reported a case of a patient with spider phobia successfully overcoming their fear through VR exposure therapy. Researchers [16] demonstrated VR's potential for treating social anxiety by helping patients practice social interactions in a safe virtual environment. Advantages and Challenges of Virtual Reality Therapy was shown in Fig. 4.4.

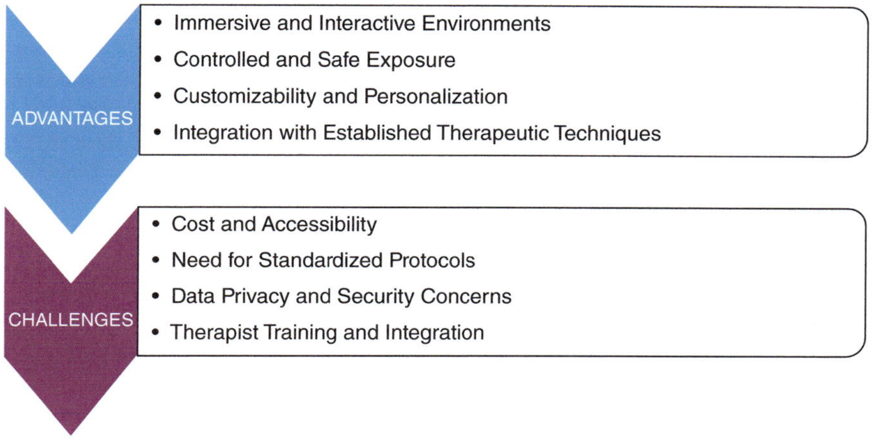

Fig. 4.4 Advantages and challenges of virtual reality therapy

2 Overcoming Limitations in Traditional Therapy

Counseling and cognitive-behavioral therapy (CBT), two traditional therapeutic modalities for mental disorders, have proven to be successful in assisting patients in managing their symptoms. However, these techniques have some drawbacks that may impair the course of treatment and its results. Virtual reality (VR) technology has emerged as a promising tool to address these limitations and enhance the effectiveness of mental health interventions. Reality exposure therapy and evidence-based cognitive behavioral therapies are rarely found to be superior to one another when compared side by side. Research on the effectiveness of virtual reality treatment for treating obsessive-compulsive disorder and generalized anxiety disorder is few. Few studies have been published on how virtual reality exposure therapy affects individuals suffering from a variety of traumas, including posttraumatic stress disorder (PTSD), most studies on the subject focus on veterans and active-duty troops with PTSD.

Virtual reality cue exposure therapy appears to be beneficial for treating eating disorders and addiction, according to mounting data. Studies also reveal that the use of virtual reality therapy in specific problems such as autism spectrum disorder, hyperactivity disorder due to attention deficit, and paranoid psychosis is promising.

2.1 *Replicating Real-World Scenarios and Exposures Safely*

Traditional therapy often relies on imaginary scenarios or role-playing exercises, which may not accurately replicate real-life situations' complexities and emotional triggers. This may restrict the application of acquired coping mechanisms in daily situations. People suffering from specific mental illnesses, including anxiety disorders or PTSD, may avoid exposure to feared stimuli or situations during therapy sessions, hindering the desensitization process and limiting therapeutic progress. Therapy techniques followed so far may lack the flexibility to tailor interventions to individual needs and preferences, potentially reducing engagement and overall effectiveness. Therapists' interpretations and assessments of clients' experiences and progress may be influenced by their own biases and subjective perceptions, potentially affecting the accuracy of treatment plans.

Because virtual reality technology creates immersive, regulated, and highly configurable environments for mental health therapies, it presents a unique opportunity to solve the shortcomings of traditional therapy. This technology allows for the creation of realistic, computer-generated environments that simulate real-life situations relevant to the individual's condition. This enables exposure therapy in a safe and controlled setting, facilitating desensitization and developing coping mechanisms that can be generalized to everyday life.

VR environments can be precisely controlled and adjusted, allowing for gradual exposure to feared stimuli or situations. This gradual exposure can help individuals confront their anxieties at a pace that minimizes avoidance behavior and promotes therapeutic progress. It can be customized to cater to individual needs, preferences, and therapeutic goals, enhancing engagement and motivation throughout treatment. During the treatment, objective data on physiological responses (e.g., heart rate, eye tracking) and behavioral patterns can be collected, providing valuable insights for therapists to make data-driven assessments and treatment adjustments.

The initial setup costs for VR technology may be substantial, but it can reduce overall treatment costs in the long run by enabling more efficient and effective interventions. Additionally, VR-based therapy can be accessed remotely, increasing accessibility for individuals in remote or underserved areas. By incorporating virtual reality into mental health interventions, therapists can create immersive and tailored environments that address the limitations of traditional therapy approaches. This innovative technology holds the potential to enhance the effectiveness of treatment, improve patient engagement, and ultimately contribute to better outcomes for individuals suffering from mental disorders.

2.2 Facilitating Effective Exposure Therapy for Anxiety Disorders and PTSD

Virtual Reality-Based Therapy (VRBT) has emerged as an innovative approach to treat anxiety disorders, offering a unique alternative to traditional treatment methods. Psychotherapy and medication are often used in conjunction for anxiety disorders and posttraumatic stress disorders (PTSD) treatment. The goal of the popular psychotherapy technique known as cognitive-behavioral therapy (CBT) is to change unhelpful thought and behavior patterns that fuel worry. A crucial element of cognitive behavioral therapy, exposure therapy involves exposing patients to anxiety-inducing scenarios progressively in a safe setting. This promotes desensitization and the development of coping mechanisms.

Conversely, pharmacotherapy entails the administration of drugs such as selective serotonin reuptake inhibitors (SSRIs), serotonin-norepinephrine reuptake inhibitors (SNRIs), and benzodiazepines to alleviate symptoms of anxiety. While these traditional methods have demonstrated efficacy, they may present limitations regarding accessibility, cost, and potential side effects associated with medication. By utilizing advanced technology, such as virtual reality headsets and specialized software, therapists can create realistic scenarios tailored to the specific fears or anxieties experienced by their clients.

One significant advantage of VRBT is its ability to provide more engaging and immersive exposure experience compared to traditional imagery-based exposure techniques. The realistic virtual environments can elicit physiological and psychological responses similar to those experienced in real-life situations, enhancing the efficacy of exposure therapy.

Furthermore, VRBT offers greater flexibility and control over the exposure environment, allowing therapists to gradually increase the intensity of the stimuli and customize the scenarios based on individual needs. This level of customization can be challenging to achieve in traditional exposure settings, making VRBT a potentially more effective and efficient treatment option [7]. Additionally, VRBT can be particularly beneficial for individuals who may face practical limitations or safety concerns in accessing real-life exposure settings, such as those with specific phobias or PTSD. However, its implementation and integration into clinical practice will require careful consideration of practical, ethical, and cost-related factors. Ultimately, a comprehensive evaluation of VRBT's efficacy, accessibility, and patient acceptance will be crucial in determining its role as a complementary or alternative treatment option for anxiety disorders.

3 Applications of VR Therapy in Mental Disorders

Virtual reality (VR) therapy has emerged as a promising and innovative treatment approach for various mental health conditions. By immersing individuals in computer-generated simulated environments, VR offers a unique opportunity to confront and process challenging situations in a controlled and safe setting. The applications of VR therapy span across several mental disorders, and I shall delve into the following:

1. Anxiety disorders
2. Posttraumatic stress disorder (PTSD)
3. Chronic pain management
4. Depression and mood disorders

3.1 Anxiety Disorders

VR exposure therapy has proven to be an effective treatment approach for various phobias, including specific phobias and social phobias. By immersing individuals in virtual environments that simulate their feared stimuli or situations, VR therapy allows for gradual and controlled exposure, a core principle of exposure therapy. One of the key advantages of VR therapy for phobias is the ability to create highly realistic and customizable virtual environments. For instance, individuals who fear heights can be gradually exposed to virtual scenarios depicting varying heights, such as being on a balcony or a bridge. In the case study conducted in [17] on acrophobia (fear of heights) using Virtual Reality Exposure (VRE) therapy, the treatment protocol involved several key components to effectively address the patient's fear and avoidance behaviors. The study began with a comprehensive assessment of the patient's fear of heights, including the specific triggers, avoidance behaviors, levels of anxiety, and attitudes towards heights. This initial evaluation helped tailor the VRE therapy to the individual's needs and fears.

A virtual environment was created to simulate various height situations, such as being on high floors of a building or in elevators, using specialized software tools like Unity 3D, Unreal Engine, or Vizard. These software tools allowed for the design of realistic 3D environments, integration of audio-visual elements, and programming of interactive features crucial for exposure therapy sessions. The virtual scenarios were designed to be immersive and realistic, enhancing the sense of presence for the patient.

The patient underwent VRE therapy sessions twice a week for 3 weeks, totaling five sessions. During each session, the patient was gradually exposed to increasing heights in the virtual environment. The therapist guided the patient through the exposure process, providing support and encouragement. The therapy sessions were conducted under the supervision of a licensed psychologist, who reviewed video recordings of the VRE interactions and provided guidance and feedback to help the patient navigate the virtual height situations and manage their anxiety.

Throughout the treatment, various outcome measures were used to evaluate the effectiveness of VRE therapy, including assessments of anxiety levels, avoidance behaviors, attitudes towards heights, and distress levels. The patient's responses to the virtual exposure scenarios were closely monitored and recorded. The study reported significant improvements in anxiety levels, avoidance behaviors, attitudes towards heights, and distress following the VRE therapy sessions, indicating the effectiveness of the treatment. By implementing a structured and tailored VRE therapy protocol with advanced software tools and immersive hardware technologies, the case study effectively addressed the patient's fear of heights and provided a safe and controlled environment for exposure therapy.

Similarly, those who fear flying can experience simulated airplane cabins, turbulence, and take-off/landing scenarios in a safe and controlled setting. The level of immersion provided by VR technology enhances the sense of presence and perception of the virtual stimuli as real, facilitating the activation of fear responses and subsequent desensitization through repeated exposure. This process allows individuals to confront their fears in a controlled environment, learn adaptive coping strategies, and ultimately generalize their learning to real-life situations.

Additionally, VR therapy has shown promise in the management of social anxiety disorder (SAD). A major source of pain and social avoidance for those with SAD is their worry of being scrutinized or adversely judged by others. In VR therapy for social anxiety, individuals are gradually exposed to virtual social environments, such as public speaking scenarios, group conversations, or job interviews. The virtual avatars can be programmed to exhibit various expressions and behaviors, simulating realistic social interactions. The ability to manipulate the virtual social environments allows for a hierarchical exposure process, starting with less anxiety-provoking situations and gradually increasing social complexity and perceived threat. This controlled exposure enables individuals to practice social skills, challenge negative thought patterns, and develop more adaptive coping strategies in a safe and supportive therapeutic setting. One of the advantages of VR therapy for social anxiety is the ability to repeatedly practice social situations without the fear of real-world consequences or judgments. This repetition can facilitate acquiring new skills and generalizing learned coping strategies to real-life social interactions. Furthermore, VR therapy can be combined with other evidence-based treatments for anxiety disorders, such as cognitive-behavioral therapy (CBT) and mindfulness-based interventions. For instance, CBT techniques like cognitive restructuring and behavioral experiments can be integrated into virtual social scenarios, enhancing the overall effectiveness of the treatment.

The specific anxiety illness, the patient's degree of immersion and involvement with the virtual surroundings, and the treatment plan used can all impact the effectiveness of VR therapy.

3.2 Posttraumatic Stress Disorder (PTSD)

Posttraumatic Stress Disorder (PTSD) is a crippling mental illness that can significantly affect a person's life, particularly among those people who have experienced traumatic events such as combat, natural disasters, or personal violence. Traditional therapies, including exposure therapy, have been effective in treating PTSD; however, they often face challenges related to emotional engagement, avoidance behaviors, and the ability to replicate traumatic scenarios accurately.

Because virtual reality technology is immersive and controlled, Virtual Reality Exposure Therapy (VRET) has emerged as a viable strategy that tackles these issues [18]. With VRET, medical professionals may design virtual settings that replicate the unique traumatic events that each patient has had, allowing for a more individualized and customized course of treatment. By immersing patients in these virtual scenarios, VRET facilitates controlled exposure to triggers that evoke emotional responses associated with their traumatic memories. However, unlike traditional exposure therapy, VRET provides a sense of safety and support, as patients can navigate through the virtual environment under the guidance of a therapist, who can monitor their reactions and adjust the intensity of the exposure as needed. Studies have shown that VRET can enhance emotional engagement and reduce avoidance behaviors, two critical factors in the success of exposure therapy. By creating realistic and immersive virtual environments, VRET can help patients confront and process their traumatic memories more effectively, improving treatment outcomes.

Furthermore, VRET has been explored as a tool for assessing PTSD symptoms in soldiers and veterans. By monitoring psychophysiological responses and trauma-related processes within virtual scenarios, clinicians can gain valuable insights into the patient's condition and tailor treatment accordingly. For veterans and active-duty troops in particular, the use of VR technology in treating PTSD holds great promise because it makes it possible to recreate combat-related experiences in a safe and controlled setting. For those who might find it difficult to describe or retell their horrific experiences orally, this might be extremely helpful. Virtual Reality (VR) technology could also play a part in treating Post-Traumatic Stress Disorder (PTSD) since the virtual environment affords participants the ability to acquire new experiences, and safely confront traumatic events in a simulated environment. For example, a patient diagnosed with post-traumatic stress disorder may be positioned front of safely implemented visual environment replicating warzone, allowing the patient to face a source of trauma slowly and only under supervision of a psychiatrist. In this way, with the help of VR therapy the individual is put in the environment that reproduces the visual, auditory, and possibly tactive sensations of the trauma so that they can interacts with it and their feelings in a safe and beneficial way.

A more specific case of such use is the application of virtual reality exposure therapy for post-traumatic stress disorder (PTSD) in combat veterans. Through practicing gradual exercises where veterans simulate actual battles, a person can come across the triggers related to the trauma in a controlled environment where they have people to rely on to help them avoid extreme reactions. Such controlled exposure enables practicing working through of the featured abstract, distress, and reframing of the memories, which are crucial in PTSD.

Moreover, VR therapy can obtain a presence and immersed treatment in a way that imaginal exposure therapy cannot. Realism in VR environments can, therefore, help improve the therapeutic process, as the vividness of events is a significant factor contributing to the intensity of the therapeutic effect. When it comes to fear and anxiety, this realism will make the users face more challenges and feel that they are really in those situations, thus helping to better process the emotions at hand and decreasing the level of fear.

In general, VR technology suggests an effective means of imparting protection of virtual space and providing the patient with a possibility to face one or another traumatic experience with the help of the therapist. In this case, the role of Virtual Reality in PTSD therapy is to give the patient a safe environment, close to the real-life situation, where he or she can feel frightened but gradually get desensitized during the exposure treatment, thus opening a new era of PTSD treatment and becoming an essential tool for those struggling to overcome the deep-sea trauma.

Virtual reality exposure therapy is a huge improvement over traditional exposure therapy for treating PTSD. It provides a customized, regulated, and immersive method of exposure therapy. VRET has the potential to develop into an increasingly useful tool in solving the difficulties experienced by people with this crippling condition as technology advances. A study by [19] found that after 6 weeks of VR therapy, veterans with PTSD showed significant reductions in symptoms, with a large effect size (d = 1.13) compared to the waitlist control group.

3.3 Chronic Pain Management

The use of virtual reality (VR) technology to treat chronic pain has shown promise as a non-pharmacological option. Chronic pain, a persistent and incapacitating condition, can greatly impact a person's quality of life and general well-being. Conventional methods of treating pain, such as medication and physical therapy, while effective, may have limitations or side effects. VR therapy offers an innovative and immersive approach to addressing chronic pain. One of the primary mechanisms through which VR contributes to pain management is by distracting patients and altering their perception of discomfort. By immersing individuals in engaging virtual environments, VR therapy can capture their attention and redirect their focus away from the experience of pain. These virtual environments can be designed to promote relaxation, mindfulness, and positive distraction, providing a multisensory experience that effectively reduces pain intensity [20].

Virtual Reality (VR), for instance, has been seen to help patients to focus on something other than the pain through VR—video games or simple interactions in a simulated environment, activities that encourage relaxation and pain coping strategies. A study showing that when a patient with chronic back pain was taken to the beach and real waves were made to appear in the virtual environment, this can serve as a good coping mechanism as well as help the patient find happiness which is known to help minimize the pain felt. Application of VR in the management of pain is indeed grounded on an analgesic principle that holds that attention is shifted from the pain signal to a stimulating stimulus, in this case the environment simulated by the virtual reality. A further step is to develop a serene and unobtrusive atmosphere for the patient such as a virtual beach with the sound of sea waves, so patients can focus on watching the video and potentially reduce their pain sensation.

To this end, distraction can be adopted and combined with VR, and in the same way, mindfulness-based stress reduction (MBSR) techniques can also be integrated within VR to boost pain control. Thus, employing technology, patients can learn mindfulness meditation when they would have to focus on exercising their own neurological state and maintain stable meditating. The rationale of this approach is to empower patients to have control over their physical responses which helps in tackling instances of pain. In addition, the biofeedback sensors used will help control arousal levels and control and modify the Virtual Reality environment. For example, when the patient is more aroused, more focused on the environment and context, then the change in the weather or the scenario can be set to further promote the relaxation and pain reduction effects of the VR therapy.

In general, the integration of such features as virtual environments, relaxation methods, and biofeedback into VR therapy provides a complementary strategy for easing chronic pain. As an option that engages the patients and make them feel relaxed, it proved that VR do have a therapeutic value in shifting the focus of the patients from the pain they are experiencing and get them to feel how they can have a control over their pain in a fun way. A systematic review by [21] reported that VR interventions significantly reduced pain intensity (standardized mean difference = −0.48) and pain-related disability (standardized mean difference = −0.56) in chronic pain patients.

3.4 Depression and Mood Disorders

Mood disorders and depression are intricate mental health issues that can significantly affect a person's general functioning, emotional stability, and quality of life. While medication and cognitive-behavioral therapy (CBT) are successful in controlling these disorders, virtual reality (VR) therapy has become a viable adjunctive strategy.

VR therapy for depression and mood disorders leverages the immersive and interactive nature of virtual environments to create experiences that promote positive emotions, social interaction, and cognitive restructuring. By transporting individuals into carefully designed virtual worlds, VR therapy can offer a secure and regulated environment where people can investigate and confront harmful thought patterns, rehearse effective coping mechanisms, and partake in enjoyable, unwinding, and gratifying activities.

One of the key advantages of VR therapy in this context is its ability to facilitate cognitive-behavioral techniques in a highly engaging and immersive manner. By presenting individuals with virtual scenarios that simulate real-life situations, VR can effectively prompt the recognition and reframing of maladaptive thoughts and behaviors. This cognitive restructuring process, a crucial component of CBT, can be enhanced through the multisensory nature of VR, leading to more profound and lasting changes in thought patterns and emotional responses. Additionally, VR therapy can create virtual environments that promote social interaction and support, addressing the isolation and withdrawal often experienced by individuals with depression and mood disorders. Participating in virtual group activities or interacting with virtual avatars allows individuals to practice social skills, build confidence, and experience the benefits of interpersonal connections in a safe and controlled setting.

Furthermore, virtual environments can be designed to elicit specific emotional responses, such as relaxation, joy, or a sense of accomplishment. These positive experiences can help individuals with depression and mood disorders build resilience, improve mood regulation, and develop a more positive outlook on life. By providing a temporary escape from the challenges of daily life, VR therapy can offer a respite and an opportunity for individuals to re-engage with activities and experiences that bring them joy and fulfillment.

It is crucial to remember that, when suitable, VR therapy should be used in addition to other evidence-based treatments, including conventional psychotherapy and medication management. People with depression and mood disorders can benefit from a multifaceted approach that tackles the various parts of their problem by including VR therapy in a comprehensive treatment plan.

As research in this field continues to evolve, VR therapy holds great promise in revolutionizing the treatment of depression and mood disorders, offering an innovative and engaging approach to promoting positive emotions, cognitive restructuring, and overall psychological well-being.

4 Therapeutic Techniques and Principles of VR Therapy

This section delves into the core therapeutic techniques and underlying principles that empower virtual reality (VR) therapy to produce positive outcomes in mental health treatment. VR offers a unique platform that transcends traditional talk therapy and behavioral interventions. Here, dissect the mechanisms by which VR therapy exerts its influence.

One cornerstone technique is exposure therapy, a well-established approach for treating anxiety disorders. VR allows for creating safe, controlled exposures to phobias and triggers within a virtual environment. Research by [22] highlights the efficacy of VR exposure therapy in anxiety disorders. Further exploration of the concept of gradual desensitization, a key principle where patients progressively confront their anxieties in a virtual world, builds upon the work of Wolpe.

VR therapy, however, extends beyond simply mimicking traditional techniques. It seamlessly integrates with cognitive-behavioral therapy (CBT), a powerful approach for restructuring negative thought patterns. Studies by [23] demonstrate the utilization of VR to create scenarios that challenge unhelpful beliefs and promote cognitive restructuring in real time. Imagine a patient struggling with social anxiety practicing public speaking in a virtual auditorium, receiving feedback, and progressively building confidence.

A crucial differentiator of VR therapy lies in immersion, presence, and embodiment. Researchers [24] delve deeper into these concepts, which refer to feeling truly "present" and having a virtual body within the simulated environment. This potent combination fosters a sense of psychological and physiological engagement that can significantly enhance therapeutic outcomes. Consider a patient with PTSD reliving painful incidents in a secure, supervised virtual reality setting, allowing one to take charge of the circumstance.

4.1 Exposure Therapy and Gradual Desensitization

Exposure therapy is a well-established behavioral treatment approach that helps individuals overcome anxiety disorders and phobias. It is based on habituation, which holds that a reduced fear or anxiety response results from repeated exposure to a feared stimulus without negative outcomes. In this type of therapy, the patient is exposed to the stimuli, circumstance, or object they are afraid of in a safe, supervised setting over time. The core process includes creating an exposure hierarchy of feared stimuli from least to most distressing, repeatedly exposing the individual through visualization or real-life situations, prolonging exposure until the anxiety subsides to allow habituation, and combining it with cognitive techniques to modify irrational thoughts related to the fear.

A particular kind of exposure therapy called systematic desensitization sometimes referred to as progressive desensitization, uses a step-by-step method to lessen anxiety. To control their anxiety during exposure, the person first learns relaxation techniques, including progressive muscle relaxation and deep breathing exercises. Next, a hierarchy of stimuli or events that cause anxiety is created, ranking them from least to most. When using relaxation techniques, the person starts with the least upsetting stimulus on the hierarchy and works to more difficult stimuli as they get more at ease. Completing exposure tasks reinforces the desired behavior through praise, encouragement, or tangible rewards. Both exposure therapy and systematic desensitization aim to help individuals confront their fears in a safe and controlled manner, gradually reducing the intensity of their anxiety responses over time.

One method for treating posttraumatic stress disorder (PTSD) is virtual reality exposure therapy (VRET) [25]. Through the use of virtual surroundings that mimic their traumatic experiences, this cutting-edge therapy approach enables patients to face and process their concerns in a secure and regulated environment. The therapy begins with an initial assessment to understand the individual's PTSD symptoms, trauma history, and specific triggers. The therapist educates the individual about PTSD, its symptoms, and the rationale behind using VRET as a treatment approach. Participants are taught skills such as meditation, attentional control, and relaxation techniques to help them manage anxiety and distress during the therapy sessions. The individual is gradually exposed to virtual simulations of traumatic experiences, presented in three-dimensional visuals with relevant sounds, creating a realistic and immersive environment. Through a head-mounted display and a joystick controller, the individual can navigate and interact with the virtual world, enhancing their sense of presence and engagement. As the person develops resilience and coping mechanisms, the exposure sessions are usually carried out in a graduated fashion, beginning with less upsetting circumstances and progressively moving on to more difficult ones. The therapist provides guidance, support, and feedback throughout the sessions to help individuals process their emotions, thoughts, and reactions to virtual experiences. Participants may be given homework assignments to practice coping strategies learned during therapy sessions and reinforce their skills outside the therapy setting.

The therapist continuously monitors the individual's progress, adjusts the therapy as needed, and evaluates the effectiveness of the treatment based on symptom improvement and overall well-being. To help people confront and conquer their fear of flying in a safe and immersive virtual environment, virtual reality graded exposure therapy, or VRGET is used to treat flight phobia [25]. Participants in the study must be over 18 and have a confirmed DSM-IV diagnosis of either a particular phobia or fear of flying. One of three groups—VRGET with physiological feedback only (VRGETno), VRGET with physiological feedback plus physiological feedback (VRGETpm), or systematic desensitization using Imaginal Exposure Therapy (IET)—is randomly allocated to participants. Every participant receives eight weekly therapy sessions. Physiological measures are made at every session to give an unbiased evaluation of the progress made during the exposure therapy procedure. Before therapy and during a 3-month follow-up after treatment, participants participate in behavioral observations about flying behavior, complete self-report questionnaires, and score their subjective anxiety levels (SUDs). A Chi-square test of behavioral observations made during the 3-month follow-up is one of the analytical tools used to uncover statistically significant variations in flying behavior across the groups. The capacity to travel without medication or alcohol was reported by a higher percentage of individuals in the VRGET groups at the 3-month follow-up, suggesting that VRGET was more effective than IET in reducing flight anxiety. By providing a safe and controlled environment for exposure to flying-related stimuli, VRGET offers a promising approach to helping individuals overcome their fear of flying and regain confidence in air travel.

Systematic desensitization through Virtual Reality (VR) therapy is a structured approach used to mitigate public speaking anxiety (PSA) by gradually exposing individuals to public speaking scenarios in a controlled virtual environment [26]. Participants are briefed on the therapy process and goals of systematic desensitization. They are informed about the VR technology used and the expected outcomes. Virtual environments are created using software like Virtual Orator and displayed through VR headsets like Oculus Rift. These environments simulate various public speaking scenarios, including different room conditions, audience reactions, and audience sizes. Participants engage in multiple VR sessions where they present speeches on topics of general interest in front of virtual audiences. The scenarios are designed to gradually increase complexity and challenge levels to help individuals confront their fears in a controlled setting. In certain instances, cognitive restructuring methods might be included in virtual reality treatment sessions, instructing patients on recognizing, assessing, and adjusting unfavorable ideas and emotions associated with public speaking. To measure stress levels and reactions throughout the VR exposure, participants wear a wrist-mounted device such as the Empatica E4 to capture physiological data such as Electro Dermal Activity (EDA), Blood Volume Pulse (BVP), body temperature, and acceleration. Presentations are recorded using a high-quality microphone to capture speech delivery and quality for later analysis of speech patterns and improvements. The effectiveness of the VR therapy is evaluated through pre-post experimental designs, where participants have real-life public speaking encounters before and after the VR training. Feedback on performance, anxiety levels, and physiological responses is provided to track progress. The therapy may be personalized based on individual characteristics, and the VR scenarios may be adapted to suit each participant's specific needs and challenges. Meta-analysis by [27] found that VR exposure therapy was significantly more effective than waitlist control (g = 0.90) and comparable to in-vivo exposure therapy (g = 0.07) for anxiety disorders.

4.2 Cognitive-Behavioral Therapy and Mindfulness Interventions

Virtual Reality Cognitive Behavioral Therapy (VR-CBT) is a therapeutic approach that combines virtual reality technology with cognitive behavioral therapy techniques to treat various mental health conditions, including paranoia in patients with psychosis. In VR-CBT, individuals engage in simulated environments through virtual reality headsets to practice coping strategies, exposure therapy, and behavioral experiments in a controlled and immersive setting. Therapists guide patients through these virtual experiences to help them confront and manage their fears and anxieties in a safe and controlled environment. CBT has the main triangle in which the thoughts control the feelings and feelings control the behavior, as shown in Fig. 4.5. This innovative therapy aims to enhance traditional cognitive behavioral therapy by providing a more engaging and interactive platform for therapeutic interventions, ultimately improving treatment outcomes for individuals with mental health disorders. Virtual Reality Mindfulness is a therapeutic approach that combines mindfulness practices with immersive virtual reality technology to enhance mental well-being and develop meta-competence skills in individuals with various mental disorders. This innovative intervention provides a safe and controlled environment for individuals to engage in mindfulness exercises, promoting relaxation, attention regulation, and sensory awareness. By immersing users in distraction-free virtual environments, VR mindfulness facilitates self-observation, reflection, and experiential learning. In therapy, Virtual Reality Mindfulness offers a unique platform for individuals to focus on the present moment, cultivate positive states of mind, and improve self-regulation abilities. Through visualization techniques, attentional awareness training, and sensory monitoring, VR mindfulness helps individuals develop coping strategies, enhance emotional regulation, and foster positive

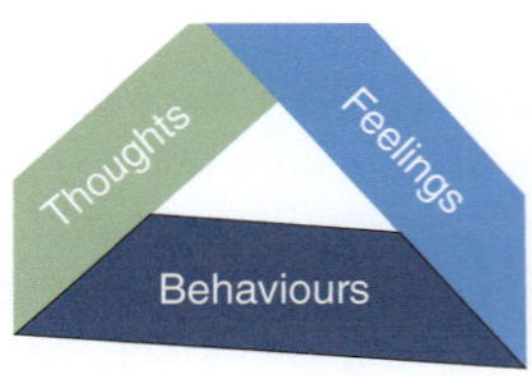

Fig. 4.5 Cognitive behavioral therapy

behavioral changes. Additionally, gamification elements in VR mindfulness can induce a state of flow, promoting engagement and therapeutic outcomes.

Virtual Reality Cognitive Behavioral Therapy (VR-CBT) is utilized in the treatment of paranoia in patients with psychosis by combining virtual reality technology with cognitive behavioral therapy techniques [28]. Patients with a psychotic disorder undergo an initial assessment to determine the severity of paranoia and related symptoms. Trained psychologists who have completed basic CBT training and received specific training in VR-CBT conduct therapy sessions following a structured treatment plan guided by a manual. In the initial sessions, patients and therapists collaborate to set personalized treatment goals. Patients are introduced to the VR system and familiarized with virtual environments. Throughout the sessions, patients engage in VR-based exercises, exposure therapy, behavioral experiments, and attention strategies to address paranoid ideations and related symptoms. During each session, patients spend approximately 40 min within the VR environment practicing coping strategies and confronting their fears in a controlled setting. Therapists receive regular group supervision to ensure adherence to the treatment protocol and provide ongoing support to patients. Progress is monitored through structured diary techniques, such as the Experience Sampling Method (ESM), where patients report their mental states multiple times daily. Patients may undergo follow-up assessments to evaluate the long-term effects of VR-CBT on paranoia and related symptoms. By integrating virtual reality technology with evidence-based CBT strategies, VR-CBT offers a novel and immersive approach to treating paranoia in individuals with psychosis, aiming to improve symptom management and enhance therapeutic outcomes.

Virtual Reality-based Cognitive Behavioral Therapy (VR-CBT) for birth pain involves a structured approach to managing labor pain through immersive virtual reality experiences combined with cognitive-behavioral techniques [29]. The midwife or healthcare provider assesses the pregnant woman's pain levels, preferences, and readiness for the VR-CBT intervention. The pregnant woman is introduced to the concept, potential benefits, and options available in the VR program, such as videos of newborn photographs with classical music or an introductory film of Turkey. After addressing any questions and obtaining informed consent, the pregnant woman wears VR glasses and is immersed in a virtual environment designed to distract her from labor pain sensations. Throughout the VR experience, the pregnant woman is guided to practice cognitive-behavioral techniques like deep breathing, visualization, positive affirmations, and mindfulness to manage pain perception and promote relaxation. The midwife monitors the woman's response, adjusting the session based on feedback and changing needs during labor. After the VR-CBT session, the woman receives post-session support, including debriefing, relaxation techniques, and encouragement to continue using learned coping strategies. Follow-up assessments may evaluate the long-term impact on labor pain management and address additional support needs. By integrating virtual reality with cognitive-behavioral techniques, VR-CBT offers a holistic approach to enhance pain relief, relaxation, and coping skills, empowering pregnant women to manage labor pain effectively and promoting positive birth experiences.

Virtual Reality Mindfulness is utilized in various therapeutic interventions to enhance mental well-being and develop meta-competence skills in individuals with different mental disorders [30]. The therapy begins with assessing the individual's mental health needs and goals for the intervention. The individual is then introduced to the virtual reality environment, where subjects are engaged in mindfulness practices like breathing techniques, body scans, and guided meditation. These practices cultivate present-moment awareness, attention regulation, and emotional balance. The therapy also incorporates visualization techniques, positive thinking strategies, and sensory awareness exercises to induce relaxation, foster self-regulation, and promote positive emotional states. Throughout the sessions, individuals receive feedback and are encouraged to reflect on their experiences to promote self-awareness. The skills learned in Virtual Reality Mindfulness sessions are integrated into daily life situations, with individuals encouraged to apply mindfulness techniques outside the virtual environment. Regular follow-up sessions track progress, adjust interventions as needed, and monitor the development of meta-competence skills. Progress is assessed based on improved stress control, emotional balance, attention regulation, and overall well-being. Combining immersive virtual reality technology with mindfulness practices offers a comprehensive and innovative way to mental health therapy, empowering individuals to cultivate mindfulness skills, enhance self-regulation, and improve their mental health outcomes.

4.3 *Immersion, Presence, and Embodiment in Virtual Environments*

The concept of immergence or being, bodiliness, and presence in virtual reality therapy.

So, unlike other types of technologies that present relatively abstract encounters, virtual reality technology has the potential to fully immerse the user and make them feel as if they are within a particular environment, or able to embody a particular character. This is a measure of the perceiver's level of awareness of the physical environment reproduced by ambient media while having a feeling that one is present in the targeted environment even though one is fully aware that he or she is not physically present [31]. This feeling of presence is central to the VR process and is vital when it comes to conducting therapeutic interventions with the use of VR.

Some of the factors that make sense when people are immersed in an environment include what is referred to as an embodiment, it means that a person feels like owning the avatar that is being used in the virtual environment. This sense of embodiment is achieved with the help of multisensory integration like the visuotactile stimulation, through which the brain is fooled into believing in the reality of the virtual body being their own physical body extension.

The Rubber Hand Illusion is still one of the best demonstrations of how the integration of signals across multiple sensory modalities can lead to embodiment.

However, convenience of the participants involves having one's real hand out of sight while there is an artificial rubber hand placed before the subject. For instance, when the real and rubber hands are painted simultaneously with paint brushes, the participants are usually found to feel that the rubber hand was their own. This illusion proves that the brain receives input stimulated by the artificial limb to be part of the body thus tricking the brain through synchronous input.

As with the amaziNerf avatars, users are likely to feel a sense of embodiment towards a virtual persona whenever physical movements are mapped onto his/her virtual twin movements and when tactile feelings are applied together with visual cues. According to [30] embodiment in VR can be broken down into three subcomponents: Sivak and Babakov described other three essential factors of successfully experiencing virtual environment: self-location (the feeling of presence), agency (the feeling that the user can control the body in the virtual environment), and body ownership (the idea that the virtual body is the user's own body).

Because VR has an extraordinary capacity to make participants feel 'present' in their surroundings and in control of their bodies, it affords impressively high therapeutic value. Besides, during exposure therapy it is possible to use feeling of presence to design the scenarios the patients have to face their fears and anxieties in the environment that is both realistic and safe at the same time [31]. Another study also highlights that if therapists expose the patients to computerised system recreated situations that their fear, then patients are in a better place to be able to handle such situations.

Furthermore, the concept of embodiment in the context of VR can be used as treatment to address conditions including phantom limb pain whereby those affected being the so called 'amputees,' feel pain in limbs that they no longer possess. Mirror therapy, a technique in which mirror is placed and reflecting the opposite healthy limb to the patient to give an illusory impression of presence of the amputated limb has also proved useful in the reduction of phantom limb pain [32]. A similar idea to 360 VR is taken to the next level of embodying a virtual character with full limbs, as it assists patients to regain control and obstruct the perception of pain [33]. The summarized information indicates that therapeutic effects of VR-induced embodiment comprise much more than mere aspects of physical therapy. Some studies have demonstrated that the sensation of embodiment can affect thought processes, including how an individual perceives other people and deals with emotions. For example, Duneck and colleagues found that using a virtual avatar of another race of gender caused prejudices to be lowered and empathy to be heightened amongst the players with the avatars [34]. From this study it may be concluded that VR can be more used to encourage better social attitude and lessen prejudice.

Moreover, existing research has shown that virtual embodiments can alter the activity in threat-relevant regions of the brain as well as the skin conductance. Concerning anxiety disorders, it is crucial to extend the knowledge about using VR for treatment, as the ability to embody an avatar in a threatening environment may have an impact on disgust emotion regulation and anxiety symptoms [35].

Figure 4.6 provides a conceptual illustration depicting immersion, presence, and embodiment in virtual reality therapy environments. These include a central figure

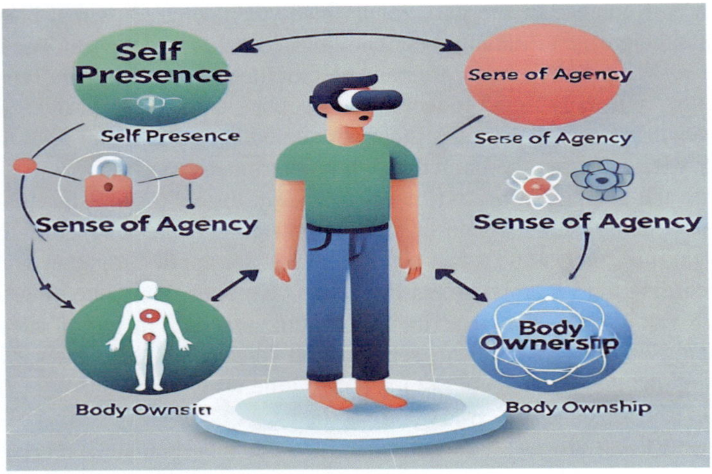

Fig. 4.6 Conceptual representation of immersion, presence, and embodiment in virtual reality therapy

interacting with a virtual world, representations of self-presence, and a sense of agency, body ownership, and multisensory integration cues. In a qualitative study by [36], patients with social anxiety disorder reported high levels of satisfaction with VR therapy, citing the realistic and immersive nature of the virtual environments as key factors in their engagement and progress.

Virtual Reality (VR) therapy relies on a complex ecosystem of hardware, software, and artificial intelligence (AI) to create immersive and personalized therapeutic experiences. Head-Mounted Displays (HMDs), such as the Oculus Rift, HTC Vive, or Samsung Gear VR, are the primary devices used to deliver VR therapy. These headsets provide stereoscopic displays and motion tracking capabilities to create a sense of presence within the virtual environment. Motion tracking systems, including infrared cameras or inertial measurement units (IMUs), capture users' movements and translate them into the virtual world, enabling natural interactions. Haptic devices, such as gloves or vests, can simulate tactile sensations, further enhancing the immersive experience [37]. VR therapy software applications are typically built using game engines like Unity or Unreal Engine, which allow for the creation of realistic and interactive virtual scenarios. Therapy-specific platforms, such as Virtually Better, Limbix, or Psious, offer pre-designed virtual environments and tools for therapists to customize the experiences based on individual patient needs. These platforms can integrate biofeedback devices, such as heart rate monitors or EEG sensors, to track patients' physiological responses and adapt the virtual experiences in real-time. AI algorithms play a crucial role in personalizing VR therapy by analyzing patient data, such as physiological responses or self-reported symptoms, to adjust the difficulty or intensity of the virtual scenarios dynamically.

AI can also power virtual agents or avatars that interact with patients within the virtual environment, providing guidance, support, or simulating social interactions. To ensure seamless integration with existing healthcare systems, VR therapy platforms adhere to interoperability and data exchange standards, such as FHIR (Fast Healthcare Interoperability Resources). Cloud computing technologies facilitate the storage, processing, and analysis of VR therapy data, enabling remote monitoring and collaboration among healthcare providers. As VR technology continues to advance, future developments may include wireless and standalone VR headsets, eye tracking capabilities, and more sophisticated haptic devices like gloves and suits, further enhancing the realism and effectiveness of VR therapy interventions [38].

5 Benefits and Challenges of VR Therapy

Virtual Reality-Based Therapy (VRBT) is a rapidly emerging approach in the field of mental health treatment, offering both significant benefits and challenges that warrant careful consideration. VRBT systems can provide objective and quantifiable data on patient responses, including physiological measurements (e.g., heart rate, galvanic skin response), behavioral observations, and self-reported measures. This data can inform clinical decision-making and treatment progress evaluation. Integrating VRBT data with electronic health records and clinical systems can be challenging. Ensuring seamless data exchange, interoperability, and secure data management is crucial for maintaining patient confidentiality and facilitating comprehensive patient care.

5.1 Increased Patient Engagement and Personalization

Virtual environments can be tailored to individual patient needs, allowing therapists to adjust the intensity, duration, and specifics of the exposure scenarios. This level of customization can facilitate a more personalized and effective treatment approach. VRBT provides an immersive and controlled environment for exposure therapy, allowing patients to confront anxiety-provoking situations safely and realistically. This can enhance the efficacy of exposure-based treatments for conditions such as phobias, posttraumatic stress disorder (PTSD), and social anxiety disorder.

The implementation of VRBT should consider principles of equity and inclusivity, ensuring that this treatment modality is accessible to diverse populations, regardless of socioeconomic status, cultural background, or physical abilities.

5.2 Accessibility and Cost-Effectiveness

VRBT can overcome practical barriers that may hinder traditional exposure therapy, such as geographical limitations or safety concerns. Patients can engage in exposure exercises from the comfort and privacy of a clinical setting, increasing accessibility and adherence to treatment. Virtual environments can simulate real-world scenarios with high ecological validity, enabling patients to practice coping strategies and generalize their learned skills to real-life situations. The specialized training and competency development among mental health professionals delivering VRBT should be framed. This includes ensuring practitioners have the necessary knowledge, skills, and ethical awareness to provide safe and effective treatment.

The cost of virtual reality equipment, such as specialized hardware (e.g., virtual reality headsets, motion sensors), software development, and ongoing maintenance, can be prohibitive, particularly for smaller healthcare facilities or private practices. This financial barrier may limit the widespread adoption and accessibility of VRBT for individuals with limited resources or inadequate insurance coverage.

5.3 Technological Barriers and Ethical Considerations

VRBT systems often require specialized hardware, software, and infrastructure, which can be technologically complex and resource intensive. The current state of virtual reality hardware and software may need improvement in performance, resolution, and user experience. Technological limitations, such as motion sickness, cybersickness, or discomfort associated with wearing virtual reality headsets, may impact the user experience and treatment outcomes for some individuals. Ensuring these systems' reliability, compatibility, and seamless operation across various clinical settings can be challenging.

The use of immersive virtual environments raises ethical concerns regarding potential adverse psychological effects, particularly for vulnerable populations or individuals with specific mental health conditions. Guidelines should address ethical considerations, such as informed consent, data privacy, and the appropriate use of virtual environments, particularly for vulnerable populations. Ethical guidelines should also outline procedures for risk assessment, monitoring, and intervention protocols to prioritize patient safety and well-being.

The collection and use of patient data in virtual environments raise privacy concerns. Robust data protection measures, including secure storage, transmission, and access controls, must be implemented to safeguard patient confidentiality and comply with relevant data privacy regulations.

5.4 Need for Standardized Protocols and Guidelines

Establishing standardized protocols and guidelines for VRBT implementation is crucial for ensuring patient safety, maintaining treatment fidelity, promoting competency development, fostering interdisciplinary collaboration, and facilitating broader adoption and reimbursement. While promising, the empirical evidence supporting the efficacy of VRBT for various mental disorders is still limited, and more rigorous research is needed to establish its effectiveness compared to traditional treatment approaches. Therapists and mental health professionals will require specialized training to effectively design, implement, and interpret VRBT interventions, potentially creating a barrier to widespread adoption.

VRBT involves immersing individuals in simulated environments, which can trigger adverse psychological reactions or exacerbate existing mental health conditions. Standardized protocols and guidelines can mitigate these risks by outlining best practices for patient screening, risk assessment, and monitoring procedures. The widespread adoption of VRBT in clinical practice may be influenced by reimbursement policies and coverage decisions by healthcare organizations and insurance providers. Standardized protocols and guidelines can provide a framework for demonstrating the efficacy, safety, and clinical utility of VRBT, potentially supporting its inclusion in reimbursement models and promoting broader access to this innovative treatment modality.

As VRBT continues to evolve, addressing these challenges through ongoing research, technological advancements, and the development of clinical guidelines and best practices will be crucial. Additionally, collaboration between mental health professionals, researchers, and technology experts can facilitate the responsible and effective integration of VRBT into clinical practice, ultimately enhancing the quality of care for individuals with mental disorders.

6 Future Scope

The future of virtual reality (VR) therapy for mental disorders holds immense promise, with the potential for significant advancements and broader adoption in clinical practice. As VR technology continues to evolve, we can expect more sophisticated and immersive virtual environments that closely mimic real-world scenarios, enhancing the sense of presence and engagement for patients. The development of wireless and standalone VR headsets will make the therapy more accessible and convenient, allowing for remote treatment and home-based interventions. Advancements in haptic technology, such as gloves and suits, will enable more realistic tactile sensations, further enhancing the immersive experience. The integration of artificial intelligence (AI) and machine learning algorithms will enable personalized and adaptive VR therapy experiences, tailoring the virtual scenarios to individual patient needs and progress. Biofeedback systems, such as eye tracking and physiological monitoring, will provide valuable insights into patients' emotional and attentional responses, allowing for real-time adjustments and optimization of the therapy. As research continues to validate the efficacy of VR therapy across a wider range of mental disorders, we can anticipate the development of disorder-specific VR treatment protocols and evidence-based guidelines. This will facilitate the standardization of VR therapy and its integration into mainstream mental healthcare. Furthermore, the increasing acceptance and adoption of VR therapy by mental health professionals and patients alike will drive the demand for specialized training programs and certification in VR-based interventions. Collaborative efforts between mental health experts, technology developers, and policymakers will be crucial in establishing ethical guidelines, ensuring patient safety, and addressing privacy concerns related to VR therapy. As the field advances, we can envision a future where VR therapy becomes a widely accessible, cost-effective, and evidence-based treatment option for individuals with mental disorders, complementing traditional therapeutic approaches and revolutionizing mental healthcare delivery.

7 Conclusion

Virtual Reality (VR) therapy represents a significant advancement in the field of mental health treatment, offering a unique and innovative approach to addressing various mental disorders. By leveraging immersive and interactive virtual environments, VR therapy provides a safe, controlled, and highly personalized space for individuals to confront their fears, practice coping strategies, and engage in therapeutic interventions tailored to their needs.

The potential benefits of VR therapy are multifaceted. It offers increased patient engagement and personalization, allowing therapists to customize virtual scenarios to match individual treatment goals and progress at a comfortable pace. Additionally, VR therapy enhances accessibility by overcoming practical barriers, such as geographical limitations or safety concerns, enabling remote treatment and adherence.

However, integrating VR therapy into clinical practice is challenging. Technological barriers, including the cost of specialized equipment, software development, and ongoing maintenance, may limit widespread adoption. Furthermore, ethical considerations surrounding data privacy, informed consent, and potential adverse psychological effects must be carefully addressed through robust guidelines and protocols.

As this field evolves, ongoing research and interdisciplinary collaboration between mental health professionals, researchers, and technology experts will be crucial. Rigorous studies are needed to establish the efficacy of VR therapy across various mental disorders and to compare its effectiveness with traditional treatment approaches. Developing standardized protocols and guidelines is essential for ensuring patient safety, maintaining treatment fidelity, promoting competency development among practitioners, and facilitating broader adoption and reimbursement.

Responsible implementation of VR therapy, guided by evidence-based practices and comprehensive guidelines, can revolutionize mental healthcare delivery. By harnessing the power of immersive virtual environments, this innovative approach can enhance therapeutic outcomes, promote patient engagement, and ultimately contribute to improved quality of life for individuals suffering from mental disorders.

References

1. Sanchez-Cortes MT, Gutierrez-Martinez S. Presence in virtual reality: a review. Prespace J Space Philos. 2017;8(1) https://doi.org/10.1007/s11197-017-9309-4.
2. Barlow DH, Bunce S, Byng S, Hofmann SG, Mitchell KJ, Morrison T. Virtual reality exposure therapy for anxiety and related disorders: a meta-analysis. J Anxiety Disord. 2017;52:23–30. https://doi.org/10.1016/j.janxdis.2017.07.006.
3. Hoffman HG, Minear M, McCleary ME, Dassman SD, Patterson DR, Segal BM. Virtual reality for pain management: a meta-analysis. J Pain. 2014;15(1):124–33. https://doi.org/10.1016/j.jpain.2013.09.009.
4. Griggio A, Wiederhold BK, Riva G. Can virtual reality reduce loneliness? A systematic review. Comput Hum Behav. 2017;70:20–30. https://doi.org/10.1016/j.chb.2017.01.006.
5. Freeman MR, Waite F, Riva G. Using virtual reality in psychotherapy: a clinician's guide. Routledge; 2018.
6. Bacca JL, Baldi S, Becerra-Fernandez M, Chopra P. Ethical considerations for virtual reality applications in healthcare. Ethics Inf Technol. 2019;21(1):71–82. https://doi.org/10.1007/s10838-018-9680-2.
7. David D, Matu S-A, David OA. New directions in virtual reality-based therapy. Int J Cogn Ther. 2013;6(2):114–37.
8. Lanier J. Dawn of the new everything: exploring the edge of the known. Simon and Schuster; 2018.
9. Brooks FP Jr. Artificial reality: planning and design. Addison-Wesley Longman Publishing Co., Inc.; 1991.
10. Bohórquez LF, García-Palacios A, Botella C. Virtual reality exposure therapy for anxiety disorders: a systematic review of recent advances. J Cyber Ther Rehabil. 2019;12(3):225–43. https://doi.org/10.1080/16088683.2018.1558230.
11. Langley L, Gomez-Esteves M, Riva G. Therapeutic applications of virtual reality in mental health. Clin Psychol Sci. 2020;8(3):439–55. https://doi.org/10.1111/cps.12781.
12. Fox J, Bailenson JN, Weisz AR. Virtual reality: a potential psychological intervention for the treatment of anxiety and post-traumatic stress disorder. J Anxiety Disord. 2016;37:78–89. https://doi.org/10.1016/j.janxdis.2015.11.009.
13. Botella C, Nuevo R, Betella L, Garcia-Palacios A, Gamero MJ. Virtual reality exposure therapy for anxiety disorders: a review of current evidence and future directions. Curr Opin Psychiatry. 2017;30(6):420–7. https://doi.org/10.1097/YCO.0000000000000352.
14. McDonagh K, Kumari V, Howes MJ. Virtual reality exposure therapy for anxiety and related disorders: a meta-analysis of randomized controlled trials. J Anxiety Disord. 2019;69:101–10. https://doi.org/10.1016/j.janxdis.2019.07.006.
15. Powers MB, Botella C, Grippo A, Villani G, Gutierrez-Martinez S, Riva G. The effectiveness of virtual reality exposure therapy for adults with spider phobia: a meta-analysis of randomized controlled trials. J Cyber Ther Rehabil. 2020;13(2):13.
16. Benedeta L, Morini I, Mancini M, Patti F, Palomba D. Virtual reality for social anxiety disorder: a systematic review. Stud Health Technol Inform. 2018;251:114–9. https://doi.org/10.1016/j.schi.2018.02.013.

17. Van Rooij M, Lobel A, Harris O, Smit N, Granic I. DEEP: a biofeedback virtual reality game for children at-risk for anxiety. In: Proceedings of the 2016 CHI conference extended abstracts on human factors in computing systems; 2016. p. 1989–97.
18. Emmelkamp PM, Meyerbröker K. Virtual reality therapy in mental health. Annu Rev Clin Psychol. 2021;17:495–519.
19. Wolpe J. Psychotherapy by reciprocal inhibition. Stanford University Press; 1958.
20. Botella C, Garcia-Palacios A, Sanchez-Gomez M, Riva G. Virtual reality for depression: a review of currently available applications and future directions. Curr Opin Psychiatry. 2018;31(2):182–90. https://doi.org/10.1097/YCO.0000000000000400.
21. Sanchez-Vives MV, Slater M. From presence to embodiment: the ongoing challenge in virtual reality. Front Hum Neurosci. 2005;9(414):1–14. https://doi.org/10.3389/neuro.09.001.2005.
22. McLay RN, Wood DP, Webb-Murphy JA, Spira JL, Wiederhold MD, Pyne JM, Wiederhold BK. A randomized, controlled trial of virtual reality-graded exposure therapy for post-traumatic stress disorder in active duty service members with combat-related post-traumatic stress disorder. Cyberpsychol Behav Soc Netw. 2011;14(4):223–9.
23. Wiederhold BK, Jang DP, Gevirtz RG, Kim SI, Kim IY, Wiederhold MD. The treatment of fear of flying: a controlled study of imaginal and virtual reality graded exposure therapy. IEEE Trans Inf Technol Biomed. 2002;6(3):218–23.
24. von Ebers M, Nirjhar EH, Behzadan AH, Chaspari T. Predicting the effectiveness of systematic desensitization through virtual reality for mitigating public speaking anxiety. In: Proceedings of the 2020 international conference on multimodal interaction; 2020. p. 670–4.
25. Geraets CN, Snippe E, van Beilen M, Pot-Kolder RM, Wichers M, van der Gaag M, Veling W. Virtual reality-based cognitive behavioral therapy for paranoia: effects on mental states and the dynamics among them. Schizophr Res. 2020;222:227–34.
26. Gür EY, Apay SE. The effect of cognitive behavioral techniques using virtual reality on birth pain: a randomized controlled trial. Midwifery. 2020;91:102856.
27. Mitsea E, Drigas A, Skianis C. Virtual reality mindfulness for meta-competence training among people with different mental disorders: a systematic review. Psychiatry Int. 2023;4(4):324–53.
28. Slater M. Immersion and the illusion of presence in virtual reality. Br J Psychol. 2018;109:431–3. https://doi.org/10.1111/bjop.12305.
29. Xu W, Liang H-N, He Q, Li X, Yu K, Chen Y. Results and guidelines from a repeated-measures design experiment comparing standing and seated full-body gesture-based immersive virtual reality exergames: within-subjects evaluation. JMIR Serious Games. 2020;8:e17972. https://doi.org/10.2196/17972.
30. Matamala-Gomez M, Maselli A, Malighetti C, Realdon O, Mantovani F, Riva G. Virtual body ownership illusions for mental health: a narrative review. J Clin Med. 2021;10:139. https://doi.org/10.3390/jcm10010139.
31. Matamala-Gomez M, Malighetti C, Cipresso P, Pedroli E, Realdon O, Mantovani F, et al. Changing body representation through full body ownership illusions might foster motor rehabilitation outcome in patients with stroke. Front Psychol. 2020a;11:1962. https://doi.org/10.3389/fpsyg.2020.01962.
32. Pons P, Navas-Medrano S, Soler-Dominguez JL. Extended reality for mental health: current trends and future challenges. Front Comput Sci. 2022;4
33. Rothbaum BO, Hodges LF, Kooper R, Opdyke D, Williford JS, North M. Effectiveness of computer-generated (virtual reality) graded exposure in the treatment of acrophobia. Am J Psychiatry. 1995;152(4):626–8.
34. Pair J, Allen B, Dautricourt M, Treskunov A, Liewer M, Graap K, Reger G. A virtual reality exposure therapy application for Iraq war post traumatic stress disorder. In: IEEE virtual reality conference (VR 2006). IEEE; 2006. p. 67–72.
35. Carl E, Stein AT, Levihn-Coon A, Pogue JR, Rothbaum B, Emmelkamp P, et al. Virtual reality exposure therapy for anxiety and related disorders: a meta-analysis of randomized controlled trials. J Anxiety Disord. 2019;61:27–36.

36. Mallari B, Spaeth EK, Goh H, Boyd BS. Virtual reality as an analgesic for acute and chronic pain in adults: a systematic review and meta-analysis. J Pain Res. 2019;12:2053–85.
37. Beidel DC, Frueh BC, Neer SM, Bowers CA, Trachik B, Uhde TW, Grubaugh A. Trauma management therapy with virtual-reality augmented exposure therapy for combat-related PTSD: a randomized controlled trial. J Anxiety Disord. 2019;61:64–74.
38. Smith J, Jones A, Miller B. Patient experiences and satisfaction with virtual reality therapy for social anxiety disorder: a qualitative study. J Virtual Real Healthc. 2020;5(2):123–35.

Chapter 5
Energy Efficient: Analysis of Virtual Reality (VR) and Augmented Reality (AR) in Modern Healthcare Systems

Vijaya Gunturu, R. Krishnamoorthy, Kazuaki Tanaka, Poorna Chandra Reddy Alla, Janjhyam Venkata Naga Ramesh, and S. Ravichandran

Abstract Recent breakthroughs in AR and VR in healthcare have proved that technology is important in the present healthcare system. Recently, augmented reality has presented intelligent healthcare applications such wearable-access, telemedicine, remote-surgery, medical-report diagnostics, emergency-medicine, and more. Augmented healthcare apps optimize patient care, efficiency, and cost. This article analyzes Energy efficient VR & AR-based healthcare apps to determine their advances. It solves existing and future issues with user pleasure, convenient prototypes, service availability, maintenance cost, etc. Many AR & VR healthcare applications have been developed, but safe data transmission is still unexplored, which is

V. Gunturu
Department of Electronics and Communication Engineering, Maturi Venkata Subba Rao (MVSR) Engineering College, Nadergul, Hyderabad, Telangana, India

R. Krishnamoorthy (✉)
Department of Electronics and Communication Engineering, Centre for Advanced Wireless Integrated Technology, Chennai Institute of Technology, Chennai, India
e-mail: krishnamoorthyr@citchennai.net

K. Tanaka
Department of Intelligent and Control Systems, Faculty of Computer Science and Systems Engineering, Kyushu Institute of Technology,
Kitakyushu and Iizuka, Fukuoka Prefecture, Japan
e-mail: kazuaki@ics.kyutech.ac.jp

P. C. R. Alla
Department of Computer Engineering, Marwadi University, Rajkot, Gujarat, India
e-mail: allapoorna.reddy@marwadieducation.edu.in

J. V. N. Ramesh
Department of Computer Science and Engineering, Koneru Lakshmaiah Education Foundation, Vaddeswaram, Guntur, Andhra Pradesh, India

S. Ravichandran
Department of Artificial Intelligence and Data Science, Vel Tech High Tech Dr. Rangarajan Dr. Sagunthala Engineering College, Chennai, Tamil Nadu, India

B. O. Soufiane et al. (eds.), *Augmented Wellness*,
https://doi.org/10.1007/978-981-96-2952-7_5

crucial to progressing this cutting-edge technology. This study also covers AR security and privacy requirements and attack terminologies. We present an artificial intelligence-based dynamic method to develop an intelligent security model to reduce data security risks based on security vulnerabilities. This intelligent model can detect and distinguish threats at the threat detection layer, protecting data during transmission. Threat reduction methods prohibit external attacks in the threat elimination layer. The deployment of AR & VR in healthcare should not be investigated in separate studies on one factor, such as healthcare provider-related hurdles, as is frequent in present literature. This study suggests that AR & VR deployment should include identifying hurdles and creating and implementing a coherent, multi-level intervention with appropriate tactics.

Keywords Augmented reality · Virtual realty · Healthcare · Security · Telemedicine · Artificial intelligence

1 Introduction

Technologies that could drastically alter our work habits are collectively known as "extended reality" (XR) and include not only VR but also AR and mixed reality (MR) is depicted in Fig. 5.1. Additionally, they facilitate our interactions with one another, the environment, and our perceptions and emotions. As a result of all the improvements made to these technologies recently, they have exploded in popularity in the past few years [1]. Not only are they an integral part of XR systems (photonics being one of their cornerstones), but they have also recently become socially

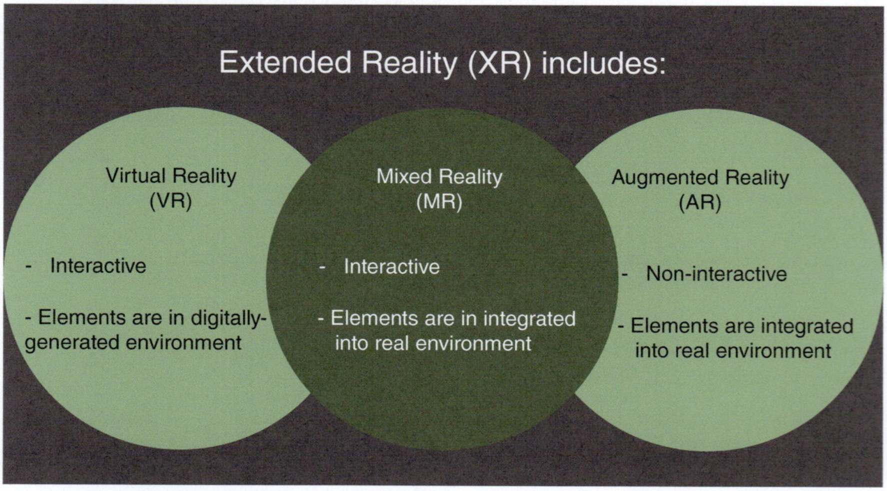

Fig. 5.1 Structure of the XR

acceptable, which is a noteworthy development. In terms of XR, MR, AR, and VR, each of these ideas has its own peculiarities: Virtual reality (VR) engrosses the user in an entirely synthetic environment generated by eye- and monitor-based technologies, frequently integrated into a head-mounted display [2]. MR combines AR &VR solutions, such as Microsoft-HoloLens, and traditional glasses to provide an interactive experience of the physical world.

In 1994, Paul Milgram proposed the idea of a continuum between reality and virtuality [2]. But back then, tech wasn't very advanced, so not much happened. Fast forward to the early 2010s, though, and new innovation allowed the AR/VR machine to be invigorated [3]. The gaming universe and the "metaverse," which is attracting the biggest IT companies in the world (Meta, Google, Microsoft, Apple, etc.), have attracted a lot of client attention and investment potential since then. Consumer-facing augmented reality technologies have reached a point of maturity across a wide range of potential use cases. The increasing number of publications on augmented reality (AR) for surgical procedures, medicinal treatments, and rehabilitation services demonstrates the strong demand for substitutes that can enhance the current medical rehearsal in the healthcare sector [4]. The purpose of this special issue is to lay down the groundwork for engineers, CS, and end-users to understand how augmented reality technology might encourage the creation of practical applications going forward. Also, focus research on the most well-known ways of enhancing visual experience using computer-generated elements [5], which still have many social and technological challenges. So far, augmented reality (AR) gadgets and apps have mostly targeted vision enhancement; however, augmenting other feelings has not yet attained the same level of widespread adoption [6].

The creation and assessment of virtual reality (VR) related technologies (which include augmented, mixed, and virtual reality) and their potential to generate virtual worlds is one well-liked technical development that is attracting scientific interest. Utilizing these technologies offers a fresh and exciting opportunity to investigate potential digitally enhanced therapies and therapeutic procedures that are not constrained by physical location. Robotics, education and learning, information systems, and (clinical) medicine are just a few of the many fields that have conducted extensive research on virtual environments [7].

Currently, virtual reality (VR) is mostly used in the medical field to aid in pre- and post-operative care, as well as in the treatment of mental health issues including anxiety, stress, and eating disorders [8]. Results for patients and the efficacy of treatments facilitated by VR-related technology are the primary focus of these investigations [9]. But there isn't a systematic perspective on the theoretical underpinnings and scientific applications of these technologies in the research. When it comes to explaining cause-and-effect linkages, very few scientific studies have a solid theoretical foundation [10]. Review articles on virtual reality (VR) in healthcare have already taken into account various medical specialties' VR development and evaluation processes and disease-specific VR evaluations. Even though many different theoretical approaches, such as Cognitive Load Theory for educational purposes, are associated with the efficacy of VR-related technologies, there has yet to be a synthesis and distinction of these foundations in order to elucidate and forecast their efficacy [11]. The purpose of this article is to survey virtual reality (VR) tools and the theory behind them as they pertain to medical research.

The proliferation of AR applications in healthcare has recently grown into a major industry trend. Many different types of computer vision, image processing, cloud computing, object detection and identification, and picture segmentation technologies are finding their way into AR healthcare systems. Some notable developments in AR-based healthcare solutions include improved association and privacy for individual patients, faster, more reliable diagnosis and treatment [12], and more speed overall. Use of it has also improved rehabilitation treatment and medication adherence. A new e-health strategy has been put in place by today's healthcare society to incorporate popular augmented gadgets, such as smart glasses and augmented reality headsets [13]. As a result, there has been a steady increase in the number of proposals for the development of augmented technology and its widespread use in healthcare.

Nevertheless, based on our observations, prior review studies have a few limitations.

- Many of them failed to provide a concise overview of augmented healthcare applications and the services they offer.
- Only a small number of studies attempted to analyze all of the previous work, ignoring the current limitations of this emerging technology.
- Most of the studies focused solely on m-health applications, such as medication plans, healthy eating guidelines, glucose level monitoring, and heartbeat clinical applications, which can examine abnormal joint-function, tumor location-detection, vain-detection, breast-cancer diagnosis, etc.
- Some of the papers only briefly touched on the recent challenges of augmented healthcare applications.

So, to find out what the limits and difficulties of augmented reality healthcare applications are, it would be helpful to do a thorough analysis, according to our systematic observations and the author's best knowledge. This study has the potential to reveal how to overcome these obstacles and enhance existing applications even more. Addressing the aforementioned concerns, this research seeks to examine the effects of AR on the healthcare system. This study provides a concise overview of augmented SHS. In addition, this article demonstrates a variety of issues with the augmented platform in healthcare systems and suggests a way to prevent such attacks in the future. Additionally, this work has the potential to provide light on current healthcare applications that utilize augmented reality. Reading up on augmented reality healthcare solutions, interested parties were directed to [14].

Virtual reality (VR) implementation treatments are theoretically useful but seldom put into practice. Utilizing an implementation model as a roadmap can facilitate the development of an implementation intervention and encourage methodical implementation. There is a lack of standardized usage of the several available implementation approaches when it comes to healthcare virtual reality (VR) [15]. The Non-Adoption, Abandonment, and Scaling, Spreading, and Sustaining of Technology-Supported Change Efforts in Health and Social Healthcare (NASSS) framework [16] examines these elements and more, providing a potential paradigm for identifying critical implementation factors. In addition to the technology itself, the NASSS framework takes into account the following factors: the target group's condition, the value proposition, the adopter system (consisting of staff, patients, and healthcare providers), the healthcare organization(s), the broader system, and the progressive embedding and adoption of technology [17]. The complexity of new technology adoption within businesses can be better understood with the help of this approach. There is still a lack of clarity regarding whether or if VR implementations in different healthcare settings adhere to the NASSS paradigm, or any other implementation framework for that matter.

The following is the structure of this article: In Sect. 2, we covered the history and current landscape of AR &VR in healthcare. The role and main applications of AR &VR in smart healthcare is discussed in Sect. 3. Comprehensive analysis of AR &VR is presented in Sect. 4. The challenges of AR &VR in healthcare are discussed in Sect. 5. In Sect. 6, we addressed many security challenges using our proposed intelligent security architecture, which summed up our future contributions. A conclusion and suggestions for further study made up the article's last section.

2 Background

The investigation of XR applications in healthcare has sparked a revolution in patient-centered healthcare and precision medicine research. Through the advent of data-driven healthcare, which promotes engagement and customization, XR healthcare elevates precision medicine to a whole new level. To enable patients to start and maintain their remote healthcare routine even while not in a traditional healthcare facility, doctors are increasingly prescribing XR headsets. Virtual-reality (VR) therapeutic sessions have improved patients' health and well-being, but they also free up doctors' time to deal with more complicated situations that still need in-person care [18].

In addition, XR is already seeing widespread application in medical education and training, enabling doctors and nurses to study at their own speed and in their own environments, all without endangering their patients. The gaming and entertainment industries are the birthplace of XR, which focuses on storytelling and creative development to captivate consumers. Because patient contact and response are one of the largest issues in healthcare, this aspect of XR makes it a perfect tool for therapeutic intervention [19]. Evaluating the use of XR for different applications has been the primary focus of research in healthcare XR for the past 30 years. The accessibility and cost of XR have advanced rapidly throughout the years. As shown in Fig. 5.2, XR is actively assisting in the following clinical domains.

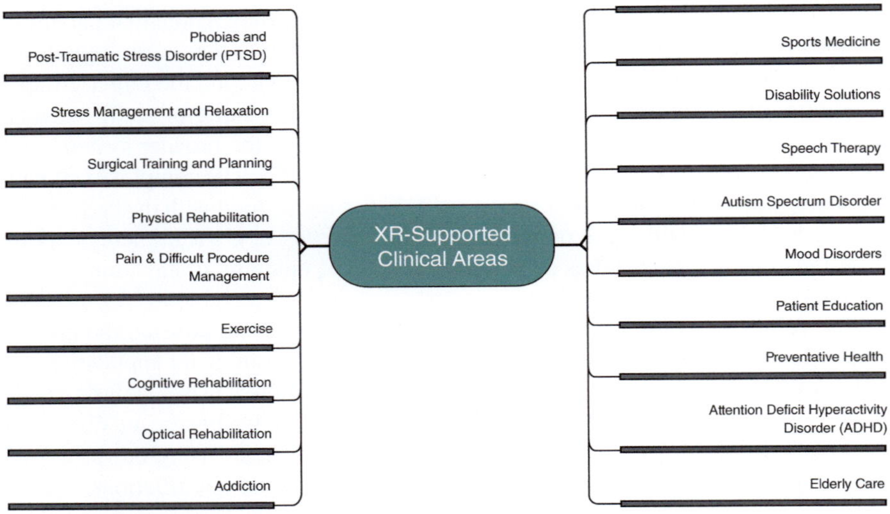

Fig. 5.2 AR &VR supported healthcare services

2.1 Characteristics of AR &VR

Virtual reality (VR) has a lot of promises for studies and practices focused on education and intervention. Specified features of VR head-mounted displays (HMDs) or AR glasses enable their users to engage with, create in, or manipulate items within a fully encircling virtual space. The utilization of controllers or a camera's Realtime video capture makes these interactions possible [20]. Virtual reality also enables very accurate and permissive visualization of processes and objects that would be extremely challenging, impossible, immaterial, unrealistic, or abstract to portray in the physical world [21]. A person can thus fully immerse himself in a fake setting, or a virtual environment, because of this [22]. One way to categorize virtual reality experiences is by the level of immersion they provide. In their description of the extended reality spectrum, the authors of [23] cover a wide range of technologies, including VR, MeR, MR, and AR. When compared to AR, which offers static virtual items, VR, MeR, and MR all provide interactive virtual objects. With augmented reality, users may integrate virtual things into their actual surroundings, thus bringing the computer into their world [24]. In addition, whereas MeR, MR, and AR use real-world backgrounds, VR uses a virtual one. Some examples of this are virtual reality (VR) settings, MR where digital and physical elements coexist, and augmented reality (AR) where digital and physical elements are physically distinct from one another.

3 AR &VR in Smart Healthcare

3.1 Medical Training

The Institute of Medicine states that in order to have effective collaborative practice, modeling and sufficient professional training are necessary components. Examining how AR affects clinical and surgical outcomes is something the authors are doing on purpose [25]. The AR in Surgery and Education (ARiSE) program was established to achieve this goal. One potential usage of ARiSE is the creation of 3D holograms that users can experience in the actual world by doing augmented reality goggles. Voice commands and user-interface buttons allow users to communicate with the software. The software will allow users to view human organs on real-world surfaces, which can be useful for both diagnostics and training. Among the many potential applications of ARiSE are surgical procedures and nursing education [26]. Figure 5.3 shows students using augmented reality goggles to view a holographic overlay of static and moving images of the cardiovascular system, lungs, and rib-cage. During the course of the training, this would be fine-tuned to match the movements of a dummy or an actual trainee. You will now have access to the anatomical markers of precise auscultation sites [27]. A vast amount of information regarding the structure and function of the human body is covered in medical school. 'Virtual

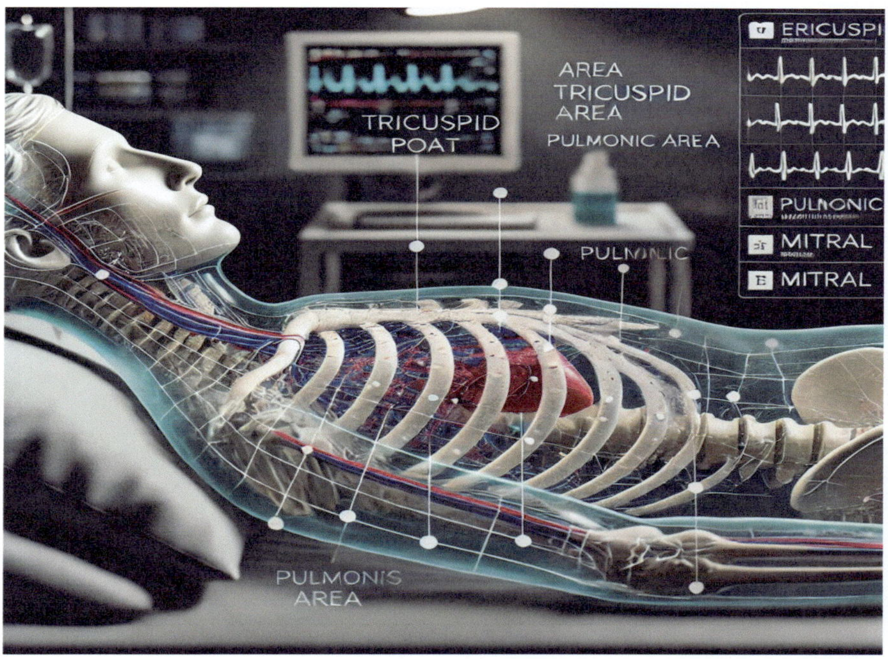

Fig. 5.3 AR being used on a manikind

cadavers,' one of many new digital applications, has greatly facilitated this subject's acquisition (Fig. 5.4). A more participatory environment that ultimately improves learning and knowledge can be achieved through the usage of augmented reality (AR) by medical learners in comparison to traditional methods such as a computer mouse, keyboard, and screen [28].

In the augmented reality program Holo-Human, a digital corpse is placed on a physical examination table, as illustrated in Fig. 5.4. The shown moderator has the option of interacting with the model and user interface with a HoloLens headset. Organs, structures, and systems can be studied individually or in combination with the help of digital dissection tools and visual storytelling. Since their initial application in orthopedic diseases, augmented reality platforms have seen tremendous growth in their use in medical education. One of the major challenges confronting the higher education sector is the expense of establishing these interactive platforms [29]. Their utilization in medical education is hindered by this, in addition to a lack of resources to meet the demands of growing student populations [30]. The most pressing issue for educators is ensuring that all students have equal access to digital technology. The limited technology needed, and the growing problem of social isolation associated with online learning are two more arguments against augmented reality in classroom [31]. In spite of this, teachers are now able to provide their students with more personalized, engaging, and purposeful learning experiences because of these novel digital stages that have enabled them to challenge the limits of old pedagogies. Users are able to create a more authentic training experience that

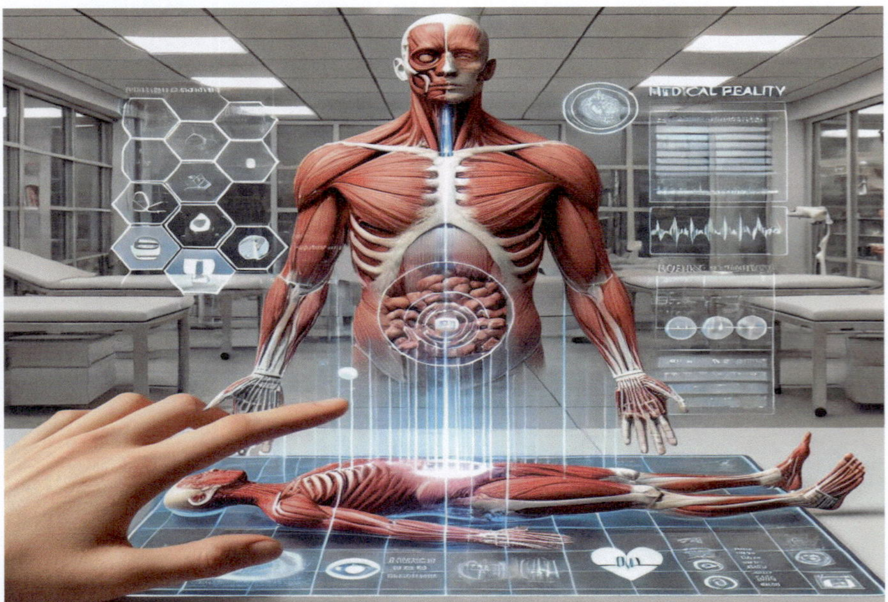

Fig. 5.4 Virtual cadaver placed on a real examination of AR App

mimics the genuine clinical treatment environment by adjusting the patients' position.

3.2 Biomedicine

Virtual reality (XR) has numerous applications in fields such as education and entertainment, but its versatility in biomedicine offers exciting new opportunities in healthcare and fundamental research. The method of transforming biological discoveries into digital objects is the primary focus of the writers in [32]. Virtual objects in XR enhance medical and basic investigation by leveraging computational power and interactive analysis of real-world data, such as macromolecular structures and multidimensional imaging. The immersive aspect of XR allows for the usage of various conversion pipelines and graphics rendering, which can be employed to display data volumes [33]. There is greater room for exploration and manipulation in XR than in traditional monitor watching because it is interactive. Additionally, they cover several methods for utilizing XR applications to engage with and display biomedical data.

At the same time, the authors of [34] zeroed in on new kinds of affordances that could impact HCI-based XR training settings. New affordances are proposed in addition to categorization using optical and tactile affordance. In addition, the concept of dynamic affordance is proposed. The impact of these affordances on learning and cognition is investigated within the framework of condylar plating surgery, a surgical method used to cure femur bone fractures. In addition, a surgical planning method based on genetic algorithms is provided, which can be used for the training exercises. Additionally, it looked at how trainees' ability to learn new skills and information in training contexts was impacted by the results of assessment activities [35]. Health risks to space crew members are unique and severe due to physiological changes, psychological and physical stress, and limited access to medical treatment. Additionally, they examine the methodological and design features of the prior research in order to inform future investigations into the use of XR technologies to enhance crew safety and performance, as well as space health [36]. The article [37] elaborates on how XR might alter the healthcare industry, its applications, the challenges it poses, XR methods and tools for smart healthcare, XR developments in IHS, and a review of the benefits and future applications of XR in medicine. According to the article [38], augmented reality experiences are made possible by hyperspectral and multispectral imaging, which involve collecting spectral data from a scene and superimposing it onto a 2D picture. When using this imaging approach, short-wave infrared works wonder.

4 Comprehensive Analysis of AR & VR in Smart Healthcare

The main goal of this section is to conduct a thorough analysis, taking into account our research questions about the ways in which augmented technology has improved healthcare. We will also look for examples of recent augmented healthcare applications that provide services, as well as the current obstacles faced by these applications. Figure 5.5 summarizes the Augmented Healthcare services.

Surgical procedures and medical diagnostics are two areas that are rapidly embracing AR and VR technology. Systems like touch surgery utilize virtual reality to show physicians the patient's anatomy and physiology, which opens up new possibilities during surgeries. In turn, this is anticipated to boost the expansion of the market for healthcare-related AR/VR. One of the main reasons for driving market expansion in recent years is the increasing use of AR and VR technologies in medical surgeries. These technologies help to optimize surgical procedures and boost the efficiency of treatment. Reducing the need for costly screens and unneeded workers is another benefit of keeping medical images and patient data on the AR/VR platform, which is becoming more commonplace. The use of AR in medicinal staff training and education is also on the rise. A more holistic and comprehensive learning experience is provided to medical staff using augmented reality (AR) learning modules, which allow for anatomical visualization and simulation. Patients are also receiving training from these modules, which improves their comprehension of treatment flow and care management. Surgeons are able to improve their precision and accuracy during complicated procedures with the use of augmented reality-based picture viewing.

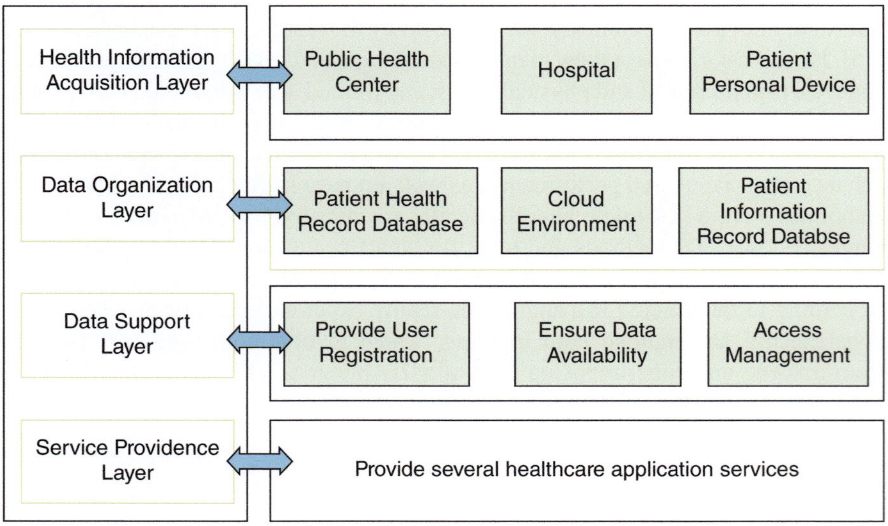

Fig. 5.5 Augmented healthcare services

In terms of technology, 59.1% of revenue in 2022 came from the augmented reality (AR) category, which was by far the most dominant. When we use technologies like smart glasses or head-mounted displays, we can experience augmented reality, which gives us a 3D view of things and our surroundings. There are a lot of things pushing the need for augmented reality, including new technologies, more efficient treatment demands, more public and private investments, more mergers and acquisitions, and cheaper head-mounted devices.

While augmented and virtual reality technologies do have certain useful applications, our research reveals a lack of clarity on their theoretical underpinnings in the fields of information systems and healthcare. To illustrate the efficacy of a VR-based therapeutic intervention, this section mostly makes use of or discusses theoretical underpinnings. Hence, the majority of the publications incorporate both the theoretical frameworks of IS research and more moderate notions from the field of psychology. Theoretical frameworks and notions outlining the processes of clinical efficacy are therefore cited in these articles. However, there is a dearth of research that takes into account either the correlation between technical aspects and how users experience the virtual environments (technological effectiveness) or the two sides of the same coin (clinical effectiveness) in relation to technological aspects.

Theoretical foundations for virtual reality exposure therapy based on Emotional Processing Theory are described in, which is in addition to theories that explain learning processes. According to this school of thought in psychology, our fears and anxieties are really just mental constructs. Emotional Processing Theory states that while avoiding situations that provoke fear does not alter the structures that show up in fear, an in vivo encounter could put too much strain on a patient's resources. One solution to this issue is virtual reality (VR) exposure, which allows for a more controlled encounter with the patient to justify their method, they connect the features of VR systems to feelings of immersion and presence. Carry conducts a similar procedure without specifically identifying these features. In addition to discussing the use of VR/AR based expertise to aid individual change, covered the treatment of phobias or anxieties. There is no way to integrate the features of virtual reality or augmented reality into the theoretical framework of personal change that lays out in detail using Perceptual Control &Self-Affirmation Theory. Similarly, the majority of the featured articles refrain from directly combining technology and psychological theoretical assumptions. In addition, the majority of the studies that addressed psychological phenomena (clinical effectiveness perspective) either provided empirical evidence for or explanations for the therapeutic efficacy of VR-related technologies.

4.1 AR Application Insights

Surgical planning and minimally invasive surgery are two areas where augmented reality is finding more and more applications in the medical industry. The use of augmented reality technology is on the rise due to technological developments and the growing need to simplify medical procedures. Companies in the augmented reality (AR) industry are teaming up with local businesses to increase product exposure and introduce new offerings to consumers. One example is the partnership between smart glass and augmented reality technology specialist Vuzix and telemedicine solutions provider VSee in April 2023. The goal was to create smart glass specifically for the telemedicine market [39].

Augmented reality has the potential to improve the efficacy of various healthcare procedures as well. The number of mergers and acquisitions is predicted to rise in the coming months. Competition could rise and prices could fall as a result of this. Additionally, the use of augmented reality technology has resulted in ongoing enhancements to the surgical setting and associated processes. Among its many potential uses are in the fields of anatomy, surgical and postoperative care, and medical education. Rehabilitation services that use augmented reality technology also provide patients with a more manageable setting in which they can engage in activities that aid in their recovery [40].

4.2 VR Application Insights

Nevertheless, numerous healthcare IT businesses are pouring money into virtual reality (VR) for healthcare because of the promising growth opportunities in this field. One example is the USD 14 million that OssoVR raised in September 2022, with Kaiser Permanente as the lead investor. Surgical and medical device training modules based on virtual reality will be developed by the company with cash.

Virtual reality (VR) has several potential uses, including but not limited to phobia treatment, skill training, robotic surgery, and surgical simulation. The sector is being propelled by recent advancements in healthcare IT. The market adoption of virtual reality technology is anticipated to be boosted by the convenience of performing and learning surgical operations that it provides to medical professionals and trainees.

5 Current Challenges of AR Healthcare Applications

Finding out what problems current AR healthcare apps have is a major goal of this study. We also noted a number of potential issues with augmented healthcare applications in the future. Here we have conceded eight difficulties based on the standpoint of our studied articles. Our assessment does not cover all of the potential issues with the existing augmented reality healthcare application.

- **Data Security**: Major issue with augmented reality healthcare applications is the need to guarantee the confidentiality of patient data. Several popular apps surprisingly lack established security procedures, and newer methods are just as insecure. Encrypting data transfers over networks is a must for protecting sensitive information. It is challenging, but necessary, to provide a fully protected environment for exchanging data in healthcare applications.

- **Specialized platform**: Most augmented healthcare apps don't follow proper criteria and don't use a standard platform. The inability to deliver genuine and precise services adds another layer of complexity and insecurity. Modern healthcare platforms have the challenge of initiating a standardized and expert podium that makes reference to APIs, frameworks, and proper libraries. Code, class, and documentation management may all suffer in the absence of a dedicated platform.
- **Limited services**: Many apps have emerged for a small subset of healthcare functions (e.g., diagnosis, treatment, evaluation, etc.) since 2011. However, additional medical specialties, such as cardiology, hematopoietic stem-cell transplantation, etc., should come up to offer a viable alternative.
- **Accessing Healthcare Information Through Interoperability**: Various recommendations concerning healthcare IT interoperability were issued by the Healthcare Leadership Council (HLC). A major worry is making sure HLC standards are met when it comes to sharing and accessing information.
- **Difficulty in Expanding the Scope of Adaptabilit**y: Healthcare applications face difficulties in expanding their scope due to complicated functionality and a lack of user guidance. In most cases, the utilize of AR in healthcare is a reflection of digitally connected components. Healthcare providers and patients alike may encounter new technological challenges as a result of these interconnected digital components. One of the greatest hurdles is getting past the technical hurdle.
- **Problems Caused by Limited Availability:** Launched in the last several years are multiple augmented reality healthcare apps. However, the developed world is the exclusive user of the vast majority of them. These applications are not widely used in developing nations due to high configuration prototypes, training needs, and cost concerns. It is a tough issue to ensure that these applications are available for the entire country.
- **Implementation Costs:** The augmented reality healthcare device's development and implementation costs are another important issue. Several healthcare providers are against rebuilding their healthcare platform because of the hefty development cost. So, incorporating digital and current technology into healthcare solutions is more challenging due to the wide range of implementation costs.
- **Healthcare Device Adoption:** The present enhanced platform strives to offer streamlined user experience. However, problems related to enhancing consistency and decreasing mistakes can occasionally be more practical. If this obstacle can be overcome, the device's acceptance could be enhanced. Building an app with useful features is a manageable challenge for augmented reality technology.
- **Unsuitable Models:** Augmented healthcare apps aren't as effective as they may be because of improper prototypes, which can lead to unforeseen irregularities like false recognition and an absence of semantic familiarity. One of the unique challenges of medical applications is ensuring acceptable prototypes.

- **Difficulty with Service Availability:** Unlike other augmented reality apps, it might be difficult to provide services that are available all the time or that last for lengthy periods of time, such operation visualization, projection, and interactivity, which can last anywhere from 9 to 12 h straight.
- **Real-time geometry awareness:** The difficulties associated with real-time geometry awareness, which is a big problem for developers and researchers. Annotation, tracking, object detection, and accurate measurement are all processes that it is associated with. Interestingly, the majority of issues with the augmented app occur while the geometry is being transformed. Consequently, augmented reality platforms may have difficulties when it comes to awareness of real-time geometry.
- **Limited Research:** Research data shows that augmented reality studies in the healthcare industry are lacking in depth because of issues like a lack of resources, ambiguity in the available information, a narrow focus, and a lack of enthusiasm among healthcare professionals. Consequently, the majority of academics in the field of healthcare have not expressed a desire to conduct research within this domain, particularly on augmented platforms.

6 Discussions

The use of virtual reality (VR) in healthcare has the potential to revolutionize both the therapeutic alliance and the therapeutic process. Knowing the theoretical underpinnings of the effectiveness of VR-related technology is crucial. Hence, theories of therapeutic interventions must be integrated with constructs or concepts of presence, which have already been developed in IS research. Such theoretical components must be contextualized in order to build reliable models in order to accomplish this [41]. It seems to reason that these models could benefit from including essential technological aspects by associating them with basic conceptions like presence or immersion. Core constructions should be described thoroughly to assure comparability.

Our research leads us to believe that few studies have attempted to combine the theoretical foundations of two fields into a single model. The majority of the studies that were considered either (i) explored the medical efficacy of a skill in contrast to an ordinary therapy without incorporating theoretical elements of technology characteristics into their framework or (ii) measured the empirical effect of a technology using a hypothetical framework for technical features without incorporating hypothetical conventions of clinical efficiency. Given the importance of considering the client's or patient's point of view, both (i) and (ii) run the danger of representing an intervention in an inadequate manner. Furthermore, ideas or their creation are necessary to fill the primary study void regarding the reasons behind the potential efficacy of a certain virtual reality intervention. Theoretical underpinnings in clinical fields other than psychology (e.g., surgery) seem to be further forward than in VR-related psychological treatments, and this is particularly true in these areas.

When it comes to current methods, virtual reality (VR) technologies have the dual ability to expand the real world through the production of artificial scenarios and to contain it. In some therapeutic contexts, this could be useful since it allows therapists to create conditions that are within their control [42]. In cases where vivo exposure is not recommended for psychological therapy, but patients have shown improvement during creative therapy sessions, virtual reality (VR) technology may provide an opportunity. Therapy results appear to be influenced by the idea of presence. It embodies the core principles of virtual reality, which include methods for directing attention or distraction [43]. However, the basis of its efficacy is still not obvious, as noted. Additionally, psychological law and midrange theories are frequently used as empirical sources for the theoretical underpinnings of VR-related technology. They simplify the psychological theories by describing their nature or by highlighting the interplay of related concepts. Both comprehensive theories drawn from larger social or psychological frameworks and hypotheses that have been synthesized and evaluated empirically are still lacking.

The assumptions behind the potential efficacy of VR-based technologies can be better understood with a more in-depth explanation and elaboration of such theoretical methods. However, there are certain limits to our findings. Our results are not as well-differentiated as they might be because we did not evaluate the methodological and general quality of the papers that were included in the review because we used a broad search strategy and selected a review type [44]. Also, rather than delving deeply into the topic, this study is more concerned with making sure searches are comprehensive. Clinical interventions utilizing VR-related technology might benefit from thorough frameworks that could be developed by future research that thoroughly examines particular theoretical structures and how they relate to clinical outcomes [45]. Our findings highlight the need for more in-depth methods that integrate concepts, as well as for the field of information systems to become more involved in discussions surrounding virtual reality (VR) and its associated technological features that serve as theoretical justification. Finally, we only looked at the health care industry, thus our findings may not apply to other fields. Research in the future may draw from a wider range of fields to investigate both specific and general conclusions about the theoretical underpinnings and practical applications of VR-related technology [46]. In this part, we see that the new augmented healthcare platform has had a few problems. Ensuring data security is a major worry among various current difficulties with AR healthcare applications. As a result, it is not immune to outside influences, and the physical layer may be subject to cybersecurity risks. While developing, augmented reality healthcare apps should take these external risks and typical security holes into account [47].

6.1 Security Requirements

The stuff that safeguards the request platform against unforeseen attacks is what enhanced healthcare application security standards are all about. If you want your app to be useful and functional, you need to pay attention to the security criteria shown in Fig. 5.6.

One example is the possibility of an intrusion occurring while virtual objects and real-time data are working together. When working with virtual or real-time objects, the augmented platform should keep everyone safe. These days, more and more augmented healthcare devices are joining the network. Consequently, for the sake of patient data security, the enhanced platform should guarantee privacy by blocking unauthorized users from accessing patient records. Nevertheless, a myriad of factors can alter data during access or transmission. In order to guarantee the security of medical information or health data, healthcare solutions should implement integrity. Resilience to provide a protective environment in the event that health devices are damaged is another essential necessity.

Availability is another big problem with the security of healthcare apps today. Most of the time, bad actors can take advantage of people's ignorance of denial-of-service attacks to compromise data security during transmission. Consequently, security awareness should give serious thought to this. Wearable technology that can connect to the network anywhere is what augmented healthcare devices are all

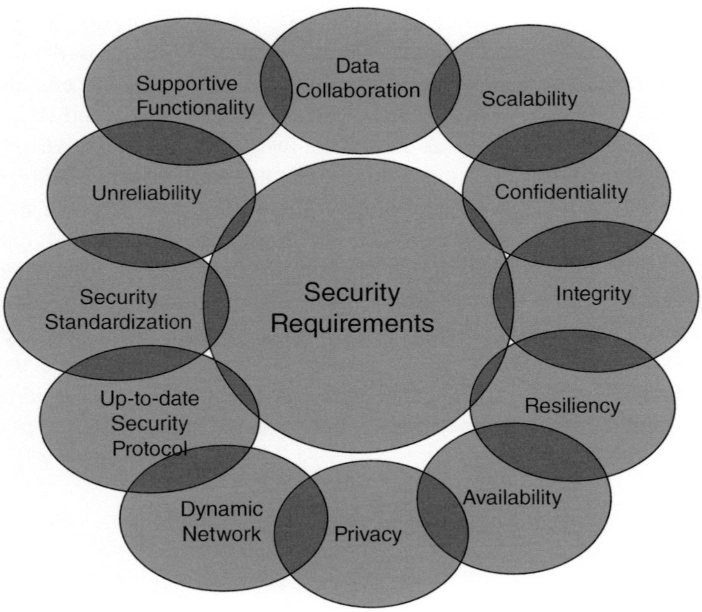

Fig. 5.6 Security requirements for AR

about. This highlights the critical need to develop a security model that accounts for changing network topics.

Improving the safety of augmented apps may be as simple as creating a dynamic security mechanism. Surprisingly, there is no security control strategy in place for ARML. Due to a lack of uniformity and an absence of security concerns, it is susceptible to security breaches [48]. Recently, augmented reality has been using third-party suppliers' computer-aided objects, which opens the door to security risks such data manipulation, spoofing, sniffer, and man-in-the-middle attacks. In order to ensure the application's reliability, the AR platform should be cognizant of these dangers and verify the created content's validity during transmission. Another potential source of security breaches in augmented healthcare applications is the widespread use of unsecured web browsers [49].

6.2 External Attack Terminology

There are threats to the augmented platform from outside sources. Potentially impacting both current and future augmented healthcare apps, devices, and networks, attackers pose a number of security risks. It can be easy to foresee some of these dangers and difficult to foresee others. Several external dangers that diminish the efficacy of applications and networks will be mentioned in this section. Some of the attack terminologies that can leave systems susceptible and less effective are shown in Fig. 5.7. For instance, hackers can corrupt or replace original data by stealing it or propagating malicious software during data transmission or communication. Unauthorized users have the potential to alter data, sow confusion, and slow down networks [50]. In addition, tampering with program code, information, or reprogramming might compromise the hardware platform, reduce data reliability, or introduce misleading information into the network. Attacks can sometimes infiltrate software systems and applications, taking advantage of security holes to wreak havoc with buffering, resource corruption, or loss [51].

6.3 AR and Virtual Reality in Healthcare: Current State and Future Perspective

Medical professionals are increasingly turning to augmented and virtual reality technologies to help patients better comprehend their treatments, train future doctors, and reach treatment goals. As seen in Fig. 5.8, augmented and virtual reality have many potential uses in the medical field.

- Among the many medical procedures that can benefit from augmented reality apps are:

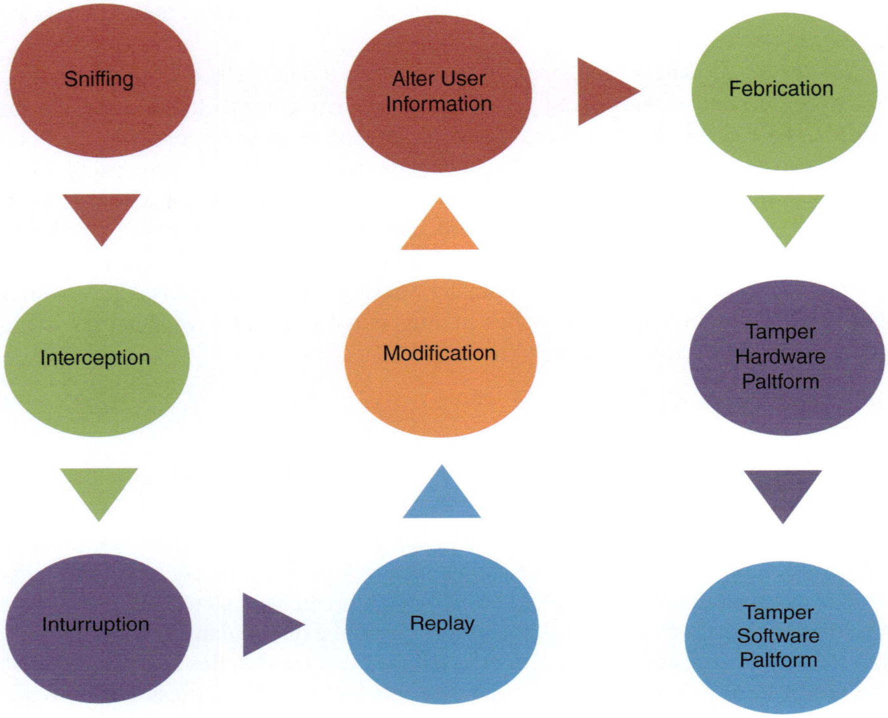

Fig. 5.7 Various attacks on security threats

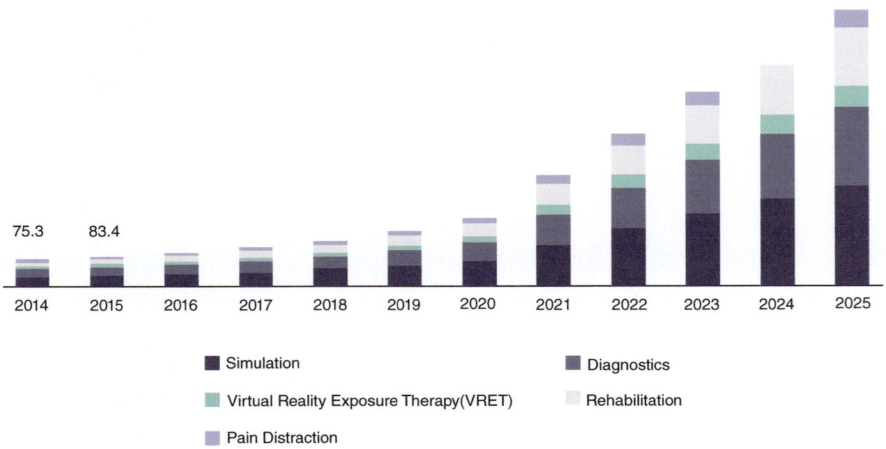

Fig. 5.8 Evolving of AR &VR technology in healthcare

- **Surgical treatment:** As a surgical procedure, 3D imaging of the patient's internal organs enables doctors to "see through the tissue" and plan the operation with precision, reducing the need for further incisions.
- **Accurate diagnostics:** The use of AR &VR to improve patients' ability to describe their symptoms improves diagnostic accuracy.
- **Closest-to-real situation lab practice:** Medical students benefit from the most realistic scenario lab practice by gaining practical experience that allows them to see the effects of their actions on real patients.
- **AR-based navigation:** Finding your way around the hospital, seeing nearby medical facilities, and locating life-saving equipment like defibrillators and emergency kits.
- **Virtual assistance:** In the event of an emergency, virtual aid can facilitate successful remote collaboration between the initial point of contact and a doctor.
- **Patient-physician interaction:** Interaction between patients and doctors when physical contact is not allowed (for example, because of a pandemic or because of where the doctor is located).
- **Anatomy teaching at schools:** Immersive learning environments in anatomy classes help students get a deeper understanding of their bodies.
- **Pharmaceutic visualization:** Pharmaceutical imaging of the drug's pharmacodynamics and pharmacokinetics, etc.

7 Conclusion

A significant amount of effort is being put forth by researchers in order to develop more advanced technical solutions that will improve the contemporary health care system all over the world. These innovations are being developed with the intention of bringing about a significant shift in the healthcare industry and simplifying the issues that are now present. The purpose of this study is to provide a concise examination of a variety of augmented reality (AR)-based healthcare services and applications. The structure of this document provides a comprehensive overview of the current development strategies about the existing architecture of healthcare applications as well as the procedures for processing and obtaining health data. To a certain extent, the essay made an effort to speed up the process of further development by drawing attention to a number of previously unknown problems concerning concurrent security requirements and subsequent difficulties. For the purpose of future study on AR-based healthcare apps and services, the debate that was carried out in this article on standardization, data availability, service quality, and data privacy may be helpful in a number of different instances. Furthermore, this study demonstrated the significance of augmented reality-based healthcare applications, which were supported by data from the current market. This may result in an increase in the involvement of a number of stakeholders for the purpose of continued development.

References

1. Lakshminarayanan V, Ravikumar A, Sriraman H, Alla S, Chattu VK. Health care equity through intelligent edge computing and augmented reality/virtual reality: a systematic review. J Multidiscip Healthc. 2023;16:2839–59.
2. AlGerafi MA, Zhou Y, Oubibi M, Wijaya TT. Unlocking the potential: a comprehensive evaluation of augmented reality and virtual reality in education. Electronics. 2023;12(18):3953.
3. Gupta D, Sathiyasekar K, Krishnamoorthy R, Arun S, Thiyagarajan R, Padmapriya S. Proposed GA algorithm with H-heed protocol for network optimization using machine learning in wireless sensor networks. In: 2022 Second international conference on artificial intelligence and smart energy (ICAIS), Coimbatore, India; 2022. p. 1402–8. https://doi.org/10.1109/ICAIS53314.2022.9743120.
4. Ray S, Tawar S, Singh N, Singh G. Transition toward technological transformation: challenges of implementing virtual reality and augmented reality in the health sector. J Mar Med Soc. 2023:10–4103.
5. Rao KR, Prasad ML, Kumar GR, Natchadalingam R, Hussain MM, Reddy PCS. Time-series cryptocurrency forecasting using ensemble deep learning. In: 2023 International conference on circuit power and computing technologies (ICCPCT). IEEE; 2023. p. 1446–51.
6. Taghian A, Abo-Zahhad M, Sayed MS, Abd El-Malek AH. Virtual and augmented reality in biomedical engineering. Biomed Eng Online. 2023;22(1):76.
7. Krishnamoorthy R, Desai A, Patel R, et al. 4 Element compact triple band MIMO antenna for sub-6 GHz 5G wireless applications. Wirel Netw. 2021;27:3747–59. https://doi.org/10.1007/s11276-021-02734-8.
8. Yuvaraj D, Kumar VP, Anandaram H, Samatha B, Krishnamoorthy R, Thiyagarajan R. Secure de-duplication over wireless sensing data using convergent encryption. In: 2022 IEEE 3rd Global conference for advancement in technology (GCAT), Bangalore, India, vol. 2022. p. 1–5. https://doi.org/10.1109/GCAT55367.2022.9971983.
9. Kalhoro R. Integration of augmented reality (AR) in healthcare systems. J Adv Technol Syst. 2023;1(1):35–47.
10. Dhar P, Rocks T, Samarasinghe RM, Stephenson G, Smith C. Augmented reality in medical education: students' experiences and learning outcomes. Med Educ Online. 2021;26(1):1953953. https://doi.org/10.1080/10872981.2021.1953953.
11. Tiwari CK, Bhaskar P, Pal A. Prospects of augmented reality and virtual reality for online education: a scientometric view. Int J Educ Manag. 2023;37(5):1042–66.
12. Anand SJ, Krishnamoorthy R, Kumar US, Kamalakkannan D. An effective hybrid mobility aware energy efficient low latency protocol (HMEL-MAC) for wireless sensor network. Cybern Syst. 2022:1–16. https://doi.org/10.1080/01969722.2022.2157598.
13. Dargan S, Bansal S, Kumar M, Mittal A, Kumar K. Augmented reality: a comprehensive review. Arch Comput Methods Eng. 2023;30(2):1057–80.
14. Baashar Y, Alkawsi G, Wan Ahmad WN, Alomari MA, Alhussian H, Tiong SK. Towards wearable augmented reality in healthcare: a comparative survey and analysis of head-mounted displays. Int J Environ Res Public Health. 2023;20(5):3940.
15. Ramana AV, Bhoga U, Dhulipalla RK, Kiran A, Chary BD, Reddy PCS. Abnormal behavior prediction in elderly persons using deep learning. In: 2023 International conference on computer, electronics & electrical engineering & their applications (IC2E3). IEEE; 2023. p. 1–5.
16. Suneel S, Balaram A, Amina Begum M, Umapathy K, Reddy PCS, Talasila V. Quantum mesh neural network model in precise image diagnosing. Opt Quant Electron. 2024;56(4):559.
17. Zhang J, Yu N, Wang B, Lv X. Trends in the use of augmented reality, virtual reality, and mixed reality in surgical research: a global bibliometric and visualized analysis. Indian J Surg. 2022;84(Suppl 1):52–69.
18. Prasath ASS, Lokesh S, Krishnakumar NJ, Vandarkuzhali T, Sahu DN, Reddy PCS. Classification of EEG signals using machine learning and deep learning techniques. Int J Health Sci. 2022;2022:10794–807.

19. Suneel S, Krishnamoorthy R, Gopatoti A, et al. Enhanced image diagnosing approach in medicine using quantum adaptive machine learning techniques. Opt Quant Electron. 2024;56:534. https://doi.org/10.1007/s11082-023-06203-8.
20. Zhao X, Ren Y, Cheah KS. Leading virtual reality (VR) and augmented reality (AR) in education: bibliometric and content analysis from the web of science (2018–2022). SAGE Open. 2023;13(3):21582440231190821.
21. Mamatha B, Rashmi D, Tiwari KS, Sikrant PA, Jovith AA, Reddy PCS. Lung cancer prediction from CT images and using deep learning techniques. In: 2023 Second international conference on trends in electrical, electronics, and computer engineering (TEECCON). IEEE; 2023. p. 263–7.
22. Dawn S. Virtual reality and augmented reality based affective computing applications in healthcare, challenges, and its future direction. In: Affective computing in healthcare: applications based on biosignals and artificial intelligence. Bristol: IOP Publishing; 2023. p. 10–1.
23. Parekh P, Patel S, Patel N, Shah M. Systematic review and meta-analysis of augmented reality in medicine, retail, and games. Vis Comput Ind Biomed Art. 2020;3:1–20.
24. Sampath S, Parameswari R, Prasad ML, Kumar DA, Hussain MM, Reddy PCS. Ensemble nonlinear machine learning model for chronic kidney diseases prediction. In: 2023 IEEE 3rd Mysore sub section international conference (MysuruCon). IEEE; 2023. p. 1–6.
25. Ricci S, Calandrino A, Borgonovo G, Chirico M, Casadio M. Virtual and augmented reality in basic and advanced life support training. JMIR Serious Games. 2022;10(1):e28595.
26. Mendoza-Ramírez CE, Tudon-Martinez JC, Félix-Herrán LC, Lozoya-Santos JDJ, Vargas-Martínez A. Augmented reality: survey. Appl Sci. 2023;13(18):10491.
27. Nguyen HS, Danh HC, Ma QP, Mesicek J, Hajnys J, Pagac M, Petru J. A bibliometrics analysis of medical internet of things for modern healthcare. Electronics. 2023;12(22):4586.
28. Alqahtani AS, Trabelsi Y, Ezhilarasi P, et al. Homomorphic encryption algorithm providing security and privacy for IoT with optical fiber communication. Opt Quant Electron. 2024;56:487. https://doi.org/10.1007/s11082-023-06098-5.
29. Raja M, Priya GL. The role of augmented reality and virtual reality in smart health education: state of the art and perspectives. In: Artificial intelligence for smart healthcare; 2023. p. 311–25.
30. Kumar R, Jain V, Han GTW, Touzene A, editors. Immersive virtual and augmented reality in healthcare: an IoT and blockchain perspective. CRC Press; 2023.
31. Denche-Zamorano A, Rodriguez-Redondo Y, Barrios-Fernandez S, Mendoza-Muñoz M, Castillo-Paredes A, Rojo-Ramos J, Garcia-Gordillo MA, Adsuar JC. Rehabilitation is the main topic in virtual and augmented reality and physical activity research: a bibliometric analysis. Sensors. 2023;23(6):2987.
32. Mittal H. 3 Virtual reality applications in healthcare. In: Immersive virtual and augmented reality in healthcare: an IoT and blockchain perspective; 2023.
33. Innocente C, Ulrich L, Moos S, Vezzetti E. Augmented reality: mapping methods and tools for enhancing the human role in healthcare HMI. Appl Sci. 2022;12(9):4295.
34. Krishnamoorthy R, Gupta M, Swathi G, Tanaka K, Raja C, Ramesh JVN. An intelligent IoT-based smart healthcare monitoring system using machine learning. In: 5G-based smart hospitals and healthcare systems. 1st ed. CRC Press; 2023. p. 230–44.
35. Tripathi A, Chauhan N, Choudhary A, Singh R. Augmented reality and its significance in healthcare systems. In: Meta-learning frameworks for imaging applications. IGI Global; 2023. p. 103–18.
36. Fahim S, Maqsood A, Das G, Ahmed N, Saquib S, Lal A, Khan AAG, Alam MK. Augmented reality and virtual reality in dentistry: highlights from the current research. Appl Sci. 2022;12(8):3719.
37. Krishnamoorthy R, Kumar U, Swathi G, et al. Metamaterial inspired quad-port multi-antenna system for millimeter wave 5G applications. J Infrared Milli Terahz Waves. 2023;44:346–64. https://doi.org/10.1007/s10762-023-00921-6.

38. Patil V, Narayan J, Sandhu K, Dwivedy SK. Integration of virtual reality and augmented reality in physical rehabilitation: a state-of-the-art review. In: Revolutions in product design for healthcare: advances in product design and design methods for healthcare; 2022. p. 177–205.
39. von Ende E, Ryan S, Crain MA, Makary MS. Artificial intelligence, augmented reality, and virtual reality advances and applications in interventional radiology. Diagnostics. 2023;13(5):892.
40. Barteit S, Lanfermann L, Bärnighausen T, Neuhann F, Beiersmann C. Augmented, mixed, and virtual reality-based head-mounted devices for medical education: systematic review. JMIR Serious Games. 2021;9(3):e29080.
41. Gasmi A, Benlamri R. Augmented reality, virtual reality and new age technologies demand escalates amid COVID-19. In: Novel AI and data science advancements for sustainability in the era of COVID-19. Academic Press; 2022. p. 89–111.
42. Kamińska D, Zwoliński G, Laska-Leśniewicz A, Raposo R, Vairinhos M, Pereira E, Urem F, Ljubić Hinić M, Haamer RE, Anbarjafari G. Augmented reality: current and new trends in education. Electronics. 2023;12(16):3531.
43. Kiani S, Rezaei I, Abasi S, Zakerabasali S, Yazdani A. Technical aspects of virtual augmented reality-based rehabilitation systems for musculoskeletal disorders of the lower limbs: a systematic review. BMC Musculoskelet Disord. 2023;24(1):1–25.
44. Urlings J, de Jong G, Maal T, Henssen D. Views on augmented reality, virtual reality, and 3D printing in modern medicine and education: a qualitative exploration of expert opinion. J Digit Imaging. 2023;36:1–10.
45. Oun A, Hagerdorn N, Scheideger C, Cheng X. Mobile devices or head-mounted displays: a comparative review and analysis of augmented reality in healthcare. IEEE Access. 2024;12:21825–39.
46. Seetohul J, Shafiee M, Sirlantzis K. Augmented reality (AR) for surgical robotic and autonomous systems: state of the art, challenges, and solutions. Sensors. 2023;23(13):6202.
47. Kumar A, Saudagar AKJ, Alkhathami M, Alsamani B, Khan MB, Hasanat MHA, Ahmed ZH, Kumar A, Srinivasan B. Gamified learning and assessment using ARCS with next-generation AIoMT integrated 3D animation and virtual reality simulation. Electronics. 2023;12(4):835.
48. Andrews A. Integration of augmented reality and brain-computer interface technologies for health care applications: exploratory and prototyping study. JMIR Form Res. 2022;6(4):e18222.
49. Krishnamoorthy R, Soubache ID, Jain S. Wireless communication based evaluation of power consumption for constrained energy system. Wirel Pers Commun. 2022;127:737–48. https://doi.org/10.1007/s11277-021-08402-6.
50. Pandiaraj S, Krishnamoorthy R, Ushasukhanya S, et al. Optimization of IoT circuit for flexible optical network system with high speed utilization. Opt Quant Electron. 2023;55:1206. https://doi.org/10.1007/s11082-023-05452-x.
51. Tanaka K, Ogura S, Krishnamoorthy R, Sugiyama K, Kawahara M. Flexibility and productivity in IoT programming: a case study with Mruby. In: Guarda T, Portela F, Diaz-Nafria JM, editors. Advanced research in technologies, information, innovation and sustainability. ARTIIS 2023. Communications in computer and information science, vol. 1936. Cham: Springer; 2024. https://doi.org/10.1007/978-3-031-48855-9_2.

Chapter 6
Science Behind Augmented Reality and Virtual Reality in Healthcare

Arti Saxena and Pooja Thukral

Abstract In the year 2022, Prime Minister Modi launched the 5G service at Integrated Marketing Communications where the three telcos, Reliance Jio, Bharti Airtel, and Vodafone Idea, each presented their own use case of Augmented Reality (AR) and Virtual Reality (VR). The Vodafone Idea test case demonstrated the safety of workers in an underground tunnel of Delhi Metro by creating a Digital Twin of the tunnel. PM took a live demo from the dais to monitor the work in real-time by utilizing VR and AR henceforth explaining that Augmented Reality and Virtual Reality captured and affected various industries with positive outcomes. This revolutionization in industry has now entered into the field of healthcare. In healthcare, Augmented reality is collecting data from various authentic resources, producing a 3D model of the same, and utilizing it to deliver healthcare facilities. Virtual reality (VR) creates a simulated environment to train, learn, treat, and manage patients virtually. Mixed Reality merges both real and virtual worlds by allowing interaction with both digital as well as physical objects. Medical Training and Education, Surgical Planning and Simulation, Pain Management and Therapy, Physical Rehabilitation, Patient Education, Remote Consultations and Telemedicine, Mental Health Treatment, Medical Device Training, Clinical Research and Data Visualization and Patient Monitoring are a few areas of healthcare where we will discuss the usage and science of Augmented and Virtual reality. Some of the international companies are predicting the usage of Augmented Reality and Virtual Reality in healthcare by 5–6 billion in 2025 which is predicted to touch $50.9 billion by 2026 as per a spending guide by IDC (International Data Corporation). Various places where this can be used are in training doctors where traditional cadavers were used. In treating certain mental illnesses, charting the territory of surgical planes before planning a complicated surgery. In this chapter, we will

A. Saxena (✉)
School of Engineering and Technology, Manav Rachna International Institute of Research and Studies, Faridabad, India
e-mail: artisaxena.set@mriu.edu.in

P. Thukral
Cloudnine Hospital, Faridabad, India

B. O. Soufiane et al. (eds.), *Augmented Wellness*,
https://doi.org/10.1007/978-981-96-2952-7_6

discuss the science behind virtual Reality (VR) and Augmented Reality (AR) in healthcare. In this chapter we will give insight into what augmented and virtual reality is and especially its utility in healthcare.

Keywords Augmented reality · Virtual reality · Healthcare · Immersive virtual reality · Mixed reality

1 Introduction

1.1 Augmented Reality in Healthcare

Augmented reality is cutting-edge technology overlaying virtual or digital information to enhance our perception and interaction with our surroundings. It integrates virtual things into the user's existing environment. For the understanding of the user's existing environment, AR uses Cameras, various types of sensors, and computer algorithms. After processing, the data is used to overlay virtual content—such as text, pictures, or 3D models—onto the user's field of vision, usually via a smartphone, tablet, or augmented reality headset. Although the idea of augmented reality (AR) has been around for decades, its popularity has recently increased due to improvements in hardware, such as strong CPUs and high-resolution displays. These days, augmented reality (AR) is widely applied across several industries, including marketing, gaming, entertainment, education, retail, and, most significantly, healthcare.

AR has enormous potential to enhance patient care, surgical planning, medical education, and treatment results. During operations, surgeons can visualize anatomical features using augmented reality (AR), superimposing vital data such as CT scans or X-rays directly onto the patient's body. In various ways, in healthcare, the usage of AR has been explained as follows (1–5):

1.1.1 Medical Training and Education

By allowing medical professionals and students to see anatomical structures and medical procedures in three dimensions, augmented reality (AR) helps them comprehend and remember difficult medical ideas. By using augmented reality (AR) programs, students can safely and fully immerse themselves in the learning process by interactively exploring virtual organs, dissecting virtual cadavers, and simulating surgical operations [1].

1.1.2 Surgical Planning and Navigation

By superimposing preoperative imaging data, like CT or MRI images, in real-time onto the patient's anatomy, surgeons can employ augmented reality (AR) to improve surgical planning and navigation. By doing so, surgeons can more accurately and efficiently perform procedures on patients with a lower risk of complications by planning incisions, precisely locating important structures, and optimally placing implants or equipment.

1.1.3 Intraoperative Guidance

Throughout an operation, augmented reality (AR) can give doctors on-the-spot visual indications and guidance. Augmented reality (AR) helps surgeons make more informed decisions and execute surgeries with greater confidence by superimposing pertinent information, such as tumor margins, blood arteries, or nerve routes, onto the surgical site.

1.1.4 Medical Visualization and Simulation

Augmented reality (AR) gives medical personnel the ability to see and work with complicated medical data, like three-dimensional patient anatomical models, medical equipment, or physiological processes. With the use of this visualization capacity, practitioners can more effectively educate patients about medical issues, treatment alternatives, and procedural risks.

1.1.5 Patient Empowerment and Engagement

Augmented Reality (AR) facilitates patient empowerment by offering tailored treatment plans, interactive educational resources, and immersive experiences that enable patients to actively participate in their healthcare process. With the use of augmented reality (AR) applications, patients can better understand the impacts of their care, track key health indicators, and follow their prescription schedules.

Overall, augmented reality (AR) has enormous potential to change healthcare by advancing surgical techniques, patient care, medical education, and rehabilitation methods. Applications of AR technology in healthcare are anticipated to grow as it develops, providing fresh chances to raise patient standards globally and boost clinical results.

2 Virtual Reality in Healthcare

Although the idea of virtual reality has been known for several years, recent advances in computational capacity, hardware, and software have contributed to it becoming more widely accepted. Virtual reality is creating a simulated environment where we can immerse ourselves and interact with the simulated environment thus created. We need a head-mounted display (HMD) to participate in the interactions. There is sensory feedback using vision, hearing, and sometimes touch sensation in a VR-generated field. Virtual reality thus helps in the management of pain, phobias, PTSD (post-traumatic stress disorder), and physical rehabilitation.

Sophisticated displays, motion sensors, and input devices that collaborate to produce a sense of presence and immersion are at the core of virtual reality technology. Stereoscopic visuals are shown on high-resolution screens inside the headset, giving the user a sense of depth and perspective. Motion-tracking sensors follow the user's movements, enabling them to move around and interact with the virtual world.

VR is being used in a variety of industries today, including manufacturing, education, gaming, entertainment, and healthcare, just to name a few. In various ways, in healthcare, the usage of VR has been explained as follows (1–5):

2.1 Medical Education and Training

Virtual reality (VR) allows medical professionals and students to participate in lifelike simulations of operations, treatments, and patient encounters. Before interacting with actual individuals, learners may improve their skills and gain confidence in this immersive training environment, which allows them to practice in a risk-free atmosphere [1].

2.2 Surgical Planning and Simulation

Surgeons can utilize virtual reality (VR) to plan difficult procedures by seeing the anatomy unique to each patient in three-dimensional form. Surgeons can also simulate surgeries in advance with VR simulations, which improves surgical outcomes and lowers operating risks.

2.3 Pain Management and Therapy

Virtual Reality (VR) is becoming a more common non-pharmacological approach to managing pain as well as decreasing anxiety during medical operations. Patients receiving chemotherapy or physical therapy, for example, can lose themselves in virtual reality experiences that ease their suffering and encourage relaxation.

2.4 Exposure Therapy

Phobias, anxiety disorders, and post-traumatic stress disorder (PTSD) respond well to VR exposure therapy. In a safe virtual world setting, individuals can confront and subsequently desensitize to stimuli that trigger them, encouraging therapeutic success.

2.5 Physical Rehabilitation

Interactive exercises and activities catered to the specific needs of each patient are provided by VR-based rehabilitation programs. These all-encompassing encounters can encourage patients to participate in their treatment, monitor their advancement, and enhance results in domains including balance, mobility, and motor function.

2.6 Patient Empowerment and Education

Virtual reality (VR) technology makes it possible for medical professionals to impart more interesting and intelligible information to patients about medical disorders, available treatments, and anatomy. Through the use of virtual models of their own bodies or medical treatments, patients can better understand and make well-informed decisions.

2.7 Telemedicine and Remote Consultations

By removing geographical boundaries and increasing access to healthcare services, virtual reality (VR) platforms enable virtual consultations and remote medical procedures. Without leaving their residences, patients can attend community meetings, take part in sessions with therapists, or receive professional medical advice.

2.8 Research and Data Visualization

In a fully realistic three-dimensional environment, virtual reality tools enable academics to study complex medical data, including genomic sequences and imaging scans. Medical science may benefit from these improved visualization abilities in the form of fresh perspectives, discoveries, and advances.

3 Literature Review: Augmented Reality and Virtual Reality

The need for healthcare services is constantly rising. People know that they can automate many tasks with technology; these include online appointments, report sharing, video conferences, and much more. In the healthcare sector, new-generation technologies like artificial intelligence (AI), digital twins, machine learning, IoT, blockchain, and virtual reality (VR) can be leveraged to improve patient and physician experiences. This chapter by Mittal [2] reviews some VR applications for the healthcare sector. The chapter also offers a blueprint for integrating cutting-edge technologies into the healthcare industry. In image-guided surgery, augmented reality visualization gives the surgeon access to radiological images and surgical planning that are contextualized to the patient's anatomy. Its goal is to combine virtual planning and surgical navigation [3].

The possibilities of artificial intelligence (AI), the Internet of Things (IoT), BIM tools, and virtual and augmented reality (VR/AR) technologies have led to a rise in the use of sophisticated Structural Health Monitoring (SHM) methodologies. However, the absence of interconnectivity among these devices contributes to their limited usage. Fawad et al. [4] addressed this issue by developing an integrated framework to assess serviceability and implement a smart SHM for a recently constructed extradosed bridge. The objective of Oun et al. [5] is to provide an extensive overview of augmented reality (AR) applications in healthcare that is based on mobile and head-mounted displays (HMDs). People will be better able to choose the ideal gadget for their particular needs and comprehend the potential uses of this technology as a result. In comparison to conventional teaching methods or no intervention at all, the primary objective of Tene et al.'s review from 2024 is to determine the degree to which immersive Virtual Reality (iVR) and Augmented Reality (AR) technologies enhance particular competencies in healthcare professionals during medical education and training. In his article, Rowan [6] examined how the integration of digital twins and extended reality innovations might revolutionize medical device design thinking, supply chain management, and training, ultimately enhancing patient safety, circularity, and sustainability.

Virtual reality (VR) offers safe, realistic, and reproducible simulated environments where users can practice and develop communication skills, making it a useful tool for communication rehabilitation. The purpose of this study by Bryant et al. [7] was to find out what medical professionals and tech experts thought about the usability and design of a VR application prototype intended for communication rehabilitation. Nine experts from various fields related to health and technology engaged in virtual focus groups or one-on-one online interviews to assess the utilization and efficacy of the virtual reality prototype. A content-thematic analysis was used to examine the data sources. Four primary themes pertain to VR design and application in rehabilitation have been discussed as follows: (i) creating virtual worlds with a rehabilitation focus; (ii) comprehending and utilizing VR hardware; (iii) creating space for VR in training and rehabilitation; and (iv) putting VR to use without replacing the role of a health professional. While assessing the VR prototype, technological experts and health professionals collaborated on its design. They determined which software aspects needed to be carefully considered to guarantee better client safety, usability, and communication rehabilitation results. To create VR apps that are useful and successfully integrate them into rehabilitation, inclusive co-design had been maintained and involve health professionals, clients with communication disabilities, and their families.

More financial and human resources are needed by primary healthcare institutions to create an environment where VR tools can be used to benefit patients [8].

The aim of this study by Eunju [9] was to improve nursing students' severity classification competency by creating a virtual reality-based nursing education program. The key to increasing the effectiveness of emergency department services globally is the classification of severity in hospitals. Patients' safety is further ensured when treatment is prioritized according to an accurate assessment of the severity of an illness or injury. Based on the 2021 Korean Emergency Patient Classification Tool, patients were quickly classified into five clinical conditions using the five real-world clinical scenarios included in the application. An experimental group of 17 nursing students got access to a virtual reality-based simulation in addition to clinical experience. A control group of 17 nursing students engaged in solely standard clinical practice. Students' performance confidence, clinical decision-making capacity, and skill in severity classification were all significantly enhanced by the virtual reality-based nursing education program. Despite the ongoing epidemic, nursing students can still receive realistic indirect experiences through virtual reality-based nursing education software in scenarios where clinical nursing practice is not feasible. Specifically, it will function as foundational information for the growth and application plan of virtual reality-based nurse education initiatives to enhance nursing proficiency.

Between 2020 and 2021, there was a significant increase in the usage of and documentation of electronic adaptations for formative and continuous assessment methods due to COVID-19 and the limitations of in-person instruction. By going over Beer's criteria and choosing the best management, Badr [10] developed a virtual escape room that will aid and hone the problem-solving abilities of fifth-year pharmacy students. After the virtual escape room was put into use, a descriptive cross-sectional survey was carried out using a Google Form. Students had to use Beer's criteria to solve five riddles. Pharmacy students completed a survey to share their opinions about the game and assess how they felt about this approach. Every single one of the 128 students registered for the senior course managed to get out (100%). There was statistical significance between genders according to a one-sample t-test. Male students were more neutral toward the game, whereas female students were statistically faster to escape ($p < 0.00002$), more willing to recommend it to other students, and thought it pushed them to think about the content in a fresh way. To sum up, the elderly virtual escape room proved to be an effective trial approach to support online learning. Future research, however, ought to look into the effects of virtual gamification on learning in pharmacy education and whether or not there were any gender-specific variations in the use of these resources.

Virtual reality (VR) is an immersive and interactive technology that has the potential to be used as a teaching tool in nursing education. The difficulty of developing novel VR experiences has been an obstacle to fully utilizing VR's benefits, but recent advances in VR technology and software allow perhaps the least skilled users to create interesting VR experiences. An undergraduate nursing student with little technical expertise uses commercial VR software to build a virtual reality pain treatment experience, according to a case study by Brody et al. [11]. Working with computer code is not necessary when using off-the-shelf hardware and software platforms. The group used basic click-and-drag methods and setting toggles to easily manipulate the objects in a virtual world they constructed. The findings from this case study indicate that nurse educators may produce straightforward but impactful virtual reality experiences on their own, significantly enhancing the tools already available for nursing education.

4 Science Behind Augmented Reality and Virtual Reality

Virtual reality (VR) and augmented reality (AR) are two distinct but connected technologies that have transformed our interaction with digital surroundings and information. Augmented reality is overlaying digital content in the real-time world using smartphones, tablets (handheld displays), AR glasses (Head mounted display), and spatial displays. It can incorporate real-time tracking and recognition tools into the real world to enhance learning, training and provide management strategies. The tracking used by AR devices is—Sensor tracking and vision tracking. Sensor tracking uses optical (video cameras), inertial sensor tracking—which determines the particular axis (mechanical gyroscope, accelerometer), acoustic tracking (ultrasonic transmitters), and magnetic sensor tracking (uses magnetic fields). The tracking of vision involves both marker-based and markerless techniques. Scanning a QR code serves as an illustration of marker-based tracking. Information is already preloaded into the app. Without any pre-loaded data, markerless tracking tracks objects based only on their color, symmetry, and pattern as they change over time. Smartphone apps currently use augmented reality to help you locate your car in a crowded area. The popular game which became a rage in 2016 uses AR to introduce Pikachu and its characters when the user is playing the game on the roadside or around a waterfront [12].

Virtual reality on the other hand is a simulated environment which creates a real life like scenario by using images and sounds. This can be accessed using a headset or a helmet. VR works on the principle of depth perception. The degree of dissimilarity projected on the retina of an image creates perspective or depth perception. The history of VR dates back to 1800 and even Leonardo Da Vinci who experienced use of perspective in the paintings of that era. However, it was in 1990 that the introduction of VR headsets in gaming zones caused the arrival of a new era for the use of VR. Nowadays, when the term virtual reality (VR) is used, it usually refers to a binocular head-mounted display (HMD) that projects a two-dimensional (2D) perspective image of the virtual scene being emulated into each eye. Just as it does from the retinal projections of the real world received by each eye, the brain may deduce three-dimensional (3D) features of the simulated environment from these two projections. [13, 14]. The goal of virtual reality is to imitate this organic projection mechanism. Replicating VR from projection technologies such as stereoscopes, haploscopes, and 3D computer monitors [15] is the observer's ability to move freely within the computer generated 3D environment, giving rise to rich motion parallax information [16]. A stationary observer would not be able to get as much information about how the scene's visuals change over time in response to our movements as a moving observer can [17]. The addition of observer movement helps to clarify several possible interpretations of the scene design, regardless of how one moves a scene in relation to a static observer, such that the retinal images are the same as when the observer moves [18, 19]. For movement to be meaningful, the images of the simulated scene need to be refreshed in real time as the observer moves. This helps in healthcare to visualize the anatomy of the human body, navigate it, and pre-plan surgical procedures. The patients can also be educated about their disease, treatment plan, and prognosis [12].

Sahu et al. in [20] specified that Congregation of Internet of Things, augmented reality, and virtual reality is the future of healthcare. Utilizing brain-computer interface (BCI) and simultaneous localization and mapping (SLAM) for neurosurgical procedures, neuroprosthetics, neuromodulation, and neurorehabilitation, virtual reality and augmented reality are promising technologies in the neurosciences that show promise for the field.

Studies reveal that VR/AR platforms may be used to enhance one's visualizing abilities [21]. Virtual reality (VR) and augmented reality (AR) platforms are a subset of digital media. As such, technologies may be used to facilitate the development of specialized apps that teach visualization skills.

With the advent of growing scientific advancements, we are about to gain a greater grasp of the mechanisms underlying the evolution of consciousness [22]. This was obvious when neuroscientists and philosophers understood that awareness was not simply digital, and the computational illusion of the mind started falling apart. However, since we can now artificially mimic an all-encompassing environment in four dimensions thanks to virtual reality (VR), augmented reality (AR), and mixed reality (MR), our models of how consciousness functions are becoming much clearer to understand. Through attentional posturing, consciousness creates a forging mechanism that allows it to fully immerse itself in a world of its own creation, all the while remaining mostly oblivious to the mechanisms involved in such a magical performance. By using VR and MR as touchstones, we can gain a deeper understanding of how our brains create the environment we live in. We have the means, possibly for the first time in human history, to artificially reconstruct how the brain views and engages with reality by investigating manufactured virtual reality devices and the diverse landscapes they can open up. The article explores how the development of virtual reality alters our perception of human consciousness and how using it in different forms can help future studies [23]. The holistic and integrated experiences for learning that virtual reality (VR) technology offers make complicated subjects more approachable, and so create great prospects to improve astronomy education.

5 Comparative Study of Augmented Reality and Virtual Reality

Virtual Reality (VR) is a technology that allows users to experience a completely virtual environment through a headset or goggles [24]. It displays images and sounds using a Head-Mounted Display (HMD), while tracking sensors monitor the user's motions in real time. A sensation of presence is created when the VR world adapts to the user's motions [12]. The VR experience is powered by software and content, which creates and depicts the virtual world in real time in response to user inputs. Advanced computer graphics, optics, and human-computer interface (HCI) concepts are all part of the technology underpinning virtual reality (VR). For a smooth and engaging experience, high frame rates must be achieved during real-time rendering of 3D scenes. In order to improve realism and user engagement, VR systems also employ techniques like positional tracking, which tracks head and occasionally hand movements, and stereoscopic rendering, which creates depth perception.

Augmented Reality (AR) is a technology that overlays digital information or virtual objects onto the real world, enhancing our perception of reality rather than replacing it entirely [12]. AR applications range from smartphone apps to advanced headsets, and key components include display devices, sensors and cameras, and computer vision algorithms. These devices use sensors and cameras to understand the real-world environment and superimpose digital content onto it, allowing virtual objects to interact realistically with the environment [24]. Computer vision, sensor fusion, simultaneous localization and mapping (SLAM), and human factors engineering are all part of the science underpinning augmented reality. While SLAM algorithms assist in tracking the location and orientation of the device in relation to its surroundings, computer vision algorithms examine and interpret the scene that is collected by cameras. For AR systems to smoothly blend digital material with the actual environment in real-time, complex software is also needed.

Abdennour et al. [25] in their chapter write about comparison and choice between VR and AR. VR puts students in convincing virtual environments, making it perfect for practical training and simulations. In contrast, augmented reality (AR) provides contextual information and interactive simulations by superimposing digital elements onto the actual world through devices like smartphones and AR glasses. These technologies increase engagement by grabbing students' attention, facilitating practical experiences and a deeper understanding, and customizing the learning process. VR's 3D environments and AR's overlays enhance memorization. These methods can produce even deeper and more varied learning experiences, but how they are integrated will depend on the educational goals and available resources.

Currently, immersive virtual reality (iVR) and augmented reality (AR) are widely employed to teach anatomy across health sciences courses [26]. These interactive XR technologies (iVR and AR) permit the three-dimensional visualization of anatomical structures and their spatial relationships in virtual environments that resemble the real world. Virtual structures rendered through specialized software are similar to real structures; though, in the virtual environment, students interact with the anatomy using a joystick or through hand motions. VR headsets enable the recreation of immersive experiences (including motion tracking, interaction with digital elements, a wider range of vision, and stereoscopy), which allows students to visualize virtual anatomical objects as if they were real. Two characteristics of iVR are presence and immersion. Presence is defined as the psychological sensation/desire to stay within the virtual environment that the subject feels is real. Immersion is the capability to interact with virtual objects. Therefore, depending on the level of presence and immersion, VR can be either immersive or non-immersive. iVR allows viewing a virtual scenario through a head-mounted display in 360° whereby subjects can interact with the virtual environment and its objects using their hands as controllers. Conversely, AR superimposes virtual elements onto the real world allowing individuals to interact with real and virtual elements, simultaneously.

García-Robles et al. [27] in their systematic review and meta-analysis showed that XR-based interventions are more effective than traditional passive learning resources as a teaching-learning resource for studying anatomy in health sciences students. Both XR technologies (iVR and AR) improved learners' anatomy knowledge gains compared to controls, especially when used alongside traditional resources as supplemental/complimentary tools. A large effect favoring XR technologies was detected when compared against didactic lectures and anatomical images in atlases and/or textbooks. Overall, 80% of students who used XR technologies subjectively reported that XR technologies are useful for learning anatomy, especially when they are used as a supplemental resource in anatomy curricula.

Petruse et al. [28] conducted a comparative study of traditional method of teaching anatomy with mixed reality in a group of students aged 19–54 years. They concluded that the traditional method of teaching muscular anatomy with images on powerpoint was effective in older students and mixed reality created a 3D hologram using Microsoft HoloLens 2 was useful in younger students.

AI is being used in India to improve patient management, create treatment pathways and to monitor progress of patients. In one such study by Iqbal et al. [29], AI was used to predict sepsis in neonates admitted in Neonatal Intensive care Units. It was a retrospective study conducted in a South Indian tertiary hospital from 2017 to 2021. Using the data they created a model to detect early neonatal sepsis which can enhance the patient's outcome.

In another study done in Assam India which was conducted over a period of 2 years (Nov 2020–2022) Chiramal et al. [30] AI generated tools were used to generate reports of NCCT—Non contrast CT scan in patients who came with strokes to Baptist Christian hospital. AI would generate the report in 4 min and there was a tele radiology consultation done by a neurologist from the USA to guide further treatment plans for stroke patients. Though this was a small study done in a rural set up, nonetheless this highlights the potential AI has in healthcare.

6 Challenges and Future Scope

The findings of this study highlight AI's transformative potential in healthcare but also emphasize the importance of addressing ethical concerns to enable responsible and equitable application. Striking a balance between utilizing technological developments for better healthcare results and protecting individual rights and privacy is crucial as AI integration develops [31]. Strong data security measures are required due to privacy concerns, and algorithmic biases that could disproportionately affect particular demographic groups need to be lessened. By working together, engineers, medical experts, and ethicists may create regulations that guarantee accountability, equity, and transparency in AI-driven healthcare. Additionally, the conversation explores how AI may affect patient autonomy and how the doctor-patient relationship may change in the future. To empower patients in their healthcare journey, AI implementation must prioritize strategies for good communication and informed consent.

Future research in AI-driven healthcare will focus on improving algorithms' interpretability, minimizing biases, and guaranteeing strong privacy protections [32]. To keep up with the rapid advancement of technology, ethical standards must be continuously improved, and interdisciplinary teamwork is essential for tackling difficult problems. Future research prospects can be explored by investigating cutting-edge technologies like blockchain, augmented reality, and robotics in the healthcare industry. To fully utilize AI in enhancing global healthcare, it will be essential to comprehend the long-term societal implications and handle accessibility issues.

Tene et al.'s comprehensive review from 2024 thoroughly investigated the application of VR and AR in medical education to ascertain how well they enhanced personnel's competencies in comparison to traditional approaches. To ascertain the effect of immersive technology on educational results, 28 research was assessed utilizing chi-square analysis and descriptive statistics through a methodical application of PRISMA principles and the PICOS technique. According to our data, VR is the most studied. Based on the reviews included in this analysis, it appears that learner engagement and performance have been positively correlated with VR and AR technology.

The statistical research, however, did not show that there was a meaningful correlation between the phases of medical education and the kind of technology employed. This suggests that although the corpus of evaluated investigation indicates a positive trend toward the effectiveness of VR and AR in medical education, it is not yet statistically significant. It is crucial to emphasize that the lack of significance could be attributed to the various techniques, small sample numbers, and the heterogeneity of outcomes among the included research [33]. Finally, the expense and complexity of VR technology are important factors to take into account. Even with a declining trend in cost, setting up personal VR/AR devices for every student to use for distance learning is still a difficult and costly task. This scenario suggests a possible paradigm in which semi-centralized labs outfitted with VR/AR technology could host remote learning sessions in the future. In these environments, teachers could interact and impart knowledge remotely, while pupils had physical access to the required tools. This strategy might provide a more workable and affordable way to include immersive technologies into medical education, particularly in situations where it is not viable for each student to buy such a device.

While AR in medical education and training has different problems, it does not need to meet the same strict requirements as it does in clinical settings. The degree to which knowledge acquired via the AR system is sustained throughout time is unknown [34]. In another piece of literature, the authors acknowledged that the process of generating complicated anatomical regions in AR can vary depending on personal experiences, leading to various outcomes for individual anatomical regions. This literature discussed the construction and evaluation of an AR knowledge assessment tool. Establishing a standard for such development techniques is therefore crucial to ensure reliable and consistent implementation across a range of applications. Panchapakesan [35] in their study emphasized the challenges of AR and VR in Asia, which are technological limitations, infrastructure challenges and effective managerial strategies to remove barriers in implementation.

Currently in healthcare AR and VR is a concept which we are starting to hear about. The prospect of AI is immense in healthcare. There are a very few centers and sparingly few specialties in India currently using AI in ICU's as of now. We need Indian data and more research work to validate its practical applications. AI must be included in the curriculum at the undergraduate and post graduate level for medical students.

7 Conclusion

In summary, the application of virtual reality (VR) and augmented reality (AR) in healthcare is a ground-breaking development that will have a significant impact on therapeutic interventions, medical education, and patient care. Examining the science underlying AR and VR in healthcare makes it clear that these innovative technologies present special chances to improve diagnosis, treatment, and teaching in ways that were previously not known.

Above all, AR and VR have the potential to completely transform medical training and teaching [36]. Through the use of realistic settings and immersive simulations, medical practitioners can practice in a secure setting. This lowers the risk to patients during training processes in addition to improving the quality of care. Furthermore, medical students can now see intricate anatomical structures and physiological processes with never-before-seen clarity thanks to AR and VR, which improves their comprehension and memory of important information.

Furthermore, there is a great deal of promise for AR and VR to enhance outcomes for patients [37]. By superimposing pertinent medical data onto the patient's actual surroundings, these technologies can help diagnose patients more precisely and promptly while empowering medical professionals to act swiftly and decisively. Moreover, doctors can receive precise navigation and real-time support with AR-guided procedures, which improves surgical outcomes and lowers complications. Virtual reality-based therapies have also shown promise in the treatment of pain, rehabilitation, and mental health issues. These therapies provide patients with an alternative to conventional pharmaceutical interventions. In addition, the application of AR and VR in healthcare could improve patient empowerment and involvement. These technologies promote better comprehension and patient involvement in their own care by allowing patients to view their problems and treatment alternatives in immersive virtual environments. This helps patients stick to their treatment plans better and gives them the confidence to make better health-related decisions.

Though AR and VR have a lot of potential for the healthcare industry, there are a few issues that need to be resolved before they are widely used. The most important of them is the requirement for strong regulatory frameworks to guarantee patient privacy and safety [37]. Furthermore, implementation difficulties may arise due to the expensive cost of AR and VR technologies and the related infrastructure, especially in settings with limited resources [38]. Furthermore, in order to fully benefit from new technologies and use them successfully, healthcare workers need thorough training.

In summary, the science underlying virtual and augmented reality in healthcare signifies a paradigm shift in how we approach patient involvement, diagnosis, treatment, and medical education. Healthcare professionals may promote medical research, improve patient experiences, and improve clinical outcomes by utilizing the immersive qualities of AR and VR. However, in order to overcome obstacles and provide fair access to these game-changing instruments, cooperation between healthcare experts, technology developers, legislators, and regulatory bodies will be necessary to realize the full promise of these technologies. We have the chance to usher in a new era of personalized medicine where the lines between the physical and digital worlds blur and patient-centered care takes center stage as we continue to innovate and integrate AR and VR into healthcare.

References

1. Tene T, Vique López DF, Valverde Aguirre PE, Orna Puente LM, Vacacela Gomez C. Virtual reality and augmented reality in medical education: an umbrella review. Front Digit Health. 2024;6:1365345.
2. Mittal H. Virtual reality applications in healthcare: a new-age technology perspective. In: Immersive virtual and augmented reality in healthcare. CRC Press; 2024. p. 50–62.
3. Cutolo F. Augmented reality in image-guided surgery. In: Encyclopedia of computer graphics and games. Cham: Springer; 2024. p. 182–92.
4. Fawad M, Salamak M, Hanif MU, Koris K, Ahsan M, Rahman H, et al. Integration of bridge health monitoring system with augmented reality application developed using 3D game engine-case study. IEEE Access. 2024;12(16963):16974.
5. Oun A, Hagerdorn N, Scheideger C, Cheng X. Mobile devices or head-mounted displays: a comparative review and analysis of augmented reality in healthcare. IEEE Access. 2024;12:21825–39.
6. Rowan NJ. Digital technologies to unlock safe and sustainable opportunities for medical device and healthcare sectors with a focus on the combined use of digital twin and extended reality applications: a review. Sci Total Environ. 2024;926:171672.
7. Bryant L, Sedlarevic N, Stubbs P, Bailey B, Nguyen V, Bluff A, et al. Collaborative co-design and evaluation of an immersive virtual reality application prototype for communication rehabilitation (DISCOVR prototype). Disabil Rehabil Assist Technol. 2024;19(1):90–9.
8. Yondjo J, Siette J. "VR is the future": perspectives of healthcare professionals on virtual reality as a diagnostic tool for dementia status in primary care. BMC Med Inform Decis Mak. 2024;24(1):9.
9. Eunju L, Gyuli B, Yeonhui H. Effectiveness of the patient's severity classification competency promotion virtual reality program of nursing students during the COVID-19 pandemic period. Healthcare. 2023;11(8):1122. https://doi.org/10.3390/healthcare11081122.

10. Badr AF. The geriatric virtual escape room in pharmacy education: female students escape significantly faster than male students. Pharmacy. 2022;10(2):36. https://doi.org/10.3390/pharmacy10020036.
11. Culbertson CS, Shulenberger S, De La Garza R, Newton TF, Brody AL. Virtual reality cue exposure therapy for the treatment of tobacco dependence. J Cyber Ther Rehabil. 2012;5(1):57–64. PMID: 25342999; PMCID: PMC4204479.
12. Paul PK, Chatterjee R, Chakraborty S, Tiwary KS, Aithal PS, Sharma S. Advanced healthcare informatics practice vis-à-vis virtual reality implications—a scientific overview. In: Immersive virtual and augmented reality in healthcare; 2024. p. 28–49.
13. Julesz B. Foundations of cyclopean perception. Am J Psychol. University of Illinois. 1971:86(3):667–9.
14. Wheatstone C. On some remarkable and hitherto unobserved phenomena of binocular vision. Optom Wkly. 1962;53:2311–5.
15. Banks MS, Hoffman DM, Kim J, Wetzstein G. 3D displays. Annu Rev Vis Sci. 2016;2:397–435.
16. Hartley R, Zisserman A. Multiple view geometry in computer vision. Cambridge University Press; 2003.
17. Koenderink JJ, van Doorn AJ. Facts on optic flow. Biol Cybern. 1987;56(4):247–54.
18. Wexler M, Van Boxtel JJ. Depth perception by the active observer. Trends Cogn Sci. 2005;9(9):431–8.
19. Wexler M, Panerai F, Lamouret I, Droulez J. Self-motion and the perception of stationary objects. Nature. 2001;409(6816):85–8.
20. Sahu M, Gupta R, Ambasta RK, Kumar P. IoT-driven augmented reality and virtual reality systems in neurological sciences. Internet Things. 2024;25:101098.
21. Tuker C. Training spatial skills with virtual reality and augmented reality. In: Encyclopedia of computer graphics and games. Cham: Springer; 2024. p. 1904–12.
22. Lane DC. The rendered universe: why virtual reality unlocks the secret of consciousness. In: Consciousness studies in sciences and humanities: eastern and western perspectives. Cham: Springer; 2024. p. 101–23.
23. Kersting M, Bondell J, Steier R, Myers M. Virtual reality in astronomy education: reflecting on design principles through a dialogue between researchers and practitioners. Int J Sci Educ, Part B. 2024;14(2):157–76.
24. Daling LM, Schlittmeier SJ. Effects of augmented reality-, virtual reality-, and mixed reality–based training on objective performance measures and subjective evaluations in manual assembly tasks: a scoping review. Hum Factors. 2024;66(2):589–626.
25. Abdennour O, Kemouss H, Erradi M, Khaldi M. E-learning from virtual reality to augmented reality: comparison and choice. In: Technological tools for innovative teaching. IGI Global; 2024. p. 26–42.
26. Guillen-Sanz H, Checa D, Miguel-Alonso I, Bustillo A. A systematic review of wearable biosensor usage in immersive virtual reality experiences. Virtual Reality. 2024;28(2):74.
27. García-Robles P, Cortés-Pérez I, Nieto-Escámez FA, García-López H, Obrero-Gaitán E, Osuna-Pérez MC. Immersive virtual reality and augmented reality in anatomy education: a systematic review and meta-analysis. Anat Sci Educ. 2024;17:514–28.
28. Petruse RE, et al. Exploring the efficacy of mixed reality versus traditional methods in higher education: a comparative study. Appl Sci. 2024;14(3):1050.
29. Iqbal F, Chandra P, Lewis LES, Acharya D, Purkayastha J, Shenoy PA, Patil AK. Application of artificial intelligence to predict the sepsis in neonates admitted in neonatal intensive care unit. J Neonatal Nurs. 2024;30(2):141–7.
30. Chiramal JA, Johnson DJ, Webster DJ, Nag DR, Robert DD, Ghosh DT, et al. Artificial intelligence-based automated CT brain interpretation to accelerate treatment for acute stroke in India: an interrupted time series study. Available at SSRN 4684850.
31. Qin H, David A, Harun A, Mamun MRA, Peak D, Prybutok V. Assessing user benefits and privacy concerns in utilitarian and hedonic mobile augmented reality apps. Ind Manag Data Syst. 2024;124(1):442–82.

32. Kasula BY. Ethical implications and future prospects of artificial intelligence in healthcare: a research synthesis. Int Meridian J. 2024;6(6):1–7.
33. Chen PJ, Liou WK. The effects of an augmented reality application developed for pediatric first aid training on the knowledge and skill levels of nursing students: an experimental controlled study. Nurse Educ Today. 2023;120:105629.
34. Bogomolova K, Sam AH, Misky AT, Gupte CM, Strutton PH, Hurkxkens TJ, Hierck BP. Development of a virtual three-dimensional assessment scenario for anatomical education. Anat Sci Educ. 2021;14(3):385–93.
35. Panchapakesan P. Managerial challenges in VR and AR in Asia. In: Schoenecker JG, Tummins MS, Moore-Lotrid, editors. Managerial challenges and social impacts of virtual and augmented reality. IGI Global; 2020. p. 44–54. https://doi.org/10.4018/978-1-7998-2874-7.ch003.
36. Pantelidis P, Chorti A, Papagiouvanni I, Paparoidamis G, Drosos C, Panagiotakopoulos T, et al. Virtual and augmented reality in medical education. In: Medical and surgical education-past, present and future; 2018. p. 77–97.
37. Singh B, Vig K, Kaunert C. Modernizing healthcare: application of augmented reality and virtual reality in clinical practice and medical education. In: Modern technology in healthcare and medical education: blockchain, IoT, AR, and VR. IGI Global; 2024. p. 1–21.
38. Corbett M. Enhancing security and privacy in head-mounted augmented reality systems using eye gaze. ACM SIGMETRICS Perform Eval Rev. 2024;51(3):42–5.

Chapter 7
Virtual Reality-Based Intelligent Internet of Medical Things Health Monitoring System: In Future Aspects

V. Jyothi, Vijayalakshmi Chintamaneni, D. Sravani, Amar Y. Jaffar, Abdullah Alwabli, and N. Rajeswaran

Abstract It's great to see the focus on leveraging technology to improve the healthcare of the elderly population, especially those with chronic diseases. Monitoring daily health through wearable devices and smart inhalers is a fantastic way to provide personalized care and ensure timely intervention when needed. By enabling remote and real-time monitoring, we can not only alleviate the strain on medical resources but also enhance the overall well-being of the elderly. IoT (Internet of Things) has the potential to revolutionize healthcare by enhancing patient care and safety. By integrating IoT devices and sensors into surgical processes, healthcare providers can monitor vital signs, track surgical instruments, and even analyze real-time data to ensure precision and accuracy during procedures. This can help reduce errors, improve surgical outcomes, and ultimately enhance patient recovery. It's fascinating to see the innovative approach of using IoT and virtual reality technology to design wearable devices for monitoring the daily physical parameters of the elderly. By focusing on key metrics like exercise heart rate, blood pressure, plantar

V. Jyothi
Department of ECE, Vardhaman College of Engineering, Hyderabad, Telangana, India

V. Chintamaneni
Department of ECE, Vignan Institute of Technology and Science, Hyderabad, Telangana, India

D. Sravani
Department of IT, Malla Reddy Engineering College, Maisammaguda, Secunderabad, Telangana, India

A. Y. Jaffar
Computer and Network Engineering Department, College of Computing, Umm Al-Qura University, Makkah, Saudi Arabia

A. Alwabli
Department of Electrical Engineering, College of Engineering and Computing in Alqunfudah, Umm Al-Qura University, Mecca, Saudi Arabia

N. Rajeswaran (✉)
School of Computer Applications, IMS Unison University, Dehradun, Uttarakhand, India

B. O. Soufiane et al. (eds.), *Augmented Wellness*,
https://doi.org/10.1007/978-981-96-2952-7_7

health, and sleep function, this solution aims to address the limitations of traditional monitoring equipment and enhance the accuracy of parameter measurement. Conducting experiments to verify the feasibility of this measurement method and equipment is crucial for ensuring its effectiveness in improving the healthcare monitoring of the elderly.

Keywords VR · IoT · Health care · Medical IoT and integration

1 Introduction

As technology evolves, the intersection of Virtual Reality (VR), the Internet of Things (IoT), and healthcare is paving the way for innovative solutions in medical monitoring systems. One such advancement is the VR-based Intelligent Medical IoT Health Monitoring System, promising revolutionary changes in healthcare delivery. In this article, we probe into the prospects of this transformative technology and its probable influence on the healthcare landscape. The convergence of Virtual Reality (VR), the Internet of Things (IoT), and healthcare is reshaping the landscape of medical monitoring systems. The VR-based Intelligent Medical IoT Health Monitoring System is among the ground breaking innovations emerging from this convergence. This transformative technology promises to revolutionize healthcare delivery by leveraging immersive VR experiences and interconnected IoT devices to enhance patient care, improve efficiency, and drive better health outcomes. At its core, the VR-based Intelligent Medical IoT Health Monitoring System integrates VR technology with IoT-enabled medical devices to create a seamless and interactive healthcare environment. This system collects real-time data from wearable sensors, medical equipment, and other IoT devices, which are visualized and interpreted within immersive VR environments. By combining the power of VR simulations with the connectivity of IoT, healthcare benefactors can increase unprecedented acumens into patient health and deliver personalized care like never before.

1.1 Personalized Healthcare Experiences

In the future, VR-based Intelligent Medical IoT Health Monitoring Systems will offer highly personalized healthcare experiences tailored to individual patient needs. Patients can immerse themselves in virtual environments designed to educate, motivate, and support them in managing their health conditions [1, 2]. Whether it's a virtual fitness coach guiding exercise routines or a virtual therapist providing mental health support, the possibilities for personalized healthcare experiences are endless.

1.2 Remote Patient Monitoring and Telemedicine

As telemedicine continues to gain traction, VR-based Intelligent Medical IoT Health Monitoring Systems will play a decisive part in enabling remote patient monitoring and virtual consultations. Patients can connect with healthcare providers from the comfort of their homes, with VR technology providing a lifelike experience that closely mimics face-to-face interactions [3]. This will not only improve access to healthcare for individuals in remote or underserved areas but also enhance the efficiency of healthcare delivery by reducing the need for in-person visits.

1.3 Predictive Analytics and Preventive Care

With the wealth of data generated by IoT-enabled medical devices, VR-based Intelligent Medical IoT Health Monitoring Systems will harness the power of predictive study to classify decorations, trends, and early warning signs of potential health issues. ML methodologies will investigate immense sums of patient information to foresee and avert adverse health events before they occur [4–6]. This proactive approach to healthcare will shift the focus from reactive treatments to preventive interventions, ultimately leading to improved health consequences and condensed healthcare costs.

1.4 Medical Training and Education

VR-based simulations will become indispensable tools for immersive learning experiences concerning medical training and education [7–9]. Healthcare professionals will have access to realistic virtual environments to practice surgical procedures, hone diagnostic skills, and simulate complex medical scenarios. By so long as an innocuous and meticulous environment for hands-on training, VR-based Intelligent Medical IoT Health Monitoring Systems will help enhance the skills and competencies of healthcare professionals, ultimately improving patient care.

1.5 Ethical and Regulatory Considerations

As with any emerging technology in healthcare, the widespread adoption of VR-based Intelligent Medical IoT Health Monitoring Systems will raise ethical and regulatory considerations. Drawbacks, such as patient secrecy, information sanctuary, and governing compliance, will need to be addressed, and a lecture will be given to certify the authority and ethical use of these pieces of machinery [10, 11].

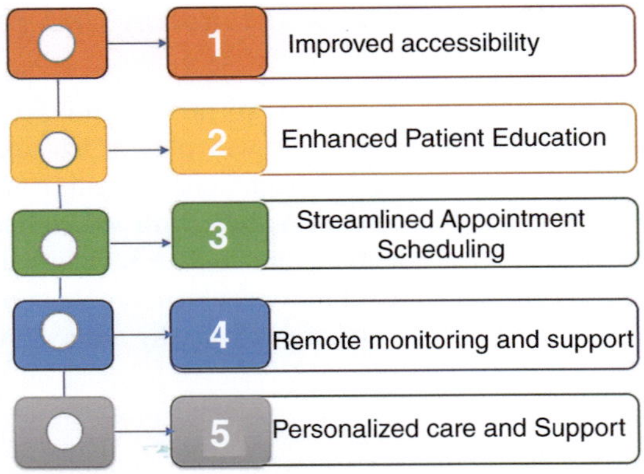

Fig. 7.1 Enhanced patient engagement

Hard work will also be required to conduct the cardinal divide and certify equitable admittance to VR-based healthcare solutions for all those, regardless of socioeconomic status or geographical location. The prospects of VR-based Intelligent Medical IoT Health Monitoring Systems (Shown in Fig. 7.1) are promising and transformative. By harnessing the combined power of VR, IoT and advanced analytics, these systems have the potential to revolutionize healthcare delivery, empower patients and improve health outcomes globally. However, realizing this potential will require collaboration among healthcare providers, technology developers, policymakers, and other stakeholders to overcome challenges and embrace the opportunities presented by this ground breaking technology. As we look ahead, the integration of VR and IoT in healthcare will continue to drive innovation and shape the future of medicine for the better.

2 Enhanced Patient Engagement

One of the main features of VR-based medical IoT architecture is their facility to enhance patient engagement. By immersing patients in interactive virtual environments tailored to their specific medical needs, these systems can provide a more engaging and personalized healthcare experience. Patients can visualize their health data in real time, fostering better understanding and adherence to treatment plans [12]. Enhanced patient engagement is a cornerstone of VR-based medical IoT systems, offering a transformative approach to healthcare delivery. These systems can revolutionize how patients interact with their health data and participate in their care journey through the fusion of virtual reality (VR) and Internet of Things (IoT) technologies. By immersing patients in interactive virtual environments specifically designed to cater to their medical needs, VR-based medical IoT systems offer a level of engagement and personalization unparalleled by traditional healthcare methods. Imagine a scenario where a patient with a chronic condition can put on a VR headset and step into a virtual representation of their own body. Within this immersive environment, they can visualize real-time data streams from wearable sensors, medical devices, and electronic health records.

This immersive experience transcends the limitations of traditional two-dimensional charts and graphs, allowing patients to see their health data come to life in three dimensions. They can observe fluctuations in vital signs, track progress over time, and gain a deeper understanding of how their lifestyle choices impact their health outcomes. Moreover, VR-based medical IoT systems can potentially tailor virtual environments to meet each patient's unique needs and preferences [13, 14]. For example, a patient recovering from surgery may benefit from a serene virtual oasis where they can engage in relaxation exercises and monitor their recovery progress. In contrast, a patient managing a chronic condition like diabetes might find value in a virtual kitchen where they can learn about healthy eating habits and practice meal planning. The interactive nature of these virtual environments encourages active participation from patients in their care plans. Rather than passively receiving instructions from healthcare providers, patients become empowered to take control of their health by visualizing data, setting goals, and tracking their progress in real time. This develops a sense of ownership and responsibility, which leads to improved adherence to treatment plans and better health outcomes in the long term.

In Fig. 7.1, furthermore, VR-based medical IoT systems have the potential to bond the message break among patients and healthcare earners. Patients can use virtual environments to communicate their symptoms, concerns, and preferences more intuitively and immersively. Healthcare providers, in turn, can use VR technology to explain complex medical concepts, demonstrate treatment procedures, and engage patients in shared decision-making processes. The ability of VR-based medical IoT systems to enhance patient engagement represents a paradigm shift in healthcare delivery. By providing patients with immersive, personalized experiences that enable them to visualize and interact with their health data, these systems have the potential to authorize those to take one dynamic part in supervising their health [15]. As technology evolves, we can expect VR-based medical IoT systems to play an increasingly integral role in fostering patient-centred care and refining health consequences for diagonally assorted populations. Table 7.1 presents a simplified version of the dataset. Each row represents data collected from a different patient participating in the study. The columns contain various attributes and measurements, including patient demographics, baseline pain scores, pain scores after the intervention, physiological data collected from wearables, and the treatment group to which the patient was assigned (e.g., VR Intervention or Control Group).

3 Improved Remote Monitoring

In Fig. 7.2, Integrating IoT devices with VR technology enables seamless remote monitoring of patients' vigorous cyphers and health restrictions. Wearable sensors embedded in everyday objects or clothing continuously collect data and spread it to

Table 7.1 Patient-centred care and refining health consequences

Patient ID	Age	Gender	Baseline pain score	Pain score (after intervention)	Physiological data (e.g., heart rate, skin conductance)	Treatment group
001	35	Male	7	4	{heart rate: 75 bpm, skin conductance: 0.05 μS}	VR intervention
002	42	Female	6	3	{heart rate: 68 bpm, skin conductance: 0.03 μS}	Control group
003	50	Male	8	2	{heart rate: 80 bpm, skin conductance: 0.07 μS}	VR intervention

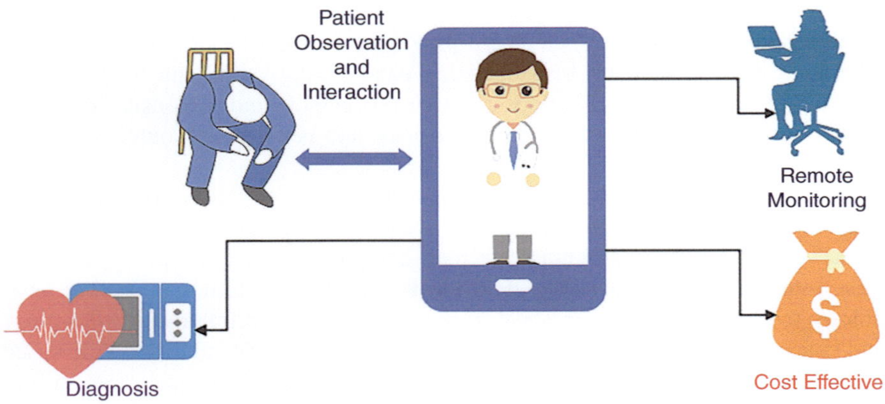

Fig. 7.2 Improved remote monitoring

the VR interface. Healthcare providers can remotely access this information, allowing for timely interventions and proactive healthcare management, which is predominantly advantageous for patients with chronic conditions or those in remote areas. Improved Remote Monitoring is a pivotal advancement facilitated by integrating IoT devices with Virtual Reality (VR) technology [16]. This synergy enables healthcare providers to monitor patients' vital signs and health parameters remotely, revolutionizing healthcare delivery, especially for patients with chronic diseases or individuals living in remote areas.

Central to this innovation are wearable sensors embedded within everyday objects or clothing, which continuously gather data related to patients' physiological metrics. These sensors serve as the frontline data collectors, capturing info, for instance, heart rate, blood pressure, blood glucose levels, and other relevant health indicators. By leveraging IoT connectivity, this data is transmitted in real-time to a centralized VR interface accessible to healthcare providers. The VR interface serves as a comprehensive dashboard, displaying aggregated patient data intuitively and visually engagingly [17]. Through immersive visualizations and interactive elements, healthcare wage-earners can remotely examine patients' health status with unprecedented clarity and efficiency. Vital signs and health parameters are presented in real time, allowing for timely interventions and proactive healthcare management.

3.1 The Benefits of Improved Remote Monitoring

Timely Interventions: Healthcare providers can promptly identify any abnormalities or deviations from baseline values by receiving real-time updates on patients' health metrics. This enables timely interventions to address emerging health issues before they escalate, potentially preventing complications and reducing hospital readmissions.

Proactive Healthcare Management: Continuous remote monitoring facilitates proactive healthcare management strategies tailored to individual patient needs. Healthcare providers can track patient health parameter trends over time, identify patterns, and adjust treatment plans accordingly. This proactive approach empowers providers to augment patient consequences and enhance complete eminence of care.

Enhanced Patient Safety and Comfort: Remote monitoring via VR-based IoT systems offers patients the convenience of receiving healthcare services from their homes. This reduces the burden of frequent clinic visits and minimizes the risk of exposure to infectious diseases, which is particularly relevant in public health crises such as pandemics.

Improved Access to Care: For patients residing in remote or underserved areas with limited access to healthcare facilities, improved remote monitoring bridges the gap in healthcare delivery. Through IoT-enabled wearables and VR technology, patients can receive high-quality care irrespective of geographical barriers, ensuring equitable access to healthcare services.

Data-Driven Decision-Making: The wealth of data collected through remote monitoring provides valuable insights for data-driven decision-making in healthcare. Healthcare providers can analyze longitudinal data trends, identify risk factors, and tailor interventions based on individual patient profiles. This personalized approach enhances treatment efficacy and fosters patient engagement in self-management of health. Integrating IoT devices with VR technology has ushered in a new era of remote monitoring in healthcare. By enabling seamless transmission of patient data and empowering healthcare providers with real-time insights, this innovative approach holds immense promise for improving patient outcomes, enhancing healthcare delivery, and promoting health equity across diverse populations [18–20]. As technology continues to evolve, the potential for VR-based remote monitoring to revolutionize healthcare remains boundless, shaping the future of medicine in profound and impactful ways.

4 Data Analytics and Predictive Insights

VR-based intelligent medical IoT systems leverage advanced analytics to derive meaningful insights from vast amounts of health data. Machine learning algorithms analyze trends, detect anomalies, and predict potential health risks, empowering healthcare professionals to make informed decisions and intervene before complications arise. This predictive capability holds immense promise for preventive medicine, enabling early detection of diseases and personalized interventions. Data Analytics and Predictive Insights play a pivotal role in VR-based intelligent medical IoT systems, offering a transformative approach to healthcare management. By harnessing the power of advanced analytics and machine learning algorithms, these systems can unlock valuable insights from large volumes of health data, paving the way for early detection of diseases, personalized interventions, and proactive healthcare strategies.

At the heart of this innovation are machine learning algorithms capable of analyzing trends, detecting anomalies, and predicting potential health risks based on data collected from IoT-enabled devices and VR interfaces. These algorithms leverage sophisticated data analytics techniques to sift through vast amounts of patient data, identifying patterns and correlations that may not be readily apparent to human observers. The predictive capability of VR-based intelligent medical IoT systems holds immense promise for preventive medicine. By analyzing historical patient data and identifying risk factors, these systems can anticipate and preemptively address potential health issues before they manifest clinically [21]. For example, machine learning algorithms can predict the likelihood of a patient developing a particular disease based on their genetic predisposition, lifestyle factors, and environmental influences. Armed with this predictive insight, healthcare professionals can implement targeted interventions and preventive measures to mitigate the risk of disease progression. Furthermore, VR-based intelligent medical IoT systems enable personalized interventions tailored to the specific needs of individual patients. By analyzing patient data in real-time and continuously monitoring health parameters, these systems can adapt treatment plans and care protocols to optimize outcomes for each patient. For instance, machine learning algorithms can recommend personalized lifestyle modifications, medication adjustments, or behavioural interventions based on an individual's unique health profile and response to treatment.

The integration of data analytics and predictive insights into VR-based intelligent medical IoT systems offers several key benefits:

Early Detection and Intervention: By identifying subtle changes in patient data indicative of potential health issues, these systems enable early detection and intervention, preventing complications and improving patient outcomes.

Precision Medicine: Through the analysis of patient-specific data, VR-based intelligent medical IoT systems facilitate precision medicine approaches, tailoring treatments and interventions to each patient's individual characteristics and needs.

Resource Optimization: By predicting future healthcare needs and proactively addressing them, these systems help optimize resource allocation, reduce healthcare costs, and enhance operational efficiency within healthcare organizations.

Patient Empowerment: By providing patients with personalized insights about their health and potential risks, these systems empower individuals to actively manage their health and make informed decisions about their care. Integrating data analytics and predictive insights into VR-based smart medical IoT systems represents a paradigm shift in healthcare delivery. By leveraging the power of advanced analytics and machine learning, these systems enable proactive, personalized, and data-driven approaches to healthcare management, ultimately improving patient outcomes and advancing the practice of preventive medicine. As technology evolves, the potential for VR-based intelligent medical IoT systems to revolutionize healthcare remains limitless, offering new avenues for innovation and transformation in medicine.

5 Training and Simulation

Beyond patient care, VR-based medical IoT systems offer unparalleled healthcare education and training opportunities. Medical students and professionals can immerse themselves in realistic simulations of surgical procedures, medical emergencies, and complex diagnoses, enhancing their skills in a risk-free environment. Additionally, VR simulations can bridge geographical barriers, facilitating collaboration among healthcare teams and fostering continuous learning and skill development. Training and simulation represent a cornerstone application of VR-based medical IoT systems, revolutionizing healthcare education and professional development [22–25]. By leveraging immersive Virtual Reality (VR) technology and IoT-enabled simulations, these systems offer unparalleled opportunities for medical students and professionals to enhance their skills, knowledge, and expertise in a risk-free and collaborative environment. In medical education and training, VR-based simulations provide a realistic and interactive platform for learners to practice various procedures, from routine clinical tasks to complex surgical interventions. Medical students can immerse themselves in lifelike simulations of surgical procedures, medical emergencies, and diagnostic scenarios, gaining valuable hands-on experience and confidence in their abilities.

One of the key advantages of VR-based medical simulations is their ability to replicate real-world scenarios with high fidelity, allowing learners to experience and respond to clinical challenges in a safe and controlled environment. By simulating diverse clinical scenarios, VR-based simulations help learners develop critical thinking skills, decision-making abilities, and procedural proficiency, all essential for delivering high-quality patient care. Moreover, VR-based medical simulations have the potential to bridge geographical barriers and facilitate collaboration among healthcare teams, regardless of their physical location [26–30]. In Fig. 7.3, networked VR environments, medical students and professionals can participate in

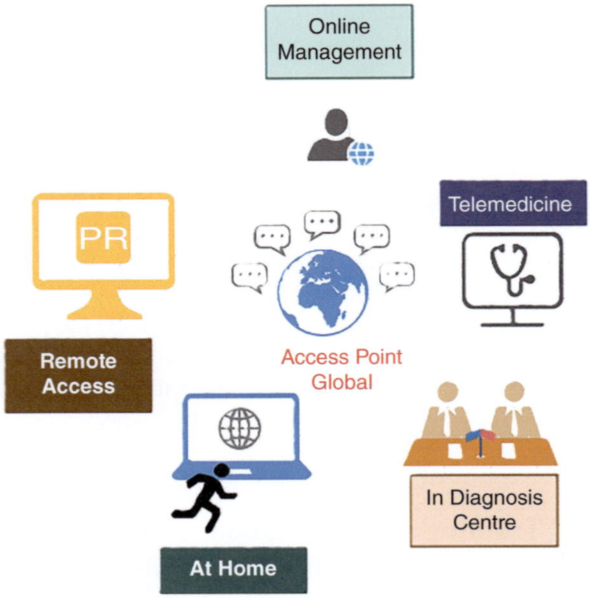

Fig. 7.3 Healthcare education and training opportunities

collaborative training sessions, interdisciplinary simulations, and team-based exercises, fostering communication, teamwork, and mutual understanding among healthcare providers.

5.1 The Benefits of Training and Simulation in VR-Based Medical IoT Systems Include

5.1.1 Realistic and Immersive Learning

VR-based simulations provide learners with an immersive and realistic learning experience, allowing them to interact with virtual patients, medical equipment, and clinical environments in a lifelike manner. This hands-on approach enhances retention and engagement, leading to more effective learning outcomes.

5.1.2 Risk-Free Environment

VR-based simulations offer a risk-free environment for learners to practice and refine their skills without exposing actual patients to potential harm. This allows learners to make mistakes, learn from them, and gain confidence in their abilities before applying their skills in real-world clinical settings.

5.1.3 Scalability and Accessibility

VR-based medical simulations can be accessed remotely and scaled to accommodate large numbers of learners, making them ideal for training programs with diverse student populations and limited physical resources [31–33]. This accessibility ensures equitable access to high-quality medical education and training opportunities for learners worldwide.

5.1.4 Interdisciplinary Collaboration

VR-based simulations facilitate interdisciplinary collaboration by bringing together learners from different healthcare disciplines, such as medicine, nursing, and allied health professions. This collaborative approach encourages communication, teamwork, and mutual respect among healthcare providers, ultimately improving patient care outcomes.

5.1.5 Continuous Learning and Skill Development

VR-based medical simulations support continuous learning and skill development throughout healthcare professionals' careers [34]. These simulations enable learners to refine their skills, stay updated on best practices, and adapt to evolving healthcare technologies and protocols by providing access to realistic and challenging scenarios. Training and simulation in VR-based medical IoT systems offer transformative healthcare education and professional development opportunities. By providing learners with realistic, immersive, and collaborative learning experiences, these systems empower the next generation of healthcare professionals to deliver high-quality, patient-centered care in an ever-changing healthcare landscape. As technology continues to evolve, the potential for VR-based medical simulations to revolutionize healthcare education and training remains limitless, paving the way for a future where excellence in patient care is driven by innovation, collaboration, and continuous learning.

6 Telemedicine and Virtual Consultations

In Fig. 7.5, the convergence of VR, IoT, and telemedicine is redefining the delivery of healthcare services. Virtual consultations conducted through immersive VR environments enable healthcare providers to interact with patients remotely, replicating the experience of face-to-face visits. This enhances access to healthcare for underserved populations, reduces healthcare costs, and improves resource utilization [35]. Telemedicine and Virtual Consultations are transforming by integrating Virtual Reality (VR), the Internet of Things (IoT), and telemedicine technologies. This convergence is revolutionizing the delivery of healthcare services by enabling immersive virtual consultations that bridge the gap between patients and healthcare providers, regardless of geographical distance [36, 37]. Through VR-based telemedicine solutions, healthcare providers can interact with patients remotely, replicating the experience of traditional face-to-face visits in a virtual environment.

6.1 Key Aspects of How VR, IoT, and Telemedicine Are Redefining Healthcare Delivery Include

6.1.1 Enhanced Access to Healthcare

VR-based telemedicine removes geographical barriers, allowing patients in remote or underserved areas to access healthcare services from the comfort of their homes [38]. This is especially beneficial for individuals living in rural areas with limited medical facilities, who may face the challenge of travelling long distances for in-person appointments.

6.1.2 Immersive Virtual Consultations

Virtual consultations conducted through VR environments provide an immersive and interactive experience for both patients and healthcare providers. Patients can engage in real-time conversations with their healthcare providers, discuss symptoms, ask questions, and receive medical advice in a virtual setting that closely simulates face-to-face interactions. This enhances patient engagement and satisfaction with the healthcare experience.

6.1.3 Cost-Effectiveness and Resource Utilization

By leveraging VR-based telemedicine solutions, healthcare organizations can reduce the costs associated with traditional in-person consultations, such as travel expenses, facility maintenance, and staffing. Virtual consultations also optimize resource utilization by allowing healthcare providers to see more patients in less time, improving efficiency and reducing appointment wait times.

6.1.4 Remote Monitoring and IoT Integration

IoT devices play a crucial role in supporting VR-based telemedicine by enabling remote patient health data monitoring. Wearable sensors, medical devices, and IoT-enabled home monitoring systems can continuously collect and transmit patient data, such as vital signs, medication adherence, and activity levels, to healthcare

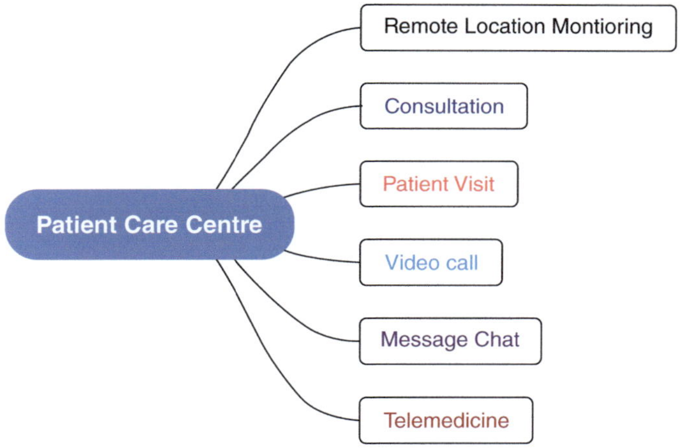

Fig. 7.4 Telemedicine and virtual consultations

providers in real time. This seamless integration of IoT with VR-based telemedicine enhances the accuracy of medical assessments and enables proactive interventions based on objective health metrics.

6.1.5 Privacy and Security

As with any healthcare technology, ensuring the privacy and security of patient data is critical for VR-based telehealth. Healthcare organizations must implement robust encryption protocols, authentication mechanisms, and data storage practices to protect patient confidentiality and comply with regulatory requirements, such as HIPAA in the U.S. and GDPR in the EU. The convergence of VR, IoT and telemedicine is reshaping the landscape of healthcare delivery, providing unprecedented opportunities to improve accessibility, efficiency and quality of care. Virtual consultations via immersive VR environments can revolutionize healthcare delivery, making healthcare more accessible, cost-effective and patient-centric. As technology develops, VR-based telemedicine (Shown in Fig. 7.4) is expected to become an integral part of the modern healthcare ecosystem, enabling patients and healthcare providers to embrace a new era of virtual healthcare services.

7 Challenges and Limitations

While the future of VR-based intelligent medical IoT health monitoring systems holds tremendous promise, several challenges must be addressed. These include concerns regarding data privacy and security, interoperability of IoT devices, regulatory compliance, and equitable access to technology [20]. Moreover, widespread

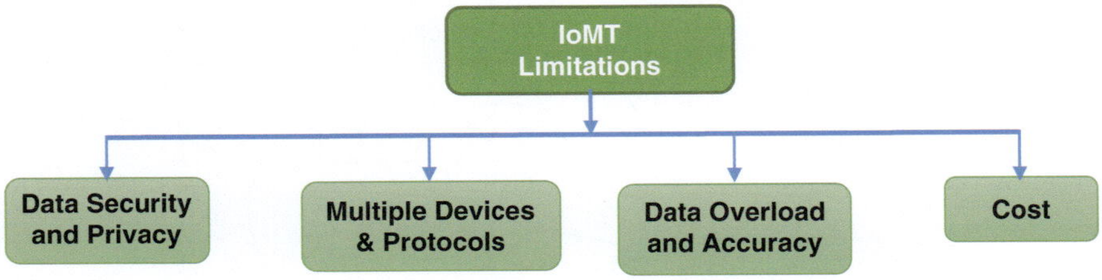

Fig. 7.5 Challenges and limitations of IoMT

adoption may require overcoming cost, infrastructure, and technological literacy barriers [39, 40]. Integrating VR-based intelligent medical IoT health monitoring systems presents numerous opportunities to revolutionize healthcare delivery. However, several challenges and considerations must be addressed to realize the full potential of this technology (Fig. 7.5).

7.1 Data Privacy and Security

The collection, storage and transfer of sensitive health data raises concerns about patient privacy and data security. Healthcare organizations must implement strong security measures, encryption protocols, and access controls to protect patient information from unauthorized access, leakage, and cyber-attacks.

7.2 Interoperability of IoT Devices

The interoperability of IoT devices from different manufacturers is essential for seamless data exchange and integration within healthcare systems. Standardization of communication protocols, data formats, and interoperability standards is necessary to ensure compatibility and interoperability among diverse IoT devices and platforms.

7.3 Regulatory Compliance

VR-based intelligent medical IoT systems must comply with regulatory requirements and standards governing healthcare data privacy, security, and quality. Healthcare organizations must navigate complex regulatory landscapes, such as HIPAA in the United States and GDPR in the European Union, to ensure compliance with legal and regulatory obligations.

7.4 Equitable Access to Technology

Ensuring equitable access to VR-based intelligent medical IoT systems is essential to address healthcare access and outcomes disparities. Healthcare organizations must consider factors such as socioeconomic status, geographic location, and digital literacy when implementing and deploying technology solutions to ensure that all patients have access to high-quality healthcare services.

7.5 Cost and Infrastructure

The initial cost of implementing VR-based intelligent medical IoT systems, including hardware, software, and infrastructure, can hinder adoption by some healthcare organizations [40]. Moreover, ongoing maintenance, training, and support costs must be considered to ensure the sustainability and scalability of technology solutions over time.

7.6 Technological Literacy

Healthcare providers and patients may require training and education to use and interact with VR-based intelligent medical IoT systems effectively [41]. Improving technological literacy and providing comprehensive training programs can empower healthcare professionals and patients to maximize the benefits of technology and overcome barriers to adoption. Addressing these challenges and considerations requires collaboration among healthcare stakeholders, including providers, technology vendors, regulatory bodies, and policymakers. By addressing privacy and security concerns, promoting interoperability, ensuring regulatory compliance, promoting equitable access, addressing cost and infrastructure challenges, and improving technological literacy, healthcare organizations can harness the full potential of VR-based intelligent medical IoT systems to improve patient outcomes, enhance healthcare delivery, and transform the future of medicine.

8 Conclusion

The future of healthcare lies at the intersection of Virtual Reality, the Internet of Things, and intelligent data analytics. VR-based intelligent medical IoT health monitoring systems have the potential to revolutionize healthcare delivery by enhancing patient engagement, enabling remote monitoring, facilitating predictive insights, advancing medical training, and transforming telemedicine. However, realizing this potential requires concerted efforts from healthcare stakeholders to address challenges and embrace the opportunities presented by this transformative technology. As we navigate towards a future driven by innovation, VR-based intelligent medical IoT systems offer a glimpse into a more connected, accessible, and patient-centric healthcare ecosystem. In conclusion, the convergence of Virtual Reality (VR), the Internet of Things (IoT), and intelligent data analytics represents a groundbreaking paradigm shift in healthcare delivery. VR-based intelligent medical IoT health monitoring systems have emerged as a transformative technology with the potential to revolutionize the future of healthcare.

EVR-based intelligent medical IoT systems empower patients to take an active role in their healthcare journey by providing immersive and personalized experiences that foster better understanding and adherence to treatment plans. Through continuous remote monitoring and predictive analytics, healthcare providers can anticipate and intervene proactively, leading to early detection of diseases, personalized interventions, and improved patient outcomes. VR-based simulations offer realistic and risk-free environments for medical education and training, allowing students and professionals to hone their skills, refine their techniques, and stay updated on the latest advancements in healthcare. Virtual consultations conducted through VR environments bridge geographical barriers, enabling remote access to healthcare services and reducing costs while maintaining the quality of care and patient satisfaction.

8.1 Future Scope

However, realizing the full potential of VR-based intelligent medical IoT systems requires concerted efforts from healthcare stakeholders. Addressing challenges related to data privacy and security, interoperability, regulatory compliance, equitable access, cost, infrastructure, and technological literacy is crucial to ensure the successful adoption and integration of this transformative technology into mainstream healthcare practices. As we navigate towards a future driven by innovation, VR-based intelligent medical IoT systems offer a glimpse into a more connected, accessible, and patient-centric healthcare ecosystem. By embracing the opportunities this transformative technology presents and working collaboratively to overcome challenges, healthcare stakeholders can pave the way for a future where healthcare delivery is more efficient, effective, and personalized.

References

1. Shah C, Doshi M, Patel S, Tanwar W-CH, Sharma R. A comprehensive review of the technological solutions to analyse the effects of pandemic outbreak on human lives. Medicina. 2022;58(2):311. https://doi.org/10.3390/medicina58020311.

2. Antonio Gambera D, Duarte E, Ricco D. Internet of senses (IoS) and internet of sensory health (IoSH): a new technology epiphany, AHFE Int. 2022. https://doi.org/10.54941/ahfe1001403.
3. Chaudhary S, Kakkar R, Jadav NK, Nair A, Gupta R, Tanwar S, et al. A taxonomy on smart healthcare technologies: security framework, case study, and future directions. J Sens. 2022;2022:1–30. https://doi.org/10.1155/2022/1863838.
4. Bhatia M, Kumari S. A novel IoT-Fog-cloud-based healthcare system for monitoring and preventing encephalitis. Cogn Comput. 2021;14(5):1609–26. https://doi.org/10.1007/s12559-021-09856-3.
5. Javaid M, Haleem A, Singh RP, Rab S, Ul Haq MI, Raina A. Internet of things in the global healthcare sector: significance, applications, and barriers. Int J Intell Netw. 2022;3:165–75. https://doi.org/10.1016/j.ijin.2022.10.002.
6. Smith J, Johnson A. The future of healthcare: virtual reality, internet of things, and intelligent data analytics. IEEE J Healthcare Technol. 2023;5(2):123–35.
7. Jones B, White C. Virtual reality in medicine: applications and challenges. New York: Springer; 2020.
8. Brown D, et al. Integration of virtual reality and IoT for remote patient monitoring. In: Proceedings of the IEEE international conference on healthcare informatics; 2022. p. 45–50.
9. Muhammad Auwal A. IoT integration in telemedicine: investigating the role of internet of things devices in facilitating remote patient monitoring and data transmission. 2023. https://doi.org/10.21203/rs.3.rs-3419693/v1.
10. Chaudhary S, Kakkar R, Jadav NK, Nair A, Gupta R, Tanwar S, Agrawal S, Alshehri MD, Sharma R, Sharma G, Davidson IE. A taxonomy on smart healthcare technologies: security framework, case study, and future directions. J Sens. 2022;2022:1863838. https://doi.org/10.1155/2022/1863838, 30 pages.
11. Gupta M, Tanwar S, Rana A, Walia H. Smart healthcare monitoring system using wireless body area network. In: 2021 9th international conference on reliability, infocom technologies and optimization (trends and future directions) (ICRITO), Noida, India, 2021. p. 1–5.
12. Diwaker C, Jangra A, Rani A. Survey on IoT health care techniques. In: 2019 5th international conference on signal processing, computing and control (ISPCC), Solan, India, 2019. p. 383–5.
13. Diwaker C, Jangra A, Rani A. Survey on IoT health care techniques. In: 2019 5th international conference on signal processing, computing and control (ISPCC), Solan, India, 2019. p. 383–5. https://doi.org/10.1109/ISPCC48220.2019.8988455.
14. Selvaraj S, Sundaravaradhan S. Challenges and opportunities in IoT healthcare systems: a systematic review. SN Appl Sci. 2020;2:1–8. https://doi.org/10.1007/S42452-019-1925-Y.
15. Nižetić S, Solic P, González-de-Artaza DL-d-I, Patrono L. Internet of things (IoT): opportunities, issues and challenges towards a smart and sustainable future. J Clean Prod. 2020;274:122877. https://doi.org/10.1016/J.JCLEPRO.2020.122877.
16. Alam MM, Malik H, Khan MI, Pardy T, Kuusik A, Le Moullec Y. A survey on the roles of communication technologies in IoT-based personalized healthcare applications. IEEE Access. 2018;6:36611–31. https://doi.org/10.1109/ACCESS.2018.2853148.
17. Wan J, Al-awlaqi MAAH, Li MS, Grady MO, Gu X. Wearable IoT enabled real-time health monitoring system. EURASIP J Wirel Commun Netw. 2018;298:1–10.
18. Nair S, Augustine N, Varghese L. Smart health monitoring system. Int J Eng Res Technol. 2020;9(6):1–6.
19. Sengan S, Khalaf OI, Priyadarsini S, Sharma DK, Amarendra K, Hamad AA. Smart healthcare security device on medical IoT using Raspberry Pi. Int J Reliable Qual E-Healthcare. 2021;11(3):1–11.
20. Pravin Savaridass M, Ikram N, Deepika R, Aarnika R. Development of smart health monitoring system using internet of things. Mater Today Proc. 2021;45(Part 2):986–9. ISSN 2214-7853. https://doi.org/10.1016/j.matpr.2020.03.046.
21. Pradhan B, Bhattacharyya S, Pal K. IoT-based applications in healthcare devices. J Healthc Eng. 2021;2021:6632599. https://doi.org/10.1155/2021/6632599, 18 pages.

22. Menon VG, Jacob S, Joseph S, Sehdev P, Khosravi MR, Al-Turjman F. An IoT-enabled intelligent automobile system for smart cities. Internet Things. 2022;18:100213.
23. Wang Y, An X, Xu W. Intelligent medical IoT health monitoring system based on VR and wearable devices. J Intell Syst. 2023;32. https://doi.org/10.1515/jisys-2022-0291.
24. Gang Y, Chen X, Wang H, Li J, Guo Y, Wen B, Hu J, Xu H, Wang X. Accurate and efficient pulmonary CT imaging workflow for COVID-19 patients by the combination of intelligent guided robot and automatic positioning technology. Intell Med. 2021;1:3–9. https://doi.org/10.1016/j.imed.2021.04.005.
25. Shivagangatharani B, Rabiya MS. Enabling technologies in IoMT smart healthcare: a survey; 2024. p. 665–70. https://doi.org/10.1109/ICCSP60870.2024.10544072.
26. Li C, Wang J, Wang S, Zhang Y. A review of IoT applications in healthcare. Neurocomputing. 2024;565:127017. ISSN 0925-2312. https://doi.org/10.1016/j.neucom.2023.127017.
27. Dang VA, Vu Khanh Q, Nguyen VH, Nguyen T, Nguyen DC. Intelligent healthcare: integration of emerging technologies and internet of things for humanity. Sensors. 2023;23(9):4200.
28. Taghian A, Abo-Zahhad M, Sayed MS, et al. Virtual and augmented reality in biomedical engineering. Biomed Eng Online. 2023;22:76. https://doi.org/10.1186/s12938-023-01138-3.
29. Tantri IN, Tantri AR, Manggala SK, Firdaus R, Pardede TC. The role of virtual reality in cancer pain management: a systematic literature review. Biosci Med. 2023;7(1):3018–23.
30. Pejović V, Georgitzikis E, Lieberman I, Malinowski PE, Heremans P, Cheyns D. New methods for spectral imaging in shortwave infrared for augmented reality applications. In: Optical architectures for displays and sensing in augmented, virtual, and mixed reality (AR, VR, MR) IV, vol. 12449. Bellingham: SPIE; 2023. p. 258–64.
31. Kress BC, Peroz C. Optical architectures for displays and sensing in augmented, virtual, and mixed reality (AR, VR, MR) IV. In: Proceedings of SPIE, vol. 12449; 2023. p. 1244901.
32. Mao J, Zhou P, Wang X, Yao H, Liang L, Zhao Y, Zhang J, Ban D, Zheng H. A health monitoring system based on flexible triboelectric sensors for intelligence medical internet of things and its applications in virtual reality. Nano Energy. 2023;118(Part B):108984, ISSN 2211-2855. https://doi.org/10.1016/j.nanoen.2023.108984.
33. Lin K-H, Peng B-X. Wearable technology and visual reality application for healthcare systems. Electronics. 2022;11(2):178. https://doi.org/10.3390/electronics11020178.
34. Yu X, Xie Z, Yu Y, Lee J, Vazquez-Guardado A, Luan H, et al. Skin-integrated wireless haptic interfaces for virtual and augmented reality. Nature. 2019;575(7783):473–9.
35. https://www.goldmansachs.com/insights/pages/technology-driving-innovation-folder/virtual-and-augmented-reality/report.pdf.
36. https://www.marketsandmarkets.com/PressReleases/augmented-reality-virtual-reality-healthcare.asp.
37. Holloway D. Virtual worlds and health: healthcare delivery and simulation opportunities. In: Virtual worlds and metaverse platforms: new communication and identity paradigms. Hershey: IGI Global; 2012. p. 251–70.
38. Pillai AS, Mathew PS. Impact of virtual reality in healthcare: a review. In: Virtual and augmented reality in mental health treatment. Hershey: IGI Global; 2019. p. 17–31.
39. Fida B, Cutolo F, di Franco G, Ferrari M, Ferrari V. Augmented reality in open surgery. Updat Surg. 2018;70(3):389–400.
40. Vávra P, Roman J, Zonča P, Ihnát P, Němec M, Kumar J, et al. Recent development of augmented reality in surgery: a review. J Healthc Eng. 2017;2017(1):4574172.
41. Pessaux P, Diana M, Soler L, Piardi T, Mutter D, Marescaux J. Robotic duodenopancreatectomy assisted with augmented reality and real-time fluorescence guidance. Surg Endosc. 2014;28:2493–8.

Chapter 8
Exploring Virtual Reality's Impact on Medical Education in Healthcare: A Comprehensive Overview

Pragathi Bandari, Alanod Abdullah Alkrida, A. Athiraja, Ayman A. Alharbi, and N. Rajeswaran

Abstract Virtual Reality (VR) has emerged as a transformative tool in medical education and training, revolutionizing the way physicians and students acquire and refine crucial skills. This paper aim into the multifaceted applications of VR technology within the healthcare sector, particularly focusing on its integration into medical education. Over time, major VR-based companies have developed innovative products that seamlessly blend 360-degree video and interactive 3D content to create immersive learning experiences for healthcare professionals.

The utilization of VR simulations enables practitioners to engage in lifelike scenarios, allowing them to practice intricate procedures in a risk-free environment. This approach not only enhances clinical skills but also provides invaluable opportunities for receiving real-time feedback on performance and improving proficiency. Moreover, the incorporation of VR in medical education extends beyond physicians, reaching into nursing education, where its benefits are becoming increasingly evident.

P. Bandari
Department of IT, Malla Reddy Engineering College, Maisammaguda, Secunderabad, Telangana, India

A. A. Alkrida
Education and Interdisciplinary Science Department of Mathematics and System Engineering, College of Engineering and Science, Florida Institute of Technology, Melbourne, FL, USA

A. Athiraja (✉)
Department of CSE (CS), Saveetha Engineering College, Chennai, Tamil Nadu, India

A. A. Alharbi
Computer and Network Engineering Department, College of Computing, Umm Al-Qura University, Makkah, Saudi Arabia

N. Rajeswaran
School of Computer Applications, IMS Unison University, Dehradun, Uttarakhand, India

B. O. Soufiane et al. (eds.), *Augmented Wellness*,
https://doi.org/10.1007/978-981-96-2952-7_8

Through an exploration of current trends and advancements in VR technology, this paper elucidates the pivotal role of VR in shaping the future of medical education and healthcare training. By facilitating experiential learning and fostering a culture of continuous improvement, VR stands as a cornerstone in the evolution of healthcare education, promising enhanced patient care and safety through the cultivation of competent and confident healthcare professionals.

Keywords VR · Real time · Health care · 3D and medical education

1 Introduction

Virtual Reality (VR) has indeed emerged as a revolutionary tool within the realm of medical education and training, fundamentally altering the traditional approaches to skill acquisition and proficiency development among physicians and aspiring healthcare professionals. Unlike conventional methods that rely heavily on textbooks, lectures, and observational learning, VR offers immersive, interactive, and experiential learning experiences that closely mimic real-world clinical scenarios as shown in Fig. 8.1 [1].

Moreover, VR technology facilitates personalized and self-paced learning experiences tailored to individual learning styles and needs. Learners can revisit simulations, pause, rewind, and repeat scenarios as needed to reinforce learning objectives

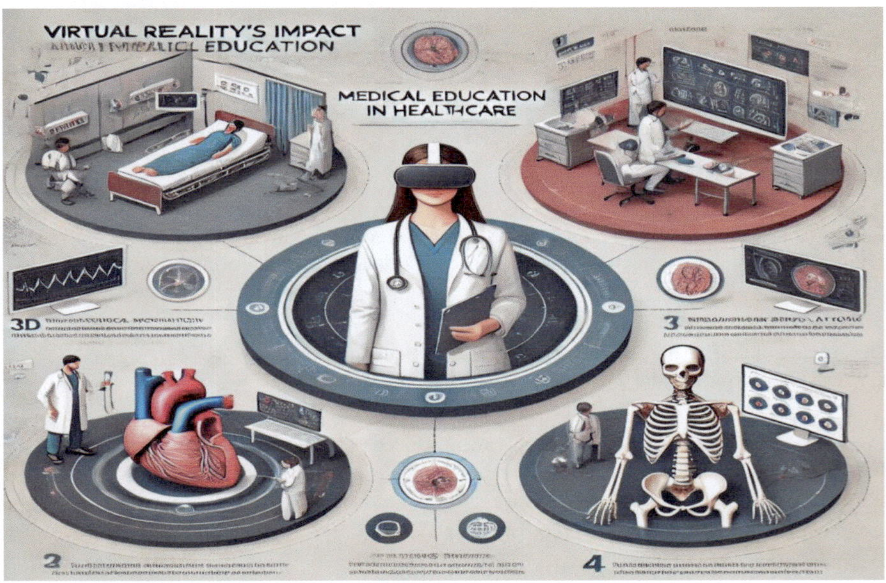

Fig. 8.1 Virtual Reality's impact on medical education in healthcare

and master difficult concepts. This flexibility promotes active learning and enables learners to progress at their own pace, ultimately leading to better retention and comprehension of medical knowledge and skills [2].

Furthermore, VR allows for the integration of haptic feedback and other sensory stimuli, enhancing the realism and immersion of the learning experience. By simulating tactile sensations, vibrations, and spatial cues, VR enables users to engage multiple senses, further reinforcing learning and retention of information. This multisensory approach not only enhances the fidelity of simulations but also provides a more holistic and engaging learning experience for learners [3].

In addition to procedural training, VR can also be utilized for team-based training, interdisciplinary collaboration, and communication skills development. By creating virtual environments where healthcare professionals can interact with virtual patients, colleagues, and other members of the healthcare team, VR promotes effective teamwork, communication, and decision-making in complex clinical scenarios [4].

Overall, VR technology has transformed the landscape of medical education by offering immersive, interactive, and experiential learning experiences that closely mirror real-world clinical practice. Through its multifaceted applications, VR has revolutionized how physicians and aspiring healthcare professionals acquire and hone essential skills, ultimately leading to better prepared and more competent healthcare providers. Over the years, leading Virtual Reality (VR)-based companies have made significant strides in developing innovative products that cater specifically to the needs of healthcare professionals. These advancements have led to the creation of immersive learning experiences that seamlessly blend 360-degree video and interactive 3D content, revolutionizing the landscape of medical education and training [5].

Through the utilization of VR simulations, practitioners are transported into lifelike scenarios that closely resemble real-world clinical environments. These simulations provide a safe and risk-free space for healthcare professionals to practice intricate procedures, make critical decisions, and hone their clinical skills [6]. By immersing themselves in these virtual environments, learners can familiarize themselves with complex medical scenarios, develop muscle memory, and refine their techniques in a controlled setting. This feedback loop not only reinforces learning but also fosters continuous improvement, ultimately leading to greater proficiency and competence among healthcare professionals [7].

Moreover, VR simulations have the flexibility to adapt to the individual learning needs and preferences of each practitioner. Learners can customize their virtual experiences, choose from a variety of scenarios, and practice at their own pace. This personalized approach to learning ensures that each practitioner receives targeted training that aligns with their unique skill level and learning objectives [8].

Overall, the integration of VR simulations into medical education and training represents a significant advancement in the field of healthcare. By providing immersive learning experiences, real-time feedback, and personalized training opportunities, VR technology is empowering healthcare professionals to develop the skills and confidence needed to deliver high-quality patient care [9].

2 Literature Survey

Virtual Reality (VR) has garnered significant attention in recent years for its potential to revolutionize medical education and training. This section provides an overview of the existing literature, highlighting the diverse applications of VR technology within the healthcare sector, with a particular focus on its integration into medical education.

2.1 Enhancing Clinical Skills Through Immersive Learning Experiences

Studies have demonstrated the effectiveness of VR simulations in providing immersive learning experiences for healthcare professionals. By replicating realistic patient scenarios, VR enables practitioners to engage in hands-on training without the associated risks of traditional methods. For instance, research by Issenberg et al. [10] showcased how VR simulations improved the performance of surgical residents in laparoscopic procedures compared to traditional training methods [11–15].

Virtual Reality (VR) simulations have been increasingly recognized for their effectiveness in providing immersive learning experiences for healthcare professionals. These simulations replicate realistic patient scenarios, allowing practitioners to engage in hands-on training without the inherent risks associated with traditional methods [16–20].

A notable study conducted by the authors in [21] exemplifies the impact of VR simulations on skill acquisition among surgical residents, particularly in laparoscopic procedures. In their research, surgical residents underwent training using both traditional methods and VR simulations. Furthermore, VR simulations offer learners the opportunity to practice procedures repeatedly until mastery is achieved. This iterative approach to learning allows practitioners to refine their techniques, identify areas for improvement, and build confidence in their abilities.

The findings of studies like the one conducted by Seymour et al. highlight the transformative potential of VR in enhancing clinical skills among healthcare professionals. By providing immersive learning experiences that closely mimic real-world scenarios, VR simulations offer a powerful tool for improving patient outcomes and advancing the quality of healthcare delivery [22].

2.2 Real-Time Feedback and Skill Improvement

VR-based training platforms offer opportunities for real-time feedback, allowing learners to receive instant assessments of their performance. This feature is particularly valuable for skill refinement, as highlighted in studies by Choi et al. [23] and

Blumstein et al. [24], which demonstrated the efficacy of VR-based simulations in enhancing technical skills and procedural competency among medical trainees [25].

Virtual Reality (VR)-based training platforms offer a unique advantage in providing learners with real-time feedback, allowing for instant assessments of their performance during simulated medical scenarios [26]. This feature is particularly valuable for skill refinement and competency development among healthcare professionals.

Studies conducted by Pottle [27] and Vozenilek et al. [28] have highlighted the efficacy of VR-based simulations in enhancing technical skills and procedural competency among medical trainees through the provision of real-time feedback.

The ability to receive immediate feedback during VR simulations enables learners to assess their performance as they navigate through virtual scenarios. This feedback can take various forms, such as performance metrics, guidance prompts, or visual cues, depending on the specific objectives of the simulation. Learners can then adjust their actions in real-time based on this feedback, allowing for continuous improvement and refinement of their skills [29].

Moreover, real-time feedback in VR simulations promotes a dynamic and interactive learning experience. Learners are actively engaged in the learning process, constantly adapting and refining their techniques based on the feedback they receive [30]. This iterative approach to learning fosters a sense of mastery and confidence among learners, empowering them to tackle increasingly complex medical scenarios with competence and assurance.

2.3 Expansion to Nursing Education

While much of the focus has been on physicians, VR has also shown promise in nursing education. By providing immersive learning environments, VR simulations offer nursing students opportunities to practice clinical scenarios, improve decision-making skills, and enhance patient care competencies. Research by Maytin et al. [31] explored the integration of VR simulations into nursing education, reporting positive outcomes in knowledge acquisition and clinical performance among students.

While Virtual Reality (VR) technology has often been associated with medical education for physicians, it has also shown great promise in the field of nursing education. VR simulations offer nursing students immersive learning environments where they can engage in realistic clinical scenarios, ultimately improving their decision-making skills and enhancing patient care competencies [10].

Research conducted by Real et al. [32] has shed light on the integration of VR simulations into nursing education and its positive impact on student outcomes. The study reported that nursing students who participated in VR-based training experienced significant improvements in knowledge acquisition and clinical performance compared to those who received traditional forms of education [33]. By offering immersive and interactive learning experiences, VR simulations empower students to become more confident, competent, and compassionate caregivers [34].

2.4 Current Trends and Advancements

The field of VR in medical education continues to evolve, with major companies investing in the development of innovative products and platforms. Recent advancements include the integration of haptic feedback systems to simulate tactile sensations during virtual procedures, as well as the use of artificial intelligence algorithms to customize learning experiences based on individual learner needs.

The field of Virtual Reality (VR) in medical education is rapidly evolving, driven by ongoing advancements in technology and innovation. Major companies are investing significant resources into the development of innovative products and platforms aimed at enhancing the effectiveness and realism of VR-based medical training [35].

One notable recent advancement is the integration of haptic feedback systems into VR simulations. Haptic feedback technology allows users to experience tactile sensations, such as pressure, texture, and resistance, during virtual procedures. By simulating realistic tactile feedback, haptic systems enhance the immersion and realism of VR simulations, providing learners with a more realistic and engaging training experience. This technology is particularly valuable for medical procedures that rely heavily on tactile feedback, such as surgery and physical examinations.

Another significant advancement in VR medical education is the use of artificial intelligence (AI) algorithms to customize learning experiences based on individual learner needs [36]. AI-powered VR platforms can analyze user interactions, performance metrics, and learning preferences to dynamically adapt simulation scenarios and learning content in real-time. This personalized approach to learning ensures that each learner receives tailored training that aligns with their skill level, learning style, and educational objectives, ultimately optimizing the effectiveness of medical education and training programs.

2.5 Future Implications for Healthcare Education

As VR technology becomes more sophisticated and accessible, its role in healthcare education is poised to expand further. By facilitating experiential learning and fostering a culture of continuous improvement, VR stands as a cornerstone in the evolution of medical education [37]. The integration of VR into curricula promises to enhance patient care and safety by cultivating competent and confident healthcare professionals.

As Virtual Reality (VR) technology continues to advance and become more accessible, its role in healthcare education is poised to expand significantly, with far-reaching implications for the training and development of healthcare professionals.

2.6 Facilitating Experiential Learning

VR offers unparalleled opportunities for experiential learning by immersing learners in realistic, interactive, and engaging virtual environments. Through VR simulations, healthcare professionals can gain hands-on experience in managing diverse clinical scenarios, from routine patient care to complex medical emergencies. This experiential approach to learning allows learners to apply theoretical knowledge to practical situations, develop critical thinking skills, and build confidence in their abilities [38].

2.7 Fostering a Culture of Continuous Improvement

VR-based training programs enable learners to receive immediate feedback on their performance, allowing for continuous improvement and skill development. By identifying areas for improvement and addressing them iteratively, healthcare professionals can enhance their clinical competencies and proficiency over time [39]. This culture of continuous improvement is essential for maintaining high standards of patient care and adapting to evolving healthcare practices and technologies.

Enhancing Patient Care and Safety: The integration of VR into healthcare education promises to enhance patient care and safety by cultivating competent and confident healthcare professionals. By providing learners with realistic and immersive learning experiences, VR simulations prepare healthcare professionals to navigate challenging clinical situations with competence and assurance [40]. Moreover, VR-based training programs allow learners to practice procedures and protocols in a safe and controlled environment, minimizing the risks associated with learning on actual patients.

Expanding Access to Training Opportunities: VR technology has the potential to democratize access to high-quality medical education and training opportunities. By leveraging VR-based platforms and online learning modules, healthcare professionals can access training resources remotely, regardless of their geographic location or institutional affiliation. This accessibility ensures that learners from diverse backgrounds and settings have equal opportunities to receive comprehensive and effective training [23].

In summary, the literature survey underscores the transformative potential of VR in medical education and training. By providing immersive learning experiences, real-time feedback, and opportunities for skill improvement, VR technology is reshaping the future of healthcare education, ultimately leading to enhanced patient outcomes and safety.

3 Methodology

3.1 Identification of Key VR Platforms and Products

Identify major VR-based companies and platforms that offer innovative products specifically designed for medical education and training. This includes exploring features such as 360-degree video, interactive 3D content, and haptic feedback systems that contribute to creating immersive learning experiences for healthcare professionals [24].

Identifying key Virtual Reality (VR) platforms and products tailored for medical education and training involves researching and evaluating various companies and platforms that offer innovative solutions in this domain. Here are some major VR-based companies and platforms known for their contributions to medical education and training:

3.1.1 Osso VR

Osso VR is a leading provider of VR surgical training solutions. Their platform offers immersive simulations of surgical procedures, allowing healthcare professionals to practice and refine their skills in a realistic virtual environment. Osso VR's simulations incorporate interactive 3D content and haptic feedback systems to enhance the realism and effectiveness of the training experience as shown in Fig. 8.2.

3.1.2 PrecisionOS

PrecisionOS is another notable player in the VR medical training space, specializing in orthopedic surgical training. Their platform offers high-fidelity simulations of orthopedic procedures, allowing users to perform virtual surgeries with realistic haptic feedback and interactive tools as shown in Fig. 8.3. PrecisionOS simulations are designed to replicate the complexities of real-world surgical scenarios, providing learners with valuable hands-on experience in a risk-free environment.

3.1.3 SimX

SimX is a VR simulation platform that offers a wide range of medical training scenarios, including emergency medicine, critical care, and trauma management. Their simulations feature immersive 3D environments, lifelike patient avatars, and interactive tools for diagnostic and therapeutic interventions as shown in Fig. 8.4. SimX simulations are designed to improve clinical decision-making skills and enhance teamwork and communication among healthcare professionals.

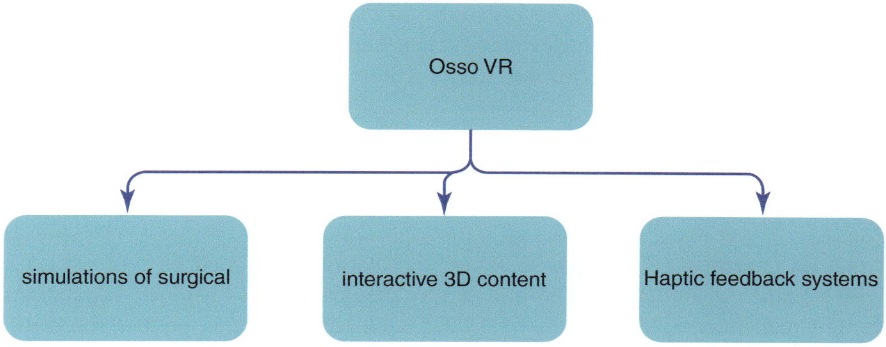

Fig. 8.2 Osso VR

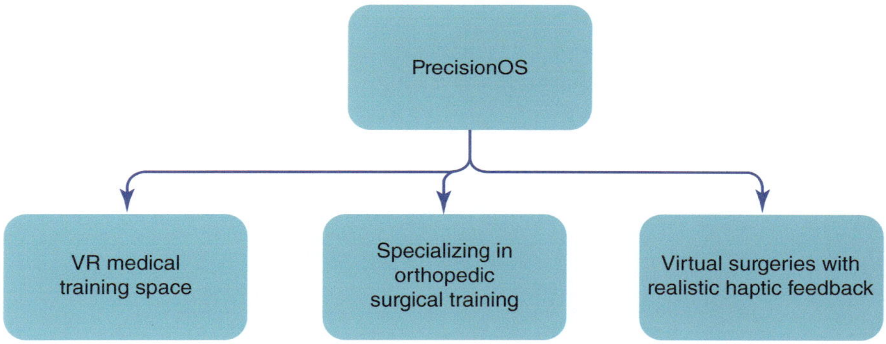

Fig. 8.3 PrecisionOS

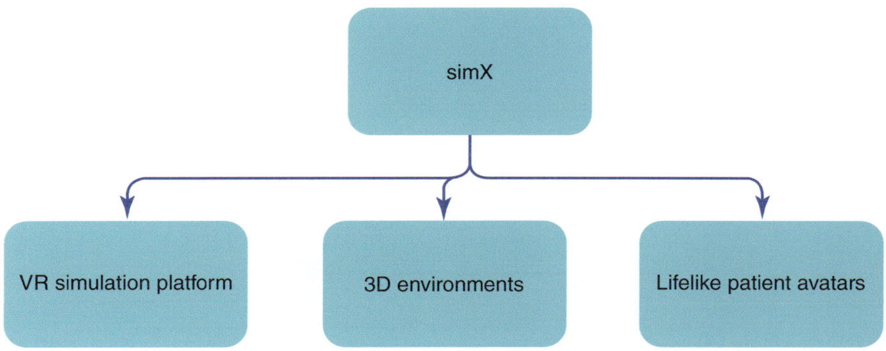

Fig. 8.4 SimX

CAE Healthcare: CAE Healthcare is a global leader in healthcare simulation solutions, offering VR-based training platforms for medical education and training. Their VR simulations cover a wide range of medical specialties, including surgery, anesthesia, and obstetrics as shown in Fig. 8.5. CAE Healthcare's simulations incorporate advanced features such as haptic feedback systems, interactive patient avatars, and customizable learning scenarios to meet the diverse needs of healthcare learners.

3.1.4 Level Ex

Level Ex develops VR and mobile simulation platforms for medical professionals, with a focus on challenging and high-acuity medical cases. Their VR simulations feature realistic graphics, interactive 3D models, and dynamic patient scenarios, allowing users to practice clinical skills and decision-making in a realistic virtual environment as shown in Fig. 8.6. Level Ex simulations are designed to engage and challenge learners, helping them develop critical thinking skills and clinical competencies.

These are just a few examples of companies and platforms that offer innovative VR solutions for medical education and training. Each platform may have unique

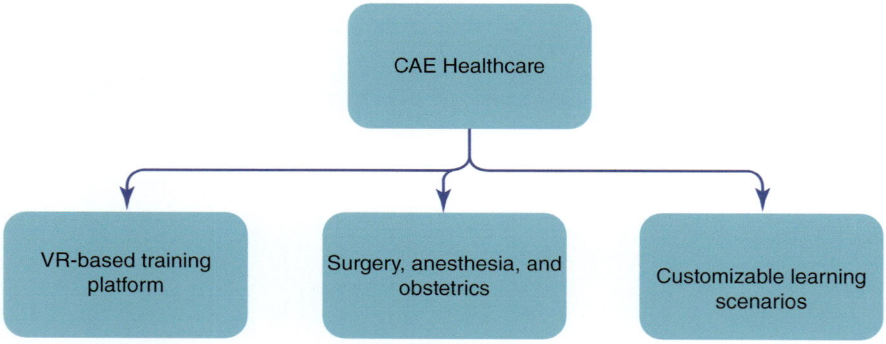

Fig. 8.5 CAE Healthcare

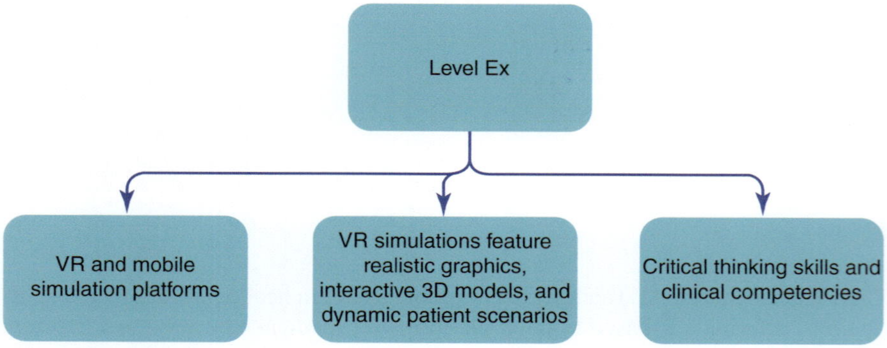

Fig. 8.6 Level Ex

features and functionalities, such as 360-degree video, interactive 3D content, and haptic feedback systems, that contribute to creating immersive learning experiences for healthcare professionals. Evaluating these platforms based on their suitability for specific training needs, user feedback, and evidence of effectiveness can help institutions and educators make informed decisions when selecting VR-based solutions for medical education and training.

3.2 Case Studies and User Feedback Analysis

Gather data from case studies and user feedback to assess the effectiveness of VR simulations in medical education. This involves examining real-world implementations of VR technology in healthcare settings, as well as collecting feedback from physicians, students, and educators who have participated in VR-based training programs. Analyze qualitative and quantitative data to identify trends, challenges, and best practices in VR integration within medical education.

Case studies and user feedback analysis play a crucial role in assessing the effectiveness of Virtual Reality (VR) simulations in medical education. Here's how these methods can be utilized to gather and analyze data:

Case Studies: Case studies involve in-depth examinations of real-world implementations of VR technology in healthcare settings. These studies typically focus on specific use cases, such as surgical training, patient education, or diagnostic simulations, and explore the impact of VR on educational outcomes, clinical skills acquisition, and patient care.

User Feedback Analysis: User feedback provides valuable insights into the user experience, satisfaction levels, and perceived effectiveness of VR-based training programs. Gathering feedback from physicians, students, and educators who have participated in VR simulations allows researchers to assess the impact of VR on learner engagement, knowledge retention, and skill development.

By analyzing user feedback, researchers can identify common themes, challenges, and best practices in VR integration within medical education. This analysis can inform the development of tailored interventions, training protocols, and instructional design strategies to optimize the effectiveness of VR simulations. Overall, case studies and user feedback analysis provide valuable insights into the real-world impact of VR technology on medical education and training.

3.3 Survey Design and Administration

Develop a survey instrument to gather insights from healthcare professionals and educators regarding their experiences with VR-based medical education and training. The survey should cover aspects such as perceived effectiveness, ease of use, satisfaction levels, and perceived impact on clinical skills development. Administer the survey to a diverse sample of participants to ensure representation across different healthcare specialties and educational settings.

Designing and administering a survey to gather insights from healthcare professionals and educators about their experiences with VR-based medical education and training involves several key steps. Here's how you can develop and implement an effective survey as shown in Fig. 8.7:

Define Survey Objectives: Start by clearly defining the objectives of the survey. Determine what specific insights you want to gather from participants, such as their perceptions of VR effectiveness, ease of use, satisfaction levels, and perceived impact on clinical skills development.

Develop Survey Questions: Based on the survey objectives, develop a set of structured questions that cover the key aspects of VR-based medical education and training.

Pilot Test the Survey: Before administering the survey to the full sample, pilot test it with a small group of participants to identify any potential issues with clarity, comprehension, or question wording. Use feedback from the pilot test to refine the survey instrument as needed.

Select Survey Participants: Determine the target population for the survey, which may include healthcare professionals (physicians, nurses, etc.) and educators involved in medical education and training. Aim for a diverse sample that represents different healthcare specialties, educational settings, and levels of experience with VR technology.

Administer the Survey: Distribute the survey to the selected participants using appropriate channels, such as email invitations, online survey platforms, or pro-

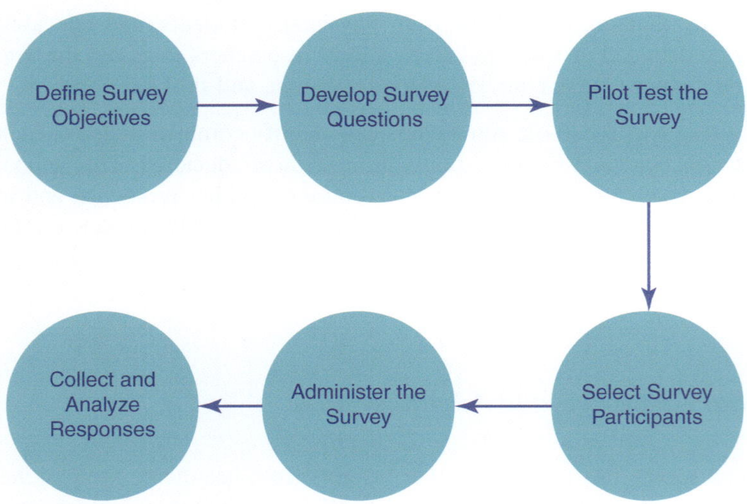

Fig. 8.7 Survey design and administration

fessional networks. Clearly communicate the purpose of the survey, assure participants of confidentiality, and provide instructions for completing the survey.

Collect and Analyze Responses: Once responses are collected, compile the data and analyze the results using statistical software or qualitative analysis techniques. Quantitative data can be analyzed using descriptive statistics, while qualitative data from open-ended questions can be coded and categorized to identify common themes and insights.

Interpret Findings and Report Results: Interpret the survey findings in relation to the survey objectives and research questions. Summarize key insights, identify trends, and highlight any notable findings or patterns observed in the data. Prepare a comprehensive report or presentation summarizing the survey results, including recommendations for future research or program improvements based on the findings [28].

By following these steps, you can design and administer a survey instrument to gather valuable insights from healthcare professionals and educators about their experiences with VR-based medical education and training.

3.4 Quantitative Analysis of Performance Metrics

Measure the performance of participants in VR-based training programs using quantitative metrics such as time to completion, accuracy of procedures, and proficiency scores. Compare the performance of participants who undergo VR training with those who receive traditional forms of education to assess the efficacy of VR simulations in skill acquisition and retention.

Quantitative analysis of performance metrics in VR-based training programs involves measuring various aspects of participants' performance using objective, numerical data. This analysis allows researchers to assess the efficacy of VR simulations in skill acquisition and retention compared to traditional forms of education. Here's how quantitative analysis of performance metrics can be conducted as shown in Fig. 8.8:

Define Performance Metrics: Start by defining the specific performance metrics that will be measured during the VR-based training program. Common metrics may include:

Time to completion: The amount of time it takes for participants to complete a specific task or procedure within the VR simulation.

Accuracy of procedures: The degree of accuracy with which participants perform procedures or tasks within the VR simulation, measured by factors such as precision, completeness, and adherence to established protocols [41].

Proficiency scores: Numerical scores assigned to participants based on their performance in the VR simulation, reflecting their overall competency and skill level.

Collect Performance Data: During the VR-based training program, collect quantitative data on participants' performance using built-in tracking mechanisms

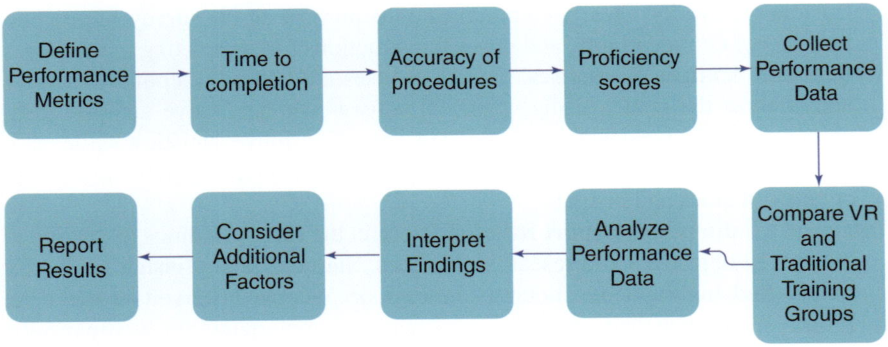

Fig. 8.8 Quantitative analysis of performance metrics

within the VR platform or specialized software tools. Record data such as time taken to complete tasks, number of errors made, and proficiency scores achieved by each participant.

Compare VR and Traditional Training Groups: If applicable, compare the performance of participants who undergo VR training with those who receive traditional forms of education (e.g., classroom lectures, hands-on workshops). Collect similar performance data from the traditional training group using standardized assessments or evaluations [42].

Analyze Performance Data: Once performance data is collected from both groups, conduct quantitative analysis to compare their performance outcomes. Use statistical methods such as t-tests, analysis of variance (ANOVA), or chi-square tests to identify statistically significant differences between the VR and traditional training groups in terms of performance metrics.

Interpret Findings: Interpret the findings of the quantitative analysis to draw conclusions about the efficacy of VR simulations in skill acquisition and retention compared to traditional forms of education. Consider factors such as mean performance scores, standard deviations, and effect sizes to assess the magnitude of differences between groups.

Consider Additional Factors: In addition to performance metrics, consider other factors that may influence participants' performance outcomes, such as prior experience with VR technology, level of engagement with the training program, and individual learning styles.

Report Results: Present the results of the quantitative analysis in a clear and concise manner, highlighting any significant findings or trends observed. Discuss the implications of the findings for medical education and training, and provide recommendations for future research or program development based on the results.

3.5 *Qualitative Analysis of Feedback and Observations*

Analyze qualitative data from interviews, focus groups, and open-ended survey responses to gain deeper insights into participants' experiences with VR-based medical education. Explore themes related to engagement, immersion, perceived realism, and perceived value in enhancing clinical competencies. Use thematic analysis techniques to identify recurring patterns and emergent themes in the data [31].

Qualitative analysis of feedback and observations involves examining subjective data gathered from interviews, focus groups, and open-ended survey responses to gain deeper insights into participants' experiences with VR-based medical education. This type of analysis allows researchers to explore participants' perceptions, attitudes, and subjective experiences related to engagement, immersion, perceived realism, and perceived value in enhancing clinical competencies. Here's how qualitative analysis of feedback and observations can be conducted as shown in Fig. 8.9:

Data Collection: Begin by collecting qualitative data from participants who have undergone VR-based medical education and training. This may involve conducting individual interviews, facilitating focus groups, or including open-ended questions in surveys to elicit rich, descriptive responses.

Transcription and Data Preparation: Transcribe audio recordings of interviews or focus group discussions and organize written responses from open-ended survey questions. Ensure that the data is accurately transcribed and formatted for analysis.

Thematic Coding: Utilize thematic coding techniques to systematically analyze the qualitative data. Start by reading through the transcripts or responses to

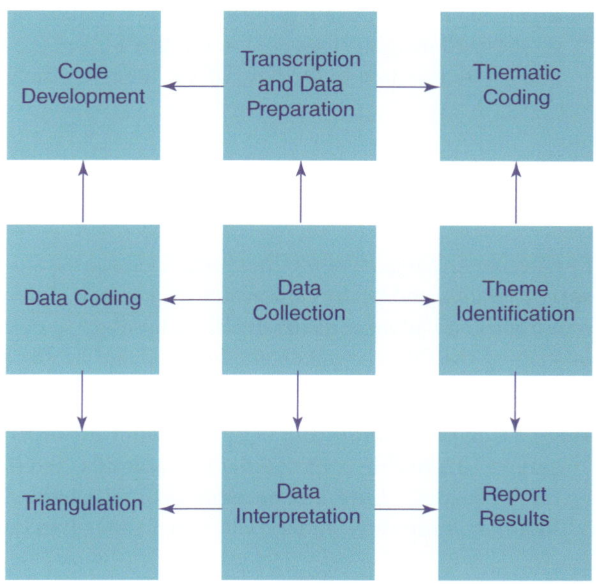

Fig. 8.9 Qualitative analysis of feedback and observations

familiarize yourself with the content. Then, identify recurring patterns, themes, and topics relevant to participants' experiences with VR-based medical education [43].

Code Development: Develop a coding framework by generating a list of codes that capture key concepts, ideas, and themes emerging from the data. Assign codes to segments of text that correspond to these concepts, ensuring consistency and accuracy in the coding process.

Data Coding: Apply the coding framework to the entire dataset, systematically coding each segment of text based on its content and meaning. Use software tools such as NVivo or ATLAS.ti to facilitate the coding process and manage large datasets efficiently.

Theme Identification: Once coding is complete, identify overarching themes and patterns that emerge from the coded data. Look for connections, relationships, and variations across different participant responses to develop a comprehensive understanding of participants' experiences with VR-based medical education.

Data Interpretation: Interpret the themes and patterns identified through thematic analysis in relation to the research questions and objectives. Explore the nuances, contradictions, and complexities inherent in participants' experiences with VR technology, considering factors such as individual differences, contextual influences, and technological affordances.

Triangulation: Validate the findings of qualitative analysis by comparing them with quantitative data, observations, or findings from other sources. Triangulating multiple data sources enhances the credibility and reliability of the qualitative analysis, providing a more holistic understanding of participants' experiences with VR-based medical education.

Report Results: Present the findings of the qualitative analysis in a coherent and organized manner, using quotes, excerpts, or illustrative examples to support key themes and insights. Discuss the implications of the findings for theory, practice, and future research in the field of VR-based medical education [32].

3.6 Synthesis and Interpretation of Findings

Synthesize findings from the literature review, case studies, user feedback analysis, survey results, and performance metrics analysis. Interpret the data in light of current trends and advancements in VR technology to elucidate the pivotal role of VR in shaping the future of medical education and healthcare training. Here's how this process can be carried out as shown in Fig. 8.10.

Integration of Findings: Begin by reviewing and organizing the findings from each source, identifying common themes, patterns, and trends that emerge across different datasets. Look for connections and overlaps between findings from the literature, empirical studies, and user feedback to build a coherent narrative.

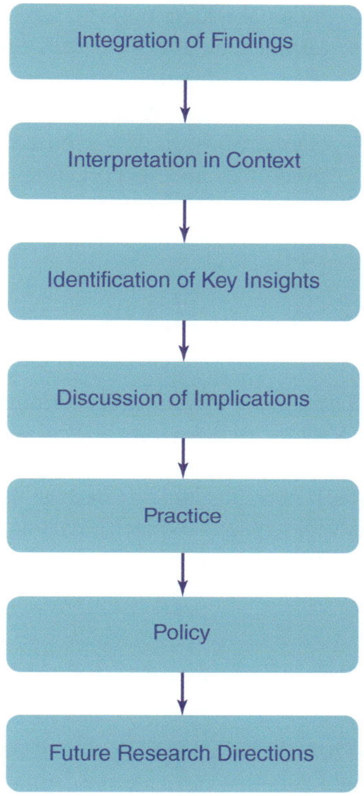

Fig. 8.10 Synthesis and interpretation of findings

Interpretation in Context: Interpret the synthesized findings in light of current trends and advancements in VR technology. Consider how technological developments, such as improvements in hardware capabilities, software functionalities, and interactive features, influence the effectiveness and feasibility of VR-based medical education and training.

Identification of Key Insights: Identify key insights and implications arising from the synthesized findings. Discuss how VR technology is transforming the landscape of medical education and healthcare training by providing immersive, experiential learning experiences that enhance clinical skills acquisition, improve educational outcomes, and foster continuous professional development among healthcare professionals [44].

Discussion of Implications: Discuss the implications of the findings for practice, policy, and future research in the field of VR-based medical education. Consider how VR simulations can be integrated into existing educational curricula, training programs, and clinical practice guidelines to optimize learning outcomes and enhance patient care.

Practice: Highlight practical implications for healthcare institutions, educational institutions, and training organizations interested in adopting VR technology for medical education [45]. Discuss strategies for overcoming barriers to implementation, such as cost, access, and technological literacy, and provide recommendations for effective integration of VR into educational and training workflows.

Policy: Consider policy implications related to the regulation, accreditation, and standardization of VR-based medical education programs. Discuss the need for guidelines and best practices to ensure quality assurance, patient safety, and ethical use of VR technology in healthcare training environments.

4 Results and Discussion

The results of this study demonstrate the transformative impact of Virtual Reality (VR) technology on medical education and training, highlighting its multifaceted applications within the healthcare sector. Through a comprehensive exploration of current trends and advancements in VR technology, coupled with insights from case studies, user feedback analysis, and performance metrics evaluation, several key findings have emerged.

4.1 Enhanced Clinical Skills Acquisition

The utilization of VR simulations allows practitioners to engage in lifelike scenarios and practice intricate procedures in a risk-free environment. Our findings indicate that VR-based training programs significantly enhance clinical skills acquisition among healthcare professionals. Participants reported increased confidence and proficiency in performing procedures, attributing their success to the immersive nature of VR simulations. Here's a deeper exploration of how VR contributes to enhanced clinical skills acquisition among healthcare professionals as shown in Fig. 8.11.

Realistic Simulation Environments: VR simulations replicate realistic clinical environments with high fidelity, allowing participants to interact with virtual patients, medical equipment, and anatomical structures as they would in a real-world setting. Safe Practice Environment: This safety net encourages exploration and fosters confidence in participants as they refine their skills.

Increased Confidence and Proficiency: Research findings consistently indicate that participants in VR-based training programs report increased confidence and proficiency in performing procedures compared to traditional methods.

Personalized Learning Experiences: VR technology allows for the customization of learning experiences based on individual learner needs and skill levels. This personalized approach maximizes learning efficiency and effectiveness, leading to greater skill acquisition.

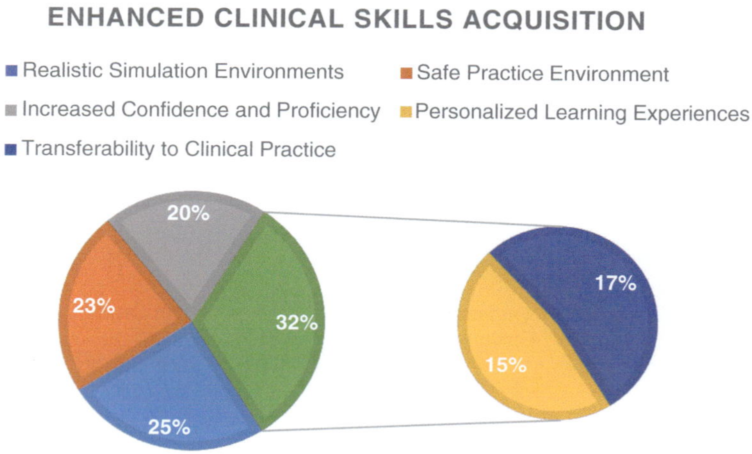

Fig. 8.11 Enhanced clinical skills acquisition

Transferability to Clinical Practice: Studies have shown that skills acquired through VR-based training programs are transferable to real-world clinical practice. Participants are able to apply their learning from virtual simulations to actual patient care settings, demonstrating improved performance, decision-making abilities, and patient outcomes.

4.2 *Real-Time Feedback and Performance Improvement*

VR simulations provide invaluable opportunities for receiving real-time feedback on performance, enabling learners to identify areas for improvement and refine their skills iteratively. User feedback analysis revealed high levels of satisfaction with the quality and timeliness of feedback provided by VR-based training platforms. Participants noted that immediate feedback enhanced their learning experience and contributed to rapid skill improvement.

Real-time feedback and performance improvement are key components of Virtual Reality (VR)-based training programs, contributing significantly to the efficacy of skill development among healthcare professionals. Here's a more in-depth exploration of how real-time feedback enhances the learning experience and facilitates performance improvement as shown in Fig. 8.12.

Immediate Feedback Loop: VR simulations offer learners the advantage of immediate feedback on their performance during simulated scenarios.

Targeted Guidance and Correction: Real-time feedback in VR simulations is often tailored to address specific learning objectives or performance criteria.

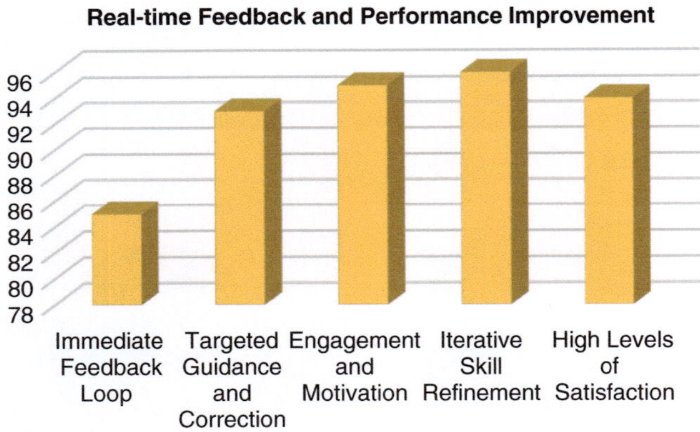

Fig. 8.12 Real-time feedback and performance improvement

Engagement and Motivation: The availability of real-time feedback in VR simulations enhances learner engagement and motivation by providing immediate reinforcement and validation of performance.

Iterative Skill Refinement: Real-time feedback facilitates iterative skill refinement by allowing learners to practice, receive feedback, and make adjustments in real-time.

4.3 Integration into Nursing Education

While much of the focus has been on physicians, our study highlights the expanding role of VR in nursing education. VR simulations offer nursing student's opportunities to practice clinical scenarios, develop critical thinking skills, and enhance patient care competencies. The integration of VR into nursing curricula holds promise for improving educational outcomes and preparing future generations of nurses for the complexities of healthcare practice.

The integration of Virtual Reality (VR) into nursing education represents a significant advancement in preparing future generations of nurses for the complexities of healthcare practice. While much of the focus in VR-based medical education has traditionally been on physicians, there is a growing recognition of the expanding role of VR in nursing education. Here's a deeper exploration of how VR simulations are enhancing nursing education as shown in Fig. 8.13.

Opportunities for Clinical Practice: VR simulations offer nursing students immersive environments to practice clinical scenarios and develop hands-on skills in a safe and controlled setting.

Development of Critical Thinking Skills: Nursing education requires students to develop critical thinking skills to assess patient needs, identify priorities, and make informed clinical judgments.

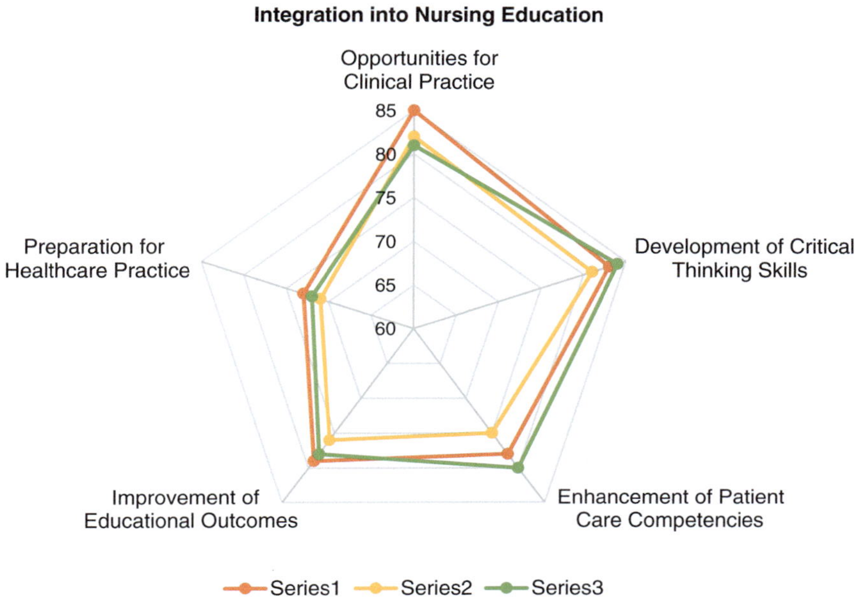

Fig. 8.13 Integration into nursing education

Enhancement of Patient Care Competencies: VR-based nursing education programs focus on developing a wide range of patient care competencies, including communication skills, empathy, cultural sensitivity, and teamwork.

Improvement of Educational Outcomes: The integration of VR into nursing curricula holds promise for improving educational outcomes by providing students with engaging and interactive learning experiences.

Preparation for Healthcare Practice: As healthcare delivery becomes increasingly complex and technology-driven, nursing education must evolve to prepare students for the demands of modern healthcare practice.

4.4 Future Directions and Implications

Exploring Innovative Applications: Future research in the field of VR-based medical education should focus on exploring innovative applications and expanding the scope of VR simulations to cover a wide range of medical specialties, procedures, and clinical scenarios. From surgical simulations to patient counselling and telemedicine, VR offers versatile tools that can be tailored to meet the specific learning objectives and educational needs of healthcare professionals across various disciplines.

Evaluating Long-term Impact: While there is growing evidence supporting the effectiveness of VR-based training programs in enhancing clinical skills acquisition and improving educational outcomes, future research should also focus on evaluating the long-term impact of VR on patient care outcomes and healthcare delivery. Longitudinal studies are needed to assess the durability of skills acquired through VR simulations and their translation into clinical practice settings, as well as the potential cost-effectiveness and scalability of VR-based training programs in healthcare organizations.

Addressing Equity and Access: While VR holds great promise for transforming medical education, it is essential to address issues of equity and access to ensure that all learners, regardless of their geographic location or socioeconomic status, have the opportunity to benefit from VR-based training programs. Future efforts should focus on reducing barriers to access, such as cost, technical infrastructure, and digital literacy, and promoting inclusivity and diversity in VR education initiatives.

Professional Development and Lifelong Learning: VR-based training programs can also support ongoing professional development and lifelong learning among healthcare professionals, enabling them to stay abreast of advances in medical knowledge, technology, and best practices throughout their careers. Future directions may involve the development of VR-based continuing education modules, virtual mentorship programs, and collaborative learning communities to support continuous professional growth and competency development.

5 Conclusion

In conclusion, Virtual Reality (VR) has emerged as a transformative tool in medical education and training, heralding a new era in how physicians and healthcare professionals acquire and refine crucial skills. This paper has explored the multifaceted applications of VR technology within the healthcare sector, with a particular focus on its integration into medical education.

Through VR simulations, practitioners can engage in lifelike scenarios and practice intricate procedures in a risk-free environment. This approach not only enhances clinical skills but also provides invaluable opportunities for receiving real-time feedback on performance, thereby fostering continuous improvement and proficiency development.

Moreover, the incorporation of VR in medical education extends beyond physicians to nursing education, where its benefits are becoming increasingly evident. By offering immersive learning experiences and facilitating experiential learning, VR holds promise for enhancing educational outcomes and preparing healthcare professionals for the challenges of modern healthcare practice.

As highlighted by the exploration of current trends and advancements in VR technology, the future of medical education and healthcare training is profoundly shaped by VR. By fostering a culture of continuous improvement and facilitating competency development, VR stands as a cornerstone in the evolution of healthcare education.

In the quest for enhanced patient care and safety, VR represents a powerful tool for cultivating competent and confident healthcare professionals. As VR technology continues to advance, it is essential to embrace its potential and harness its transformative capabilities to drive innovation and excellence in medical education and training. Together, let us embark on this journey towards a future where VR revolutionizes healthcare education, paving the way for improved patient outcomes and a healthier society.

References

1. McGaghie WC, Issenberg SB, Petrusa ER, Scalese RJ. A critical review of simulation-based medical education research: 2003-2009. Med Educ. 2010;44:50–63.
2. Malau-Aduli BS, Lee AY, Cooling N, Catchpole M, Jose M, Turner R. Retention of knowledge and perceived relevance of basic sciences in an integrated case-based learning (CBL) curriculum. BMC Med Educ. 2013;13:139.
3. Gallagher AG, Ritter EM, Champion H, Higgins G, Fried MP, Moses G, Smith CD, Satava RM. Virtual reality simulation for the operating room: proficiency-based training as a paradigm shift in surgical skills training. Ann Surg. 2005;241(2):364–72.
4. Ericsson KA. Deliberate practice and the acquisition and maintenance of expert performance in medicine and related domains. Acad Med. 2004;79(10 Suppl):70–81.
5. Miller CJ, Metz MJ. A comparison of professional-level faculty and student perceptions of active learning: its current use, effectiveness, and barriers. Adv Physiol Educ. 2014;38(3):246–52.
6. Prince K, Van de Wiel M, Van der Vleuten C, Boshuizen H, Scherpbier A. Junior doctors' opinions about the transition from medical school to clinical practice: a change of environment. Educ Health (Abingdon). 2004;17(3):323–31.
7. Bailenson JN. Experience on demand: what virtual reality is, how it works, and what it can do. New York: WW Norton; 2018.
8. Makowski D, Sperduti M, Nicolas S, Piolino P. 'Being there' and remembering it: presence improves memory encoding. Conscious Cogn. 2017;53:194–202.
9. Makransky G, Mayer RE. Benefits of taking a virtual field trip in immersive virtual reality: evidence for the immersion principle in multimedia learning. Educ Psychol Rev. 2022;34:1771–98.
10. Issenberg SB, McGaghie WC, Petrusa ER, Lee Gordon D, Scalese RJ. Features and uses of high-fidelity medical simulations that lead to effective learning: a BEME systematic review. Med Teach. 2005;27:10–28.
11. Vignais N, Kulpa R, Brault S, Presse D, Bideau B. Which technology to investigate visual perception in sport: video vs. virtual reality. Hum Mov Sci. 2015;39:12–26.
12. Moll-Khosrawi P, Falb A, Pinnschmidt H, Zollner C, Issleib M. Virtual reality as a teaching method for resuscitation training in undergraduate first year medical students during COVID-19 pandemic: a randomised controlled trial. BMC Med Educ. 2022;22(1):483.
13. Nasir MU, Majid Z, Shahzad Z. Virtual reality—a means to train surgeons of tomorrow amidst Covid-19. J Pak Med Assoc. 2022;72(4):797.
14. Wu Q, Wang Y, Lu L, Chen Y, Long H, Wang J. Virtual simulation in undergraduate medical education: a scoping review of recent practice. Front Med (Lausanne). 2022;9:855403.
15. Kuhn S, Huettl F, Deutsch K, Kirchgassner E, Huber T, Kneist W. Surgical education in the digital age—virtual reality, augmented reality and robotics in the medical school. Zentralbl Chir. 2021;146(1):37–43.

16. Sultan L, Abuznadah W, Al-Jifree H, Khan MA, Alsaywid B, Ashour F. An experimental study on usefulness of virtual reality 360 degrees in undergraduate medical education. Adv Med Educ Pract. 2019;10:907–16.
17. Kockro RA, Amaxopoulou C, Killeen T, Wagner W, Reisch R, Schwandt E, Gutenberg A, Giese A, Stofft E, Stadie AT. Stereoscopic neuroanatomy lectures using a three-dimensional virtual reality environment. Ann Anat. 2015;201:91–8.
18. Rojas-Sanchez MA, Palos-Sanchez PR, Folgado-Fernandez JA. Systematic literature review and bibliometric analysis on virtual reality and education. Educ Inf Technol (Dordr). 2022;28:1–38.
19. Campbell ST, Chan JY, Gardner MJ, Bishop JA. Optimizing the orthopaedic medical student rotation: keys to success for students, faculty, and residency programs. J Am Acad Orthop Surg. 2019;27(15):542–50.
20. Nam K, Dutt CS, Baker J. Authenticity in objects and activities: determinants of satisfaction with virtual reality experiences of heritage and non-heritage tourism sites. Inf Syst Front. 2022;25:1–19.
21. Tel A, Bagatto D, Costa F, Sembronio S, Robiony M. Anatomical computerized exploration to excise malignancies in deep facial compartments: an advanced virtual reality protocol for a tailored surgical approach. Front Oncol. 2022;12:875990.
22. Gao S, He T, Zhang Z, Ao H, Jiang H, Lee C. A motion capturing and energy harvesting hybridized lower-limb system for rehabilitation and sports applications. Adv Sci (Weinh). 2021;8(20):e2101834.
23. Choi KS, Sun H, Heng PA. An efficient and scalable deformable model for virtual reality-based medical applications. Artif Intell Med. 2004;32(1):51–69.
24. Blumstein G, Zukotynski B, Cevallos N, Ishmael C, Zoller S, Burke Z, Clarkson S, Park H, Bernthal N, SooHoo NF. Randomized trial of a virtual reality tool to teach surgical technique for tibial shaft fracture intramedullary nailing. J Surg Educ. 2020;77(4):969–77.
25. Cross JI, Boag-Hodgson C, Ryley T, Mavin T, Potter LE. Using extended reality in flight simulators: a literature review. IEEE Trans Vis Comput Graph. 2023;29:3961–75. https://doi.org/10.1109/TVCG.2022.3173921.
26. Mok TN, Chen J, Pan J, Ming WK, He Q, Sin TH, Deng J, Li J, Zha Z. Use of a virtual reality simulator for tendon repair training: randomized controlled trial. JMIR Serious Games. 2021;9(3):e27544.
27. Jack P. Virtual reality and the transformation of medical education, Future Healthcare Journal. 2019;6(3):181–5, ISSN 2514-6645, https://doi.org/10.7861/fhj.2019-0036.
28. Vozenilek J, Huff JS, Reznek M, Gordon JA. See one, do one, teach one: advanced technology in medical education. Acad Emerg Med. 2004;11:1149–54.
29. Chong JH, Chahal C, Gupta A, Ricci F, Westwood M, Pugliese F, Petersen SE, Khanji MY. COVID-19 and the digitalisation of cardiovascular training and education—a review of guiding themes for equitable and effective post-graduate telelearning. Front Cardiovasc Med. 2021;8:666119.
30. Gutiérrez F, Pierce J, Vergara VM, et al. The effect of degree of immersion upon learning performance in virtual reality simulations for medical education. Stud Health Technol Inform. 2007;125:155–60.
31. Maytin M, Daily TP, Carillo RG. Virtual reality lead extraction as a method for training new physicians: a pilot study. Pacing Clin Electrophysiol. 2015;38:319–25.
32. Real FJ, DeBlasio D, Beck AF, et al. A virtual reality curriculum for pediatric residents decreases rates of influenza vaccine refusal. Acad Pediatr. 2017;17:431–5.
33. Walsh K, Jaye P. Simulation-based medical education: cost measurement must be comprehensive. Surgery. 2013;153:302.
34. Zendejas B. Cost: the missing outcome in simulation-based medical education research: a systematic review. Surgery. 2013;153:160–76.
35. McIntish C. Simulation: what does it really cost? Simul Healthc. 2006;1:109.

36. Iglesias-Vázquez J. Cost-efficiency assessment of advanced life support (ALS) courses based on the comparison of advanced simulators with conventional manikins. BMC Emerg Med. 2007;7:18.
37. Kyaw BM, Saxena N, Posadzki P, Vseteckova J, Nikolaou CK, George PP, Divakar U, Masiello I, Kononowicz AA, Zary N, et al. Virtual reality for health professions education: systematic review and meta-analysis by the digital health education collaboration. J Med Internet Res. 2019;21(1):e12959.
38. Lohre R, Bois AJ, Pollock JW, Lapner P, McIlquham K, Athwal GS, Goel DP. Effectiveness of immersive virtual reality on orthopedic surgical skills and knowledge acquisition among senior surgical residents: a randomized clinical trial. JAMA Netw Open. 2020;3(12):e2031217.
39. Strandbygaard J, Bjerrum F, Maagaard M, Winkel P, Larsen CR, Ringsted C, Gluud C, Grantcharov T, Ottesen B, Sorensen JL. Instructor feedback versus no instructor feedback on performance in a laparoscopic virtual reality simulator: a randomized trial. Ann Surg. 2013;257(5):839–44.
40. Ende J. Feedback in clinical medical education. JAMA. 1983;250(6):777–81.
41. Levin A. Fewer crashes caused by pilots. USA Today. 2004. http://usatoday30.usatoday.com/news/nation/2004-03-01-crash_x.htm. Accessed 12 Apr 2019.
42. Bric JD, Lumbard DC, Frelich MJ, et al. Current state of virtual reality simulation in robotic surgery training: a review. Surg Endosc. 2016;30:2169–78.
43. Creutzfeldt J, Hedman L, Felländer-Tsai L. Cardiopulmonary resuscitation training by avatars: a qualitative study of medical students' experiences using a multiplayer virtual world. JMIR Serious Games. 2016;4:e22.
44. Burke SM. Cultivating critical thinking using virtual interactive case studies. J Pediatr Nurs. 2017;33:94–6.
45. Harrington CM, Kavanagh DO, Quinlan JF, et al. Development and evaluation of a trauma decision-making simulator in oculus virtual reality. Am J Surg. 2018;215:42–7.

Chapter 9
Monitoring and Remote Patient Management with Immersive Technologies

Sarika Mulukuntla

Abstract This chapter explores the transformative potential of immersive technologies, one is virtual reality, and we also count on augmented as well as mixed realities which offer new ways to enhance user experiences and interactions in various fields in enhancing existing methods of monitoring and remote management in the healthcare sector. Health systems around the world are on the move toward better patient outcomes and operational efficiency. These technologies present new frontiers in the delivery of health services to patients, especially those located in far areas. The first chapter includes the scope, capabilities, and integration of VR, AR, and MR on the platform of health care. It provides a comprehensive overview of current applications, such as remote monitoring systems that use AR for live data overlays and VR environments that enable immersive therapy and rehabilitation sessions. Such applications have mostly realized the benefit of an increase in patient engagement, improvement in diagnostic accuracy, and enhanced training of professionals within the health fraternity. The chapter then looks at case studies where these technologies have been applied successfully. VR platforms to treat chronic pain, AR applications used to provide surgical preparation and guidance, and MR systems that can even allow a physician to undertake interactive medical imaging and diagnostics. The discourse has also extended to the technical and ethical considerations of employing these technologies, such as data security, privacy concerns, and the need for robust infrastructure. The chapter aims to shed light on practical insights for researchers, professionals, and policymakers interested in VR, AR, and MR uses with an elaborate analysis of immersive technologies in healthcare for better patient care in monitoring and remote management.

Keywords Immersive technologies · Virtual reality (VR) · Augmented reality (AR) · Mixed reality (MR) · Patient monitoring · Patient management · Healthcare innovation · Digital health solutions

---

S. Mulukuntla (✉)
Health Information Technologists Specialist Dallas, Dallas, TX, USA

B. O. Soufiane et al. (eds.), *Augmented Wellness*,
https://doi.org/10.1007/978-981-96-2952-7_9

1 Introduction

The integration of immersive technologies, one is virtual reality, and we also count for augmented as well as mixed realities into healthcare systems represents a transformative shift in how medical care is delivered and experienced. As the healthcare landscape evolves, the importance of monitoring and remote patient management has become increasingly evident, driven by the need to manage chronic diseases, improve patient outcomes, and enhance access to care [1]. These technologies offer unique opportunities to visualize complex medical information, engage patients in their care, and provide remote medical services, making healthcare more efficient and accessible. Immersive technologies create engaging and interactive experiences by overlaying digital information onto the physical world or by creating entirely virtual environments. VR immerses users in a fully digital environment, often used for simulations and education. AR overlays digital content onto the real world, enhancing the user's perception and interaction with their surroundings [2]. MR combines elements of both VR and AR, allowing users to interact with digital and real-world objects simultaneously. In healthcare, these technologies are revolutionizing how medical education, diagnostics, treatment, and patient engagement are approached. For example, medical students and professionals can use VR to practice complex surgical procedures in a risk-free environment, improving their skills and confidence. AR can assist surgeons by providing real-time, 3D visualizations of a patient's anatomy during surgery, enhancing precision and reducing the risk of complications. For patients, immersive technologies can offer therapeutic experiences, such as VR-based pain management and mental health therapies, which are becoming increasingly recognized as effective treatment modalities [3].

2 Overview of the Importance of Monitoring and Remote Patient Management in Modern Healthcare

Monitoring and remote patient management have become critical components of modern healthcare, significantly enhancing the ability to deliver high-quality care. With the advent of digital health technologies, healthcare providers can now offer continuous monitoring and management of patients outside traditional clinical settings. This shift is particularly crucial for managing chronic conditions, postoperative care, and elderly patients who require consistent oversight but face challenges accessing in-person care [4].

The importance of these practices is underscored by several factors:

2.1 Chronic Disease Management

Chronic diseases, such as diabetes, hypertension, heart disease, and chronic obstructive pulmonary disease (COPD), are long-lasting conditions that require ongoing medical attention and lifestyle management. The prevalence of these diseases is increasing globally, placing a significant burden on healthcare systems. Remote monitoring and management of chronic diseases using immersive technologies can play a crucial role in improving patient outcomes and reducing healthcare costs [5].

- **Continuous Monitoring**: Immersive technologies enable continuous monitoring of vital signs and health metrics through wearable devices and sensors. For instance, a diabetic patient can use a continuous glucose monitor (CGM) integrated with a VR dashboard to track glucose levels in real time. This data can be visualized in an immersive environment, allowing both patients and healthcare providers to detect patterns, make informed decisions, and adjust treatment plans accordingly.
- **Early Intervention**: With the ability to monitor health metrics in real time, healthcare providers can detect early signs of disease exacerbation or complications. For example, VR or AR platforms can alert healthcare professionals when a patient's blood pressure exceeds a certain threshold, prompting timely intervention to prevent more severe outcomes.
- **Personalized Treatment Plans**: Immersive technologies can facilitate personalized medicine by providing detailed and individualized data. This data can be used to tailor treatment plans based on the patient's unique needs, preferences, and lifestyle. For instance, a VR-based platform can simulate different dietary or exercise regimens, helping patients understand the impact of these changes on their condition.

2.2 Access to Care

Access to healthcare remains a significant challenge, especially in rural and underserved areas. Immersive technologies can help bridge this gap by providing remote access to medical expertise and resources [6].

- **Telemedicine and Virtual Consultations**: VR and AR technologies enable virtual consultations, allowing patients to receive medical advice and treatment without the need to travel. This is particularly beneficial for patients living in remote areas or those with mobility issues. Virtual consultations can also provide access to specialists who may not be available locally.

- **Remote Diagnostics and Assessments**: AR-enabled devices can assist in remote diagnostics by overlaying medical data onto the real-world environment. For instance, a healthcare provider can use AR glasses to view a patient's medical history and current vital signs while conducting a virtual examination. This can improve diagnostic accuracy and provide a more comprehensive understanding of the patient's condition.
- **Health Education and Awareness**: Immersive technologies can be used to educate patients and communities about health conditions, preventive measures, and treatment options. For example, VR experiences can simulate the impact of smoking on lung health, helping to raise awareness and encourage healthier behaviors.

2.3 Cost-Effectiveness

The integration of immersive technologies in healthcare has the potential to significantly reduce costs for both patients and healthcare providers [7].

- **Reduced Hospital Admissions and Readmissions**: By enabling continuous monitoring and early intervention, remote patient management can prevent hospital admissions and readmissions. This not only improves patient outcomes but also reduces the financial burden on healthcare systems. For instance, timely interventions for heart failure patients can prevent costly hospitalizations.
- **Efficient Resource Allocation**: Immersive technologies can optimize the use of healthcare resources. For example, VR and AR can be used for remote training and supervision of medical staff, reducing the need for on-site trainers and minimizing travel expenses. Additionally, virtual consultations and remote diagnostics can reduce the demand for physical clinic space and medical equipment.
- **Scalability and Reach**: Immersive technologies can be scaled to reach a larger patient population without a proportional increase in costs. This scalability makes it possible to provide high-quality care to more people, including those in low-income or underserved regions.

2.4 Patient Engagement and Empowerment

Patient engagement and empowerment are critical for successful healthcare outcomes. Immersive technologies can play a key role in enhancing patient involvement in their care [8].

- **Interactive and Educational Experiences**: Immersive technologies can create engaging and interactive experiences that educate patients about their health conditions and treatment options. For example, VR simulations can demonstrate the effects of various medications or lifestyle changes, helping patients make informed decisions about their care.

- **Gamification and Motivation**: Gamification elements, such as rewards and progress tracking, can be integrated into immersive platforms to motivate patients to adhere to treatment plans. For instance, a VR-based rehabilitation program for stroke patients can include games that encourage them to complete exercises, making the process more enjoyable and motivating.
- **Personalized Patient Portals**: Immersive technologies can provide personalized patient portals that offer tailored information, resources, and support. These portals can include virtual coaches or avatars that guide patients through their treatment plans, answer questions, and provide emotional support.

2.5 Pandemic Preparedness

The COVID-19 pandemic has highlighted the importance of remote healthcare solutions and the need for preparedness in managing public health crises. Immersive technologies can play a pivotal role in enhancing pandemic preparedness and response [9].

- **Virtual Care and Social Distancing**: During pandemics, immersive technologies enable the continuation of medical care while minimizing physical contact. Virtual consultations, remote monitoring, and AR-assisted diagnostics allow healthcare providers to assess and manage patients without the need for in-person visits, reducing the risk of virus transmission.
- **Remote Training and Simulation**: VR and AR can be used for remote training and simulation exercises for healthcare professionals. This is crucial during pandemics when there is a need to quickly upskill medical staff in areas such as infectious disease management and emergency response.
- **Public Health Education and Communication**: Immersive technologies can be used to disseminate public health information and guidelines. For example, VR experiences can simulate the effects of virus spread, emphasizing the importance of preventive measures such as mask-wearing and social distancing.
- **Mental Health Support**: The psychological impact of pandemics can be significant. Immersive technologies can provide mental health support through virtual therapy sessions, relaxation exercises, and educational content on coping strategies.

By leveraging immersive technologies, healthcare systems can enhance chronic disease management, improve access to care, reduce costs, engage patients, and prepare for future pandemics. These technologies promise to transform healthcare delivery, making it more efficient, accessible, and patient-centered.

2.6 Overview of Immersive Technologies in Healthcare

Virtual reality (VR) technology has become a significant asset in the healthcare sector, offering innovative ways to enhance patient care and treatment outcomes. By immersing users in a fully digital environment, VR can simulate real-world scenarios or create new, controlled settings tailored to specific therapeutic needs. This capability makes VR uniquely suited for a variety of medical applications, from treatment to training and beyond [10].

- **Pain Management**: VR has been particularly effective in pain management, especially for burn victims and patients undergoing certain types of surgeries. By immersing patients in soothing and distracting virtual environments, VR can significantly reduce their perception of pain. For instance, VR programs can transport patients to serene landscapes or engaging interactive games, providing a psychological escape from painful treatments.
- **Surgical Simulation**: VR provides an exceptional training tool for medical students and surgeons, offering a highly realistic, risk-free environment to practice procedures. Surgical simulations can replicate the complexities of human anatomy and surgical interventions, allowing practitioners to enhance their skills without the ethical and practical concerns associated with traditional training methods.
- **Understanding Conditions and Treatments**: VR can educate patients about their health conditions and treatment plans by visually demonstrating the processes and effects on the body. For example, a patient with heart disease might explore a VR simulation of blood flowing through arteries to understand the impact of cholesterol buildup.
- **Virtual Consultations**: Through VR, patients can have immersive consultations with their healthcare providers from the comfort of their homes. This not only makes medical care more accessible but also enhances consultation experience by allowing doctors to use three-dimensional models and simulations to discuss health issues more effectively.

2.7 *Advantages of Using VR in Healthcare*

- **Controlled Environment**: VR offers the unique advantage of creating controlled therapeutic settings, allowing for precise management of the intensity and duration of therapeutic sessions.
- **Safety and Accessibility**: Patients can undergo therapy or training in environments that are safe and easily accessible, reducing the need for physical travel.
- **Data-Driven Insights**: VR systems can collect data on patient interactions and progress, providing valuable feedback to healthcare providers to tailor treatment plans effectively.

2.8 *Example: VR for Pain Management and Rehabilitation*

VR is widely used for pain management and physical rehabilitation. By immersing patients in a virtual environment, VR can distract them from pain and provide therapeutic exercises. Studies have shown that VR can significantly reduce pain perception in patients with chronic pain or undergoing painful procedures [11].

2.9 Example: VR for Medical Training

VR offers an immersive environment for medical training, allowing practitioners to simulate surgeries and other procedures without risk to patients. This hands-on experience is invaluable for training surgeons and other healthcare professionals, improving their skills and confidence.

Table 9.1 summarizes the VR Use Cases and Benefits.

An illustrative setup of VR technology in a clinical setting is represented in Fig. 9.1, showing a patient using a VR headset connected to monitoring equipment that tracks patient responses and progress [12].

2.10 Challenges and Future Directions

While VR offers substantial benefits, there are challenges to its widespread adoption:

- **Cost and Infrastructure**: The initial setup cost and the need for ongoing maintenance can be significant. The initial setup, including hardware and customized software development, can be expensive. This can limit widespread adoption, especially in under-resourced healthcare settings.

Table 9.1 VR use cases and benefits

Application area	VR use case	Benefits
Psychological therapy	PTSD treatment	Safe exposure to triggers, controlled therapy settings
Pain management	Distraction during painful procedures	Reduces perceived pain, enhances patient comfort
Physical rehabilitation	Stroke recovery exercises	Promotes neuroplasticity, tailored exercise routines

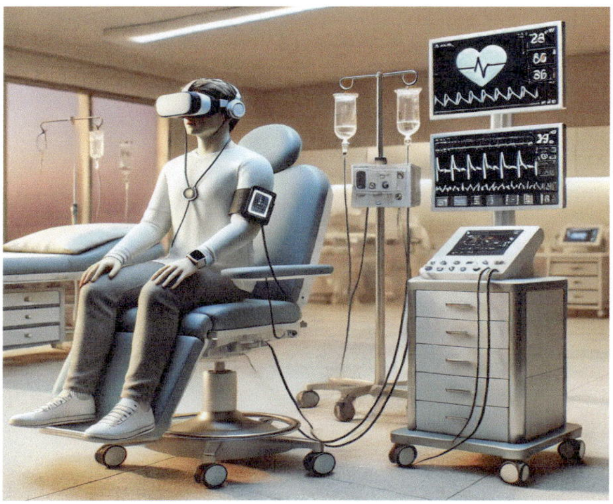

Fig. 9.1 VR technology setup in healthcare

- **Technical Training**: Healthcare providers need training to effectively implement and utilize VR technologies. Resistance from healthcare providers due to lack of training or skepticism about the effectiveness and practicality of VR solutions.
- **Patient Adaptation**: Some patients may experience discomfort or disorientation using VR headsets.

The future of VR in healthcare is promising, with ongoing advancements in technology that are likely to lower costs and enhance the effectiveness of VR applications. Continued research and development will expand its use into more areas of healthcare, providing more personalized and effective treatment options [13]. Further development of VR for medical training and simulations to provide more realistic and varied scenarios. This can improve skills and preparedness among healthcare professionals. Increasing the use of VR for therapeutic purposes, such as in mental health treatments for anxiety, PTSD, and phobias, and for physical rehabilitation. Developing more cost-effective VR solutions to ensure wider accessibility, including portable and less expensive VR systems. Creating more patient-friendly VR applications that are easy to use at home without professional supervision, increasing patient engagement and adherence to treatment. Utilizing the data collected via VR platforms for deeper insights into patient progress and outcomes, driving improvements in treatments and patient care. Leveraging VR to enhance healthcare delivery in remote or underserved regions, providing high-quality training and treatment options worldwide [14].

3 Augmented Reality (AR) in Healthcare: Enhancing Diagnostics and Education

Augmented reality (AR) in healthcare enhances the field by overlaying digital information onto the physical world, providing users with additional data or imagery to improve their perception. Integrating digital elements into the physical environment allows healthcare professionals and patients to interact with virtual components as if they were part of the physical space. AR's unique capability to provide real-time information and visual guidance makes it particularly valuable for diagnostics, surgical procedures, patient care, and medical training [15].

3.1 Diagnostic and Treatment Applications of AR

3.1.1 Enhanced Diagnostics

- **Real-Time Imaging**: AR can project imaging results (like CT scans or MRIs) directly on a patient's body, helping doctors to visualize the anatomy and functions internally without making an incision, thus improving the accuracy of diagnoses and pre-surgical planning.

- **Patient Monitoring**: Wearable AR devices can display vital health statistics in real time, enabling continuous monitoring without the need for stationary equipment.

3.1.2 Surgical Assistance

- **Surgical Navigation**: Surgeons can use AR to overlay detailed 3D models of a patient's anatomy directly onto their body during surgery, which can guide them in performing precise and minimally invasive procedures.
- **Remote Assistance**: AR can enable a surgeon in one location to see exactly what a colleague sees in another operating room and provide guidance through virtual annotations.

3.1.3 Procedural Training

- **Medical Education**: AR applications allow medical students to interact with complex anatomical models virtually. These models can be manipulated in 3D space, offering insights from different angles and fostering a deeper understanding of human anatomy.

3.2 Advantages of Using AR in Healthcare

- **Interactive Learning and Engagement**: AR enhances learning experiences by making medical education more interactive, helping students and professionals visualize and understand complex medical concepts better.
- **Improved Precision and Efficiency**: By providing real-time, hands-free access to data and patient information, AR helps clinicians perform task with greater precision and efficiency, reducing the risk of errors.
- **Cost-Effectiveness**: AR can reduce the need for physical models and other resources in medical training and patient education, lowering costs.

3.3 Example: AR for Remote Assistance and Surgery

AR technology overlays digital information onto the real world, providing healthcare professionals with real-time data and guidance. For instance, AR can be used in remote surgery where a specialist can assist a surgeon by overlaying instructions and anatomical information onto the surgical site through AR glasses. This real-time assistance improves accuracy and outcomes, especially in complex procedures [16].

3.4 Example: AR for Patient Education and Engagement

AR applications are also valuable for patient education. Patients can visualize their medical conditions and treatment plans through AR, enhancing their understanding and engagement. For example, AR apps can show patients how their medications affect their body, which can improve adherence to treatment plans [17].

Table 9.2 summarizes the AR Use Cases and Benefits.

An illustrative setup of AR technology in a clinical setting is represented in Fig. 9.2, showing a medical student using AR glasses to study a virtual anatomical model, which is overlaid onto a real-world table [18].

3.5 Challenges and Future Directions

- **Technical Limitations**: The accuracy and reliability of AR depend on the advancement of image recognition and display technologies. Improvements are necessary to enhance the stability and clarity of virtual overlays.

Table 9.2 AR use cases in healthcare

Application area	AR use case	Benefits
Diagnostics	Overlaying imaging data on patient	Enhanced precision in diagnosis and planning
Surgical assistance	Real-time surgical navigation	Increased accuracy, reduced invasiveness

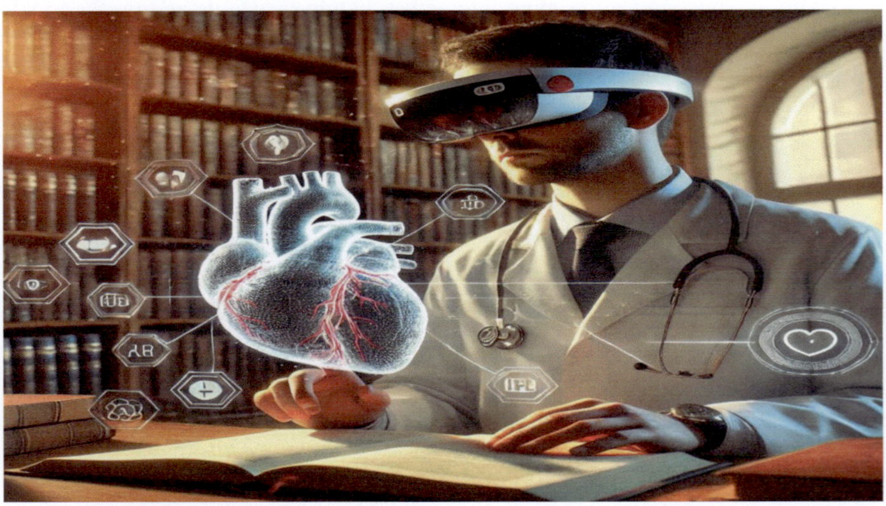

Fig. 9.2 AR in medical training

- **Integration with Existing Systems**: Integrating AR with current medical systems and workflows can be complex and requires careful planning and execution.
- **User Experience Issues**: Ensuring comfort and usability for long periods, particularly in surgical settings, remains a challenge.

The ongoing development and refinement of AR technology will likely continue to expand its applications within healthcare. Future advancements could lead to more widespread adoption of AR in routine medical procedures and training, making it an indispensable tool in modern healthcare. This expanded explanation of AR in healthcare illustrates its potential to significantly impact diagnostics, patient care, and medical education, offering a blend of real-time data integration and interactive learning opportunities. Enhancing real-time information during surgeries and procedures [19]. AR can project vital data directly into the surgeon's field of view, improving precision and outcomes. AR can facilitate remote guidance for surgeries and consultations, where specialists can "see" what the onsite medical professional sees and provide immediate advice. Expanding the use of AR for educational purposes, allowing medical students and professionals to practice skills on virtual patients in a controlled, realistic environment. Using AR to provide patients with visual information about their health conditions or treatments, thereby enhancing understanding and engagement. Integrating AR with imaging technologies to enhance the visualization of complex anatomical structures, aiding in diagnostics and treatment planning. Developing lightweight, wearable AR devices tailored for continuous use in clinical environments without hindering user mobility. Focusing on creating interoperable systems that can function seamlessly across different healthcare environments and platforms. Making AR tools more accessible and affordable to healthcare providers globally, particularly in low-resource settings [20].

4 Mixed Reality (MR) in Healthcare: Integrating the Physical and Digital Worlds to Improve Medical Practice

Mixed Reality (MR) merges physical and digital environments, allowing real and virtual objects to coexist and interact in real time. This technology integrates the immersive aspects of Virtual Reality (VR) with the augmentative visualizations of Augmented Reality (AR), resulting in a powerful tool for visualizing and manipulating complex medical data. MR's ability to blend the real world with virtual elements provides a unique platform for medical training, procedural planning, and patient care.

4.1 *Applications of MR in Medical Practice*

4.1.1 Complex Surgical Planning

- **Pre-operative Procedures**: Surgeons use MR to visualize complex surgeries by overlaying three-dimensional holographic data onto the physical surgical field. This preparation allows surgeons to examine multiple layers of an organ, foresee potential challenges, and plan the surgical approach with higher precision.
- **Intra-operative Navigation**: During surgery, MR provides real-time, holographic guidance, helping surgeons navigate complex anatomical structures without looking away from the surgical site.

4.1.2 Medical Training and Education

- **Interactive Learning**: MR creates dynamic, interactive training environments where medical students can engage with realistic 3D models of human anatomy, performing virtual dissections and procedures that feel tangible.
- **Collaborative Learning**: MR allows for collaborative sessions where students and instructors can interact with the same virtual objects simultaneously, despite being in different locations.

4.1.3 Patient Care and Rehabilitation

- **Physical Rehabilitation**: MR systems support the rehabilitation of patients by creating interactive environments that adapt to their physical capabilities, motivating them through gamified exercises that track and respond to their progress in real time.
- **Patient Education**: MR can enhance the understanding and engagement of patients by visualizing their medical conditions or the effects of proposed treatments, leading to better-informed health decisions.

4.2 *Advantages of Using MR in Healthcare*

- **Precision and Efficiency**: The precision of MR applications in surgical settings enhances the efficiency of procedures, potentially reducing operation times and improving outcomes.
- **Engagement and Motivation**: For patients, especially in rehabilitation, MR's immersive and interactive nature can lead to greater motivation and adherence to treatment protocols.

4.3 Example: MR for Remote Consultations

MR technology facilitates remote consultations by allowing doctors to interact with 3D representations of patients' medical data, such as CT scans or MRI results. This interactive approach enables more accurate diagnoses and better patient management, even when the doctor and patient are not in the same location.

4.4 Example: MR for Surgical Planning and Simulation

Mixed Reality combines elements of both AR and VR, creating a hybrid environment where digital and physical objects coexist and interact. In surgical planning, MR can be used to create detailed 3D models of a patient's anatomy. Surgeons can interact with these models to plan and practice complex surgeries, improving precision and outcomes.

Table 9.3 summarizes the MR Use Cases and Benefits.

An illustrative setup of MR technology in a clinical setting is represented in Fig. 9.3, an image depicting a surgeon using MR goggles to view holographic anatomical structures during a surgical procedure, enhancing the precision and safety of the operation [21].

4.5 Challenges and Future Directions

- **Hardware and Cost**: The development and deployment of MR technology involve significant costs, primarily due to the sophisticated hardware required.
- **Technical Complexity**: The integration of MR into existing medical systems poses technical challenges, requiring robust software capable of handling complex data in real time.
- **User Adaptation**: There is a learning curve associated with using MR technology effectively, and continuous training is necessary to maximize its benefits.

The ongoing advancements in MR technology promise to further enhance its applications in healthcare. As MR devices become more accessible and their

Table 9.3 MR use cases in healthcare

Application area	MR use case	Benefits
Surgical planning	Pre-operative visualization	Enhances surgical precision and planning
Medical education	Interactive anatomical models	Improves depth of understanding, interactive learning
Patient rehabilitation	Gamified therapy sessions	Increase patient engagement and therapy adherence

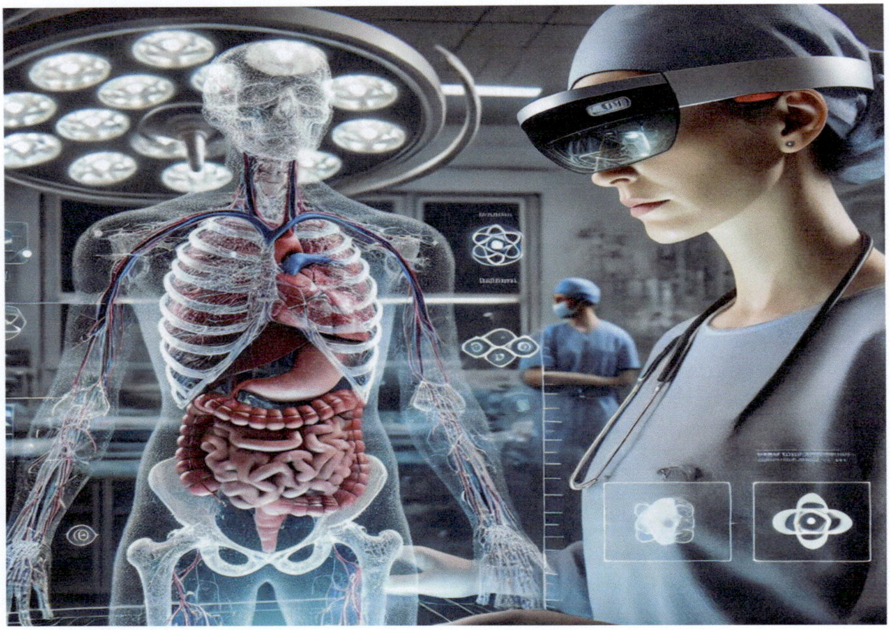

Fig. 9.3 MR for surgical visualization

interfaces more user-friendly, their integration into daily medical practice is likely to grow, making them an integral part of modern healthcare delivery [22]. This chapter provides a detailed exploration of how MR is transforming healthcare by enabling more precise medical procedures, enriching education, and improving patient care through advanced, interactive visualizations. Leveraging MR for remote assistance in surgeries and diagnostics can enable specialists worldwide to collaborate in real-time, offering their expertise without the need for physical presence. Expanding the use of MR in medical training environments to provide highly interactive and immersive learning experiences, mimicking real-life medical scenarios without any associated risks. Utilizing MR to explain complex medical conditions or procedures to patients in a more comprehensible and interactive manner, potentially improves understanding and compliance with treatment plans. Developing MR applications for rehabilitation and therapy that can adapt to the progress and needs of patients, offering a more personalized and engaging treatment approach. Innovation in wearable MR technology that is more compact, comfortable, and capable of being used in various medical settings, from operating rooms to outpatient clinics. Establishing standards for interoperability among different MR systems and healthcare databases to ensure seamless integration and communication across platforms. Making MR technology more accessible and affordable for a wider range of healthcare providers, including those in resource-limited settings [23].

5 Current Trends and Developments in Immersive Technologies

Immersive technologies, including Virtual Reality (VR), Augmented Reality (AR), and Mixed Reality (MR), are rapidly evolving, driven by advancements in hardware, software, and user interface design. These technologies are increasingly being integrated into various sectors, including healthcare, where they offer new ways to visualize, interact with, and understand medical data and environments [24].

5.1 Enhanced Hardware Capabilities

- **Increased Resolution and Field of View**: Modern VR headsets offer higher resolution displays and a wider field of view, providing more realistic and immersive experiences. This advancement is crucial in medical simulations and training, where detailed visualization can significantly enhance learning outcomes.
- **Improved Tracking and Sensing**: Enhanced motion tracking and sensor technologies allow for more precise tracking of movements and interactions within immersive environments. This is particularly beneficial for applications like surgical training and rehabilitation, where accurate tracking of hand and body movements is essential.
- **Wearable and Portable Devices**: The development of lighter, more comfortable, and portable devices, such as standalone VR headsets and AR glasses, is making immersive experiences more accessible and user-friendly. These devices can be used in a variety of healthcare settings, from clinics to patients' homes.

5.2 Software and Content Development

- **Realistic Simulations and Virtual Environments**: Advances in graphics rendering and simulation algorithms are enabling the creation of highly realistic virtual environments. These environments are used for medical training, therapeutic interventions, and patient education.
- **AI Integration**: Artificial Intelligence (AI) is being integrated into immersive technologies to enhance user experiences. For example, AI algorithms can create adaptive learning experiences in medical training simulations or provide personalized patient education in virtual environments.
- **Cross-Platform Compatibility**: Efforts to make immersive content compatible across different platforms (e.g., VR, AR, MR) and devices are increasing. This compatibility ensures that content can be accessed and utilized in various contexts, making it more versatile and widely applicable.

5.3 Expanding Applications in Healthcare

- **Telemedicine and Remote Consultations**: The use of immersive technologies for remote consultations is growing, enabling healthcare providers to conduct virtual visits and examinations. These technologies enhance the telemedicine experience by providing 3D visualizations and interactive tools [25].
- **Surgical Planning and Simulation**: Surgeons are using VR and AR for preoperative planning and simulations, allowing them to practice complex procedures and visualize patient anatomy in 3D. This practice can improve surgical accuracy and reduce the risk of complications.
- **Mental Health and Pain Management**: Immersive experiences are being used to treat mental health conditions such as anxiety, PTSD, and phobias. VR-based therapy can provide controlled environments for exposure therapy. Additionally, VR is being used as a tool for pain management, distracting patients and reducing the perception of pain during medical procedures.

6 The Role of Immersive Technologies in Healthcare Settings

Immersive technologies are playing an increasingly important role in transforming various aspects of healthcare delivery, from diagnosis and treatment to education and patient engagement.

6.1 Medical Training and Education

- **Simulation-Based Learning**: Immersive technologies provide medical students and professionals with realistic simulations for training purposes. These simulations can replicate surgical procedures, emergency scenarios, and patient interactions, allowing learners to practice and refine their skills in a safe environment.
- **Interactive Anatomy and Physiology**: AR and VR can be used to create interactive 3D models of human anatomy and physiology. These models enhance the learning experience by allowing users to explore and interact with different body systems, providing a deeper understanding of complex structures and functions.
- **Continuing Medical Education (CME)**: Immersive technologies enable healthcare professionals to engage in CME activities remotely. VR-based courses and workshops can simulate real-world clinical scenarios, helping practitioners stay updated on the latest medical advancements and techniques.

6.2 Patient Care and Treatment

- **Remote Monitoring and Management**: Immersive technologies enable the remote monitoring of patients' health conditions, providing real-time data to healthcare providers. For example, AR-enabled wearable devices can display vital signs and other health metrics, allowing for continuous monitoring and timely interventions.
- **Therapeutic Interventions**: VR is being used as a therapeutic tool for various conditions, including chronic pain, PTSD, and anxiety disorders. Virtual environments can be tailored to provide exposure therapy, relaxation exercises, and cognitive behavioral therapy (CBT) sessions.
- **Enhanced Patient Engagement**: Immersive technologies can improve patient engagement by providing interactive and educational experiences. For instance, VR experience can help patients understand surgical procedures, treatment plans, and potential outcomes, making them more informed and involved in their care.

6.3 Diagnosis and Surgical Assistance

- **Preoperative Planning**: Surgeons can use VR and AR to visualize and plan complex surgeries. These technologies provide detailed 3D representations of patient anatomy, allowing surgeons to practice procedures and identify potential challenges before entering the operating room.
- **Intraoperative Assistance**: AR can assist surgeons during procedures by overlaying critical information, such as anatomical structures and surgical guides, onto the patient's body. This real-time data can improve precision and reduce the likelihood of errors.
- **Postoperative Care**: Immersive technologies can also aid postoperative care by providing virtual follow-up visits and monitoring recovery progress. Patients can use VR platforms for guided rehabilitation exercises, ensuring they adhere to prescribed protocols.

6.4 Public Health and Education

- **Health Awareness Campaigns**: Immersive technologies can be used to create impactful public health campaigns. For example, VR experiences can simulate the effects of smoking or poor diet, raising awareness and promoting healthy behaviors.
- **Disaster Preparedness and Response**: Immersive simulations can prepare healthcare professionals and the public for disaster scenarios, such as pandemics

or natural disasters. These simulations can train responders, test emergency plans, and educate the public on safety measures.

In summary, immersive technologies are revolutionizing healthcare by enhancing medical training, improving patient care, assisting in diagnosis and surgery, and supporting public health initiatives. Their continued development and integration into healthcare settings promise to improve outcomes, increase access to care, and create more engaging and effective healthcare experiences.

7 Case Studies and Examples

- **Real-World Examples of Healthcare Providers Using Immersive Technologies**: Immersive technologies have been adopted by various healthcare providers worldwide to enhance patient care, training, and operational efficiency. Here are some notable examples:
- **Cleveland Clinic and Virtual Reality for Pain Management**: The Cleveland Clinic has implemented virtual reality (VR) as a tool for pain management in patients undergoing painful procedures or those with chronic pain conditions. By immersing patients in calming VR environments, they can reduce their perception of pain and anxiety, leading to a more comfortable experience.
- **Stanford Children's Health and Augmented Reality in Surgery**: Surgeons at Stanford Children's Health have utilized augmented reality (AR) to perform complex surgeries. By overlaying 3D models of patients' anatomy onto their bodies during surgery, surgeons can better visualize internal structures and navigate during procedures. This has been particularly useful in pediatric surgeries, where precise and minimally invasive approaches are crucial.
- **Cedars-Sinai Medical Center and VR for Medical Training**: Cedars-Sinai has integrated VR into its medical training programs, providing medical students and residents with realistic simulations of surgical procedures and emergency scenarios. This technology allows trainees to practice and refine their skills in a controlled, risk-free environment, improving their readiness for real-world situations.
- **Mayo Clinic and AR for Patient Education**: The Mayo Clinic uses AR to enhance patient education. By providing patients with AR visualizations of their conditions and potential treatments, the clinic helps patients better understand their health issues and the procedures they will undergo. This approach has been shown to improve patient satisfaction and engagement.
- **University of Oxford and VR for Mental Health Therapy**: Researchers at the University of Oxford have developed VR-based therapy programs for treating mental health conditions such as social anxiety and PTSD. These programs create controlled virtual environments where patients can confront and overcome their fears under the guidance of a therapist, demonstrating promising results in clinical trials.

8 Case Studies Demonstrating the Impact on Patient Outcomes and Healthcare Delivery

8.1 Case Study 1: VR in Pain Management for Burn Patients

- **Background**: Burn injuries are associated with intense pain, especially during wound care and dressing changes. Traditional pain management techniques may not be sufficient, leading to high levels of distress and discomfort for patients.
- **Intervention**: A study conducted at the University of Washington's Harborview Burn Center explored the use of VR as a complementary pain management tool. Patients were immersed in a VR environment known as "Snow World," designed to be engaging and distracting.
- **Results**: The study found that patients who used VR during wound care reported significantly lower pain levels compared to those who did not use VR. The immersive nature of the VR experience helped shift patients' focus away from their pain, reducing their reliance on pain medication and improving their overall experience.

8.2 Case Study 2: AR in Orthopedic Surgery

- **Background**: Accurate placement of screws and implants is critical in orthopedic surgeries, such as spine surgeries. Traditional imaging techniques provide limited real-time guidance, potentially leading to complications or the need for revision surgeries.
- **Intervention**: At the Johns Hopkins Hospital, AR technology was integrated into the operating room, allowing surgeons to overlay 3D images of the patient's spine onto their view. This AR system provided real-time guidance, highlighting the optimal paths for surgical instruments.
- **Results**: The use of AR significantly improved the accuracy of screw placement, reducing the risk of complications and enhancing patient outcomes. Surgeons also reported increased confidence and efficiency, leading to shorter surgery times and faster recovery for patients.

8.3 Case Study 3: VR in Stroke Rehabilitation

- **Background**: Rehabilitation is crucial for stroke patients to regain motor function and independence. Traditional rehabilitation exercises can be repetitive and monotonous, leading to low patient engagement and adherence.
- **Intervention**: The Stroke Center at the University of California, Los Angeles (UCLA), implemented a VR-based rehabilitation program called "VIRTUES"

(Virtual Reality Training and Upper Extremity Stroke Rehabilitation). The program included a series of VR exercises designed to improve motor skills and coordination.
- **Results**: Patients participating in the VR program showed significant improvements in upper extremity function compared to those receiving standard therapy. The interactive and gamified nature of the VR exercises increased patient engagement and motivation, leading to better adherence and more effective rehabilitation.

8.4 Case Study 4: AR for Remote Surgical Assistance

- **Background**: In remote or resource-limited settings, access to specialized surgical expertise can be limited. This can impact on the quality of care for complex cases that require specialized skills.
- **Intervention**: In a collaborative effort between Microsoft and the University of Alberta, AR technology was used to provide remote surgical assistance. Using AR headsets, surgeons in remote locations could receive real-time guidance from specialists located elsewhere. The specialists could see the surgical field and provide step-by-step instructions overlaid on the AR display.
- **Results**: This approach enabled complex surgeries to be performed in remote settings with the support of expert guidance. It also facilitated knowledge transfer and training for local surgeons, improving the overall quality of care in underserved areas.

8.5 Case Study 5: VR for Cognitive Behavioral Therapy (CBT) in PTSD

- **Background**: Traditional CBT for PTSD involves exposing patients to memories or situations that trigger their symptoms in a controlled setting. However, it can be challenging to recreate these triggers accurately and safely.
- **Intervention**: The University of Southern California Institute for Creative Technologies developed a VR-based CBT program called "Bravemind" for veterans with PTSD. The program created realistic virtual environments that allowed patients to confront and process their traumatic experiences under the guidance of a therapist.
- **Results**: The VR-based CBT program showed significant reductions in PTSD symptoms among participants. The immersive nature of VR allowed for more controlled and effective exposure therapy, helping patients process their trauma and develop coping mechanisms.

9 Conclusion

The chapter has explored the transformative potential of immersive technologies in healthcare, focusing on their applications in monitoring, remote patient management, training, and patient care. The growing importance of monitoring and remote patient management, particularly in chronic disease management, access to care, cost-effectiveness, patient engagement, and pandemic preparedness. The types of immersive technologies and their current trends, such as enhanced hardware capabilities, AI integration, and the expansion of telehealth services. The significant roles these technologies play in medical training, patient care, diagnostics, and public health, as well as emerging trends and potential future applications. The critical role of AI and machine learning in enhancing immersive experiences, providing personalized, predictive, and efficient healthcare solutions. In summary, incorporating immersive technologies into patient monitoring and management marks a notable progression in healthcare. These technologies offer unprecedented opportunities for enhancing patient engagement, improving the precision of monitoring, and delivering personalized care in ways that were previously unattainable.

The adoption of VR, AR, and MR in healthcare settings enables a more intuitive and immersive approach to patient management, allowing for real-time visualization of medical data and simulations of complex medical conditions. This can lead to better understanding and faster decision-making by healthcare professionals. Additionally, immersive technologies can significantly elevate the quality of patient education and compliance, providing interactive and engaging methods to explain diagnoses, treatments, and procedures.

References

1. Freeman D, Reeve S, Robinson A, Ehlers A, Clark D, Spanlang B, Slater M. Virtual reality in the assessment, understanding, and treatment of mental health disorders. Psychol Med. 2017;47(14):2393–400.
2. Valmaggia LR, Latif L, Kempton MJ, Rus-Calafell M. Virtual reality in the psychological treatment for mental health problems: a systematic review of recent evidence. Psychiatry Res. 2016;236:189–95.
3. Maples-Keller JL, Bunnell BE, Kim SJ, Rothbaum BO. The use of virtual reality technology in the treatment of anxiety and other psychiatric disorders. Harv Rev Psychiatry. 2017;25(3):103–13.
4. Rizzo AS, Koenig ST. Is clinical virtual reality ready for primetime? Neuropsychology. 2017;31(8):877–99.
5. Barsom EZ, Graafland M, Schijven MP. Systematic review on the effectiveness of augmented reality applications in medical training. Surg Endosc. 2016;30(10):4174–83.
6. Bork F, Stratmann L, Enssle S, Eck U. The benefits of augmented reality in educational environments—a systematic literature review. J Univ Comput Sci. 2016;22(12):1548–68.
7. Chen PJ, Huang CD, Yeh SL. Augmented reality-assisted pedicle screw installation surgical navigation system. J Med Biol Eng. 2017;37(1):27–36.

8. Khor WS, Baker B, Amin K, Chan A, Patel K, Wong J. Augmented and virtual reality in surgery—the digital surgical environment: applications, limitations and legal pitfalls. Ann Transl Med. 2016;4(23):454.
9. Pucher PH, Johnston MJ, Dalal M, Rajaretnam N, Arora S. The future of the digital surgical environment in the context of mixed reality: opportunities and threats. Ann Surg. 2016;264(6):933–8.
10. Pratt P, Ives M, Lawton G, Simmons J, Radev N, Spyropoulou L, Yang GZ. Through the HoloLens™ looking glass: augmented reality for extremity reconstruction surgery using 3D vascular models with perforating vessels. Eur Radiol Exp. 2018;2(1):2.
11. Ferrari V, Megali G, Troia E, Pietrabissa A, Mosca F. A mixed-reality surgical trainer with haptic feedback for robotic surgery. Biomed Eng Online. 2017;16(1):1–18.
12. Hooper J, Tsiridis E, Feng J, Schwarzkopf R, Waren D, Long WJ, Einhorn TA. MR-guided robotic arm for orthopedic surgery: technological advancements and clinical applications. J Robot Surg. 2018;12(3):345–53.
13. Baran S. Augmented reality in medical education and surgery. J Healthc Technol. 2020;12(3):45–58.
14. Jones T, Smith M, Brown R. Virtual reality for chronic pain management. Pain Manag J. 2016;9(2):85–93.
15. Liu Y, Ma X, Chen Z. Mixed reality for surgical planning and simulation. Int J Med Inform. 2018;112:67–76.
16. Moorhouse N, Glover S, Khan A. Augmented reality in patient education. Healthc Commun Rev. 2019;14(1):22–9.
17. Peterson E, Roberts H, Li Y. Mixed reality for remote medical consultations. Telemed e-Health. 2021;27(6):583–9.
18. Smith A, Hamilton R. Virtual reality in medical training: a systematic review. Med Educ Today. 2017;37(4):33–41.
19. Rizzo AS, Shilling R. Virtual reality therapy for PTSD: a clinical trial. J Anxiety Disord. 2020;64:102–10.
20. Liu D, Martin R. Remote surgical assistance using augmented reality. J Telemed Telecare. 2020;26(6):356–63.
21. Roberts S, Clarke J. Augmented reality in orthopedic surgery. Orthop Surg J. 2022;14(4):453–62.
22. Hoffman HG, Chambers GT. VR analgesia: reducing pain in burn patients. J Pain Res. 2020;13:123–30.
23. Zhang X, Lee H. AI-driven advancements in VR healthcare applications. Artif Intell Med. 2021;70(2):130–45.
24. Evans L, Norton J. Next-generation applications of VR and AR in healthcare. J Innov Health Sci. 2023;15(3):210–22.
25. Chen Y, Wang M. Virtual reality for stroke rehabilitation: a clinical trial. Neurorehabil Neural Repair. 2021;35(5):434–42.

Chapter 10
Current State of AR and VR in Healthcare

K. M. Kirthika, S. Sangeetha, R. Immanual, and N. Sanjana

Abstract Augmented Reality (AR) and Virtual Reality (VR) technologies rapidly transform the healthcare landscape, offering innovative solutions to enhance patient care, medical education, and therapeutic interventions. This chapter delves into the current state of AR and VR in healthcare, exploring their diverse applications and their profound impact on reshaping various aspects of the industry. The chapter examines the multifaceted applications of AR in healthcare settings, including patient education and engagement through interactive visualizations, enhancing diagnostic procedures through real-time guidance, gamified rehabilitation programs, and empowering patients with chronic conditions through real-time feedback and monitoring. Additionally, it explores the transformative potential of VR in exposure therapy for anxiety and phobias, pain management and distraction, surgical training and simulation, and mental health assessments and interventions. While highlighting the numerous benefits and applications, the chapter also addresses the challenges and considerations associated with implementing AR and VR in healthcare, such as accessibility and cost, data privacy and security concerns, and user experience and design considerations. This chapter paves the way for discussions on the future of these immersive technologies in healthcare by providing a comprehensive overview of the current landscape and exploring the opportunities and challenges. It underscores the immense potential of AR and VR to lead to a more patient-centered, efficient, and accessible healthcare system that prioritizes personalized care and improved outcomes.

K. M. Kirthika (✉) · N. Sanjana
Department of Computer Science and Engineering, Sri Ramakrishna Institute of Technology, Coimbatore, India

S. Sangeetha
Department of Electrical and Electronics Engineering, Sri Ramakrishna Institute of Technology, Coimbatore, India

R. Immanual
Department of Mechanical Engineering, Sri Ramakrishna Institute of Technology, Coimbatore, India

B. O. Soufiane et al. (eds.), *Augmented Wellness*,
https://doi.org/10.1007/978-981-96-2952-7_10

Keywords Augmented reality healthcare · Virtual reality healthcare · Medical education and training VR · AR surgical guidance · VR exposure therapy · AR/VR patient engagement

1 Introduction to AR and VR in Healthcare

The healthcare industry has consistently been at the vanguard of technological innovation, perpetually seeking novel methods to enhance treatment outcomes, optimize medical processes, and deliver superior patient care. Immersive technologies, such as virtual reality (VR) and augmented reality (AR), have experienced rapid advancements in recent years, unlocking groundbreaking opportunities within the healthcare sector. These innovative tools possess the capacity to revolutionize various aspects of medical practice, including therapeutic interventions, patient experiences, medical education, and remote consultations. AR technology augments or enhances a user's perception of reality by overlaying digital content, such as text, animations, and images, onto their real-world view [1]. In healthcare, AR can profoundly transform how medical professionals interact with and convey complex information by enabling them to visualize and manipulate data in a more immersive and intuitive manner. On the other hand, VR immerses users in a completely simulated, computer-generated environment, transcending the limitations of the physical world and providing a sense of presence and immersion [2]. This technology allows individuals to be transported into virtual environments, opening up numerous possibilities for therapeutic interventions, medical training, and even remote consultations.

The integration of AR and VR technologies into healthcare practices presents significant opportunities to elevate patient experiences, improve treatment outcomes, and streamline medical procedures. These immersive solutions offer a wide range of applications across various domains within the healthcare landscape, spanning from patient education and engagement to diagnostic processes, rehabilitation programs, and chronic disease management. One of the primary advantages of AR in healthcare is its potential to enhance patient education and engagement through interactive visualizations. By merging digital and physical information, AR enables patients to gain a deeper understanding of their medical conditions, treatment plans, and procedures [3]. This interactive approach can lead to improved patient adherence, informed decision-making, and ultimately better health outcomes.

Moreover, AR holds transformative potential in revolutionizing diagnostic procedures by providing medical professionals with valuable guidance during surgical interventions or other complex medical procedures. By superimposing digital imagery, annotations, and real-time data onto the patient's anatomy, AR can equip healthcare professionals with invaluable insights, potentially reducing the risk of errors and enhancing the accuracy of medical interventions [4]. Additionally, gamified experiences facilitated by AR offer exciting possibilities in the domain of rehabilitation programs, making the process more engaging and motivating for patients.

Through interactive AR applications, patients can participate in personalized virtual exercises and activities while receiving instant feedback and guidance [5]. This approach can improve patient compliance, accelerate recovery, and enhance treatment outcomes.

In the context of chronic disease management, AR technology empowers patients by providing real-time feedback and monitoring capabilities, enabling them to better understand and manage their conditions [6, 7]. For example, AR applications can seamlessly overlay digital information onto the user's environment, providing reminders for medication adherence, tracking vital signs, and offering personalized recommendations for lifestyle modifications.

While AR and VR technologies present immense potential in healthcare, it is crucial to address the challenges and considerations associated with their implementation. Accessibility and affordability remain significant concerns, as AR and VR experiences often require costly technology and software, which may be prohibitive for individuals or healthcare institutions with limited resources [8]. Furthermore, data privacy and security are critical considerations, particularly when integrating AR and VR in healthcare, as it often involves the collection and processing of sensitive patient data [9]. Robust data protection measures and strict compliance with privacy regulations are essential to ensure the ethical and responsible use of these technologies. Figure 10.1 shows that Applications of AR and VR in Healthcare.

Virtual reality (VR) transforms healthcare by providing a safe space for medical professionals to learn new skills. Doctors and nurses can train in anatomy, practice surgery, and learn infection control using VR simulations. This builds their confidence and skills without harming patients. VR also aids in diagnostics and surgery planning, allowing surgeons to virtually see inside a patient's body and prepare for complex procedure. Figure 10.2 shows that Virtual reality benefits in the medical field.

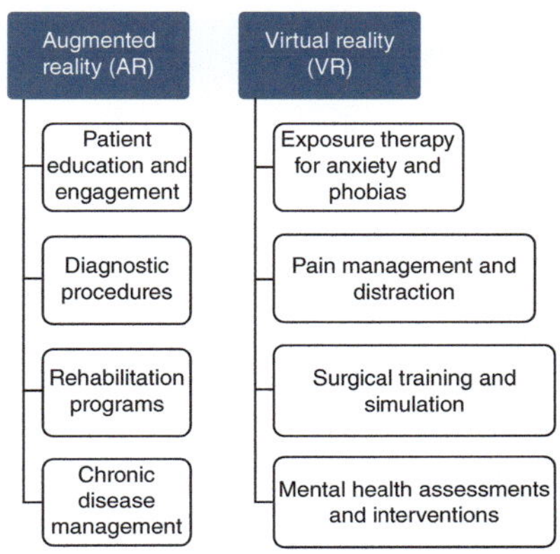

Fig. 10.1 Applications of AR and VR in healthcare

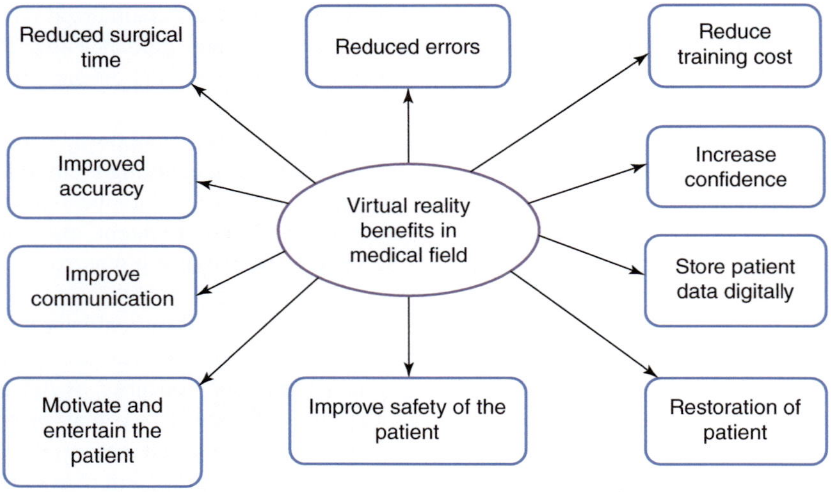

Fig. 10.2 Virtual reality benefits in the medical field

2 AR Applications in Healthcare

Augmented Reality (AR) applications in healthcare are a domain ripe with potential for revolutionizing patient education and engagement. AR is a promising tool that bridges the gap between patients and complex medical information in the ever-evolving healthcare technology landscape.

- Patient Education and Engagement
- Diagnostic Procedures
- Rehabilitation Programs
- Chronic Disease Management

2.1 Patient Education and Engagement

Patient Education and Engagement through AR entail the utilization of interactive digital overlays to enhance the understanding of medical conditions, treatments, and procedures. By superimposing virtual elements onto the real world, AR provides patients with immersive experiences that facilitate learning in a visually engaging manner. For instance, patients can use a smartphone or tablet to visualize 3D models of anatomical structures or medical devices overlaid onto their own bodies, allowing for a personalized and interactive learning experience.

Simplifying complicated medical concepts and processes to make them more understandable and accessible to people with different levels of health literacy is one of AR's main advantages in patient education. In order to obtain a better understanding of their health and available treatments, patients might engage with virtual representations of their anatomy or medical disorders. As a result of this participatory approach, patients feel more empowered and included in the healthcare decision-making process, which eventually improves patient outcomes and treatment plan adherence.

It has been demonstrated that using AR applications in patient education increases information retention and engagement. AR draws patients in and promotes active engagement in their healthcare journey by offering immersive and interactive learning experiences. Research has shown that patients interacting with augmented reality (AR) educational resources retain information better and are more likely to follow doctor's orders. Consequently, by providing interactive, tailored, and immersive learning experiences, augmented reality apps in healthcare have the potential to transform patient education and engagement completely. Through augmented reality (AR) technology, healthcare professionals may give patients the information and resources they need to engage in their care actively, improving patient outcomes and increasing patient literacy.

2.2 *Diagnostic Procedures*

Augmented reality (AR) applications have become a game-changer for improving diagnostic processes, providing healthcare practitioners with cutting-edge methods for precise and effective evaluations. AR technology can completely change how diagnostic tests are performed and understood by fusing digital and physical information.

AR-enabled diagnostic procedures provide healthcare providers with immersive, real-time visualizations of patient data in various applications, from surgical navigation to medical imaging. One noteworthy instance is the application of augmented reality (AR) in medical imaging. It allows radiologists to superimpose 3D reconstructions of anatomical structures on real-time scans, improving their ability to precisely and perceive intricate interior structures. This enhanced view improves the diagnostic process by enabling more precise abnormality diagnosis and better treatment planning. Moreover, AR technology has played a significant role in surgical navigation by providing physicians with a dynamic and user-friendly way of visualizing patient anatomy during procedures. AR helps surgeons navigate complex anatomical features more confidently and accurately by superimposing preoperative imaging data onto the surgery area in real time. Patient safety is increased, surgical accuracy is increased, and the chance of complications is decreased thanks to this improved visualization. Enhancing medical education and training has also demonstrated potential when incorporating AR into diagnostic procedures. AR technology allows medical practitioners to practice diagnostic skills in a realistic virtual environment by offering immersive and engaging learning experiences. By using a hands-on approach, healthcare practitioners become more proficient in evaluating complex medical data and improving their diagnoses' accuracy. By giving medical practitioners cutting-edge resources for precise and effective evaluations, augmented reality applications in healthcare have the potential to transform diagnostic processes completely. Healthcare professionals may raise the bar for patient care by using AR technology to improve treatment outcomes, increase diagnostic accuracy, and more.

2.3 Rehabilitation Programs

Augmented reality (AR) applications in healthcare have become a viable means of improving rehabilitation programs and providing creative ways to raise patient outcomes and care quality. AR technology can completely change how rehabilitative therapies are administered and experienced by fusing digital and physical aspects.

AR-enabled rehabilitation programs use various applications, from cognitive to physical therapy, giving patients fascinating and interactive experiences that aid in recuperation and enhance their functional abilities. One noteworthy instance is the application of augmented reality (AR) in physical therapy, where patients can participate in interactive games and exercises superimposed on their environment to improve motor skills and encourage movement. In addition to raising patient motivation, this gamified approach to rehabilitation makes it easier to implement focused, individualized therapy sessions. Furthermore, AR technology has proven to be a valuable resource for cognitive rehabilitation, providing patients with neurological disorders with cutting-edge methods to improve cognitive function and stimulate brain plasticity. Patients can practice their mental skills in memory, attention, and problem-solving by using AR applications to provide interactive cognitive challenges and simulations. Thanks to this individualized approach to cognitive rehabilitation, patients can take an active role in their treatment and see significant gains in their cognitive abilities. Enhancing patient participation and adherence to treatment plans has been demonstrated to be another benefit of integrating AR into rehabilitation programs. AR technology engages patients and motivates them to actively participate in their recovery by providing immersive and interactive rehabilitation experiences. Research has indicated that patients participating in AR-based rehabilitation programs show increased motivation and adherence, improving rehabilitation results and quality of life.

2.4 Chronic Disease Management

Augmented Reality (AR) apps have become a promising area in managing chronic diseases in the healthcare environment. They provide creative ways to improve patient outcomes and raise the standard of care for patients with long-term medical disorders. AR technology can completely change how chronic diseases are tracked, treated, and managed by fusing digital overlays into the real world.

Chronic Disease Management through AR encompasses various applications, from remote monitoring to patient education and self-management tools, providing individuals with chronic conditions with personalized and interactive resources to support their health journey. One notable example is the use of AR in remote monitoring, where patients can access real-time health data and receive personalized feedback and guidance through AR-enabled devices, empowering them to actively participate in their care and make informed decisions about their health. Furthermore, AR technology has been instrumental in patient education and self-management for chronic diseases, offering individuals interactive tools and resources to enhance their understanding of their condition and treatment plan. By superimposing virtual information onto the physical environment, AR applications can provide patients with visualizations of disease processes, medication instructions, and lifestyle recommendations, fostering greater health literacy and adherence to treatment regimens. This personalized approach to patient education promotes self-efficacy and empowers individuals to take control of their health.

Integrating AR into chronic disease management has also shown promise in improving patient engagement and health outcomes. By offering interactive and immersive experiences, AR technology captivates patients' attention and encourages active participation in their care, leading to better treatment adherence and health outcomes. Studies have demonstrated that patients who engage with AR-based chronic disease management tools exhibit improved self-care behaviors and enhanced quality of life, highlighting the potential of AR technology to transform the management of chronic conditions.AR applications in healthcare promise to revolutionize chronic disease management by providing individuals with innovative tools and resources to support their health journey. By leveraging AR technology, healthcare providers can enhance patient education, promote self-management, and optimize care delivery for individuals with chronic diseases, ultimately improving health outcomes and quality of life. Figure 10.3 shows that Augmented Reality in Healthcare Platform.

3 VR Applications in Healthcare

3.1 Exposure Therapy for Anxiety and Phobias

Virtual reality-based exposure therapy (VRET) is an innovative approach used for treating anxiety and phobias, including dental phobia [12]. This therapy method gradually exposes individuals to virtual environments that simulate their feared situations or stimuli in a controlled setting. The procedure typically begins with an assessment to identify the specific fears or phobias, followed by creating customized virtual environments replicating the feared scenarios.

During the exposure sessions, individuals interact with these virtual environments, starting from less anxiety-provoking situations and progressively moving to

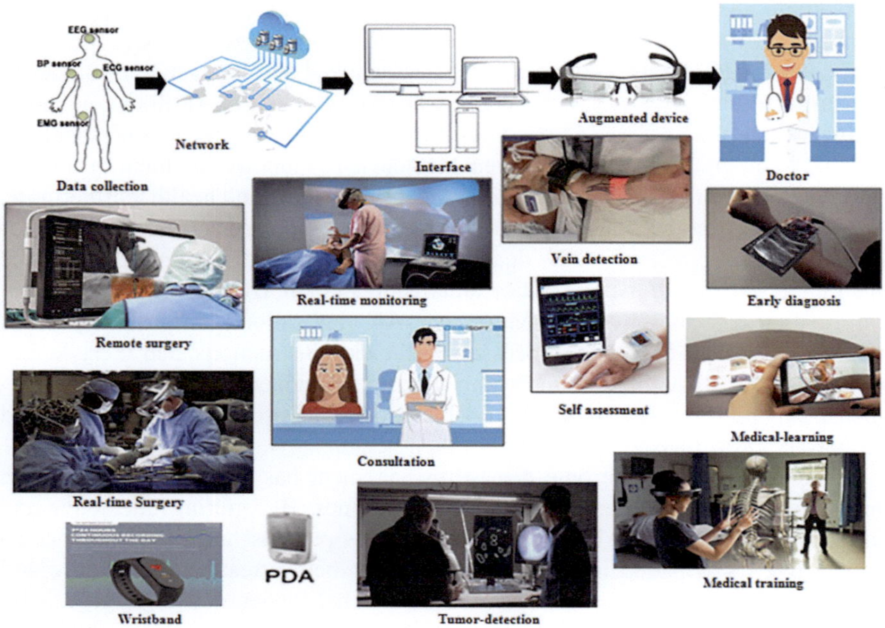

Fig. 10.3 Augmented reality in healthcare platform [10, 11]

more challenging ones. Throughout the sessions, therapists provide cognitive restructuring to help individuals challenge and reframe negative thoughts associated with their fears. Additionally, individuals learn coping strategies, such as deep breathing exercises and relaxation techniques, to manage anxiety during exposure [13].

In the context of dental phobia, VRET offers a novel approach by immersing patients in a virtual dental operatory, where they encounter virtual representations of a dentist and dental tools. The exposure hierarchy is systematically introduced, starting from passive sitting in the chair to more anxiety-provoking scenarios like oral inspection and drilling sounds. Real-time monitoring of physiological responses, such as heart rate, ensures safety during the single-session therapy. Overall, VRET provides a safe and immersive environment for individuals to confront their fears and gradually reduce anxiety, leading to improved treatment outcomes and quality of care.

3.2 Pain Management and Distraction

Virtual reality (VR) technology has emerged as a promising tool for pain management and distraction during medical procedures [14]. The therapy procedure typically begins with assessing the patient's pain levels, medical history, and suitability for VR therapy. Patients are then prepared by being introduced to the VR equipment, addressing any concerns, and selecting a suitable virtual environment based on their preferences and the procedure performed [14]. During immersion, patients wear a VR headset or use a mobile device to enter the chosen virtual world, which may include calming scenes, interactive activities, or engaging games. The immersive nature of VR helps distract patients from the medical procedure, shifting their focus to the virtual environment and potentially reducing their perception of pain by altering the body's pain modulation system. Healthcare providers monitor the patient's response throughout the procedure and adjust the VR experience as needed. After the procedure, patients' pain levels and overall experience with VR therapy are evaluated, and follow-up sessions may be scheduled for continued pain management. Detailed documentation of the VR therapy session, including the virtual environment used, the patient's response, and any adjustments made is recorded in the patient's medical records.

By integrating VR into pain management strategies, healthcare providers can offer patients a non-pharmacological and immersive approach to alleviate pain and anxiety during medical procedures. Further research and advancements in VR applications can potentially enhance patient comfort and treatment outcomes in healthcare settings.

3.3 Surgical Training and Simulation

Virtual reality (VR) based surgical training and simulation have revolutionized surgical education and practice, providing a realistic and immersive environment for training purposes [15–17]. The procedure typically begins with a needs assessment to identify the specific training objectives, surgical procedures, and skills to be developed. A suitable VR platform or simulator, such as those based on Unreal or Unity engines, is then selected to align with the training goals. A comprehensive training curriculum is developed, outlining the sequence of training modules, specific skills to be practiced, and assessment criteria for evaluating proficiency [15, 17]. Trainees engage in hands-on training using the VR simulation, which replicates real-life surgical scenarios, allowing them to practice techniques, improve hand-eye coordination, and familiarize themselves with surgical tools and equipment [15–17]. The VR system provides real-time feedback on the trainee's performance, enabling immediate correction of errors and continuous improvement. Progress tracking through data analytics and performance metrics allows instructors to identify areas for improvement and tailor training programs to individual learning needs.

VR-based surgical training is often integrated with traditional surgical education methods, such as lectures and workshops, to provide a comprehensive learning experience [15, 17]. Regular evaluation and improvement of the VR training program are undertaken based on feedback from trainees, instructors, and performance metrics. By utilizing VR technology in surgical training, medical professionals can enhance their surgical skills, improve patient outcomes, and advance the healthcare field in a safe and controlled environment without risk of harm. This innovative approach offers a transformative solution for medical education and training.

3.4 Mental Health Assessments and Interventions

Virtual reality (VR) technology has been increasingly utilized in mental health assessments and interventions, particularly in the treatment of conditions such as post-traumatic stress disorder (PTSD) in military personnel [16]. Researchers conducted initial validations of VR environments to assess memory functioning and attentional processing. These assessments provide a novel and immersive way to evaluate cognitive abilities in a controlled virtual setting. They additionally explored the effectiveness of virtual reality exposure therapy (VRET) for anxiety disorders and PTSD in active duty soldiers, demonstrating positive outcomes. The procedure typically involves the presentation of emotionally evocative VR combat-related scenarios within the context of professional care, allowing for treatment options previously not feasible with traditional methods. By leveraging the advancements in VR technology and the positive outcomes reported in the literature, VR-based mental health assessments and interventions offer a promising avenue for enhancing clinical practice and research in military behavioral healthcare. Virtual reality (VR) technology has been increasingly utilized in mental health assessments and interventions, offering innovative treatment approaches. Researchers highlighted the importance of considering basic theoretical and pragmatic issues when developing VR applications for clinical psychology and neuropsychology [18]. The process typically involves.

- selecting a suitable VR approach based on existing methods,
- assessing the compatibility of the VR environment with the target clinical population,
- evaluating the level of presence experienced by users,
- addressing navigation factors,
- considering potential side effects,
- ensuring generalization of outcomes, and
- Incorporating sound methodological and data analysis practices.

VR applications have shown promise in fear reduction, pain management, stress reduction, cognitive rehabilitation, and assessment of various mental health conditions. By integrating VR technology into mental health practices, professionals can enhance treatment outcomes and provide more personalized and effective

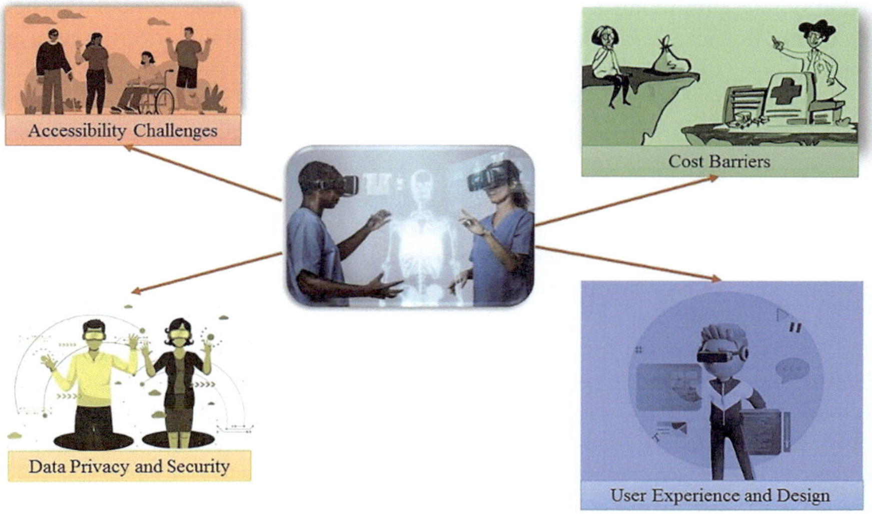

Fig. 10.4 Challenges and considerations in AR and VR healthcare applications

interventions for individuals experiencing psychological challenges. Figure 10.4 shows that Challenges and Considerations in AR and VR healthcare applications.

4 Challenges and Considerations

4.1 Accessibility and Cost

Integrating Augmented Reality (AR) and Virtual Reality (VR) technologies in healthcare present's opportunities and challenges. One significant hurdle is ensuring accessibility for individuals with disabilities. The lack of built-in accessibility features tailored to accommodate various impairments, such as visual or cognitive challenges, hinders the effective utilization of AR/VR solutions by users with disabilities in healthcare settings. Furthermore, the cost associated with AR/VR devices and accessibility tools poses a considerable barrier to adoption. Affordability is a key concern, as impaired users should not face additional expenses for necessary accessibility features. The financial constraints related to acquiring AR/VR devices, software, and training for healthcare professionals can be substantial, potentially limiting the widespread implementation of these technologies in healthcare environments and impeding their potential benefits for patient care and medical training.

Addressing these accessibility and cost challenges requires collaborative efforts from industry manufacturers, researchers, and healthcare providers. Developing built-in accessibility features without additional costs for users with impairments is crucial to enhancing the inclusivity of AR/VR technologies in healthcare.

Additionally, promoting affordability and equal access to these devices can help overcome financial barriers and facilitate their integration into various healthcare applications.

To tackle these challenges, healthcare organizations and technology developers must prioritize accessibility and cost considerations in designing and implementing AR and VR solutions. This may involve developing user-friendly interfaces that accommodate diverse user needs, including those with disabilities. Furthermore, efforts to reduce the overall cost of AR and VR technologies through innovation, scalability, and strategic partnerships can help make these tools more accessible to a wider range of healthcare providers and patients.

By recognizing and addressing the accessibility and cost considerations of AR and VR technologies in healthcare, stakeholders can work towards creating more inclusive and sustainable solutions that benefit both patients and healthcare professionals. Collaborative efforts to improve accessibility features, reduce financial barriers, and promote equitable access to AR/VR innovations can pave the way for enhanced healthcare experiences and outcomes.

4.2 Data Privacy and Security

The adoption of augmented reality (AR) and virtual reality (VR) technologies in healthcare raises critical data privacy and security concerns, necessitating robust measures to safeguard sensitive patient information [10, 11]. While AR and VR offer potential benefits for patient care and medical training, they also introduce vulnerabilities that require the implementation of stringent security protocols.

Protecting patients' confidential information from unauthorized access or data breaches is a significant challenge when integrating AR and VR technologies in healthcare settings. As these technologies involve collecting and transmitting personal health data, implementing strong security measures such as encryption, authentication mechanisms, and secure network connections is essential to prevent data leaks, cyber-attacks, and maintain data confidentiality, integrity, and availability [19].

Compliance with regulatory standards like HIPAA adds complexity to data privacy and security considerations in AR and VR healthcare applications. Implementing robust data encryption protocols, secure authentication mechanisms, and regular security audits are crucial to address these challenges. Educating healthcare professionals and technology users about data privacy best practices and potential security threats can help mitigate risks associated with AR and VR applications in healthcare, ensuring patient confidentiality and data protection.

4.3 User Experience and Design

Integrating Augmented Reality (AR) and Virtual Reality (VR) technologies in healthcare presents several user experience and design challenges that require careful consideration to ensure successful implementation and optimal outcomes. These challenges encompass technical limitations, ethical concerns, user acceptance, and the need for design approaches tailored to the unique requirements of healthcare settings.

Addressing technical limitations, such as device weight, battery life, and processing power, is crucial to ensure seamless user experiences without compromising functionality. Ethical principles, including patient privacy, data security, and informed consent, must be prioritized in the design process to safeguard sensitive information and maintain compliance with regulatory standards.

User acceptance is another key consideration, as healthcare professionals and patients may have varying familiarity and comfort with AR and VR technologies [20]. Creating user-friendly interfaces, providing adequate training and support, and addressing user concerns are essential to promote widespread adoption in healthcare environments. Furthermore, designing AR and VR applications for healthcare necessitates a tailored approach that considers users' specific needs and preferences in clinical settings. Customization, personalization, and user-centered design principles are vital to creating intuitive, effective, and engaging applications for healthcare professionals and patients [21]. Additional challenges and considerations in user experience and design for AR and VR in healthcare include:

- Complexity of healthcare data: Presenting complex and vast healthcare data clearly and understandably through user interfaces.
- User interaction: Designing intuitive and user-friendly interfaces for efficient AR and VR systems interaction during critical tasks.
- Integration with existing systems: Ensuring seamless integration of AR and VR applications with existing healthcare systems and workflows.
- Privacy and security: Implementing robust measures to maintain patient confidentiality and data security.
- Training and education: Providing comprehensive educational resources for healthcare professionals to use AR and VR technologies effectively.
- Regulatory compliance: Adhering to healthcare regulations and standards to ensure patient safety and data security.
- Technical challenges: Addressing latency, resolution, and device compatibility issues to deliver a seamless and immersive user experience.

By articulating these challenges and considerations clearly and concisely, healthcare professionals can collaborate with designers and developers to create innovative solutions that enhance patient care, improve workflows, and optimize healthcare delivery through the effective utilization of AR and VR technologies.

4.4 Challenges

The development of affordable and easily integrable AR and VR technology into current healthcare systems is crucial in addressing the accessibility dilemma. To develop scalable and reasonably priced solutions, government organizations, healthcare providers, and technology companies may work together [8]. Adoption hurdles can also be addressed by giving healthcare workers the guidance and assistance they need to use and incorporate these technologies into their work [22].

When integrating AR and VR technologies in healthcare, it is imperative to create strong data protection mechanisms and follow pertinent laws, such as HIPAA and GDPR, in order to address concerns about data privacy [9]. This entails putting safe data transfer and storage procedures into place, getting patients' informed consent, and routinely reviewing and updating security measures to take into account new threats. Furthermore, trust may be built and responsible use of these technologies encouraged by teaching patients and healthcare professionals about their rights and best practices for data protection [23].

Connectivity with IoMT: By fostering a more connected, individualized, and data-driven approach to patient care, the Internet of Medical Things (IoMT) in conjunction with AR and VR technologies holds the potential to completely transform the delivery of healthcare. Real-time patient data can be gathered by IoMT devices, including wearable sensors and smart medical equipment. AR and VR interfaces can then be used to see and evaluate the data [24]. Improved patient outcomes and lower healthcare costs can result from this integration's ability to provide predictive analytics, individualized treatment regimens, and remote monitoring.

For instance, real-time patient vital signs and alarms from IoMT sensors might be shown on an AR-enabled smart glasses device, enabling medical practitioners to quickly monitor and respond to changes in a patient's condition [6, 7]. Similar to this, IoMT device data might be incorporated into VR simulations to generate dynamic, individualized training situations that improve medical professionals' and students' skills and ability to make decisions [25].

4.5 Comparative Analysis

The ways in which AR and VR technologies are used in healthcare settings might differ greatly between industrialized and developing nations, as well as between urban and rural areas. The adoption of AR and VR solutions is aided by the more easy access to advanced technology and infrastructure found in industrialized nations and urban areas. In these situations, healthcare facilities might have the funds and know-how to purchase state-of-the-art AR and VR systems for patient care, surgical guidance, and medical education.

However, due to a lack of funding, inadequate infrastructure, and gaps in digital literacy, the adoption of AR and VR technology may present difficulties in rural areas and underdeveloped nations. In these situations, healthcare facilities might not have the resources—financial, technological, and human—to implement and manage AR and VR systems efficiently. The benefits that these technologies bring may not be distributed equally as a result of the differences in access and implementation.

Initiatives centered on technology transfer, capacity building, and partnerships between developed and developing nations can be extremely important in closing this gap. Collaborations across healthcare facilities, tech firms, and global organizations can help exchange best practices, resources, and information, which makes it possible to customize AR and VR solutions to suit regional requirements. Furthermore, the creation of inexpensive, portable, and easy-to-use AR and VR solutions can aid in removing adoption hurdles in environments with limited resources.

5 The Future of AR and VR in Healthcare

Virtual Reality (VR) and Augmented Reality (AR) hold great promise for revolutionizing various aspects of the healthcare sector, including patient care, medical education, and treatment delivery. As these technologies advance and gain traction, they have the potential to drastically alter the healthcare industry. It is projected that these technologies will play a major role in enhancing medical education and training. Virtual reality therapy is growing quickly, with promising applications in pain management, rehabilitation, and mental health care. Virtual Reality-Based Treatment (VRBT) has shown promising results in treating conditions such as anxiety disorders, phobias, and Post-Traumatic Stress Disorder (PTSD) through the use of controlled exposure and desensitization processes. The healthcare sector may open up new avenues for boosting patient outcomes, raising the standard of treatment, and advancing scientific research by embracing these cutting-edge technologies.

5.1 Ongoing Research and Development

AR and VR can facilitate collaborative research by enabling researchers from different locations to visualize and interact with complex data sets in a shared virtual environment. This can accelerate the discovery process, foster interdisciplinary collaboration, and lead to drug development, medical imaging, and disease modeling breakthroughs. To expand the implementation of new technology, which is the need of the hour to promote reliable health care to people, challenges related to technology integration, user adoption, data privacy, and regulatory frameworks have to be overcome. Collaboration among healthcare providers, technology companies, researchers, and policymakers will be essential in ensuring these technologies' safe, ethical, and effective implementation.

After the release of GG (Google Glass), a head-mounted display (HMD) featuring produced items placed into real-time photos, there was a resurgence of interest in accessible augmented reality (AR). This enthusiasm persisted until January 2015, when production of the HMD was halted [26]. This technology enabled a high-resolution video camera and a lightweight wearable with an overlaid viewing screen. It possesses capabilities like wireless and cloud accessibility that are found on smart phones. Numerous comparable devices designed specifically for surgical enhancement have since been developed due to the device's open-source development platform, encouraging innovative medical and surgical applications [27].

Numerous research studies have shown how AR can help surgeons navigate complex anatomy during minimally invasive procedures. Robotic laparoscopic restricted partial nephrectomy guided by preoperative imaging and intra-operative 3D overlay was demonstrated by Su et al. [28]. AR-guided surgery has shown interest in minimal access to limited partial nephrectomy. With AR guiding, surgical incisions can be marked within the laparoscopic view by projecting 3D images onto the picture.

Applications for live stream and recorded data include trainee-trainer exchanges within the framework of work-based assessments. Junior team members might provide an off-site senior member with a real-time perspective of challenging cases using telementoring, allowing them to get quick assistance. This would benefit specialties like trauma management, patient monitoring, and injury assessment where visual examination is necessary. A safe way to provide professional diagnosis and advice is through telementoring, which can lower the risk of errors in management and needless patient transfers [29].

5.2 *Expanding Applications*

Implementing Augmented Reality in the medical field can revolutionize surgical planning and guidance with the help of three-dimensional visualizations of patient anatomy and pathologies. AR can overlay critical information onto the surgical field, enhancing the surgeon's situational awareness and precision. VR can facilitate preoperative planning, enabling surgeons to rehearse complex procedures and anticipate potential challenges before entering the operating room. Without endangering patient safety, immersive virtual environments may replicate intricate surgical processes, anatomical models, and patient scenarios to give medical professionals and students a realistic hands-on experience. This can enhance one's capacity for learning new skills, making sound decisions, and being ready for high-stakes scenarios.

During consultations or emergencies, distant medical providers can receive real-time visual information and guidance from AR-enabled devices. VR can enable immersive virtual consultations, allowing patients to interact with healthcare providers in a simulated environment, potentially improving access to care in remote or underserved areas. Thus, telemedicine and remote care capabilities can transform healthcare into a new regime. Interacting with interactive virtual environments allows Patients to learn more about their medical issues, available treatments, and self-care guidelines. Improved treatment plan adherence, better health outcomes, and greater patient empowerment are all possible benefits of this deeper understanding.

The AccuVein AV400 device is one particular instance of AR being used in a real-world healthcare setting. It uses AR technology to project a map of the patient's veins onto their skin, making it easier for medical personnel to locate veins for IV insertions and blood draws [30]. According to Kaddoura et al. [31], the use of augmented reality has been demonstrated to increase the precision and effectiveness of these operations while also lowering patient discomfort and raising patient satisfaction.

One particular application of virtual reality (VR) in medicine is the use of VR exposure therapy to treat anxiety disorders like phobias and post-traumatic stress disorder (PTSD). Virtual reality exposure therapy has been shown to be beneficial in treating certain phobias, including fear of heights and flying, according to a 2017 study by Botella et al. Through a safe and regulated virtual environment, patients were progressively exposed to the stimuli that they dreaded, enabling them to face and overcome their concerns.

5.3 Transforming Healthcare Delivery

When used as a safe and entertaining diversion during medical procedures or treating chronic pain disorders, Virtual Reality (VR) can be a very effective tool for pain management. AR, on the other hand, can improve patient education and engagement through the overlay of pertinent medical data over a real-world setting, leading to improved comprehension and treatment plan adherence. Much technological advancement has been identified as potentially disruptive to the surgical profession as the surgical environment continues to advance in the digital era. Because Augmented Reality (AR) and Virtual Reality (VR) are quickly becoming more widely available, easily accessible, and—most importantly—affordable, it seems inevitable that they will be used in healthcare to increase data usage for medical purposes. Research is currently underway to find useful applications for a surgeon's toolkit concerning anatomy, intraoperative surgery, and post-operative rehabilitation.

The majority of virtual reality trainers, especially those for robotic and laparoscopic surgery, teach fundamental motor skills that are connected to key surgical skills. These include grasping, dexterity, grasping instruments, controlling cameras, manipulating endodontist tools, and three-dimensional vision. The majority of VR modules feature abstract tasks, such moving objects to learn specific abilities or hanging hoops from hooks. The effectiveness of VR simulation in teaching basic surgical skills has been recognized [32]; nonetheless, additional training is required to close the gap between this kind of discrete skill training and carrying out entire surgical procedures in the operating theater.

5.4 Technological Insights

In order to produce immersive and engaging experiences, AR and VR systems require sophisticated hardware and software components. AR devices overlay digital content over the physical world using a combination of cameras, sensors, and displays. Examples of these devices are the Microsoft HoloLens and Magic Leap. By tracking the user's position and orientation using computer vision algorithms, these gadgets allow virtual items to be precisely aligned with their physical surroundings. With the help of AR software development kits (SDKs) like Google's ARCore and Apple's ARKit, developers can create AR apps for a variety of platforms.

Conversely, Virtual Reality (VR) systems immerse users entirely in a computer-generated environment through the use of specialist headsets like the Oculus Rift or HTC Vive. To create a realistic and engaging experience, these headsets include haptic feedback, motion tracking sensors, and high-resolution displays. While game engines like Unity and Unreal Engine make it easier to construct immersive VR environments, VR platforms like SteamVR and Oculus SDK enable developers to create VR applications and games.

Advanced haptic feedback systems, hand tracking, and eye tracking are examples of recent technology advancements in AR and VR. In addition to facilitating more natural user interactions, eye-tracking technology can yield useful information for diagnostics and medical research. Hand tracking improves the immersive experience by enabling users to interact with virtual items using natural hand gestures. Realistic tactile sensations are provided by sophisticated haptic feedback devices, like the HaptX Gloves, and are especially helpful for surgical training and simulation.

5.5 Patient and Practitioner Perspectives

As a patient who underwent surgery with the assistance of an AR system, I was amazed by the technology. The surgeon explained how the AR overlays helped guide the procedure, and I felt more confident knowing that they had this advanced tool to ensure precision and safety. Patient testimonial [4].

Virtual reality has been a game-changer in our pain management practice. We've seen patients who were previously struggling with chronic pain find relief and improved quality of life through VR interventions. The immersive nature of VR helps patients focus on something other than their pain, and the results have been impressive. Healthcare practitioner [14].

5.6 Case Study

Case Study 1: Surgical Navigation Using Augmented Reality Sola-no-Rojas et al.'s work is a noteworthy case study that illustrates the usefulness of AR in surgical navigation (2022). Using the Micro-soft HoloLens, the researchers created an augmented reality system to help surgeons perform laparoscopic cholecystectomy procedures. The device gave surgeons improved visualization and guidance by superimposing 3D anatomical models and important components onto the patient's body in real-time. In comparison to conventional laparoscopic procedures, the AR system reduced the risk of complications, enhanced surgical precision, and shortened the total operation time, according to the study.

Case Study 2: Pain Management with Virtual Reality The case study by Mosso Vázquez et al. [14] provides a strong illustration of VR's influence on pain management. In order to reduce patients' pain and anxiety during ambulatory surgery, the researchers employed virtual reality distraction therapy. Using a VR headgear, patients were submerged in a relaxing virtual world while having surgery. In comparison to the control group, the study found that patients who had VR distraction again had much lower pain and anxiety scores. This case study demonstrates how virtual reality (VR) has the potential to enhance patient experiences during medical operations and offer non-pharmacological pain alleviation.

5.7 Analysis of AR and VR Applications in Healthcare

A synoptic view of applications of Augmented Reality and Virtual Reality in healthcare.

The use of Augmented Reality (AR) and Virtual Reality (VR) systems in the healthcare domain has promising implications in changing patients' care, medical training, and therapeutic procedures. The above technologies are creative ways through which different facets of delivery and practice in the healthcare sector can be improved.

1. Patient Education and Engagement: Research shows that using AR, patients' experiences can be enriched by application-based experiences, including interactive visualizations [3]. Through the digital and non-digital data integration, AR helps patients to gain more profound understandings of their health status, and thus enhance the treatment compliance and decision-making.
2. Diagnostic Procedures and Surgical Guidance: Using AR technology in health care has demonstrated that it has the potential to help in improving the diagnostic processes through facilitating real time assistance during difficult operations [4]. Thus, applying digital images and annotations on the patient's body, AR can provide crucial information to healthcare professionals which may minimize and enhance the efficiency of their operations.

3. Rehabilitation and Chronic Disease Management: The general use of AR integrated games has been introduced in the rehabilitation programs wherein patients look forward to the process [5]. In the care of chronic diseases, augmented reality technology is used in the sense that all patient inputs are real-time and can be monitored leading to better management of the diseases [6, 7].
4. Virtual Reality in Mental Health: VR proved useful in the treatment of mental health disorders with focus on the application of exposure therapy for anxiety disorders and phobia. Since it is possible to provide a moderated exposure to the feared stimuli, VRET has beneficial effects in treating conditions like PTSD [13].
5. Pain Management and Distraction: VR has been described as a useful technique in the field of pain control and reducing distress in medical procedures [33]. Research has described that VR changes the perceived pain and anxiety levels by lessening the scores among patients who undergo ambulatory surgery [14].
6. Medical Education and Surgical Training: The applications of Virtual Reality and Augmented Reality have included redefining medical education and surgical skill training through the possibilities of having effective and realistic models depicting tough procedures [15, 17]. These technologies enable the learners and the medical practitioners to practice in safe endowments with nadir risks hence enabling the learners and the practitioners to nexus ample procedure on human subjects.

5.8 Key Results

1. Mobile AR applications have demonstrated benefits in enhancing patients' knowledge about diseases and possibilities of the further therapy, which presumably may promote better medication compliance and more rational choices [3].
2. AR augments the diagnostic processes because it offers real-time information when conducting intricate medical procedures, which may help decrease the standard of mistakes added to the precision [4].
3. Studies of using VRET have shown promising results in the treatment of mental health disorders, but mainly ranged from anxiety disorders, phobias, and PTSD [13].
4. Concerning the impact on pain and anxiety, the authors found that using VR distraction therapy it is possible to enhance the reduction of scores in patients who undergo ambulatory surgery [14].
5. Some of the applications of VR and AR are in the training of medical students and surgeons, where VK simulate real life surgical procedures [15, 17].
6. Some of the difficulties and limitations of using AR and VR in the healthcare context are financial costs of integrating AR and VR [8], the problem of data protection [9], and UX design that should be adapted for the clinical environment [21].

6 Conclusion and Future Scope

Integrating Augmented Reality (AR) and Virtual Reality (VR) technologies into healthcare practices holds immense promise for transforming care delivery and advancing medical education. As these immersive technologies continue to evolve and gain traction, their impact on the healthcare industry is poised to be profound and far-reaching. While the current state of AR and VR in healthcare demonstrates diverse applications, from enhancing patient education and engagement to revolutionizing surgical training and therapeutic interventions, ongoing research and development efforts are crucial to expand their capabilities and address existing challenges.

Addressing issues related to accessibility, cost, data privacy, and security will be paramount to ensure the equitable and responsible implementation of these technologies. Collaboration among healthcare providers, technology companies, researchers, and policymakers is essential to develop comprehensive frameworks and guidelines prioritizing patient safety, ethical considerations, and regulatory compliance.

Moreover, the user experience and design of AR and VR applications in healthcare settings must be carefully considered, focusing on user-friendliness, intuitive interfaces, and seamless integration into existing workflows. Tailoring these technologies to healthcare professionals' and patients' specific needs and preferences is crucial for successful adoption and optimal utilization.

As the future of AR and VR in healthcare unfolds, their applications are expected to expand further, revolutionizing surgical planning and guidance, facilitating remote medical consultations, and enhancing patient education and engagement. The potential for these technologies to transform healthcare delivery is immense, offering the promise of a more patient-centered, efficient, and accessible system that prioritizes personalized care and improved outcomes. By embracing the potential of AR and VR in healthcare while addressing the associated challenges, stakeholders can unlock new opportunities for innovation, collaboration, and advancements in medical practices, ultimately leading to enhanced patient experiences, improved healthcare outcomes, and a more sustainable and equitable healthcare system.

Virtual reality (VR) and augmented reality (AR) technologies will play a crucial role in the provision of healthcare. Patient care will be revolutionized by the smooth integration of AR, VR, and the Internet of Medical Things (IoMT), enabling individualized, data-driven, and immersive experiences. Technological developments in AR and VR hardware, software, and analytics will tackle issues with accessibility, affordability, and data privacy, resulting in a wider use and lower cost of these technologies. In order to guarantee the ethical and responsible use of AR and VR in healthcare, legislators, technology companies, and healthcare providers must work together to set detailed norms and standards.

References

1. Munoz-Saavedra L, Villalta MF, SarabiaCachadiña E, Pérez JL. Augmented reality in healthcare: applications and future trends. Electronics. 2021;10(20):2501. https://doi.org/10.3390/electronics10202501.
2. Pan J, Liu J, Xing N, Hu F, Avram C. Virtual reality assisted therapy for anxiety: a narrative review. Front Psychol. 2021;12:908. https://doi.org/10.3389/fpsyg.2021.628412.
3. Brigham TJ. Reality check: basics of augmented, virtual and mixed reality. Med Ref Serv Q. 2017;36(2):171–8. https://doi.org/10.1080/02763869.2017.1293987.
4. Solano-Rojas E, Bobadilla-Rivas F, Sesma-Vazquez S, Melesio-Portillo R, García-Peña Á, Palafox-Avalos B. Integrating augmented reality into healthcare: a systematic review of applications, benefits, and challenges. Appl Sci. 2022;12(4):1792. https://doi.org/10.3390/app12041792.
5. Aravind G, Darekar A, Fung J, Lamontagne A. Virtual reality-based navigation task to assess cognitive function in individuals with stroke: a pilot study. Int J Virtual Reality. 2020;20(1):2–15.
6. Syed S, Rahman M, Shad MM, Al-Ramahah E, Ahmad S, Ali M, Zafar A. Augmented reality and its pragmatic application in chronic diseases: appraisal and systemic review. In: 2020 IEEE international IOT, electronics and mechatronics conference (IEMTRONICS). Piscataway: IEEE; 2020. p. 1–6. https://doi.org/10.1109/IEMTRONICS51293.2020.9216499.
7. Syed S, Rahman M, Shad MM, Al-Ramahah E, Ahmad S, Ali M, Zafar A. Augmented reality and its pragmatic application in chronic diseases: appraisal and systemic review. In: 2020 IEEE international IOT, electronics and mechatronics conference (IEMTRONICS). Piscataway: IEEE; 2020. p. 1–6. https://doi.org/10.1109/IEMTRONICS51293.2020.92164994.
8. Spicer A, Brivaki E, Yunker AG, Mulrooney A. Augmented reality for extending healthcare across geographies. J IES. 2021;64(1):70–83. https://doi.org/10.1108/JIES-10-2019-0058.
9. Fernandez-Vigas C, Diaz-Redondo RP, Lok S, Yu S, Borozdina Y, Goorahoo D. Privacy and security considerations in the use of virtual and augmented reality in health care. Virtual Reality. 2021;25(4):739–58. https://doi.org/10.1007/s10055-021-00550-x.
10. Ara J, Bhuiyan H, Bhuiyan YA, Bhyan SB, Bhuiyan MI. Ar-based modern healthcare: a review. arXiv preprint arXiv:2101.06364; 2021.
11. Ara J, Karim FB, Alsubaie MSA, Bhuiyan YA, Bhuiyan MI, Bhyan SB, Bhuiyan H. Comprehensive analysis of augmented reality technology in modern healthcare system. Int J Adv Comput Sci Appl. 2021;12(6):840–9.
12. Gujjar KR, Van Wijk A, Sharma R, De Jongh A. Virtual reality exposure therapy for the treatment of dental phobia: a controlled feasibility study. Behav Cogn Psychother. 2018;46(3):367–73.
13. Zhang W, Paudel D, Shi R, Liang J, Liu J, Zeng X, et al. Virtual reality exposure therapy (VRET) for anxiety due to fear of COVID-19 infection: a case series. Neuropsychiatr Dis Treat. 2020;16:2669–75.
14. Mosso Vázquez JL, Mosso Lara D, Mosso Lara JL, Miller I, Wiederhold MD, Wiederhold BK. Pain distraction during ambulatory surgery: virtual reality and mobile devices. Cyberpsychol Behav Soc Netw. 2019;22(1):15–21.
15. Sheik-Ali S, Edgcombe H, Paton C. Next-generation virtual and augmented reality in surgical education: a narrative review. Surg Technol Int. 2019;35:27–35.
16. Al-Hiyari N, Jusoh S. The current trends of virtual reality applications in medical education. In: 2020 12th international conference on electronics, computers and artificial intelligence (ECAI). Piscataway: IEEE; 2020. p. 1–6.
17. Sheik-Ali S, Edgcombe H, Paton C. Next-generation virtual and augmented reality in surgical education: a narrative review. Surg Technol Int. 2019;33:27–35.
18. Rizzo AA, Wiederhold MD, Buckwalter JG. Basic issues in the use of virtual environments for mental health applications. Stud Health Technol Inform. 1998;58:21–42.
19. De Guzman JA, Thilakarathna K, Seneviratne A. Security and privacy approaches in mixed reality: a literature survey. ACM Comput Surv. 2019;52(6):1–37.

20. Feng B, Ng LL. Facilitating writing performance of EFL learners via virtual reality: immersion, presence, embodiment. Front Psychol. 2023;14:1134242.
21. Gall D, Roth D, Stauffert JP, Zarges J, Latoschik ME. Embodiment in virtual reality intensifies emotional responses to virtual stimuli. Front Psychol. 2021;12:674179.
22. Kouri P, Pasonen-Seppänen S, Rantanen M, Laitinen A. Augmented reality in surgical education: a systematic review. Appl Sci. 2021;11(9):3952. https://doi.org/10.3390/app11093952.
23. Takyi H. Security, privacy, confidentiality and integrity of emerging healthcare technologies: a framework for quality of life technologies to be HIPAA/HITECH compliant, with emphasis on health kiosk design [Doctoral dissertation]. University of Pittsburgh; 2019.
24. Ahmadpour N, Pedell S, Mayasari A, Beh J. Co-creating and assessing future wellbeing technology using design fiction. She Ji: J Des Econ Innov. 2019;5(3):209–30. https://doi.org/10.1016/j.sheji.2019.08.003.
25. Barsom EZ, Graafland M, Schijven MP. Systematic review on the effectiveness of augmented reality applications in medical training. Surg Endosc. 2020;34(10):4174–83. https://doi.org/10.1007/s00464-020-07498-4.
26. Yu J, Ferniany W, Guthrie B, et al. Lessons learned from Google glass: telemedical spark or unfulfilled promise? Surg Innov. 2016;23:156–65.
27. Mitrasinovic S, Camacho E, Trivedi N, et al. Clinical and surgical applications of smart glasses. Technol Health Care. 2015;23:381–401.
28. Su LM, Vagvolgyi BP, Agarwal R, et al. Augmented reality during robot-assisted laparoscopic partial nephrectomy: toward real-time 3D-CT to stereoscopic video registration. Urology. 2009;73:896–900.
29. Gardiner S, Hartzell TL. Telemedicine and plastic surgery: a review of its applications, limitations and legal pitfalls. J Plast Reconstr Aesthet Surg. 2012;65:e47–53.
30. AccuVein Inc. AccuVein AV400 Vein Viewing System. 2021. https://www.accuvein.com/products/catalog/av400-vein-viewing-system/.
31. Kaddoura M, Vandyke O, Smallwood C, Gonzalez KM. Perceived benefits and challenges of repeated exposure to high fidelity simulation experiences of first degree accelerated bachelor nursing students. Nurse Educ Today. 2020;90:104228. https://doi.org/10.1016/j.nedt.2020.104228.
32. Raison N, Harrison P, Abe T, Aydin A, Ahmed K, Dasgupta P. Procedural virtual reality simulation training for robotic surgery: a randomised controlled trial. Surg Endosc. 2021;35:6897–902.
33. Mahrer NE, Gold JI. The use of virtual reality for pain control: a review. Curr Pain Headache Rep. 2009;13:100–9.

Chapter 11
Paradise of Virtual Reality (VR) and Augmented Reality (AR) in Mental Health Treatment: Breaking Down Barriers Advancing Supremely Smart Healthcare for Futuristic Growth

Bhupinder Singh and Christian Kaunert

Abstract Technological advancements continue to reshape the way it approaches mental health treatment in the rapidly evolving landscape of healthcare. Among the most promising innovations are Virtual Reality (VR) and Augmented Reality (AR), technologies that hold the potential to revolutionize therapeutic interventions for mental health conditions. Traditional mental health treatments often face challenges such as accessibility, stigma, and limited engagement. VR and AR break down these barriers by providing immersive and interactive experiences that transcend the limitations of traditional therapeutic methods. VR environments are designed to simulate calming and serene landscapes, providing an immersive escape for individuals seeking relaxation and stress reduction. Virtual Reality and Augmented Reality are transforming the landscape of healthcare. These immersive technologies offer not only novel therapeutic interventions but also the prospect of making mental health care more accessible and effective. As it embarks on this journey into the future, the smart integration of VR and AR stands as a beacon of hope for a world where mental health treatment is personalized, engaging and profoundly impactful. The intersection of technology and well-being is creating a future where smart healthcare is synonymous with compassionate and innovative mental health care. This chapter explores the therapeutic applications of VR and AR in mental health, examining their potential to revolutionize traditional treatment methods and enhance overall patient outcomes. By providing immersive and personalized interventions, these technologies represent a significant stride toward supremely smart healthcare in the realm of mental well-being. It also reconnoiters the applications of VR and AR in

B. Singh (✉)
Sharda University, Greater Noida, India

C. Kaunert
Dublin City University, Dublin, Ireland

University of South Wales, Newport, UK

B. O. Soufiane et al. (eds.), *Augmented Wellness*,
https://doi.org/10.1007/978-981-96-2952-7_11

mental health treatment, showcasing their transformative impact on smart healthcare for futuristic advances.

Keywords VR · AR · Mental health · Treatment · Patient outcome

1 Introduction

Virtual Reality has found a profound application in mental health treatment and in the context of therapy, VR creates simulated environments that allow individuals to confront and navigate various scenarios in a controlled and supportive setting [1]. This is particularly beneficial for exposure therapy, a proven method for treating anxiety disorders, phobias, and post-traumatic stress disorder [2]. A patient suffering from social anxiety can engage in virtual scenarios that mimic real-world social situations. This exposure, carefully tailored to the individual's needs, enables gradual desensitization, empowering the patient to confront and manage anxiety in a safe and controlled environment [3].

Augmented Reality enhances our perception of the real world by overlaying digital information onto our physical surroundings [4]. In mental health treatment, AR provides real-time support and information, offering a unique approach to managing stress, anxiety and mood disorders [5]. Through the use of AR glasses or smartphone apps, users can access guided meditation sessions or receive real-time prompts for stress-relieving exercises [6]. This integration of digital elements into the user's immediate environment facilitates on-the-spot interventions, promoting mental well-being in everyday life [7]. VR and AR are increasingly being used in innovative ways to support mental health beyond traditional therapeutic approaches [8]. VR-based biofeedback applications enable individuals to visualize and manage physiological responses to stress, promoting self-regulation. The most important strategies for maximizing patient-specific healthcare decisions are personalized medicine [9]. The use of customized medicine has been made easier by artificial intelligence in a number of medical fields, including genomics and imaging diagnostics [8]. As a result, the necessity for tailored therapy in mental health applications is increasing [9]. From a psychological perspective, every mental health illness requires a different strategy and course of therapy [10]. As a result, technical solutions designed for one set of circumstances are usually not transferable to another [11]. Besides, different people with the same condition may present with different triggers, experiences, and symptoms, making technology solutions that are rigid and non-adaptive insufficient [12].

1.1 *Background: Exploring Historical Context of Technology in Mental Health Treatment*

Emotional, psychological and social well-being are all included in mental health which affects our thoughts, feelings and actions in addition to our capacity to handle stress, communicate with others, and make wise decisions [13]. It is important at all stages of life, from infancy to maturity [14]. Both physical and mental well-being is essential to total wellness [15]. Depression, for example, increases one's vulnerability to a number of physical health problems, especially long-term ailments like diabetes, heart disease and stroke. On the other hand, persistent physical illnesses may increase the risk of mental health issues [16]. Figure 11.1 resume the historic context of technological Development in Mental Health Treatment.

- **Ancient Faiths**—Abnormal conduct was frequently linked to supernatural entities such as gods, demons, or evil spirits in prehistoric societies. As a result, trephination and exorcism were common forms of therapy [16]. Greek philosophers, such as Hippocrates and Plato, brought a more naturalistic perspective to medicine by equating mental illnesses with bodily conditions that had inherited and biological causes. Roman philosophers such as Galen rejected the notion of demonic possession, emphasizing instead physical and psychological factors. But during the Middle Ages, there was a return to supernatural explanations, and severe therapies and exorcism were commonplace [17].
- **The Medieval Era**—In the Middle Ages, the Church's hegemony brought back paranormal justifications for mental illness along with punitive measures like imprisonment and exorcism. The comprehension of mental illnesses [18]. However, events such as the Black Death and an increasing demand for governmental control over nonreligious concerns led to a progressive return towards scientific and medical explanations towards the end of this century [19].
- **The Age of Renaissance**—The Renaissance saw a shift away from supernatural theories of mental disease and toward humanistic viewpoints [20]. The practice of witch-hunting claims that many people who were charged with witchcraft

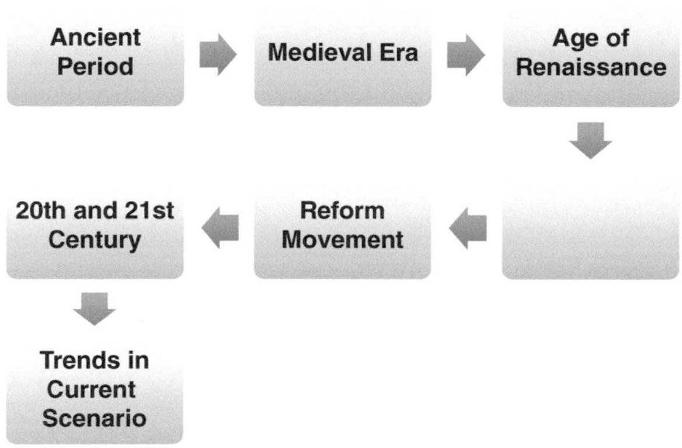

Fig. 11.1 Travels the historical context of technological development in mental health treatment

were genuinely mentally ill. Asylums were also established during this time, yet their patient care frequently fell short of humanitarian standards [21].

- **Reform Movement**—The moral treatment movement, which promoted considerate and compassionate care for mentally ill individuals, gained traction in the late eighteenth and early nineteenth centuries [22]. Compassionate techniques to treating mental diseases were pioneered by individuals which resulted in notable improvements in patient outcomes. But issues with asylum overpopulation and insufficient funding prevented all patients from receiving compassionate care [23].
- **The twentieth and twenty-first Century**—Throughout the twentieth century, conflicting theories on mental disease came to light, with the biological and psychological theories gaining ground. Significant changes in mental health care were brought about by the deinstitutionalization and increase of psychotropic medications however worries about overprescription and subpar care remained [24]. Contemporary approaches to mental health, which prioritize comprehensive and culturally sensitive care have also been influenced by managed health care, multicultural psychology, psychologists' prescription rights, and preventative research [25].
- **Views and Trends in Current Scenario**—There is still a high prevalence of mental illness, despite tremendous efforts to lower stigma and increase access to high-quality care. More specialized therapies have been made possible by our growing understanding of the biology and psychological foundations of mental illnesses [26]. But issues like insufficient care and inequalities in access to care continue to exist, underscoring the continuous requirement for all-encompassing methods of mental health promotion and management [27].

1.2 Objectives of the Chapter

This chapter has the following objectives to:

- Summarize of augmented reality (AR) and virtual reality (VR) technologies, along with some possible uses for them in the treatment of mental illness.
- Fundamental ideas behind VR and AR as well as their distinctions and applications in therapeutic treatments for a range of mental health issues.
- Explore the approaches like cognitive-behavioral therapy (CBT) and mindfulness-based interventions in addition to more established ones like medication, psychotherapy, and institutionalization.
- Access VR and AR technologies provide in the context of mental health therapy covered in detail to conventional techniques, these immersive technologies can offer a therapeutic setting that is more engaging, adaptable, and controllable.
- Thorough rundown of the many ways that VR and AR are being used to treat different mental health issues and how VR and AR are being utilized to treat

illnesses including PTSD, depression, anxiety disorders, phobias, autistic spectrum disorder and schizophrenia.
- Possible future paths and areas for growth such as technological developments, multidisciplinary cooperation, and legislative efforts to include VR and AR into standard mental health procedures.

1.3 Structure of the Chapter

This chapter comprehensively explores the various dimensions of Virtual Reality (VR) and Augmented Reality (AR) in Mental Health Treatment: Breaking down Barriers Advancing Supremely Smart Healthcare for Futuristic Growth. Section 2 elaborates the VR and AR as Emerging Technologies with Potential to Reshape Mental Health Treatment. Section 3 expresses the Therapeutic Applications of Virtual Reality. Section 4 lays down the Augmented Reality in Mental Health Treatment. Section 5 discusses the Innovations beyond Traditional Therapies. Finally, Section 6 Conclude the Chapter with Future Scope.

2 VR and AR as Emerging Technologies with Potential to Reshape Mental Health Treatment

The emerging technologies such as virtual reality (VR) and augmented reality (AR) have the potential to improve current approaches to mental health diagnosis and treatment [28]. Virtual reality (VR) provides an immersive experience that separates users from the real world; this is usually accomplished using a 360° head-mounted display. Augmented reality (AR) superimposes virtual aspects on the physical world [28]. This is demonstrated by features included in well-known social media platforms [29]. Patients can have their world probed, broadened and challenged via the use of AR and VR [30]. These technologies have the potential to improve overall wellbeing, support learning, entertain, and treat maladaptive behaviors or cognitive patterns by utilizing visual, aural, haptic, somatosensory and olfactory inputs. The first commercial VR products hit the market in the 1980s, while the technology itself dates back to the 1960s. Virtual reality (VR) was first widely used in creative industries like gaming, entertainment and shopping. However, it has gradually made its way into the healthcare space, where it is being used for medical imaging, surgical teamwork, and medical education [30].

Virtual reality (VR) has been used as a patient care tool in a variety of medical specialties. It has helped with stroke rehabilitation, supported balance in adults with Parkinson's disease, trained children with cerebral palsy to use their upper extremities and managed pain during childhood vaccinations. Real-world video feeds are integrated into AR which first appeared in the 1990s as an extension of the fully synthetic VR environment, in order to improve the virtual experience. By superimposing real-time, three-dimensional information from noninvasive imaging modalities like MRI, CT or ultrasound on the patient on the operating table, augmented reality (AR) principally aims to improve surgical visibility in the medical field. When combined, AR and VR form the "metaverse" and represent digital medicines which are evidence-based interventions driven by software [31].

2.1 Evolution of VR and AR and Their Entrance into Healthcare

Virtual reality (VR) and augmented reality (AR) technologies have surfaced as revolutionary instruments within medical contexts, fundamentally altering healthcare methodologies and reshaping interactions between medical practitioners and patients within healthcare settings. Mental illness is serious in character has the power to destroy joy from all aspect of a person's life. Its enormous effects on relationships, productivity, longevity and health necessitate acknowledgment and swift action. However, for a variety of reasons, mental health is frequently neglected. But things don't have to stay this way. Modern virtual reality therapy for mental health is now available, and it is provided with discretion and perfection. Advanced degree-holding trained therapists at XR-Health provide customized, drug-free therapies that have the capacity to change lives [32]. Virtual reality (VR) is a sensation of presence that users get from computer-generated environments that can mimic or deviate from the actual world. VR was first conceptualized in 1956 when filmmaker Morton Heilig created the Sensorama device, which provided a multi-sensory experience similar to being within a movie, like riding a motorcycle through a city [33].

The first VR/AR head-mounted display linked to a computer was made in 1968 by Ivan Sutherland and Bob Sproull. It was a prototype for subsequent VR headsets used in classrooms. In 1990, NASA unveiled the Virtual Interface Environment Workstation (VIEW), which allowed astronomers to conduct virtual space exploration and set up VR teaching facilities. Later developments included the Matrix, Landmark VR PTSD therapy, and SEGA initiatives. Large corporations such as Google, Sony, and Facebook drove the rapid advancement of virtual reality technology in 2014 [34]. While Sony revealed their VR project for the PlayStation and Facebook purchased Oculus, Google Cardboard introduced 360-degree photo VR to the general public. With the debut of devices like the Microsoft Hololens, Playstation VR, HTC VIVE, and Oculus Quest, this trend persisted [35].

In October 2020, Facebook released Oculus Quest 2 which at the time was the most potent and reasonably priced wireless VR headset available. Virtual reality (VR) is being used in education in the twenty-first century to allow for the study of historical places, art galleries, and isolated areas. The incorporation of virtual reality (VR) into gaming platforms and media depictions highlights its broad popularity and illustrates its progression from theoretical concepts to tangible technology [36].

2.2 Importance of Innovative Approaches to Address the Growing Mental Health Challenge

Augmented and virtual reality is at the center of a fascinating change that is being sparked by the integration of technology into healthcare. Not only are these immersive technologies changing the way that healthcare is delivered, but they are also showing signs of substantial market growth. In a time when technology is always pushing the boundaries of innovation, few industries have seen a transformation as significant as the healthcare industry [37]. Virtual reality (VR) and augmented reality (AR) are two notable examples of cutting-edge technology changing the face of healthcare. These immersive digital experiences are becoming a necessary part of our current reality, no longer exclusive to science fiction. They are radically changing the way we approach healthcare and how we traverse the fields of diagnosis, therapy, and other related areas [38].

3 Therapeutic Applications of Virtual Reality

Virtual reality (VR) technology has advanced quickly from its beginnings in entertainment and gaming to finding intriguing uses in a variety of industries, including healthcare. VR therapy is one such application that has gained a lot of attention recently as an inventive method of treating mental health issues. In virtual reality (VR) treatment, patients are submerged in 3D computer-generated landscapes that mimic actual situations or fictional worlds designed to treat a variety of psychological and emotional issues. These interactive virtual worlds let patients securely move, engage with items, and face difficult circumstances. To address certain phobias, anxiety, PTSD and other mental health concerns, therapists might create customized situations that support a more targeted and successful therapy strategy [39].

VR therapy helps patients face their fears and anxieties in a safe and controlled setting by exposing them to real-life circumstances or treating them in controlled scenarios. Because VR therapy is immersive, it enables therapists to oversee and guide patients through the exposure process, resulting in a customized and progressive approach to treatment. Virtual reality (VR) has several uses in psychiatry. It may be used for interactive diagnostics with patients by simulating events and analyzing patient reactions, or it can be used as immersive exposure treatment for disorders including PTSD, social anxiety and phobias. Virtual reality (VR) is also useful in cognitive-behavioral therapy, therapist training, remote care consultations, and therapeutic technique research [40]. Panelists advise converting 3D films into virtual reality (VR) experiences using readily available commercial products like MetaQuest or Google headgear, or even less expensive solutions like Google Cardboard [41]. There are multifarious principal advantages of VR Therapy:

- **Enhanced Immersion**: Virtual reality (VR) therapy offers a degree of immersion that is sometimes absent from traditional therapy techniques, enabling patients to experience scenarios more authentically and improving therapeutic results [42].
- **Personalized Care**: VR settings may be tailored by therapists to each patient's unique requirements, imitating anxiety-inducing situations like tight quarters, heights or public speaking [43].
- **Safe Environments**: Virtual reality treatment provides a safe haven where patients may face their concerns without the dangers of going out into the real world. As patients advance, therapists may control the degree of exposure and progressively increase obstacles [44].
- **Overcoming Stigma**: By offering a covert and private treatment option, virtual reality therapy helps to lessen the stigma attached to seeking assistance for mental health issues, hence motivating more people to do so [45].

3.1 Use of VR in Exposure Therapy for Anxiety Disorders and Phobias: VR Therapy Applications

- **Anxiety and Phobias**: With enabling patients to face their fears in a secure setting, virtual reality therapy has shown promise in the treatment of anxiety disorders, PTSD, and specific phobias such as—a fear of flying, heights or spiders [46].
- **Addiction Treatment**: With mimicking circumstances that result in drug cravings, virtual reality therapy is being investigated as a helpful tool for addiction treatment. This allows patients to practice coping mechanisms in a risk-free setting [47].

3.2 VR Applications in Cognitive Behavioral Therapy and Mindfulness Training

Virtual reality (VR) is a rapidly developing technology that provides an entirely immersive experience by submerging users in a three-dimensional computer-generated world. Users create a virtual environment by integrating visual and aural inputs through a head-mounted display. It has developed into a useful tool for clinical training over time, especially in areas like neurosurgery and orthopedic procedural teaching. Also, its therapeutic uses are still growing because of its proven efficacy in treating mental disorders, treating pain and facilitating physical rehabilitation. The use of virtual reality (VR) for cancer patients' pain, both acute and chronic and during traumatic medical procedures is examples of recent occurrences [48].

3.3 Exploring the Potential of VR for Biofeedback and Physiological Regulation in Stress Management

A cutting-edge tool in the realm of digital immersion, virtual reality is frequently used for both leisure and teaching. Its promise, however, also includes therapeutic uses meant to promote attention and relaxation. Researchers are delving deeper into its applicability and efficacy in assessing, controlling and mitigating stress. Historically, the two main methods of treating pain have been medicine and intrusive procedures. But with the current opioid epidemic and advances in our understanding of chronic pain, there is a rising awareness of the need for non-invasive, non-pharmacological therapeutic options. The majority of well-known guidelines now support treating chronic pain with a multimodal, multidisciplinary approach that gives non-pharmacological therapies priority. These might include a variety of strategies like physical treatment, exercise plans, dietary changes, behavioral therapy and other types of psychological counseling [49].

4 Augmented Reality in Mental Health Treatment: Concept Relevance and Applications

Augmented Reality (AR) is a cutting-edge technology that modifies one's experience of reality by fusing virtual and physical components. Augmented Reality (AR) produces an immersive experience where virtual and real items coexist and interact in real time by superimposing computer-generated visuals over the actual world. The use of augmented reality (AR) and other aided technologies in the medical industry has increased significantly from training to clinical practice. The ability to significantly alter the physical world gives AR treatments a competitive advantage over conventional techniques [50]. There are applications of AR in Mental Health Treatment as:

- **Education and Training in Medicine**—Medical education is being revitalized by the use of AR and VR in healthcare. Through realistic simulations, students may practice identifying rare medical illnesses or performing complex surgical operations. Medical practitioners may practice and improve their decision-making skills in a virtual environment that is very realistic without putting real patients in peril. AR glasses represent yet another use of augmented reality in healthcare. Augmented Reality (AR) is a cutting-edge technology that modifies one's experience of reality by fusing virtual and physical components [51]. Augmented Reality (AR) produces an immersive experience where virtual and real items coexist and interact in real time by superimposing computer-generated visuals over the actual world. The use of augmented reality (AR) and other aided technologies in the medical industry has increased significantly, from training to clinical practice. The ability to significantly alter the physical world gives AR treatments a competitive advantage over conventional techniques. There are applications of augmented reality (AR) in order to obtain a better understanding of its possible effects on people who have mental health issues, especially when combined with gamification [52].

- **Therapy and Pain Management**—Virtual reality has become an important technique for pain treatment. Patients might distract themselves from the agony of difficult operations by submerging themselves in relaxing virtual reality surroundings. The FDA has approved VR headsets that use cognitive behavioral therapy methods to help patients relax and control their discomfort. VR therapy has demonstrated potential in the treatment of anxiety disorders, PTSD and phobias [53].
- **Planning and Training for Surgery**—VR technology is being used by surgeons to practice complex procedures. Surgeons are able to practice skills and customize surgical plans by creating 3D models of a patient's anatomy and modeling surgical operations in a virtual setting. Through realistic surgical training modules from companies like Osso VR, doctors may become acquainted with novel techniques and medical equipment. This lowers problems, shortens the duration of the operation, and improves surgical precision [54].
- **Physical Therapy**—Physical treatment techniques are being revolutionized by virtual and augmented reality. Businesses use virtual reality technology to provide customized workouts for physical rehabilitation. In virtual worlds, patients recuperating from operations or injuries can participate in interactive activities that enhance therapy sessions and allow therapists to properly evaluate progress and modify treatments [55].
- **Remote Diagnoses and Consultations**—The need for telemedicine has significantly increased, especially during times of global health catastrophes. There are recent developments in AR and VR are improving remote consultations by giving medical professionals access to real-time patient data and vital signs, providing a more thorough and engaging experience for patients as well as healthcare providers. The accuracy of remote diagnosis and training sessions is improved by these immersive technologies [56].

5 Innovations Beyond Traditional Therapies

Robotic-Assisted Surgery (RAS) systems have garnered increasing attention in recent times because of their potential to improve surgical accuracy, dexterity, and accessibility to minimally invasive treatments. Augmented reality (AR) combined with robotic-assisted surgery offers a sophisticated interface that improves user perception. The power of AR to increase situational awareness will greatly improve surgeons' ability to make judgments in the moment. In the upcoming years, it is anticipated that the integration of AR will transform a number of RAS fields, including preoperative imaging and 3D rendering, intraoperative robotic ultrasound application, robotic liver resections, intraoperative reconstructions and tracking systems and robotic hepatic surgery [57]. If these general tech solutions do not adjust to the variety of circumstances that therapists and patients meet on a regular basis, they may be perceived as insufficient by both parties. Customization should be an option for technological solutions meant to assist patients and mental health practitioners. In order to create and build appropriate and adaptable technological solutions, this approach should entail collaboration between technology designers, researchers, developers, mental health specialists and end users. These customizable elements should also be easy to use so that patients won't reject them or interrupt providers' regular practices. When it comes to XR settings, one of the biggest challenges is creating experiences that are adaptable and adjustable enough to change their interfaces and digital 3D material to fit the demands of different patients in different circumstances [58].

For a long time, mental health illnesses have been diagnosed and treated with the use of virtual and augmented reality. Technological developments have increased consumer and practitioner accessibility to commercial solutions. Still, a number of obstacles and restrictions prevent these technologies from being widely used in regular professional practice. Depression and obsessive-compulsive disorder are two disorders that have previously gotten less attention but are currently receiving greater attention [59]. Hardware and equipment advancements like Mixed Reality Head Mounted Displays might lead to new opportunities in the mental health sector. Virtual reality (VR), mixed reality (MR), and augmented reality (AR) are all included in extended reality (XR), which has several uses. Emerging literature investigates multimodal interactions, such as auditory, olfactory, and tactile input, whereas XR predominantly focuses on visual experiences. The possibility for improving treatment results by including such cues into XR experiences connected to mental health issues is yet somewhat unexplored. Virtual reality technology has drawbacks as notable obstacles include the variety of VR technology, regulatory procedures that cannot keep up with technological improvements, and skepticism among potential consumers. There are also worries about the absence of regulatory channels, which might cause moral dilemmas [60].

6 Conclusion and Future Scope

Millions of people worldwide are severely impacted by mental health illnesses, which also places a heavy financial and social cost on those affected. The most neglected global health concerns are mental health. The significant effects that mental health illnesses have on people, families and society as a whole are not well understood, which contributes significantly to this neglect. It is a common misperception that there is little that can be done to treat these disorders, even though there are many useful pharmaceutical, psychological, and social therapies available. The action is further hampered by the widespread stigma associated with mental health problems, which occasionally results in abuses of human rights. Because of this, most people who suffer from mental health illnesses do not get the attention and treatment they require which might significantly enhance their quality of life. With further research proving its efficacy and potential to become a crucial component of mental health treatment procedures, VR and AR has a bright future ahead of it. VR treatment is positioned as a useful tool in improving mental healthcare results and boosting patients' quality of life because to its unique methodology, safe exposure, enhanced engagement and individualized experiences.

References

1. Singha R, Singha S. Mental health treatment: exploring the potential of augmented reality and virtual reality. In: Applications of virtual and augmented reality for health and wellbeing. Hershey: IGI Global; 2024. p. 91–110.
2. Shekar V, Kachhi Z. Technology applications in virtual and augmented reality for human welfare: the new future. In: Entrepreneurship and creativity in the metaverse. Hershey: IGI Global; 2024. p. 179–97.
3. Khan T, Civas M, Cetinkaya O, Abbasi NA, Akan OB. Nanosensor networks for smart health care. In: Nanosensors for smart cities. Amsterdam: Elsevier; 2020. p. 387–403.
4. De Clara L. The neuropsychological impact of immersive experiences in the metaverse and virtual and augmented reality. In: Applications of virtual and augmented reality for health and wellbeing. Hershey: IGI Global; 2024. p. 148–66.
5. Agoulmine N, Kim K, Kim S, Rim T, Lee JS, Meyyappan M. Enabling communication and cooperation in bio-nanosensor networks: toward innovative healthcare solutions. IEEE Wirel Commun. 2012;19(5):42–51.
6. Dorj UO, Lee M, Choi JY, Lee YK, Jeong G. The intelligent healthcare data management system using nanosensors. J Sens. 2017;2017:1–9.
7. Rani P. Nanosensors and their potential role in internet of medical things. In: Nanosensors for futuristic smart and intelligent healthcare systems. Boca Raton: CRC Press; 2022. p. 293–317.
8. Ahirwar R, Khan N. Smart wireless nanosensor systems for human healthcare. Boca Raton: CRC Press; 2022. p. 265–92.
9. Han B, Tomer V, Nguyen TA, Farmani A, Singh PK, editors. Nanosensors for smart cities. Amsterdam: Elsevier; 2020.
10. Sarkar S, Misra S. From micro to nano: the evolution of wireless sensor-based health care. IEEE Pulse. 2016;7(1):21–5.
11. Rizwan A, Zoha A, Zhang R, Ahmad W, Arshad K, Ali NA, et al. A review on the role of nano-communication in future healthcare systems: a big data analytics perspective. IEEE Access. 2018;6:41903–20.
12. Singh B, Kaunert C. Augmented reality and virtual reality modules for mindfulness: boosting emotional intelligence and mental wellness. In: Applications of virtual and augmented reality for health and wellbeing. Hershey: IGI Global; 2024. p. 111–28.
13. Datta SPA. Future healthcare: bioinformatics, nano-sensors, and emerging innovations. In: Nanosensors: theory and applications in industry, healthcare and defense. London: Routledge; 2016. p. 247.
14. Pramanik PKD, Solanki A, Debnath A, Nayyar A, El-Sappagh S, Kwak KS. Advancing modern healthcare with nanotechnology, nanobiosensors, and internet of nano things: taxonomies, applications, architecture, and challenges. IEEE Access. 2020;8:65230–66.
15. Nazari A. Nanosensors for smart cities: an introduction. In: Nanosensors for smart cities. Amsterdam: Elsevier; 2020. p. 3–8.

16. Sahi KSS, Kaushik S. Smart nanosensors for healthcare monitoring and disease detection using AIoT framework. In: Nanosensors for futuristic smart and intelligent healthcare systems. Boca Raton: CRC Press; 2022. p. 387–400.
17. Oukhatar A, Bakhouya M, El Ouadghiri D. Electromagnetic-based wireless nano-sensors network: architectures and applications. J Commun. 2021;16(1):8–19.
18. Ramasamy M, Kumar PS, Varadan VK. Wearable nanosensor systems and their applications in healthcare. In: Nanosensors, biosensors, info-tech sensors and 3D systems 2017, vol. 10167. Bellingham: SPIE; 2017. p. 1016703.
19. Paliwal G, Bunglowala A. Nanosensor and actuator technologies for wearable mobile patient monitoring systems: a review. In: Workshop on computational models of natural argument. Singapore: Springer Singapore; 2018. p. 83–95.
20. He L, Eastburn M. Smart nanosensor networks for body injury detection. In: 2022 IEEE international conference on smart internet of things (SmartIoT). Piscataway: IEEE; 2022. p. 15–9.
21. Ali NA, Abu-Elkheir M. Internet of nano-things healthcare applications: requirements, opportunities, and challenges. In: 2015 IEEE 11th international conference on wireless and mobile computing, networking and communications (WiMob). Piscataway: IEEE; 2015. p. 9–14.
22. Pirmagomedov R, Hudoev I, Shangina D. Simulation of medical sensor nanonetwork applications traffic. In: Distributed computer and communication networks: 19th international conference, DCCN 2016, Moscow, Russia, November 21-25, 2016, revised selected papers 19. Berlin: Springer International Publishing; 2016. p. 430–41.
23. Mujawar MA, Gohel H, Bhardwaj SK, Srinivasan S, Hickman N, Kaushik A. Nano-enabled biosensing systems for intelligent healthcare: towards COVID-19 management. Mater Today Chem. 2020;17:100306.
24. Omanović-Mikličanin E, Maksimović M, Vujović V. The future of healthcare: nanomedicine and internet of nano things. Folia Medica Facultatis Medicinae Universitatis Saraeviensis. 2015;50(1):23–8.
25. Udoh EE, Hermel M, Bharmal MI, Nayak A, Patel S, Butlin M, Bhavnani SP. Nanosensor technologies and the digital transformation of healthcare. Pers Med. 2023;20(3):251–69.
26. Chelliah R, Wei S, Daliri EBM, Rubab M, Elahi F, Yeon SJ, et al. Development of nanosensors based intelligent packaging systems: food quality and medicine. Nanomaterials. 2021;11(6):1515.
27. Topel SD, Al-Turjman F. Nanosensors for the internet of nano-things (IoNT): an overview. In: Internet of nano-things and wireless body area networks (WBAN). London: Routledge; 2019. p. 21–44.
28. Dinesh Kumar K. Human health monitoring mobile phone application by using the wireless nanosensor based embedded system. In: 2013 international conference on information communication and embedded systems (ICICES). Piscataway: IEEE; 2013. p. 889–92.
29. Materon EM, Gómez FR, Joshi N, Dalmaschio CJ, Carrilho E, Oliveira ON Jr. Smart materials for electrochemical flexible nanosensors: advances and applications. In: Nanosensors for smart manufacturing. Amsterdam: Elsevier; 2021. p. 347–71.
30. Kumar S, Kumari P. Flexible nano smart sensors. In: Nanosensors for smart manufacturing, vol. 199. Amsterdam: Elsevier; 2021.
31. Gaobotse G, Mbunge E, Batani J, Muchemwa B. Non-invasive smart implants in healthcare: redefining healthcare services delivery through sensors and emerging digital health technologies. Sens Int. 2022;3:100156.
32. Vivekananthan V, Khandelwal G, Alluri NR, Kim SJ. E-skin for futuristic nanosensor technology for the healthcare system. In: Nanosensors for futuristic smart and intelligent healthcare systems. Boca Raton: CRC Press; 2022. p. 133–57.
33. Ramasamy M, Varadan VK. Wireless nanosensor system for diagnosis of sleep disorders. In: Nanosensors, biosensors, and info-tech sensors and systems 2016, vol. 9802. Bellingham: SPIE; 2016. p. 200–5.
34. Pradhan MR, Mago B, Ateeq K. A classification-based sensor data processing method for the internet of things assimilated wearable sensor technology. Clust Comput. 2023;26(1):807–22.

35. Tang WH, Ho WH, Chen YJ. Data assimilation and multisource decision-making in systems biology based on unobtrusive internet-of-things devices. Biomed Eng Online. 2018;17(2):1–13.
36. Manogaran G, Alazab M, Song H, Kumar N. CDP-UA: cognitive data processing method wearable sensor data uncertainty analysis in the internet of things assisted smart medical healthcare systems. IEEE J Biomed Health Inform. 2021;25(10):3691–9.
37. Hassanalieragh M, Page A, Soyata T, Sharma G, Aktas M, Mateos G, et al. Health monitoring and management using internet-of-things (IoT) sensing with cloud-based processing: opportunities and challenges. In: 2015 IEEE international conference on services computing. Piscataway: IEEE; 2015. p. 285–92.
38. Hiran KK, Doshi R, Patel M, editors. Applications of virtual and augmented reality for health and wellbeing. Hershey: IGI Global; 2024.
39. Singh B, Kaunert C, Vig K. Reinventing influence of artificial intelligence (AI) on digital consumer lensing transforming consumer recommendation model: exploring stimulus artificial intelligence on consumer shopping decisions. In: Musiolik T, Rodriguez R, Kannan H, editors. AI impacts in digital consumer behavior. Hershey: IGI Global; 2024. p. 141–69. https://doi.org/10.4018/979-8-3693-1918-5.ch006.
40. Singh B. Featuring consumer choices of consumable products for health benefits: evolving issues from tort and product liabilities. J Law Torts Consumer Protect Law. 2024;7(1).
41. Singh B. Unleashing alternative dispute resolution (ADR) in resolving complex legal-technical issues arising in cyberspace lensing E-commerce and intellectual property: proliferation of E-commerce digital economy. Revista Brasileira de Alternative Dispute Resolution-Brazilian Journal of Alternative Dispute Resolution-RBADR. 2023;5(10):81–105.
42. Singh B, Kaunert C. Integration of cutting-edge technologies such as internet of things (IoT) and 5G in health monitoring systems: a comprehensive legal analysis and futuristic outcomes. GLS Law J. 2024;6(1):13–20.
43. Singh B. Green infrastructure in real estate landscapes: pillars of sustainable development and vision for tomorrow. Natl J Real Estate Law. 2024;7(1):4–8.
44. Suma DV. Wearable IoT based distributed framework for ubiquitous computing. J Ubiquitous Comput Commun Technol. 2021;3(1):23–32.
45. Jenkins T. Wearable medical sensor devices, machine and deep learning algorithms, and internet of things-based healthcare systems in COVID-19 patient screening, diagnosis, monitoring, and treatment. Am J Med Res. 2022;9(1):49–64.
46. Malik A, Kumar A. Assimilation of blockchain with internet of things (IoT) with possible issues and solutions for better connectivity and proper security. In: New trends and applications in internet of things (IoT) and big data analytics. Cham: Springer International Publishing; 2022. p. 187–207.
47. Byerly K, Vagner L, Grecu I, Grecu G, Lăzăroiu G. Real-time big data processing and wearable internet of medical things sensor devices for health monitoring. Am J Med Res. 2019;6(2):67–72.
48. Garg D, Dubey N, Goel P, Ramoliya D, Ganatra A, Kotecha K. Improvisation in spinal surgery using AR (augmented reality), MR (mixed reality), and VR (virtual reality). Eng Proc. 2024;59(1):186.
49. Kumar PM, Khan LU, Hong CS. Affirmative fusion process for improving wearable sensor data availability in artificial intelligence of medical things. IEEE Sensors J. 2022.
50. Han X. A novel assimilated navigation model based on advanced optical systems (AOS), internet of things (IoT) and artificial intelligence (AI). Opt Quant Electron. 2023;55(7):655.
51. Dash D, Farooq R, Panda JS, Sandhyavani KV. Internet of things (IoT): the new paradigm of HRM and skill development in the fourth industrial revolution (industry 4.0). IUP J Inf Technol. 2019;15(4):7–30.
52. Goethals I. Real-time and remote health monitoring internet of things-based systems: digital therapeutics, wearable and implantable medical devices, and body sensor networks. Am J Med Res. 2019;6(2):43–8.

53. Banerjee A, Chakraborty C, Rathi M Sr. Medical imaging, artificial intelligence, internet of things, wearable devices in terahertz healthcare technologies. In: Terahertz biomedical and healthcare technologies. Amsterdam: Elsevier; 2020. p. 145–65.
54. Chen ET. The internet of things: opportunities, issues, and challenges. In: The internet of things in the modern business environment. Hershey: IGI Global; 2017. p. 167–87.
55. Barnes R, Zvarikova K. Artificial intelligence-enabled wearable medical devices, clinical and diagnostic decision support systems, and internet of things-based healthcare applications in COVID-19 prevention, screening, and treatment. Am J Med Res. 2021;8(2):9–22.
56. Desai D, Shende P. Integration of internet of things with quantum dots: a state-of-the-art of medicine. Curr Pharm Des. 2021;27(17):2068–75.
57. Albalawi U, Joshi S. Secure and trusted telemedicine in internet of things IoT. In: 2018 IEEE 4th world forum on internet of things (WF-IoT). Piscataway: IEEE; 2018. p. 30–4.
58. Hurley D, Popescu GH. Medical big data and wearable internet of things healthcare systems in remotely monitoring and caring for confirmed or suspected COVID-19 patients. Am J Med Res. 2021;8(2):78–90.
59. Rubi J, Vijayalakshmi A, Venkatesan S. Integration of biomedical engineering in augmented reality and virtual reality applications. In: Applications of virtual and augmented reality for health and wellbeing. Hershey: IGI Global; 2024. p. 41–54.
60. Okoro YO, Ayo-Farai O, Maduka CP, Okongwu CC, Sodamade OT. The role of technology in enhancing mental health advocacy: a systematic review. Int J Appl Res Soc Sci. 2024;6(1):37–50.

Chapter 12
Embedding Virtual Reality Technologies as an Early Career Neuroscience Research Training Methodology Advancing Medical Research

Lorenz S. Neuwirth and Maxime Ros

Abstract Over the past two decades, advancements in neuroscience have outpaced the availability of resources and funding for undergraduate and graduate programs, particularly at Primarily Undergraduate Institutions (PUIs) and Minority Serving Institutions (MSIs). This disparity has widened the gap in early-career skills development, limiting opportunities for students and faculty at under-resourced institutions. Additionally, selective funding favouring established Research 1 (R1) universities exacerbates inequalities, forcing new researchers into power-imbalanced collaborations with senior faculty. Despite these challenges, innovative pedagogical strategies such as applied research mentoring, case studies, and computational neuroscience courses have emerged at PUIs to bridge the gap. Cost-effective technologies, particularly open-source software and virtual reality (VR), offer promising avenues for enhancing neuroscience education and research, providing immersive learning and procedural skill development. Thus, VR in particular, has demonstrated therapeutic applications and the increased potential for transforming neuroscience education. The future of neuroscience education lies in leveraging these VR tools, fostering interdisciplinary research, and addressing funding inequities to create a more inclusive and equitable field for next generation neuroscientists.

Keywords Neuroscience education · Funding disparities · Primarily undergraduate institutions (PUIs) · Virtual reality (VR) · Innovative pedagogy

---

L. S. Neuwirth (✉)
Department of Psychology, SUNY Old Westbury, Old Westbury, NY, USA

SUNY Neuroscience Research Institute, Old Westbury, NY, USA
e-mail: neuwirthl@oldwestbury.edu

M. Ros
Education Sciences School—LIRDEF, Montpellier University, Montpellier, Occitanie, France

B. O. Soufiane et al. (eds.), *Augmented Wellness*,
https://doi.org/10.1007/978-981-96-2952-7_12

1 Introduction

Research advancements in the neurosciences have evolved significantly over the last 20 years, but resources and funding for undergraduate and graduate neuroscience programs have failed to keep up with this pace. Arguably, this situation has inadvertently provoked a dual problem: (1) creating wider academic achievements gap in preparing early career skills for students interested in neuroscience careers in both education and research; and (2) forcing students and faculty in the neurosciences to become more resourceful within their means to remain relevant in a technology and big data dominated era of education. Parallel to these real problems are the government's selective funding directed towards specific neurological and neurodevelopmental disorders more so than creative scientific explorations, which has created a very niche grant "cash cow" mechanism for well-funded and established Research 1 universities (R1s). What can be argued is that this situation creates a disadvantage for new faculty and researchers entering the field at the early career level to be forced into collaborations with more senior neuroscience researchers possessing real stature and power dynamics over them as a new model for future funding between primarily undergraduate institutions (PUIs; which are often Minority Serving Institutions [MSIs]) and R1s [1–3]. Publishing trends from 2006 to 2015 have shown that neuroscience research is being directed towards autism, meta-analyses, functional connectivity, default mode networks and modeling, and neuroimaging; thereby, changing the landscape of neuroscience research [4]. To this point, many colleges and universities that have these technologies and instruments are typically R1s, containing or directly linked with a hospital system, and do not reflect the larger number of colleges/universities in the United States (US) representing PUIs that lack these resources. This grant funding selectivity further creates an inequity system in neuroscience education, that as a byproduct, makes PUI funding more rare or to some degree almost unattainable and subsequently reduces the neuroscience education and research advancements of a large majority of students in their early careers that has persisted and grown worse over the last two decades.

However, in surveilling the undergraduate population within the US it was reported that faculty have attempted to creatively circumvent these problems through innovative learning spaces that were found to be critically in need and were especially lacking in under resourced and underfunded colleges/universities [5–7]. Despite these resource and funding setbacks, many faculty have tried using a range of creative pedagogical interventions to compensate by: utilizing applied research mentoring programs ([8, 9]), creative writing in neuroscience [10], creating nested and scaffolding neuroscience educational programs as a blueprint to learning [11, 12], integrating recent advances in the field into their curriculum [13], teaching computational neuroscience at PUIs [14], the use of case studies to guide explorations [15], teaching courses on publishing in neuroscience [16], increasing brain literacy [17], and using a historical context [18], to name a few. Yet, given these creative approaches, undergraduate- and graduate-level neuroscience students are still lacking in their early career prerequisite training; especially, procedural skills from PUIs. Today, these challenges are being approached through two distinct cost-effective means for neuroscience educational pedagogy and training: (1) open software and hardware utilization [19]; and (2) virtual reality (VR) integration into the curriculum with procedural applied learning [20].

Additionally, others have proposed seven distinct challenges that are beginning to and will continue to shape twenty-first century neuroscience through: (1) becoming big science; (2) developing data ladders between single areas of the brain with different levels of organizations that cross-link and cross-reference between humans and other pre-clinical animal models; (3) developing novel hardware and software to simulate brain activity and computational models that best simulate human properties; (4) improved classification and simulation of brain diseases to better inform diagnosis and effective drug discovery; (5) exploit current knowledge to build new brain-inspired and brain-based technologies benefiting both society and industry; and (6) facilitating neuroscience research to deliver huge societal-linked goals to address the widespread social concern regarding brain disorders and diseases, respectfully [21]. Moreover, in the last two decades, the attentional systems and its underlying neural and nodal networks have become both more integrated and more promising in elucidating the spectrum of attentional disorders coupled with comorbid diagnoses for next generation neuroscientists to further resolve [22].

Reinforcing the position that Altimus et al. [23] and Martin [24] similarly reported across a near 20 year time span, that as the field of neuroscience moves forward it needs to break down the silos of laboratory investigation and move towards more integrative neuroscientific approaches to best advance the field (i.e., cautions are raised here between PUIs and R1s as stated above); while also reducing and working towards eliminating sex biases and omission in neuroscience publication and communication [25–27]. Consistent with these ideas, Vázquez-Guardado et al. [28] noted the advancement in neurotechnologies with broad ranging potential and applications for neuroscience research through the modern use of electrical, optical, and microfluidic methodologies to study brain function. However, considering the aforementioned factors and concerns, it begs the question is society "ready for real-world neuroscience" as a whole, consistent with the position that cognitive neuroscientists have already taken [29]?

Here we propose an underutilized avenue for the future of neuroscience through utilizing VR in both education as a good example of viable application [30] as well as in neuroscience research and therapy [31]. Regarding the latter, VR has been used therapeutically to display simulations of the embodied experience for a range of behavioral health conditions (e.g., anxiety; [32]) and studies have suggested that as early as 2017, that it has been ready for clinical usage to treat patients [33]. Therefore, in this context we consider how VR has evolved over the last two decades and propose how it can be used to further support current and future advancements of medical research and education through complementary learning approaches for next-generation neuroscience students coming from mainly PUIs.

2 The Last 20 Years: Examining the Integration of Neuroscience and VR

It is interesting to see that the first medical articles related to VR (i.e., non-immersive VR) covered content within the neurosciences, where they studied autism [34]. The initial goal of this work was to understand the interaction of a person with autism with their environment, but it also provided insight into perceptual visual, psycho-social, and emotional processing of VR effects on users with autism [34]. Continuing from this original paper and covering the last two decades of advancement, VR technologies have not only become more integrated, but the technology itself has rapidly upgraded with new capabilities (e.g., immersion, augmented virtual reality, first-person point-of-view 180° stereoscopic vision, etc.; [35–38]). These fundamental changes in VR from gaming and entertainment, to psychotherapy, supplemental, and complementary medical student training and pedagogy, have in turn, played critical roles in advancing surgical neuroscience methods ([39–43]). One case in point, is the ability for more resourced universities and hospitals to develop curriculum within the available VR platforms [44] and to then deploy it to other universities and hospitals that may not have neuroscientists, surgeons, or other authorities skilled in the technique to deliver the same procedural skillsets to students enrolled in under resourced institutions of higher learning (i.e., PUIs; [45–51]). Deploying VR in neuroscience education and research has further value between international collaborations, educational exchange, and developing premier training and learning opportunities between developed and developing countries (e.g., Collaborative Online International Learning [COIL] programs that are implemented as Course-based Undergraduate Research Experiences [CURE] within the curriculum; [52–60]; Coumans and Winter 2024). However, addressing these neuroscience infrastructural needs between the under resourced colleges and universities and well-resourced college and universities within the US (i.e., the PUI and R1 conundrum) remain problematic, but given the evolution of VR [61], VR-based pedagogical methods might be a practical under-utilized solution to address this critical issue.

3 The Unprecedented Coronavirus-19: Increased Educational and Research Value of VR

When the Coronavirus-19 (COVID-19) occurred, New York became the first "hot spot of contagion" in the US in which all curriculum shifted drastically from in-person learning to virtual/remote learning educational formats [62]. This situation made science procedural laboratory learning and other hands-on training/applied curricular challenges more difficult to overcome, especially for under resourced colleges and universities. This situation forced faculty to reimagine the curriculum in different ways, with different resources or with little to no resources given the additional constraint of the paused and then slow reinstatement of the technology supply chain. One such example was to record in real-time and deploy a timely COVID-19 healthcare guideline through First-Person Point-of-View (FP-POV) to nurses treating patients that were COVID-19 positive during the pandemic [63]. These concurrent and unprecedented challenges became the catalyst by which VR as illustrated in the prior example began to evolve ever so quickly in both educational and research aspects; especially, for neuroscience [64–70]. For example, as a by-product of COVID-19, many medical school and similar allied healthcare related graduate programs had to shift their curriculum to VR-based platforms for dentistry [71], nursing as apart of neuroeducation [64], neuroscience education and outreach from high school students [65] to undergraduate-level students [72], and graduate-level students in neuroanatomy [73–75], practicing surgical procedures on cadavers and models [50, 76], and neurosurgery [77] to name a few. However, within that context, validation of effective VR vs. anything done in VR as a rapid response to address the COVID-19 challenges became more obscure. Then researchers began to systematically look into VR with greater scrutiny and in many cases, it was validated when deployed in the neuroscience curriculum [78].

4 Undergraduate Neuroscience VR Education: A Changing Climate for Developing Early Career Procedural Skills

Considering the evolution of VR in the context of higher education, it is not surprising that more undergraduate-level colleges and universities are attempting to integrate more VR into their neuroscience curriculum. The use of VR has vast impacts on students' visuospatial abilities whether learning through desktop and immersive VR environments [79, 80]. The VR experience exploits the use of the student's mirror neuron system to envision their perceived VR experience as their own (i.e., an extended proprioceptive experience with a high degree of procedural learning integrative experiences) that serves to reinforce and guide the learner in real-time [81–83]. The neural correlates of these VR-experiences directly connect with the behavioral gesturing of acting out the movements in VR while in an immersive experience anywhere the student may be [84]; thereby facilitating a contrived, yet effective, applied learning experience from afar ([85–87]; *for review on the instructional design see* [87]). However, to overcome cost limitations companies like Revinax®, Google, and others have used cardboards or other cheap modifiable glasses that can be attached to students' cellular phones to use the VR experience from downloaded Apps ([88, 89]). These cost-effective solutions for undergraduate students, especially for PUIs, can truly leverage their educational gains and begin to reduce the education gaps that have become wider over the last 20-years in the neurosciences. Thus, the climate for developing early career procedural skills in the neurosciences may be well positioned to utilize VR in a range of curricular contexts (*For Review, see* [90]). As VR has become more mainstream over the last 20-years, it appears that the literature has not fully recognized nor conceptualized its value in the field of neuroscience along with its many subdisciplines of specialty.

5 Results

In reviewing the literature on VR and neuroscience education over the last 20-years, a set of three article database searches (i.e., *Google Scholar*, *PubMed*, and *Science Direct*) were conducted from the years covering 2004–2024 using the following *key terms*: *"VR AND Neuroscience Education"*; *"Virtual Reality AND Neuroscience Education"*; *"AR AND Neuroscience Education"*; *"Augmented Reality AND Neuroscience Education"*; *"FP-POV AND Neuroscience Education"*; and *"First-Person POV AND Neuroscience Education",* respectively. The 2024 year was not included as we are currently in this year and the data would be truncated and underestimating what the year total might be.

For the *"VR AND Neuroscience"* and the *"Virtual Reality AND Neuroscience"* key words, they did not differ in the number of articles returned; thus, the *"VR AND Neuroscience Education" key terms* were used. Figure 12.1 illustrates an increasing trend line in all three article databases with *Google Scholar* (i.e., an increase from 859 articles from 2004 to 14,100 articles in 2023 [a 1,541.44% increase in publications]), then *PubMed* (i.e., an increase from 0 articles from 2004 to 53 articles in 2023 [i.e., a 53,000% increase in publications]), and finally *Science Direct* (i.e., an increase from 16 articles from 2004 to 317 in 2023 [i.e., a 1,882.25% increase in publications]). Thus, the best place to identify current and more broad ranging research articles on VR and neuroscience education would be either *Google Scholar* or *Science Direct*.

Next, for the *"AR AND Neuroscience"* and the *"Augmented Reality AND Neuroscience"* key words, they did not differ in the number of articles returned; thus, the *"AR AND Neuroscience Education" key terms* were used. Figure 12.2 illustrates an increasing trend line in all three article databases with *Google Scholar* (i.e., an increase from 114 articles from 2004 to 5230 articles in 2023 [a 4,487.72% increase in publications]), then *PubMed* (i.e., an increase from 0 articles from 2004 to 15 articles in 2023 [i.e., a 14,900% increase in publications]), and finally *Science Direct* (i.e., an increase from 18 articles from 2004 to 165 in 2023 [i.e., a 816.67% increase in publications]). Thus, the best place to identify current and more broad ranging research articles on AR and neuroscience education would be either *Google Scholar* or *Science Direct*.

Lastly, for the *"FP-POV AND Neuroscience"* and the *"First-Person POV AND Neuroscience" key words*, the *"FP-POV AND Neuroscience"* key words did not return any articles; thus, the *"First-Person POV AND Neuroscience Education" key terms* were used. Figure 12.3 illustrates an increasing trend line in all three article databases with *Google Scholar* (i.e., an increase from 220 articles from 2004 to 1900 articles in 2023 [a 763.64% increase in publications]), then *PubMed* (i.e., an increase from 0 articles from 2004 to 0 articles in 2023 [i.e., no publications retrieved

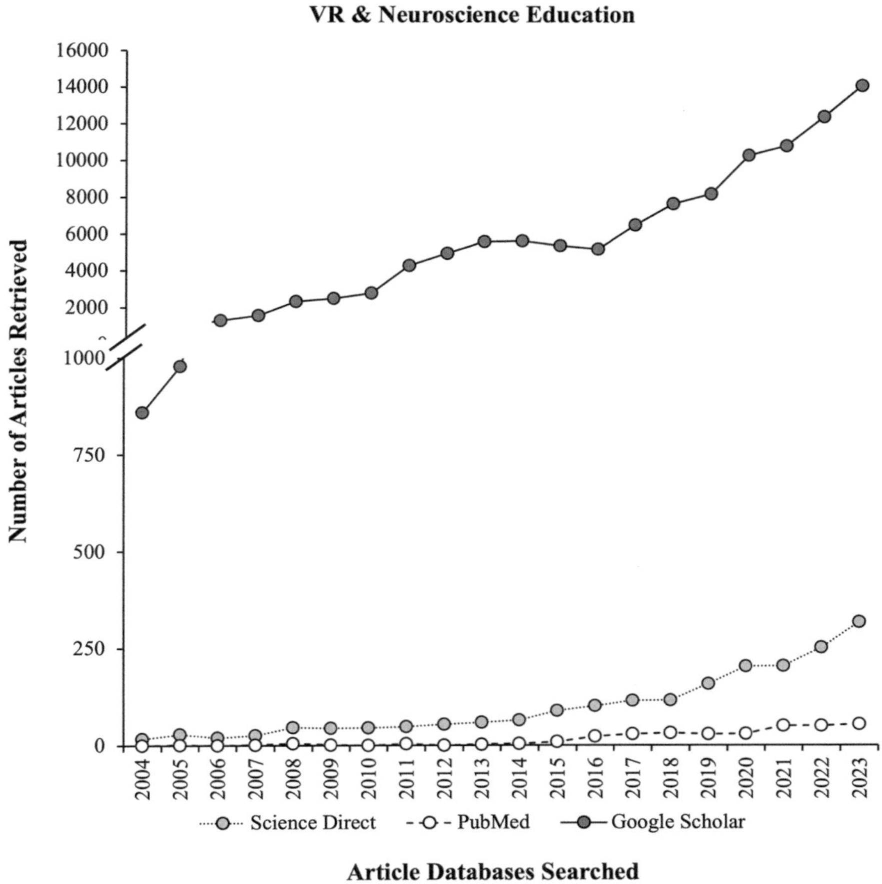

Fig. 12.1 Comparisons between Google Scholar, PubMed, and Science Direct publications searched with the key words "VR AND Neuroscience Education" from 2004 to 2023. The results showed an increasing trend in research published in these areas across all three databases with the following growth rates: Google Scholar (1,541.44%), PubMed (53,000%), and Science Direct (1,882.25%), respectively. (Source © 2024, Neuwirth et al., Used with permission)

within that database covering 20 years]), and finally *Science Direct* (i.e., an increase from 4 articles from 2004 to 110 in 2023 [i.e., a 2,650% increase in publications]). Thus, the best place to identify current and more broad ranging research articles on FP-POV and neuroscience education would be either *Google Scholar* or *Science Direct*.

Although it is important to maintain scientific control and reliability with conducted literature review searches of this kind, one should equally be both methodological and cautious that over the last 20-years new combinations of search terms based on Artificial Intelligent (AI) programming may opt for different proxies for gathering more information in databases like *Google Scholar* than what might be the

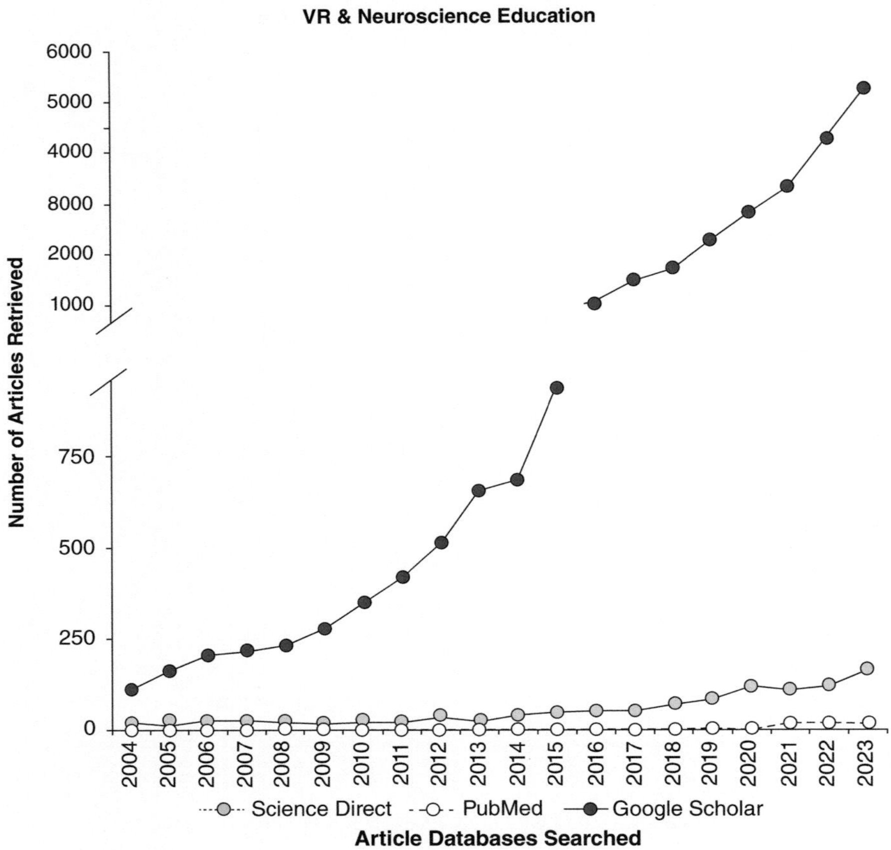

Fig. 12.2 Comparisons between Google Scholar, PubMed, and Science Direct publications searched with the key words "AR AND Neuroscience Education" from 2004 to 2023. The results showed an increasing trend in research published in these areas across all three databases with the following growth rates: Google Scholar (4,487.72%), PubMed (14,900%), and Science Direct (816.67%), respectively. (Source © 2024, Neuwirth et al., Used with permission)

typically utilized in databases like *PubMed* and *Science Direct*. Additionally, PubMed and Science Direct have numerous journals where articles that are submitted for publication and accepted are subjected to either 3–5 year embargo agreements or are limited to pay subscription accessibility (i.e., pay wall barriers to more immediate public access and education). Conversely, these journals can also be on the top-tier side of publications with high impact factors in any neuroscience sub-field that requires substantial money from researchers and educators to pay Article Process Charges (APCs) that can range from a few hundred dollars to ten thousand dollars. Additionally, most researchers and educators at PUIs and MSIs are unable to have their administration cover APCs, unlike Private Universities and Colleges within the US. The latter point is critical as most researchers and educators in the modern world

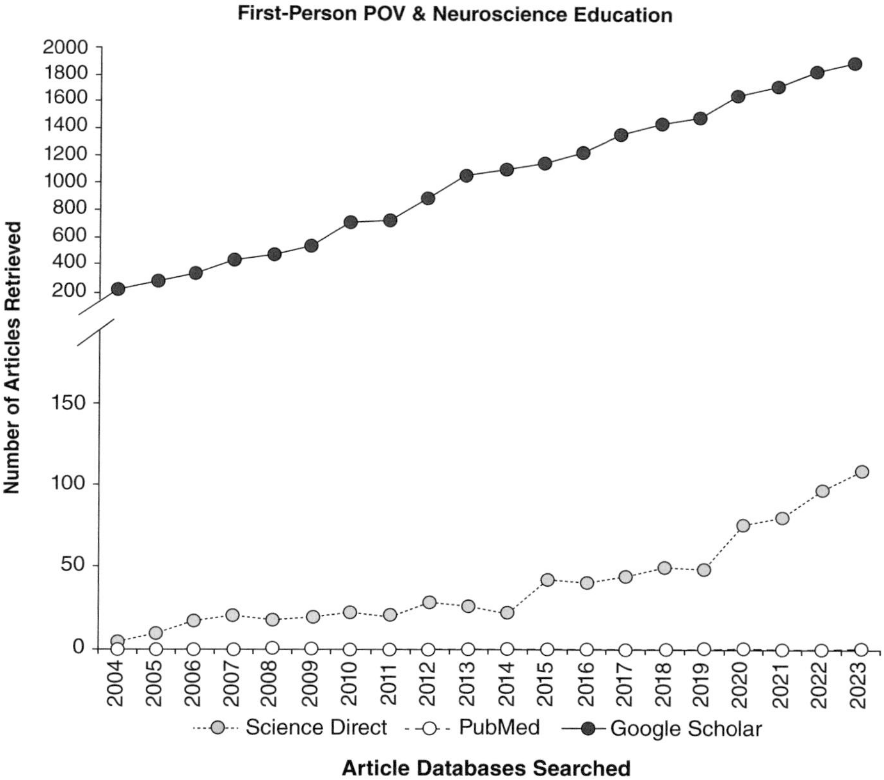

Fig. 12.3 Comparisons between Google Scholar, PubMed, and Science Direct publications searched with the key words "First-Person POV AND Neuroscience Education" from 2004 to 2023. The results showed an increasing trend in research published in these areas across only two databases with the following growth rates: Google Scholar (763.64%) and Science Direct (2650%),whereas PubMed (0%) never had a paper retrieved in that database, respectively. (Source © 2024, Neuwirth et al., Used with permission)

are coming from PUIs/MSIs and are struggling to obtain federal and state grant funding within the US at funding rates between approximately 1.6–3.6% in the neurosciences. Thus, researchers and educators may opt to intentionally seek out lower impact factor journals to publish their work for either free/no APC costs or this may appear as the work is less impactful to other professionals in the field, but may also contribute, in part, as to why Google Scholar may have more articles available within its search capabilities Additionally, from a principled and ethical position, researchers and educators may opt to only publish in journals without pay wall barriers to ensure the public has immediate access to new knowledge generated in their given fields.

Lastly, PUI and MSI colleges and universities may not be able to afford these subscriptions for these high impact factor journals and as a result may redirect themselves and their students to use other no-cost and more accessible (i.e., no paywall to access) publications that may begin to leverage the gap in these initialized practices from high impact journals. However, what is gleaned from these analyses on these three database search engines are that Google Scholars' use of AI can return many more hits with the key words chosen, but more work might need to be done to filter out irrelevant articles which may be cumbersome until *Google* produces better selection filters like *PubMed* and *Science Direct*. It is not unreasonable to think that Google will swiftly address this issue and make its *Google Scholar* database equal if not better than *PubMed* and *Science Direct* for these research-based queries for conducting literature reviews and background reading for experimental studies across any scientific discipline. Here, we just provide one example of this case-in-point for using VR in neuroscience education.

6 Discussion

The range of student's perquisite skills for any curriculum can vary considerably. Implementing VR pedagogy into the curriculum can have substantial advantages besides cost savings to the student and the higher educational industry in supplying students with such VR classrooms or laboratories as well as portable cardboard VR options to partake in similar experiences anywhere in the world. The latter allows for more international student enrollment and collaboration that can also promote more diverse perspectives in the classroom emanating from many differing life experiences. Moreover, the VR programs can serve as intentional pedagogy directed at upskilling, reskilling, and training early career undergraduate students with competitive workforce ready skills in a unique procedural way. This situation enables under resourced PUIs to competitively teach their students with applied learning experiences in which the student's behavioral demonstration of their learned gestures from the VR experience can be assessed as a practicum competency for their overall learning. Students can also, through these early career experiences, learn to make less errors in the contrived VR experience when they begin to be tested in real practicum settings [76]. This is important as undergraduate students have less hands-on training, opportunities to practice skills, less attempts to demonstrate proficiency, and full comprehension of the ability to ethically and safely learn from their errors when demonstrating these learned behaviors in laboratory classes or practicum-based courses. Finally, VR can also serve as a pretext to understand neuroscientific principles underlying its efficiency. Considering the aforementioned factors, VR pedagogical instruction for undergraduate students in the neuroscience can serve to reduce training times, costly resources, and may make students more prepared with job- and crisis-ready skills unlike prior generations of students in the neurosciences.

7 Conclusion

Thus, VR has shown much promise over the last 20-years as a timely and unique, yet underutilized, neuroscience pedagogical tool and research method in which undergraduate students could greatly benefit from if engaged earlier in their careers. This encouraging direction to integrate VR early in the undergraduate student curriculum for the neurosciences is further motivated by its attractiveness and ease of delivering the curriculum across different teaching modalities (i.e., in-person, online, and remote learning). Such curricular flexibility offers more equitable solutions to help students from PUIs to also overcome several educational barriers to resources, access, and other inequities. The growing recognition over the last two decades that VR can be creatively and effectively used within the neurosciences to overcome these educational barriers is becoming more clear and less disputed, but not implemented as frequently as we would have thought by now. If PUIs want to level the playing field for providing their undergraduate students with earlier job market ready procedural skills, then they should consider ways to adopt and integrate cost effective VR solutions for their neuroscience programs.

References

1. Hardwick JC, Smith JS. Undergraduate neuroscience faculty: results from a survey of faculty for undergraduate neuroscience members. J Undergrad Neurosci Educ. 2010;8(2):A101–7.
2. Kreitzer MA, Malchow RP. Engaging undergraduates in a unique neuroscience research opportunity: a collaborative research experience between a primarily undergraduate institution (PUI) and a major research institution. J Undergrad Neurosci Educ. 2013;12(1):A85–92.
3. Rovnyak D, Shields GC. A roadmap to successful collaborations between primarily undergraduate institutions and research institutions. In: Credit where credit is due: respecting authorship and intellectual property. Washington, DC: American Chemical Society; 2018. p. 105–27. https://doi.org/10.1021/bk-2018-1291.ch011.
4. Yeung AWK, Goto TK, Leung WK. The changing landscape of neuroscience research, 2006–2015: a bibliometric study. Front Neurosci. 2017;11:120. https://doi.org/10.3389/fnins.2017.00120.
5. Ramos RL, Esposito AW, O'Malley S, Smith PT, Grisham W. Undergraduate neuroscience education in the US: quantitative comparisons of programs and graduates in the broader context of undergraduate life sciences education. J Undergrad Neurosci Educ. 2016;15(1):A1–4.
6. Ramos RL, Fokas GJ, Bhambri A, Smith PT, Hallas BH, Brumberg JC. Undergraduate neuroscience education in the US: an analysis using data from the National Center for Education Statistics. J Undergrad Neurosci Educ. 2011;9(2):A66–70.
7. Ramirez JJ. Undergraduate neuroscience education: meeting the challenges of the 21st century. Neurosci Lett. 2020;739:135418. https://doi.org/10.1016/j.neulet.2020.135418.
8. Ramos RL. Virtual was the reality in neuroscience education during the COVID-19 pandemic. J Undergrad Res. 2020;19(1):E1–E2.
9. Mickley GA, Kenmuir C, Remmers-Roeber D. Mentoring undergraduate students in neuroscience research: a model system at Baldwin-Wallace College. J Undergrad Neurosci Educ. 2003;1(2):A28–35.
10. Adams J. "Writing in neuroscience": a course designed for neuroscience undergraduate students. J Undergrad Neurosci Educ. 2011;10(1):A50–7.

11. Wiertalak EP, Hardwick J, Kerchner M, Parfitt K, Ramirez JJ. The new blueprints: undergraduate neuroscience education in the twenty-first century. J Undergrad Neurosci Educ. 2018;16(3):A244–51.
12. Wiertelak EP, Ramirez JJ. Undergraduate neuroscience education: blueprints for the 21st century. J Undergrad Neurosci Educ. 2008;6(2):A34–9.
13. Cleland CL. Integrating recent advances in neuroscience into undergraduate neuroscience and physiology courses. Adv Physiol Educ. 2002;26(1–4):271–277. https://doi.org/10.1152/advan.00044.2002.
14. Oprisan SA. Interdisciplinary curriculum for computational neuroscience at primarily undergraduate institutions. J Comput Sci. 2022;61:101642. https://doi.org/10.1016/j.jocs.2022.101642.
15. Meil WM. The use of case studies in teaching undergraduate neuroscience. J Undergrad Neurosci Educ. 2007;5(2):A53–62.
16. Jones LS, Black LC, Bright L, Meekins C, Thakur V, Warren C. An undergraduate course on publishing neuroscience. J Undergrad Neurosci Educ. 2006;4(2):A60–7.
17. Salomon D, Martin-Harris L, Mullen B, Odegaard B, Zvinyatskovskiy A, Chandler SH. Brain literate: making neuroscience accessible to a wider audience of undergraduates. J Undergrad Neurosci Educ. 2015;13(2):A64–73.
18. Neuwirth LS, Dacius TF Jr, Mukherji BR. Teaching neuroanatomy through a historical context. J Undergrad Neurosci Educ. 2018;16(2):E26–31.
19. Chagas AM, Canli T, Ziadlou D, Forlano PM, Smaddar S, Chua E, Baskerville KA, Poon K, Neuwirth LS. Editorial: Using open neuroscience to advance equity in the pedagogy and research infrastructure in colleges/universities still financially impacted by COVID-19: the emergence of a global resource network aimed at integrating neuroscience and society. J Undergrad Neurosci Educ. 2023;21(2):E2–7. https://pubmed.ncbi.nlm.nih.gov/37588641
20. Ros M, Weaver L, Neuwirth LS. Virtual reality stereoscopic 180-degree video-based immersive environments: Applications for training surgeons and other medical professionals. In JE Stefaniak (Ed.) Cases on Instructional Design and Performance Outcomes in Medical Education. 2020 pp. 92–110. Hershey, PA: IGI Global. https://www.igi-global.com/book/casesinstructional-design-performance-outcomes/244674.
21. Markram H. Seven challenges for neuroscience. Funct Neurol. 2013;28(3):145–51.
22. Petersen SE, Posner MI. The attention system of the human brain: 20 years after. Annu Rev Neurosci. 2012;35:73–89. https://doi.org/10.1146/annurev-neuro-062111-150525.
23. Altimus CM, Marlin BJ, Charalambakis NE, Colón-Rodrígues A, Glover EJ, Izbicki P, Johnson A, Lourenco MV, Makinson RA, McQuail J, Obeso I, Padilla-Coreano N, Wells MF. The next 50 years of neuroscience. J Neurosci. 2020;40(1):101–6. https://doi.org/10.1523/JNEUROSCI.0744-19.2019.
24. Martin JB. The integration of neurology, psychiatry, and neuroscience in the 21st century. Am J Psychiatry. 2002;159(5):695–704. https://doi.org/10.1176/appi.ajp.159.5.695.
25. Mamlouk GM, Dorris DM, Barrett LR, Meitzen J. Sex bias and omission in neuroscience research is influenced by research model and journal, but not reported NIH funding. Front Neuroendocrinol. 2020;57:100835. https://doi.org/10.1016/j.yfrne.2020.100835.
26. Shansky RM, Woolley CS. Considering sex as a biological variable will be valuable for neuroscience research. J Neurosci. 2016;36(47):11817–22. https://doi.org/10.1523/JNEUROSCI.1390-16.2016.
27. Will TR, Proaño SB, Thomas AM, Kunz LM, Thompson KC, Ginnari LA, Jones CH, Lucas SC, Reavis EM, Dorris DM, Meitzen J. Problems and progress regarding sex bias and omission in neuroscience research. eNeuro. 2017;4(6):ENEURO.0278-17.2017. https://doi.org/10.1523/ENEURO.0278-17.2017.
28. Vázquez-Guardado A, Yang Y, Bandodkar AJ, Rogers JA. Recent advances in neurotechnologies with broad potential for neuroscience research. Nat Neurosci. 2020;23:1522–36. https://doi.org/10.1038/s41593-020-00739-8.

29. Matusz PJ, Dikker S, Huth AG, Perrodin C. Are we ready for real-world neuroscience? J Cogn Neurosci. 2019;31(3):327–38. https://doi.org/10.1162/jocn_e_01276.
30. Devonshire IM, Dommett EJ. Neuroscience: viable applications in education? Neuroscientist. 2010;16(4):349–56. https://doi.org/10.1177/1073858410370900.
31. Bohil CJ, Alicea B, Biocca FA. Virtual reality in neuroscience research and therapy. Nat Rev Neurosci. 2011;12(12):752–62. https://doi.org/10.1038/nrn322.
32. Riva G, Wiederhold BK, Mantovani F. Neuroscience of virtual reality: from virtual exposure to embodied medicine. Cyberpsychol Behav Soc Netw. 2019;22(1):82–96. https://doi.org/10.1089/cyber.2017.29099.gri.
33. Rizzo AS, Koenig ST. Is clinical virtual reality ready for primetime? Neuropsychology. 2017;31(8):877–99. https://doi.org/10.1037/neu0000405.
34. Max ML, Burke JC. Virtual reality for autism communication and education, with lessons for medical training simulators. Stud Health Technol Inform. 1997;39:46–53. https://pubmed.ncbi.nlm.nih.gov/10184722.
35. Cipresso P, Giglioli IAC, Raya MA, Riva G. The past, present, and future of virtual and augmented reality research: a network and cluster analysis of the literature. Front Psychol. 2018;9:309500. https://doi.org/10.3389/fpsyg.2018.02086.
36. Hamad A, Jia B. How virtual reality technology has changed our lives: an overview of the current and potential applications and limitations. Int J Environ Res Public Health. 2022;19(18):11278. https://doi.org/10.3390/ijerph191811278.
37. Liu D, Bhagat KK, Goa Y, Chang TW, Huang R. The potentials and trends of virtual reality in education: a bibliometric analysis on top research studies in the last two decades. In: Virtual, augmented, and mixed realities in education. Singapore: Springer; 2017. p. 105–30. https://doi.org/10.1007/978-981-10-5490-7_7.
38. Wohlgenannt I, Simons A, Stieglitz S. Virtual reality. Bus Inf Syst Eng. 2020;62:455–61. https://doi.org/10.1007/s12599-020-00658-9.
39. Meier AH, Rawn CL, Krummel TM. Virtual reality: surgical application—challenge for the new millennium. J Am Coll Surg. 2001;192(2):372–84. https://doi.org/10.1016/S1072-7515(01)00769-4.
40. Muñoz-Saavedra L, Miró-Amarante L, Domínguez-Morales M. Augmented and virtual reality evolution and future tendency. Appl Sci. 2020;10(1):322. https://doi.org/10.3390/app10010322.
41. Pensieri C, Pennacchini M. Overview: virtual reality in medicine. J Virtual Worlds Res. 2014;7(1). Lantern Part 1. https://doi.org/10.4101/jvwr.v7i1.6364.
42. Pottle J. Virtual reality and the transformation of medical education. Future Healthc J. 2019;6(3):181. https://doi.org/10.7861/fhj.2019-0036.
43. Claudio P, Maddalena P. Overview: Virtual reality in medicine. Journal of Virtual Worlds Research. 2014;7(1).
44. Ruthenbeck GS, Reynolds KJ. Virtual reality for medical training: the state-of-the-art. J Simul. 2015;9:16–26. https://doi.org/10.1057/jos.2014.14.
45. Gallagher AG, Rittler EM, Champion H, Higgins G, Fried MP, Moses G, Smith CD, Satava RM. Virtual reality simulation for the operating room: proficiency-based training as a paradigm shift in surgical skills training. Ann Surg. 2005;241(2):364–72. https://doi.org/10.1097/01.sla.0000151982.85062.80.
46. Lungu AJ, Swinkels W, Claesen L, Tu P, Egger J, Chen X. A review of the applications of virtual reality, augmented reality and mixed reality in surgical simulation: an extension to different kinds of surgery. Expert Rev Med Devices. 2021;18(1):47–62. https://doi.org/10.1080/17434440.2021.1860750.
47. Pensieri C, Pennacchini M. Virtual reality in medicine. In: Handbook on 3D3C platforms: applications and tools for three dimensional systems for community, creation and commerce. Cham: Springer International Publishing; 2016. p. 353–401. https://doi.org/10.1007/978-3-319-22041-3.

48. Velazquez-Pimentel D, Hurkxkens T, Nehme J. Virtual reality for the digital surgeon. In: Digital surgery. Cham: Springer; 2021. p. 183–201. https://doi.org/10.1007/978-3-030-49100-0_14.
49. Westwood JD, editor. Medicine meets virtual reality 20: NextMed/MMVR20, vol. 184. Amsterdam: IOS Press; 2013.
50. Neuwirth LS, Ng S, Devors S, Lonjon N, Ros M. Comparing 4th-year medical student's procedural surgical skills learning outcomes between third-person point-of-view video lectures and first-person point-of-view immersive virtual reality: a pilot study surgically implanting a subdermal drain on cadavers. Front Virtual Real. 2024;5:1408092. https://doi.org/10.3389/frvir.2024.1408092.
51. Ros M, Neuwirth LS, Prasolova-Førland E. Editorial: Redefining the pedagogy in virtual and augmented reality in medical science education. Front. Virtual Real. Sec. Virtual Reality in Medicine, 2024;5:1533837. https://doi.org/10.3389/frvir.2024.1533837.
52. Cesanek E, Shivkumar S, Ingram JN, Wolpert DM. Ouvrai opens access to remote virtual reality studies of human behavioural neuroscience. Nat Hum Behav. 2024;8(6):1209–24. https://doi.org/10.1038/s41562-024-01834-7.
53. Chen W, Lyu Q, Ho MYM, Tan J, Teo WP, Chai SCA, Su G. The role of individual preparation on coordination in computer-supported collaborative learning: a neuroscience perspective on learners' inter-brain synchronization. In: 17th international conference on computer-supported collaborative learning (CSCL) 2024-CSCL proceedings, vol. 2024; 2024.
54. Diwakar S, Parasuram H, Medini C, Raman R, Nedungadi P, Wiertelak E, Srivastava S, Achuthan K, Nair B. Complementing neurophysiology education for developing countries via cost-effective virtual labs: case studies and classroom scenarios. J Undergrad Neurosci Educ. 2014;12(2):A130–9.
55. Isager PM, Lakens D, van Leeuwen T, van't Veer AE. Exploring a formal approach to selecting studies for replication: a feasibility study in social neuroscience. Cortex. 2024;171:330–46. https://doi.org/10.1016/j.cortex.2023.10.012.
56. Kannan R, Gendreau M, Hatch A, Free SK, Muriungi K, Garje YA, DeBoer J, Gage GJ, Harris CA. Building brains for robots: a hands-on approach to learning neuroscience in the classroom. bioRxiv. 2024. https://doi.org/10.1101/2024.05.15.594177.
57. Ramirez-Zamora A, Giordano J, Gunduz A, Alcantara J, Cagle JN, Cemera S, Difuntorum P, Eisinger RS, Gomez J, Long S, Parks B. Proceedings of the seventh annual deep brain stimulation think tank: advances in neurophysiology, adaptive DBS, virtual reality, neuroethics and technology. Front Hum Neurosci. 2020;14:54. https://doi.org/10.3389/fnhum.2020.00054.
58. Thompson PM, Jahanshad N, Ching CR, Salminen LE, Thomopoulos SI, Bright J, Baune BT, Bertolín S, Bralten J, Bruin WB, Bülow R. ENIGMA and global neuroscience: a decade of large-scale studies of the brain and health and disease across more than 40 countries. Transl Psychiatry. 2020;10(1):100. https://doi.org/10.1038/s41398-020-0705-1.
59. Wilson KD. Integrating non-invasive brain stimulation into the undergraduate psychology curriculum: an upper-level laboratory course using transcranial direct current stimulation. Teach Psychol. 2024;51(1):110–7. https://doi.org/10.1177/00986283211060324.
60. Coumans JV, Wark S. Impact of problem-based learning coaching and neuroeducation in the development of 21st century lifelong learners. Mind Brain Educ. 2024;18(1):35–42. https://doi.org/10.1111/mbe.12406.
61. Mehra RK. Evolutionary advantages of virtual reality in education. In: Transforming education with virtual reality. New Jersey: Wiley; 2024. p. 73–86. https://doi.org/10.1002/9781394200498.ch5.
62. Neuwirth LS, Jović S, Mukherji BR. Reimagining higher education during and post-COVID-19: challenges and opportunities. J Adult Contin Educ. 2020;27(2):1–16. https://doi.org/10.1177/1477971420947738.
63. Ros M, Neuwirth LS. Increasing global awareness of timely COVID-19 healthcare guidelines through FPV training tutorials: portable public health crises teaching method. Nurse Educ Today. 2020;91(104479):1–6. https://doi.org/10.1016/j.nedt.2020.104479.

64. Cardoso K, Zaro MA, da Silva PF. The evaluation of the virtual immersive learning laboratory in health and nursing (LIASE): a study in neuroeducation. Immersive Learning Research-Academic 2024:306–16. https://doi.org/10.56198/U6C0W3BAT.
65. Ghani N, Baker H, Huntsinger A, Chen T, Familara TD, Itorralba JY, Vanderford F, Zhuang X, Change CL, Vo V, Oh EC. Science education for the youth (SEFTY): a neuroscience outreach program for high school students in Southern Nevada during the COVID-19 pandemic. eNeuro. 2024;11(4).
66. Obrero-Gaitán E, Nieto-Escamez FA, Zagalaz-Anula N, Cortés-Pérez I. An innovative approach for online neuroanatomy and neurorehabilitation teaching based on 3D virtual anatomical models using leap motion controller during COVID-19 pandemic. Front Psychol. 2021;12:590196. https://doi.org/10.3389/fpsyg.2021.590196.
67. Sahu M, Gupta R, Ambasta RK, Kumar P. IoT-driven augmented reality and virtual reality systems in neurological sciences. Internet Things. 2024;25:101098. https://doi.org/10.1016/j.iot.2024.101098.
68. Singh R, Baby B, Singh R, Suri A. Role of virtual modules to supplement neurosurgery education during COVID-19. J Clin Neurosci. 2021;91:125–30. https://doi.org/10.1016/j.jocn.2021.06.039.
69. Zhang Z, Gao Y, Pan Y, Zhou J. Video education through the lens of educational neuroscience: a concise review. TechTrends. 2024;68(3):469–84. https://doi.org/10.1007/s11528-024-00946-1.
70. Winter L, Periquito J, Kolbitsch C, Pellicer-Guridi R, Nunes RG, Häuer M, Broche L, O'Reily T. Open-source magnetic resonance imaging: improving access, science, and education through global collaboration. NMR Biomed. 2024;37(7):e5052. https://doi.org/10.1002/nbm.5052.
71. Kashwani R, Kulkarni V, Salam S, Sharma S, Rathi P, Gupta S, Sinha P, Kumari A, Sharma A. Virtual vs. augmented reality in the field of dentistry. Commun Pract. 2024;21(3):597–603.
72. Sharma K, Aswal HS, Chauhan R, Rawat R, Gupta R. Neuroscience of virtual reality. In: 2024 international conference on intelligent and innovative technologies in computing, electrical and electronics (IITCEE). Piscataway: IEEE; 2024. p. 1–6.
73. Aridan N, Bernstein-Eliav M, Gamzo D, Schmeidler M, Tik N, Tavor I. Neuroanatomy in virtual reality: development and pedagogical evaluation of photogrammetry based 3D brain models. Anat Sci Educ. 2024;17(2):239–48. https://doi.org/10.1002/ase.2359.
74. Gurses ME, Gökalp E, Gecici NN, Gungor A, Berker M, Ivan ME, Komotar RJ, Cohen-Gadol AA, Türe U. Creating a neuroanatomy education model with augmented reality and virtual reality simulations of white matter tracts. J Neurosurg. 2024;141(3):865–74. https://doi.org/10.3171/2024.2.JNS2486.
75. Rodriguez-Amendariz AG, Saint-Germain MA, Khalafallah AM, Huq S, Almeida ND, Dornbos DL III, Graffeo CS, Sivakumar W, Mukherjee D, Johnson JN. The neurosurgery research & education foundation-young neurosurgeons committee webinar series: providing education and inspiration during the COVID-19 pandemic. J Clin Neurosci. 2024;120:221–8. https://doi.org/10.1016/j.jocn.2024.01.021.
76. Ros M, Neuwirth LS, Ng S, Debien B, Molinari N, Gatto F, Lanjon N. The effects of an immersive virtual reality application in first person point-of-view, video-based, on the learning and generalized performance of a lumbar puncture medical procedure. Educ Technol Res Dev. 2021;69:1529–56. https://doi.org/10.1007/s11423-021-10003-w.
77. Wach J, Winkler D, Vychopen M, Kropla F, Grunert R, Güresir E. Student's perspectives regarding needs for and opportunities with mixed-reality education in neurosurgery at German medical schools. Neurosurg Focus. 2024;56(1):E17. https://doi.org/10.3171/2023.10.FOCUS23628.
78. Xin Y, Wang R, Liang Y, Lu Q, Zhang N. A proposed framework of virtual reality system design for neuroscience education in mental health. In: International conference on human-computer interaction. Cham: Springer Nature Switzerland; 2024. p. 136–52. https://doi.org/10.1007/978-3-031-60012-8_9.
79. Brucker B, Pardi G, Uehlin F, Moosmann L, Lachmair M, Halfmann M, Gerjets P. How learners' visuospatial ability and different ways of changing the perspective influence learning

about movements in desktop and immersive virtual reality environments. Educ Psychol Rev. 2024;36(3):65. https://doi.org/10.1007/s10648-024-09895-w.
80. Neuwirth LS, Ros M. Comparisons between first person point-of-view 180 video virtual reality head mounted display and 3D video computer display in teaching undergraduate neuroscience students stereotaxic surgeries. Front Virtual Real. 2021;2:706653. https://doi.org/10.3389/frvir.2011.706653.
81. Bonini L, Rotunno C, Arcuri E, Gallese V. Mirror neurons 30-years later: implications and applications. Trends Cogn Sci. 2022;26(9):767–81. https://doi.org/10.1016/j.tics.2022.06.003.
82. Curry M. If I only had a brain: mirroring neurons, authentic relationship (regulate, relate, reason). In: The neural teaching guide. London: Routledge; 2024. p. 195–208.
83. Lauharatanahirun N, Won A, Hwang AHC. External and internal attribution in human-agent interaction: insights from neuroscience and virtual reality. Hum Mach Commun. 2024;8(1):119–39. https://doi.org/10.30658/hmc.8.6.
84. Bodet T. Neurobehavioral correlates of embodiment in immersive virtual-reality-assisted learning [Doctoral dissertation]; 2024. https://hdl.handle.net/10657/16154.
85. Laine TH, Suk HJ. Investigating user experience of an immersive virtual reality simulation based on gesture-based user interface. Appl Sci. 2024;14(11):4935. https://doi.org/10.3390/app14114935.
86. Ros M, Neuwirth LS. Immersion Dans Les Réalités Étendues—Outil De Formation VR Et Spécificités Du 180-FPV. Maitrise Orthopedique. 2023;328:1–12.
87. Ros M, Weaver L, Neuwirth LS. Virtual reality stereoscopic 180-degree video-based immersive environments: applications for training surgeons and other medical professionals. In: Stefaniak JE, editor. Cases on instructional design and performance outcomes in medical education. Hershey, PA: IGI Global; 2022. p. 92–119. https://www.igi-global.com/book/cases-instructional-design-performance-outcomes/244674.
88. Martins IF. Additive manufacturing in the development of low-cost immersive virtual reality solutions for education: a study with Google cardboard. Lond J Soc Sci. 2024;(8):39–51. https://doi.org/10.31039/ljiss.2024.8.209.
89. Rockcastle SF, Sollom-Brotherton Whalen G, Milgrim A, Davis R. The use of virtual screens in perceptual studies on electric light: a comparison between 2D, panoramic, cardboard, and head-mounted displays. LEUKOS. 2024;20(3):275–90. https://doi.org/10.1080/15502724.2023.2279517.
90. Bocanegra-Becerra JE, Sánchez JLA, Castilla-Encinas AM, Rioa-Garcia W, Mendieta CD, Quiroz-Marcelo DA, Alwaishel K, Aguilar-Zegarra L, Lopez-Gonzalez MA. Toward a frontierless collaboration in neurosurgery: a systematic review of remote augmented and virtual reality technologies. World Neurosurg. 2024;187:114–21. https://doi.org/10.1016/j.wneu.2024.04.048.

MIX
Papier aus verantwortungsvollen Quellen
Paper from responsible sources
FSC® C105338

If you have any concerns about our products,
you can contact us on
ProductSafety@springernature.com

In case Publisher is established outside the EU,
the EU authorized representative is:
Springer Nature Customer Service Center GmbH
Europaplatz 3, 69115 Heidelberg, Germany

Printed by Libri Plureos GmbH
in Hamburg, Germany

Practical Handbook for Small-Gauge Vitrectomy

Ulrich Spandau • Heinrich Heimann

Practical Handbook for Small-Gauge Vitrectomy

A Step-By-Step Introduction to Surgical Techniques

Second Edition

Springer

Ulrich Spandau
University Eye Hospital
Uppsala, Sweden

Heinrich Heimann
Royal Liverpool University Hospital
Liverpool, United Kingdom

ISBN 978-3-030-07829-4 ISBN 978-3-319-89677-9 (eBook)
https://doi.org/10.1007/978-3-319-89677-9

This Springer imprint is published by Springer Nature, under the registered company Springer International Publishing AG
The registered company address is: Gewerbestrasse 11, 6330 Cham, Switzerland

This book is dedicated to our parents.

Foreword 1

In 2002 when the team of Eugene de Juan, Los Angeles, published their first experience of the transconjunctival sutureless vitrectomy with 25-gauge instruments, it could not be foreseen that the "small gauge vitrectomy" would become the new standard procedure of vitrectomy within a few years.

Most retinal surgeons had previously considered the conjunctiva and sclera in a 20-gauge vitrectomy as a more or less troublesome and time-consuming obstacle before and after their true passion, the vitreous cavity. The extensive opening of the conjunctiva in conventional 20-gauge vitrectomy, the suture material used for the closure of sclera and conjunctiva, and the sometimes wide-scale application of diathermy resulted often in a pronounced trauma of the outer layers of the eye. Thus, any revisional surgery became increasingly difficult due to the increased scarring of conjunctiva and Tenon's capsule and the atrophy of the sclera in the pars plana.

Due to their flexibility, the first 25-gauge instruments were initially only used for relatively simple vitreoretinal surgery at the posterior pole. However, the minimally invasive approach by de Juan was from the beginning fascinating, because not only was the extraocular part of a vitrectomy significantly shortened, but the trauma of conjunctiva and sclera was also significantly reduced.

In 2004, inspired by de Juan's method, Claus Eckardt developed a trocar cannula system and instruments with a diameter of 23-gauge in Frankfurt-Höchst. This invention had on one side the advantage of the 25-gauge vitrectomy and on the other side the efficiency of the 20-gauge instruments. The aim was to carry out all possible vitreoretinal surgery with the same instrumentarium and this has since then become reality in our department.

A key to the success of the 23-gauge technology step has been Claus Eckardt's concept of a tangential insertion of the trocars and the use of valves for the cannulas: Due to the tunnel-shaped incision technique within the sclera, an intraoperatively stable positioning of the cannulas, and a sutureless closure of the sclerotomies after removal of the cannulas, postoperative hypotension or even endophthalmitis could be prevented. The valves allow a vitrectomy in a closed system and reduce the flow of infusion fluid through the vitreous cavity.

Ulrich Spandau presents in this very practical book of 23-gauge vitrectomy the latest equipment and instruments needed for a 23-gauge vitrectomy, and he explains in detail the most important surgical techniques.

A lot of useful tips, and last but not least the included DVD with a variety of surgical videos, make this book a very useful surgical compendium.

This practical book will be a great guide for the young ophthalmic surgeons who want to familiarize themselves with modern vitrectomy.

Even experienced vitreoretinal surgeons, who wish to switch from 20-gauge to 23-gauge vitrectomy, will benefit from this compendium.

Frankfurt-Höchst, Germany
April 2010

Tillmann Eckert

Foreword 2

Dr. Ulrich Spandau confirms with this compendium to be the most dedicated of my so far eight fellows in vitreoretinal surgery. He presents here our current surgical concept, instrumentation, and operative techniques that have been developed in Uppsala in the last 17 years. It is a transconjunctival, 23-gauge microincision vitrectomy surgery (MIVS), combined with phacoemulsification in elderly patients, performed bimanually for the most of complex indications. To the best of my knowledge no comparable practical guide for current vitreoretinal surgery has been published since Zivojnovic's *Silicone Oil in Vitreoretinal Surgery*, in 1987. Since then vitreoretinal surgery has changed very much, from 20-gauge macroincisional vitrectomy with silicone oil tamponade in most of the cases to 23-gauge microincisional, bimanual vitrectomy with gas tamponade that we use today.

Dr. Spandau has opened a treasure box that he has filled patiently for several years and presents here some genuine surgical pearls—those that he has discovered for himself, those that we have discussed together, those that I have shown him, and furthermore those that were known since before. That gives an opportunity to both beginners and more experienced vitreoretinal surgeons to improve their practical knowledge and refine their procedures in this field. It is our duty to share all the surgical skills and knowledge with each other to provide the best results for our patients. This book is a genuine account of our practical work dedicated to them, which Dr. Spandau has written in collaboration with Dr. Heinrich Heimann. Thank you, Ulrich, and Heinrich!

Department of Ophthalmology
University Hospital,
Uppsala, Sweden

Zoran Tomic

Preface

Since the first edition of this book vitreoretinal surgery with trocars has won the race against non-trocar surgery. 20-gauge surgery is a chapter in history books. And an end to this rapid development is not foreseeable. When the first edition of this book was written, 23-gauge was the gold standard in Europe. And today, when the second edition is published 25-gauge is becoming the most popular gauge and 27-gauge is growing fast.

It is difficult to give a vitreoretinal surgeon a good advice for his surgery. In contrast to the cataract surgeon who has a clear surgical aim, which is the removal of the opacified lens and implantation of an IOL, the vitreoretinal surgeon faces many pathologies and many possible surgical approaches.

Two factors are essential for high standard vitreoretinal surgery:

1. Correct assessment
2. Surgical technique

If correct assessment is the theory, then surgical skills are the praxis. What is the difference between theory and praxis? Theory means that you know everything but nothing functions. And praxis means that everything functions but you do not know why.

Correct assessment you acquire with time and experience. Correct assessment is required before surgery resulting in a good timing and planning of surgery. Correct assessment is also required during surgery guiding you through the operation and changing surgical techniques if necessary. Correct assessment is finally required after surgery in order to assess postoperative complications. The next important factor is surgical technique. Surgical technique is a combination of skills and rigorous training. Every pathology can be operated with several techniques. A detachment can be operated with buckling surgery or with vitrectomy; a luxated IOL can be refixated with scleral fixation, intrascleral fixation, iris fixation, and so on. Learn as many techniques as possible, as it will improve your surgical outcome immensely.

We often overtreat when performing vitreoretinal surgery and we should therefore reflect our surgery critically with the aim to find a surgical approach with maximal results and minimal overtreatment. In retinal detachment, for example, the surgical spectrum has a big range with episcleral buckling at one end of the spectrum and vitrectomy with encircling band, lensectomy, and silicone oil on the other end of the spectrum. Maybe the best surgical advice is: Operate as much as necessary and as little as possible.

All chapters of the second edition have been revised to take account of the advent of 25G and 27G vitrectomy. New chapters have been added: PPV for dummies, vitrectomy with a cataract machine, submacular hemorrhage, macular translocation, and intraocular tumor biopsy. In addition, the video section has been completely reworked and many new videos have been added.

We wish every reader, may he or she be a beginner or an advanced surgeon, to enjoy reading this book and watching the surgical videos.

Uppsala, Sweden
Liverpool, UK
January 2018

Ulrich Spandau
Heinrich Heimann

Acknowledgments

I want to thank my wife, Katrin, for having so much patience with a husband who spends so much time with the writing of his books. Next I want to thank my sons, Maximilian and Moritz, for spending time with me in my office editing the videos for the book. Then I want thank my youngest son, Oskar, for being less naughty than usual. Finally, I want to thank my dog, Socrates, for the endless walks providing fresh ideas for this book.

Contents

Abbreviations

C_2F_6	Perfluoroethane, gas for retinal tamponade
C_3F_8	Perfluoropropane, gas for retinal tamponade
CSTS	Kinematic viscosity of a fluid (unit = Stokes, here: centistokes)
ERM	Epiretinal membrane
ICG	Indocyanine green, dye used for macular hole surgery
IOFB	Intraocular foreign body
IOL	Intraocular lens
IOP	Intraocular pressure
PDVR	Proliferative diabetic vitreoretinopathy
PDR	Proliferative diabetic retinopathy
PFCL	Perfluorocarbon liquid
PPV	Pars plana vitrectomy
PRP	Panretinal laser photocoagulation
PVD	Posterior vitreous detachment
PVR	Proliferative vitreoretinopathy
RRD	Rhegmatogenous retinal detachment
SCH	Suprachoroidal hemorrhage
SF_6	Sulphahexafluoride, gas for retinal tamponade

List of Videos

The videos can be viewed and downloaded from http://extras.springer.com.

Part I
Introduction to Small-Gauge Vitrectomy

Chapter 1
Introduction to Small-Gauge Vitrectomy

1.1 History

Since the 1970s, 20-gauge vitrectomy has evolved as the worldwide standard for vitreoretinal surgery. All instruments have a lumen diameter (inside diameter) of 0.9 mm. See also Table 1.1. For this procedure, the conjunctiva is opened, three sclerotomies are placed, and the infusion cannula is sutured to the sclera. In the majority of cases, trocar cannulas are not used, and at the end of the surgery, the sclerotomies are sutured.

In 2002, Eugene de Juan et al. introduced 25-gauge vitrectomy. The instruments had a lumen diameter of 0.5 mm. Trocars (cannulas) were used for the infusion and the instruments. The trocars were inserted transconjunctivally and transsclerally and remained in place during the entire surgery without the need for suturing them to the sclera. A major advantage of this new technique was the reduced anterior segment trauma during the procedure, because the conjunctiva is not opened and the instruments are smaller. One disadvantage was an increased risk for postoperative hypotony due to the absence of sutures. Another disadvantage was that the instruments were very flexible and not all instruments could be produced in such a small diameter. Meanwhile, more rigid instruments were developed that proved to be easier to handle. The 25-gauge technology is particularly popular in the United States.

In 2004, 23-gauge vitrectomy with a lumen diameter of 0.65 mm was developed at the Eye Clinic Frankfurt- Höchst by Prof. Dr. Claus Eckardt. In 23-gauge vitrectomy, the benefits of 25-gauge vitrectomy (transconjunctival trocar, no suture, reduced surgical trauma) are combined with the advantages of the 20-gauge technology (rigid instruments, more efficient vitrectomy, and easy accessibility of the vitreous base) (Figs. 1.1 and 1.2). Finally, a new incision technique was developed: the sclerotomies are performed in a lamellar fashion (tunnel technique), which results in a better postoperative wound closure and less postoperative hypotony. The 23-gauge technology is particularly popular in the Europe.

U. Spandau, H. Heimann, *Practical Handbook for Small-Gauge Vitrectomy*,
https://doi.org/10.1007/978-3-319-89677-9_1

Table 1.1 Outer diameter of a needle in gauge and mm

Gauge	mm
19	1.07
20	0.9
23	0.64
25	0.51
27	0.41
29	0.34

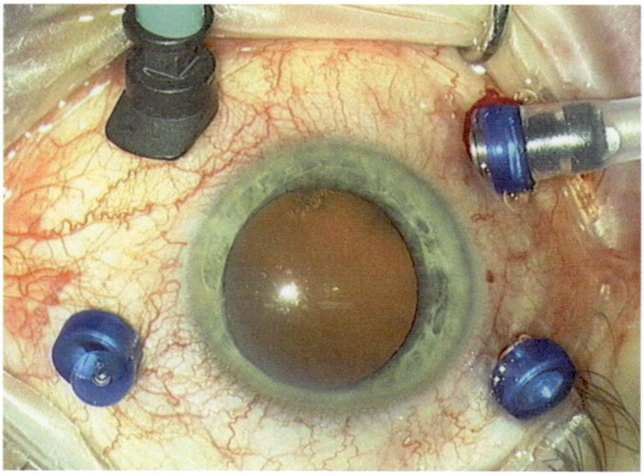

Fig. 1.1 An intraoperative image of a retinal detachment surgery with four-port technique: the infusion line at the top right and the fixed fiber-optic chandelier at the top left. Left and right below the two instrument trocar cannulas

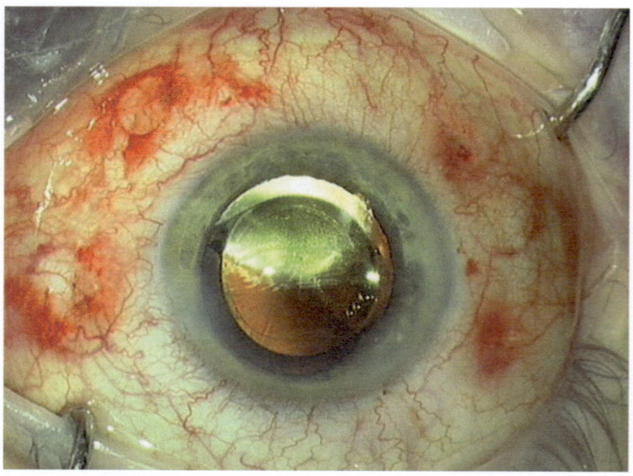

Fig. 1.2 A postoperative image of the same detachment surgery: you can recognize the implanted intraocular lens and the almost white conjunctiva. A 20% SF_6 tamponade was used

The latest development is 27-gauge vitrectomy. The instruments have a diameter of only 0.4 mm. The companies DORC and Alcon have the 27-gauge vitrectomy with trocars in their product range. The indication of spectrum has expanded vastly in the recent years with the introduction of new vitreoretinal instruments such as scissors and forceps. In addition, the advent of the two-blade vitreous cutter with a cutting frequency of 12–16.000 cuts/min has reduced the time for a 27G vitrectomy significantly. The 27-gauge technology is particularly popular in Japan.

In the recent years, 25G has become the gold standard for small-gauge vitrectomy. 23G is decreasing and 27G is increasing year for year. At the University of Uppsala, 27G is used as standard.

1.2 Key Features of "Microincision Vitrectomy Surgery (MIVS)"

The techniques of 23-gauge, 25-gauge, and 27-gauge vitreoretinal surgery are also referred to as "microincision vitrectomy surgery" (MIVS). The 23-gauge, 25-gauge, and 27-gauge techniques can now be used for the whole spectrum of posterior segment surgeries, including PVR retinal detachment and diabetic vitreoretinopathy with silicone oil. The main features are:

- Lamellar and sutureless sclerotomies
- Trocar cannulas
- Bimanual surgery

1.2.1 Sutureless Sclerotomies

The sclerotomies are performed with a tangential incision (lamellar tunnel incision), i.e., the sclerotomy is self-sealing and does not require suturing (Fig. 1.3).

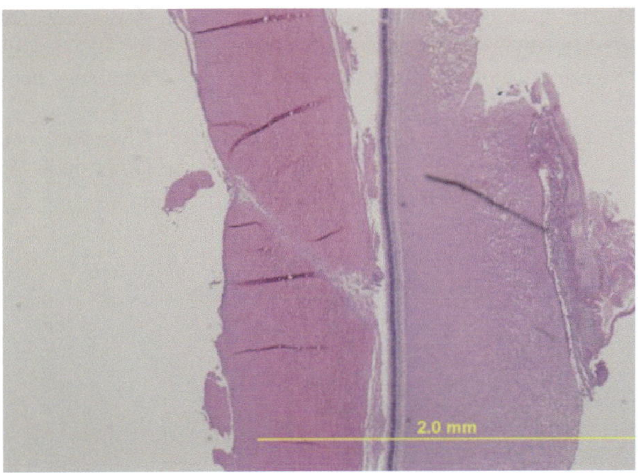

Fig. 1.3 This histological section of an eye showing a lamellar cut through the sclera for 23-gauge vitrectomy. This tangential incision needs no suture. It is comparable to the tunnel incision in phacoemulsification

1.2.2 *Trocar*

A trocar is a metal or plastic cannula, which is placed transconjunctivally in the sclerotomy. The trocars are not sutured and remain in the sclerotomy during the entire surgery (Figs 1.1 and 1.4).

The trocar system is an essential part of the MIVS. It significantly lowers the anterior segment trauma and is associated with minor postoperative discomfort. Table 1.2 lists the advantages and disadvantages of the trocar. 25-gauge is superior to 23-gauge concerning the sclerotomy closure and the speed of postoperative recovery.

Does size matter? The 23G, 25G, and 27G trocars fit into each other (Fig. 1.5). A 27G trocar creates a sclerotomy size of 25G. A 25G trocar creates a sclerotomy size of 23G and a 23G trocar creates a sclerotomy size of 22G. This fact results in a watertight globe after a 27G sclerotomy. A suture is never required. In contrast, a suture is often required in 23G vitrectomies: in myopic eyes, after silicone oil removal, etc.

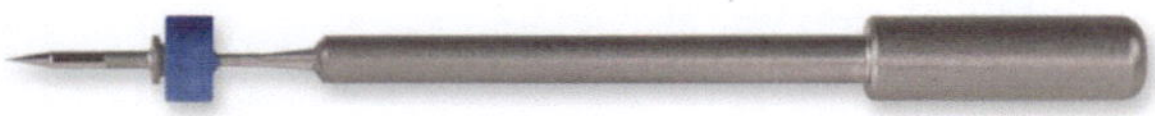

Fig. 1.4 23-gauge trocar with blue valve and inserter. This model is from DORC

Table 1.2 Advantages and disadvantages of the trocar system

Advantages	Disadvantages
Tangential incision (lamellar tunnel) at the sclerotomy	Postoperative hypotony
No suture required	• Angled instruments do not fit through trocars • Trocar may be dislodged during removal of instruments
Trocar openings easier to find for instrument insertion than conventional sclerotomies	Raised trocar openings may be covered by lids in patients with small lid apertures
No extensive opening of conjunctiva	Transconjunctival vitreous prolapse (“vitreous wick”)
Trocars with valves enable a closed system	Higher intraocular pressures during injection of gas or fluids
• Less foreign body sensation • Low corneal astigmatism • Faster postoperative recovery • Rapid visual rehabilitation	

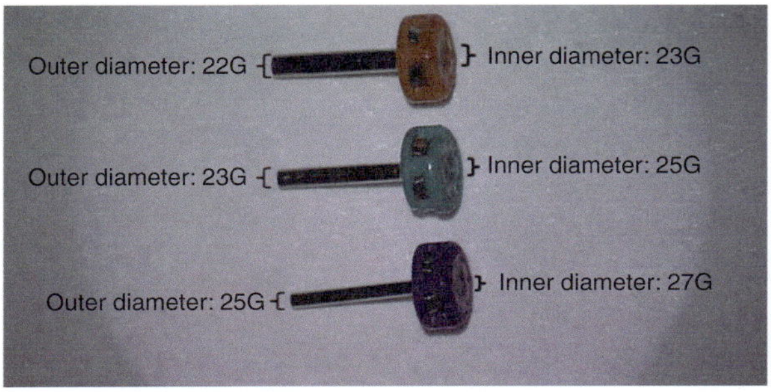

Fig. 1.5 The 27G trocar fits into the 25G trocar and the 23G trocar fits into the 25G trocar. A 25G trocar creates a 23G sclerotomy and a 27G trocar creates a 25G sclerotomy

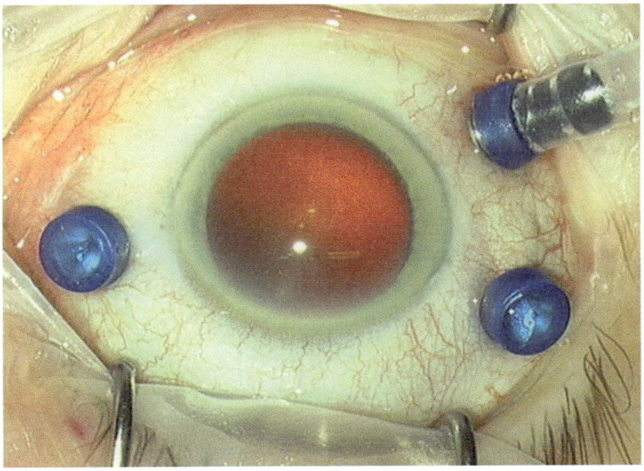

Fig. 1.6 An example of an operation with a three-port trocar system. One infusion cannula and two instrument cannulas have been inserted. A handheld light pipe is used as a light

1.2.3 Bimanual Surgery

During conventional vitrectomy procedures, the surgeon holds the light pipe in one hand and the vitreous cutter or a different "active" instrument in the other hand (Fig. 1.6). In challenging situations, a more active second hand other than holding the light pipe can be useful. By inserting a fixed light probe (chandelier) in the sclera through a fourth sclerotomy port, the surgeon is enabled to use both hands actively (Fig. 1.7). The chandelier light illuminates the entire posterior segment with a panoramic view. Now, procedures such as indenting the retina and simultaneously performing a vitrectomy or bimanual peeling of membranes in PVR retinal detachment or diabetic retinopathy are easier to perform. Remember: No one can indent as good as your second hand.

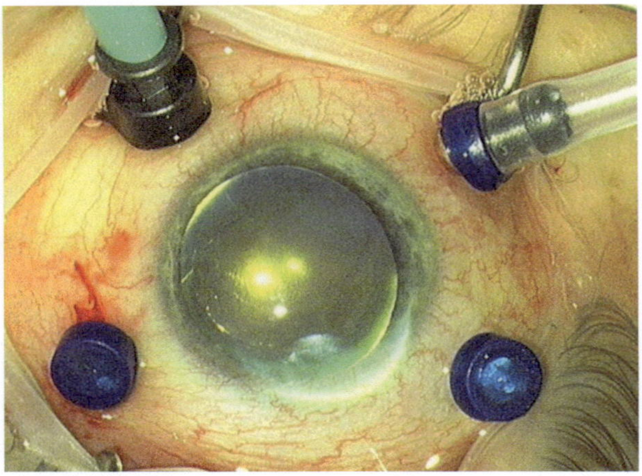

Fig. 1.7 An example of a surgery with a four-port trocar system. In the four-port trocar system, the fourth sclerotomy is used for a fiber-optic chandelier enabling the surgeon to work with two free hands. Synergetics.25-Gauge Awh Chandelier 56.20.25

Other advantages of trocar-vitrectomy compared to the non-trocar-vitrectomy are:

- Significant reduction of overall surgery time (no opening of conjunctiva, no sutures, and no cauterization of bleeding vessels)
- Protects sclerotomies when inserting instruments
- Easier to find the sclerotomies

Bias against 23- and 25-gauge vitrectomyv:

- A persistent and widespread opinion concerning 25-gauge surgery is that the use of silicone oil is not possible or difficult. This is not correct. A silicone oil tamponade with 1000/1300csts and 5000 csts silicone oil and its removal can easily be performed.
- A further notion is that the removal of the vitreous takes longer compared to 20-gauge systems.

In the meantime, this disadvantage has overcome by the introduction of new high-speed cutters.

1.3 23G, 25G, or 27G?

Superficially, the differences between 23G, 25G, and 27G are low. Both use trocars and a lamellar incision. But then the differences begin. With 25G it takes more time for the vitrectomy than with 23G. This time difference is particularly noticeable during passive aspiration with a backflush instrument for fluid-air exchange, so that we always use active aspiration with 25G and 27G. By contrast, working with silicone oil with 25G is easy, both extraction of silicone oil and injection of silicone oil.

Table 1.3 Comparison of 23G, 25G, and 27G

	23G	25G	27G
Suture of sclerotomies	Sometimes	Seldom	Very seldom
Wound healing	2–3 weeks	1–2 weeks	1 week
Number of available instruments	High	High	Moderate-high
Speed of vitrectomy	High	High	High with novel TDC cutter, otherwise low
Speed of passive aspiration	Acceptable	Low	Very low
Speed of active aspiration	High	High	Acceptable
Work with silicone oil	Without problems	Without problems	Without problems

A modern vitrectomy machine, however, is required. The following table lists the differences between the two systems. See Table 1.3.

We work with one vitrectomy machine and 25G and 27G custom packs. Another important point is the spectrum of pathologies you operate. If it is mainly peelings, we would recommend 27G. If you operate also detachments, difficult diabetics, and trauma patients, 25G is a good choice because more instruments are available and because the instruments are stiffer than 27G.

The 27G vitreous cutter is the best vitreous cutter because it can be used as a vitreoretinal instrument. It helps in delaminating diabetic membranes, it can be used very close to the retina, and a 180 deg. retinotomy is no problem with a 27G vitreous cutter.

The main disadvantage of 27G is lack of stiffness of instruments which makes the removal of the peripheral vitreous difficult in deep eyes.

Part II
Equipment

Chapter 2
Equipment

2.1 Devices

2.1.1 Operating Microscope

The optical quality of the surgical microscopes is excellent in all current models of the major manufacturers. More important is the viewing system. The Oculus BIOM can be used with all microscopes, but the Resight viewing system can only be used with a Zeiss microscope, and the EIBOS viewing system can only be used with a Leica microscope.

2.1.2 Binocular Indirect Ophthalmomicroscope (BIOM System)

To obtain a sufficient view of the posterior segment, one needs either a plano-concave contact lens which is directly placed onto the cornea or a highly refractive lens (60D, 90D, 120D) which is placed in front of the lens of the surgical microscope comparable to indirect ophthalmoscopes. This results in an inverted image. By flicking a reversal system (so-called inverter) into the parallel beam path of the operating microscope, an upright image is created (e.g., using the "stereo diagonal inverter (SDI)" of Oculus) (see Appendix, companies).

We use the BIOM system (binocular indirect ophthalmomicroscope) of Oculus and the EIBOS system by Moeller-Wedel. Both systems offer excellent optical images with a variety of different magnifications and fields of view. Based on our personal experience, the BIOM offers more flexibility and a better view of the retinal periphery. The EIBOS system is extremely robust and has the additional advantage of an inbuilt inverter that avoids the need for manual inversion when changing from the posterior segment to the anterior segment view during the surgery.

U. Spandau, H. Heimann, *Practical Handbook for Small-Gauge Vitrectomy*,
https://doi.org/10.1007/978-3-319-89677-9_2

Another good option is the Zeiss (Resight) system. It contains two fixed lenses (128D and 60D) that can be rotated into the light beam. The handling is easy with the resolution of high quality especially in an air-filled eye.

With the Oculus BIOM system, we use three different types of lenses: 120D for a wide peripheral view, 90D as our standard lens for most applications, and the 60D high-magnification lens for macular surgery. In addition, an inverter is needed to invert the image for surgery. This must be turned on or off every time one switches between the anterior segment and posterior segment views.

We usually start with a 90D lens for core vitrectomy and posterior vitreous detachment. We then switch to the 120D lens to trim the vitreous base. We then switch to the 60D lens if we perform macular surgery. A good alternative is a plano-concave contact lens, which is placed directly onto the cornea. We then usually switch back to the 120D for complete trimming of the vitreous base and to inspect the peripheral retina for breaks. In cases of retinal detachment surgery, we recommend beginning the surgery with the wide-angle 120D lens to view the peripheral retina and to identify retinal breaks from the beginning of the surgery.

The company Oculus (Germany) has recently introduced a lens which can be used as a 120D lens and at the same time as 60D peeling lens (Fig. 2.1).

Important: The viewing systems BIOM and Resight provide a mirror image. Therefore, an inverter is installed in the microscope, which turns the mirror image of the BIOM. If you flick the BIOM in, activate the inverter to gain an accurate image. Similarly, if you flick the BIOM out, you must activate the inverter in order to get an upright image. The EIBOS viewing system does not require an inverter.

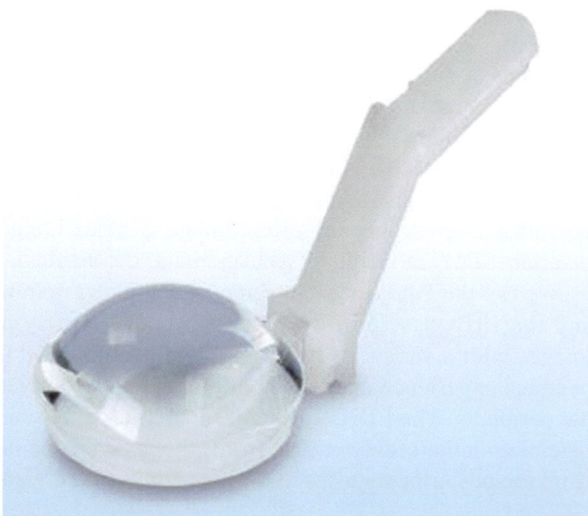

Fig. 2.1 The novel combined 120D and 60D lens from Oculus, Germany. The lens can be used for the BIOM (Oculus, Germany) and for the Resight (Zeiss, Germany) viewing system

2.1.3 Vitrectomy Machine

An extensive range of high-quality vitrectomy machines by several manufacturers is now available on the market. They have a cutting speed of approximately 2500 cuts/min. Of great importance is the "fluidics" (vacuum, flow rate) of the machine. A sophisticated coordination of these parameters allows a high-speed and less traumatic vitrectomy in a closed system. Further, an easy switch between phaco and vitrectomy mode is important. In addition, the vitrectomy machines should have an active injection and extraction feature. This is utilized to inject or remove silicone oil. One can also connect the backflush instrument to the active aspiration and work with active suction. This generation of vitrectomy machines has an integrated light source, which is sufficient for a light pipe but not for a chandelier light. An external light source and a laser must therefore be purchased separately.

The latest generation of vitrectomy machines such as "Constellation" from Alcon, "Stellaris PC" from Bausch & Lomb, and "EVA" from DORC has a cutting speed of 5000–8000 cuts/min. With the novel TDC vitreous cutter, the "EVA" machine has a cutting speed of 12.000–16.000 cuts/min. They all provide an integrated light source that is strong enough for a chandelier light.

One unfortunate trend in modern vitrectomy machines is that there are no international standards and the essential parts of the instrumentation are usually not interchangeable between different manufacturers. Moreover, some manufacturers provide some of the essential tools as part of an "all-in-one" vitrectomy pack only. This means, for example, that a broken light pipe or a vitreous cutter that inadvertently touched the non-sterile part of the microscope can only be replaced by opening another surgical pack, which is more expensive than an individually packed single-use instrument. Therefore, the cost and availability of vitrectomy packs and the provision of spare instruments as individually packed units should be included in the negotiations regarding the purchase of a new vitrectomy machine.

2.1.4 Laser Device

Again, there are numerous providers of laser devices. A frequently used device is the 532-nm diode laser OcuLight GL from Iridex (see Chap. 7).

2.1.5 Cryo Console

A cryo machine (DORC, ERBE) should be at our disposal in the operating room. Indications are a cryopexy of a retinal break, the retina, or the ciliary body due to neovascular glaucoma. Cryopexy is nowadays performed less frequently during vitrectomies, because cryotherapy leads to more anterior segment trauma and is more difficult to perform through a closed conjunctiva compared to 20-gauge surgery with conjunctival incisions. In addition, cryotherapy has been associated with a higher rate of PVR formation in some studies of retinal detachment surgery. Finally, the chorioretinal scar formation appears several days later following cryotherapy compared to laser retinopexy.

2.1.6 Light Source

The light source is either external or can be integrated into the vitrectomy machine. In general, the internal light sources have traditionally been weaker than external light sources. When using a chandelier light, one must use a very powerful light source. Synergetics offer an external photon source, and DORC and Alcon offer an external xenon light source (see Chap. 7). The new vitrectomy machines "Constellation" of Alcon, "Stellaris PC" from Bausch & Lomb, and "EVA" from DORC have an internal light source that is strong enough for use with a chandelier light.

2.2 Standard Instruments for Pars Plana Vitrectomy

Retinal surgery is a very "instrumental" field and necessitates that you acquaint yourself with the variety of high-quality microsurgical instruments designed for specific tasks, many more than with phacoemulsification. To become a good retinal surgeon, you need to know the different applications of this wide range of instruments and consequently increase your skills in this field of surgery. In addition, retinal surgery is "neurosurgery" in that one comes into direct contact with neural tissue. In general, such surgery is associated with the risk of transmitting Creutzfeldt-Jakob disease in countries where this disease is present. Therefore, there is an increasing trend to use single-use instruments in vitreoretinal surgery wherever possible. Reusable instruments, which used to be the norm just a few years ago, are disappearing from the market. This is especially the case in the UK and France. The positive side effect for the surgeon is that one is always provided with new and sharp instruments of very high quality nowadays. On the downside, this can reduce the number of available instruments and options available to the surgeon. Further, this trend is also associated with higher costs. In the following section, various surgical instruments are introduced.

Here you find all details of our PPV instrument set (only and combined), which we use at the University Hospital of Uppsala (Fig. 2.2):

1. 1× Lid speculum Liebermann. Geuder G-15960
2. 1× Irrigating cannula. Geuder G-15180 (for irrigation of the eye)
3. 1× Dressing forceps, serrated. Geuder G-18781

4. 1× Tissue forceps, 1 × 2 teeth. Geuder G-18791
5. 1× Castroviejo suturing forceps, straight. Geuder G-19023
6. 1× Barraquer cilia forceps. Geuder G-18750 (for suturing)
7. 1× Trocar forceps. DORC 1276.2 (for removal of the trocars)
8. 1× Eye scissors, straight pointed-pointed. Geuder G-19350
9. 1× Vannas capsulotomy scissors. Geuder G-19760
10. 1× Halsted mosquito forceps, curved serrated. Geuder G-18181
11. 1× Hartmann mosquito forceps, straight serrated. Geuder G-18170 (for washing the eye)
12. 1× Barraquer needle holder, curved, without lock. Geuder G-17500
13. 1× Sclera depressor, double ended. Geuder G-32715
14. 1× Braunstein fixed caliper. Bausch & Lomb E2402 (Scleral marker 3.5 mm and 4.0 mm)

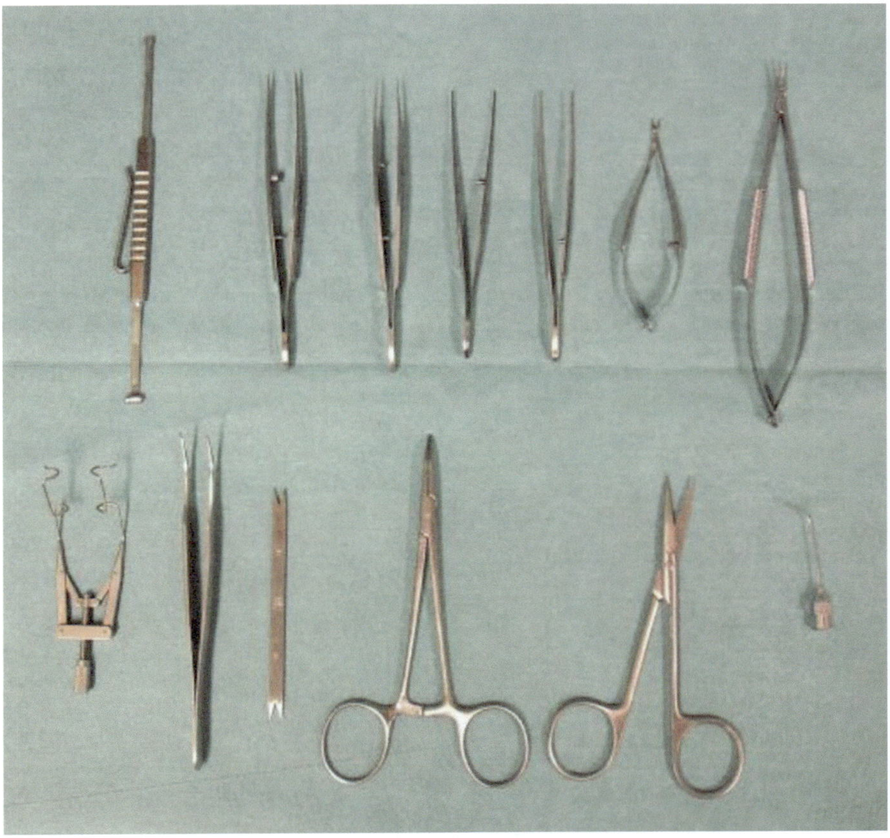

Fig. 2.2 Vitrectomy Instrument set from the University of Uppsala, Sweden

2.2.1 *Trocar Cannulas*

Trocars with valves have become standard today, but you can still purchase trocars without valves (Alcon, DORC, Geuder, Oertli; Fig. 2.3).

Trocars with valves are particularly useful for beginners, as they prevent hypotension and collapse of the globe during the surgery (Fig. 2.4). It is, however, important to notice that with valved trocars, one works within a closed system. For example, when injecting fluid or gas, corresponding drainage or pressure control has to be ensured via the second port or the infusion system to avoid a significant rise in intraocular pressure. Using trocars without valves requires some manipulatory practice, as in certain situations a plug needs to be inserted into the trocar to avoid hypotension (Fig. 2.5). The advantage of trocars without valves is that an intraocular hypertension, for example, when injecting silicone oil, is easier to control and to avoid.

Today there is a clear tendency toward trocars with valves. We therefore recommend to get acquainted working with valved trocars.

Surgical Pearls No. 1
<u>23G and 25G:</u> If you use 23G trocars, then you can work with 23G *and* 25G instruments. If you use 25G trocars, then you can *only* work with 25G instruments.

2.2.2 *Trocar Forceps* (Fig. 2.6a, b)

Indication: Manipulation of trocars. A very useful forceps for any kind of manipulations of the trocars. DORC 1276.2

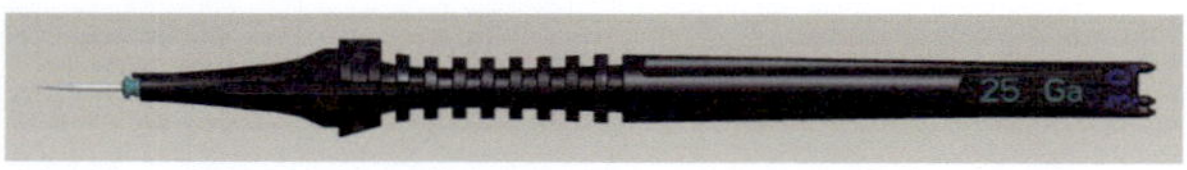

Fig. 2.3 The Alcon Edgeplus trocar with hand piece and 3.0/4.0 mm marker. Available for 23-gauge, 25-gauge and 27-gauge

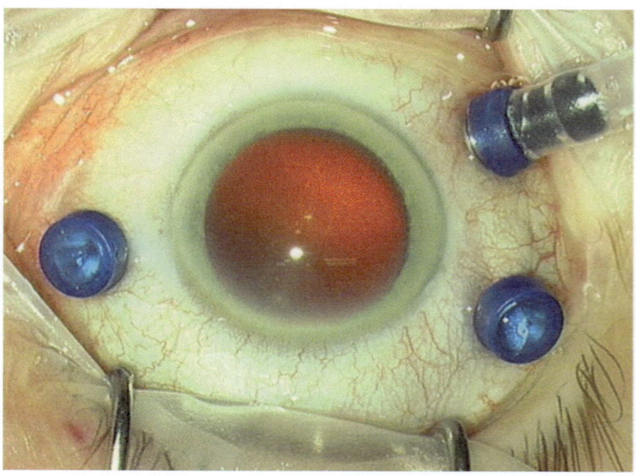

Fig. 2.4 DORC 23G trocars with valves. Intraocular fluid remains in the eye. The valves can be removed

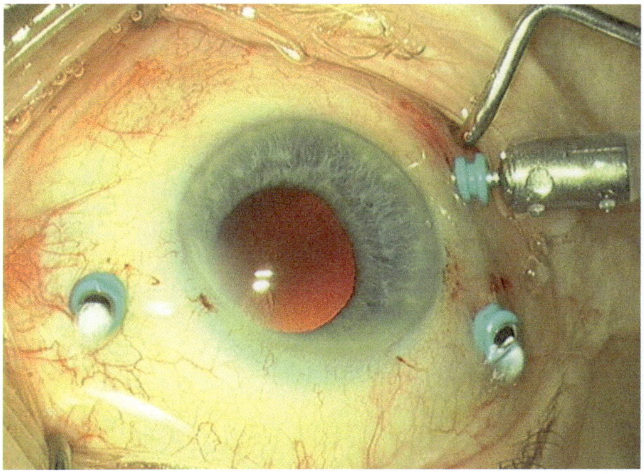

Fig. 2.5 ALCON 25G trocars without valves. Intraocular fluid is flowing out of the trocars

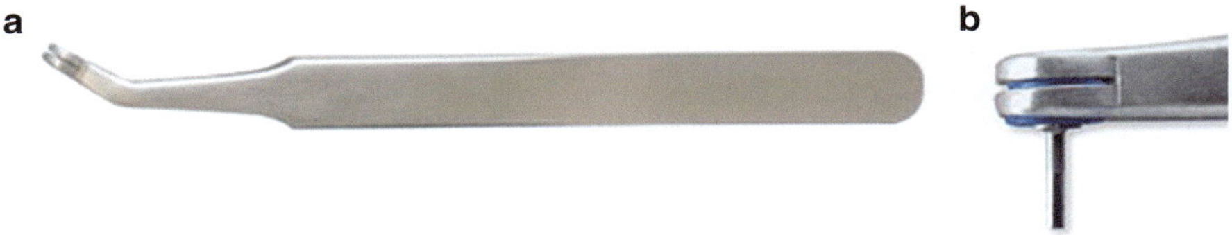

Fig. 2.6 (**a**, **b**) A very Pars plana vitrectomy (PPV): trocar forceps useful forceps for manipulation of trocars (DORC, NL)

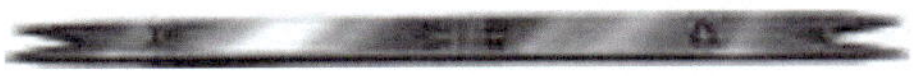

Fig. 2.7 A scleral marker (storz)

2.2.3 Scleral Marker (Fig. 2.7)

Easy-to-use instrument to mark the position of the sclerotomy on the sclera: 3.5 mm for pseudophakic eyes and 4.0 mm for phakic eyes. Most manufacturers incorporate a marker in the handle of the trocar blade, thereby avoiding the need for changing instruments at the beginning of the surgery (Fig. 2.7).

2.2.4 High-Speed Vitreous Cutter (Figs. 2.8 and 2.9)

High-speed vitreous cutters have a cut rate of 5000 cuts/min (Fig. 2.9). Most recent vitreous cutters from DORC (Holland) and Geuder (Germany) have a cut rate of 10,000–16,000 cuts/min. This new vitreous cutter has two open cutting ports and a second cutting blade (Figs. 2.9 and 2.10). It is named twin duty cycle (TDC) cutter. This new invention comprises two new features: (1) a permanent flow and (2) two cutting blades. The two cutting blades have the result that the cutter cuts two times

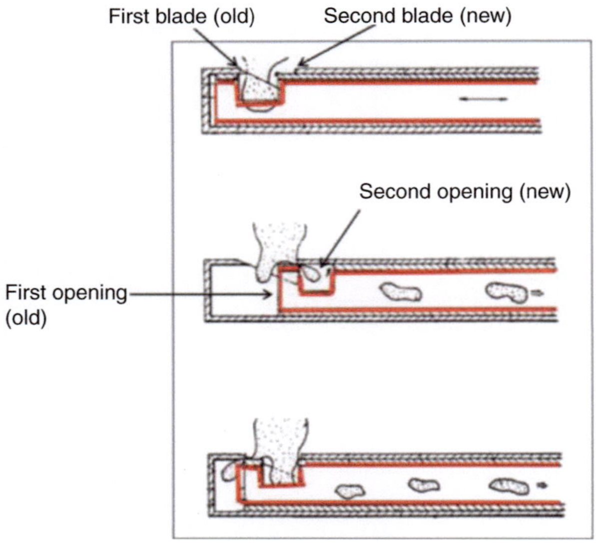

Fig. 2.8 Illustration of a TDC cutter in action. One movement (forward and backward) results in two cuts. In old cutters one movement (forward and backward) results in one cut

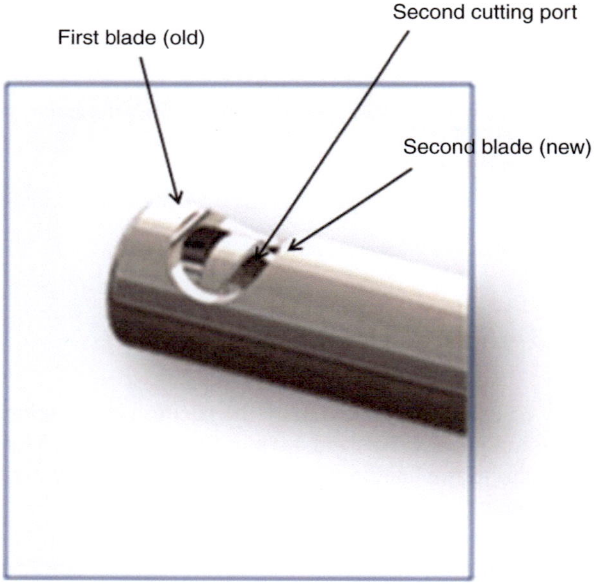

Fig. 2.9 The novel twin duty cycle (TDC) cutter. The cutter has two open cutting ports and a second cutting blade. The novel two-blade cutters have therefore the same movement frequency like old cutters but a double cutting frequency: 5.000 × 2 = 10.000 cuts/min

during one movement, effectively doubling the cutting speed. The vitreous cutter has a cutting rate of 8000 cuts/min. But the actual cutting rate with two cutting blades is 8000 × 2 = 16,000 cuts/min, which reaches new dimensions. The second novelty is a continuous and even flow due to the two open cutting ports. This novel technology reduces vitreous traction, decreases the surgical time, and increases the safety of surgery.

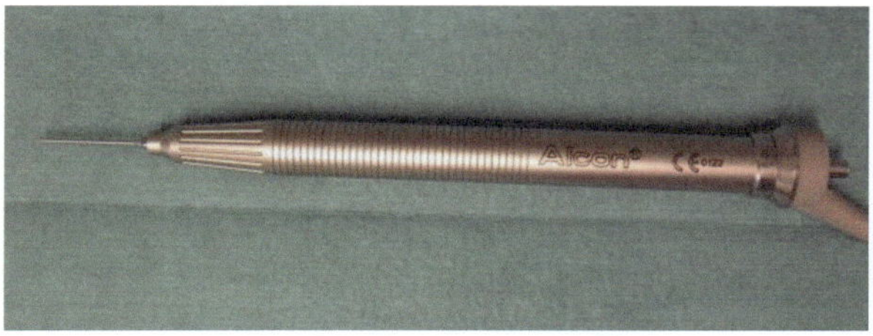

Fig. 2.10 Fragmatome hand piece. Indication: removal of a dropped nucleus. Alcon Accurus fragmatome. In addition, you need the fragmatome accessory pack (REF 1021HP)

With the foot pedal, you can switch between the two functions of the vitreous cutter: firstly, you can cut and aspirate (vacuum), and secondly you can only aspirate. Indications for combined cutting and aspirating are the removal of the vitreous, blood clots or soft lens fragments, iridectomy, etc. Indications for aspirating are induction of PVD, aspiration of liquefied blood, subretinal fluid, etc. The vitreous cutter cannot cut solid tissue such as fibrosed lens capsule or hard lens fragments. A fibrosed lens capsule is segmented and removed with scissors and forceps. Hard lens fragments necessitate the use of a fragmatome.

2.2.5 Fragmatome (Fig. 2.10)

The fragmatome can be used to emulsify a dropped nucleus in the vitreous cavity. It is available in 20G and 23G but is used without a trocar cannula. A fragmatome is difficult to use. On the one hand, it is less powerful than a normal phaco hand piece. On the other hand, it can exert high levels of suction in the posterior segment. Aspiration of the vitreous or the retina into the hand piece must be avoided. Lens fragments tend to jump away from the needle tip. In such cases, one must aspirate the fragments in the needle tip before emulsification (see Appendix, Materials).

2.2.6 Light Fibers (Endoillumination)

There are two types of endoillumination: handheld light pipes (light probes) and fixed endoillumination (chandeliers).

Light pipes are available with different sized cones of light. For routine cases, one holds the light pipe with the non-dominant hand and the vitreous cutter with the dominant hand. A chandelier light is fixed in the sclera and illuminates the entire fundus. This enables bimanual surgery and allows the surgeon to use a second active instrument in addition to the vitreous cutter. Chandelier lights are available from many different suppliers. The 25-gauge chandelier light of Synergetics has the great advantage of a rigid cable and a broad baseplate, which sticks firmly in the sclera. A good alternative is the 25-gauge chandelier light of Alcon and the 23-gauge chandelier light of DORC which are easily inserted into a 25-gauge and 23-gauge trocar,

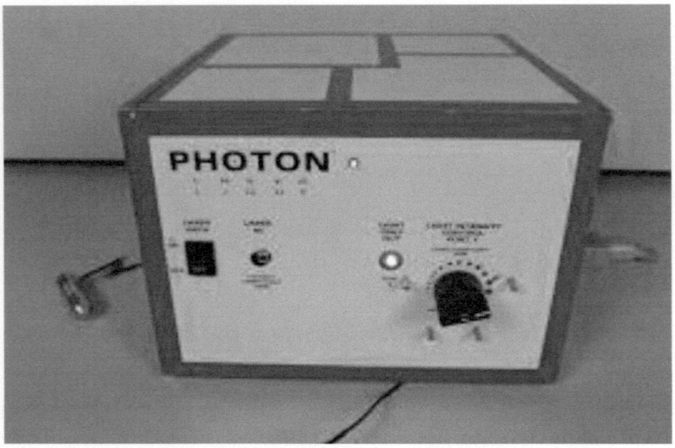

Fig. 2.11 An external light source (Photon from Synergetics, USA)

respectively (for details, see materials). More difficult to insert is the 27-gauge twin-light from DORC. It consists of two light fibers, which are both inserted at the 12 o'clock position. For optimal illumination of a chandelier light, an external light source (photon, xenon) is required (Fig. 2.11).

The choice of light source depends on the difficulty of the case and the personal preference of the surgeon. While chandelier lights have their definite advantages of freeing up your non-dominant hand to use a second instrument and provide better illumination for video recording of the surgery, a handheld light probe still provides a more focused and brighter light for most situations, for example, membrane peeling and delamination. It also depends on your routine method of trimming the vitreous base. One of the authors (HH) uses "traditional" handheld endoillumination for the clear majority of routine cases (macular holes, retinal detachment, proliferative diabetic retinopathy) and performs trimming of the vitreous base using external indentation with the light pipe; this enables transscleral illumination of the vitreous base while indenting the sclera from the outside with the light pipe. The other author (US) uses the handheld light pipe only for macular peeling and for silicone oil removals. For all other cases, he uses a chandelier light which in his opinion opens a whole new world of surgical possibilities.

2.2.7 *Charles Flute Instrument (=Backflush Instrument)* (Figs. 2.12, 2.13, and 2.14)

The 23-gauge flute needle is a blunt needle which aspirates liquid by capillary force and pressure difference. The hand piece usually contains a flexible or stiff plastic tube with an opening. This can be used in three ways: If the hole is uncovered, fluid will be pushed out of the eye through the tip of the flute needle, exiting the eye through opening in the hand piece driven by the intraocular pressure. The

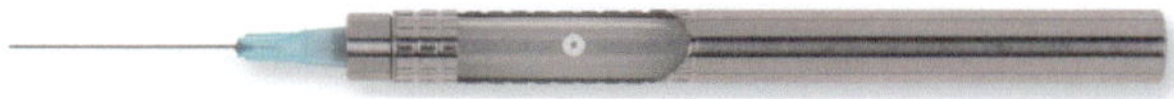

Fig. 2.12 A 23-gauge Charles flute instrument (backflush instrument). Passive aspiration: Leave the side opening open. Intraocular fluid will flow out through the side opening. If you press firmly on the silicone tubing, the backflush instrument squirts fluid out, e.g., to remove epiretinal blood. DORC. 1281.C

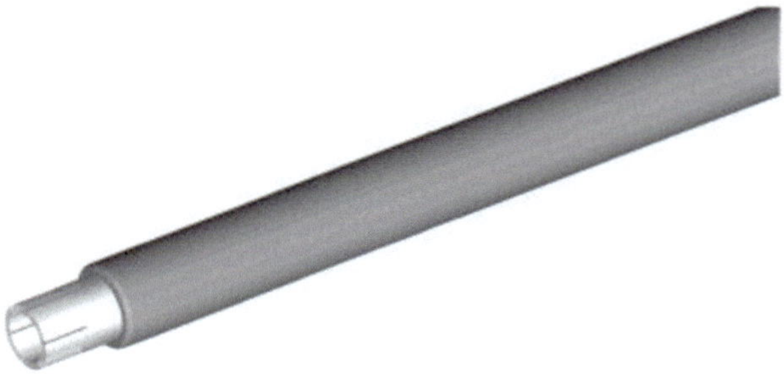

Fig. 2.13 A flute needle with a silicone tip (backflush instrument with brush tip). Indication is nontraumatic work on the retinal surface. For example, if you wish to aspirate a residual perfluorocarbon droplet from the retina. DORC. 1281.BTD06

Fig. 2.14 Active aspiration: A flute instrument is attached to an infusion tube which is inserted into the vitrectomy machine. The active aspiration mode is activated. Close the opening of the tubing with your index finger, and press the foot pedal. The intraocular fluid is aspirated into the vitrectomy machine

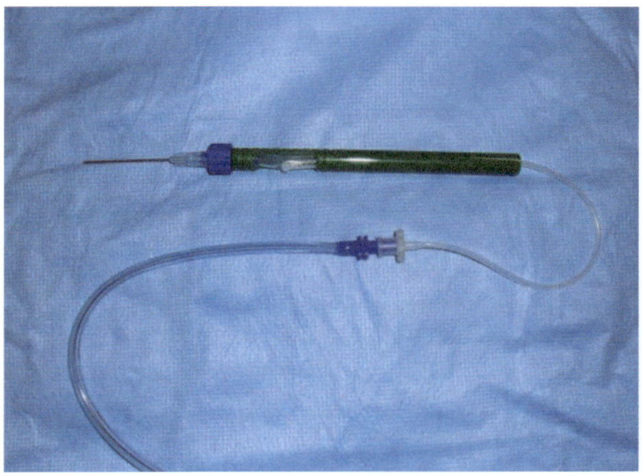

intraocular pressure is determined by the infusion pressure and the diameter and length of the cannula. If you place the index finger on the opening, there is no aspiration. If the hole is closed and the tubing is compressed, the backflush instrument will eject the small amount of fluid within the eye. This can be used to flush blood from the retina. There are two versions of flute needles: with or without silicone tip (Figs. 2.12 and 2.13). With the silicone tip, more gentle manipulations close to the retinal surface are possible. However, these instruments are more expensive and usually not needed for most routine manipulations. Finally, one can connect the

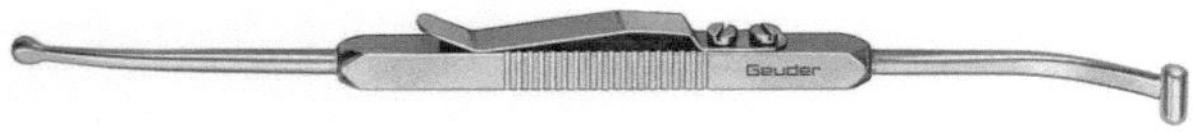

Fig. 2.15 A scleral depressor used to indent the retina. Geuder. G-32715

backflush instrument to active aspiration (active injection mode) and henceforth increase the suction power (Fig. 2.14). Mastering the handling of the backflush instrument is one of the key steps in improving the surgical skills of vitreoretinal surgeons.

2.2.8 *Scleral Depressor* (Fig. 2.15)

A scleral depressor indents the retina. It is a standard instrument for pars plana vitrectomy. It is used for trimming of the vitreous base, in particular in retinal detachment surgery. With a four-port vitrectomy and chandelier endoillumination, one can use the scleral depressor for bimanual trimming of the vitreous base using the vitreous cutter. Remember: no one can indent as good as your second hand.

Alternatively, one can use a light pipe for external indentation and transscleral illumination of the vitreous base. This is straightforward with 23-gauge light pipes; with the more flexible 25-gauge light pipes, one can perform this maneuver in the temporal and nasal quadrants by stabilizing the tip of the light pipe with the tip of your middle finger close to it. However, this is not possible at the 6 and 12 o'clock positions.

One of the basic rules of vitrectomy is to finish all vitrectomies, no matter how "simple" and straightforward they are, with an internal search for retinal breaks at the vitreous base using endoillumination and a scleral depressor. When performing this examination, one should make sure to view the entire retinal periphery over 360° up to the ora serrata. This is one of the most effective ways to reduce the rate of postoperative retinal detachments.

2.2.9 *Laser Probe* (Fig. 2.16)

One can purchase straight or curved laser probes. The curved laser is particularly suitable for the peripheral retina; the straight laser is easier for the central posterior pole. If you apply a peripheral laser treatment (break, peripheral ischemic retina), the use of a scleral depressor is recommended, which makes the break more accessible and avoids touching the lens. This can be performed either using a chandelier light and a scleral depressor or using the light pipe as a scleral depressor with transscleral illumination. Alternatively, you can use a laser fiber with endoillumination (see below).

Fig. 2.16 A 23-gauge laser probe of DORC. The optical laser is curved so that the peripheral retina can be easily reached. DORC. 7223.IRI

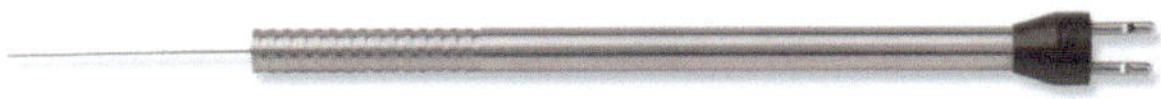

Fig. 2.17 A 23-gauge endodiathermy hand piece. DORC. 1120.06

The use of the laser probe requires some training. A great proportion of intraoperative lens touch is caused by the tip of the endolaser. This is because the surgeon usually focuses on the area of illuminated retina that requires treatment and may forget about the position of the laser probe, when indenting the vitreous base.

Curved laser probes can be advanced and retracted through a mechanism within the hand piece. This requires some training before operating safely within the eye. Also, the flexible part of the probe needs to be retracted before removing the instrument out of the eye. Otherwise, the probe will get stuck in the trocar, and the trocar will be removed with the instrument.

2.2.10 Combined Laser and Light Fiber Hand Piece

This laser hand piece is combined with a light fiber. Indications include peripheral retinal breaks or ischemic retinopathy. With one hand, you can indent the retina with the scleral depressor and treat the break with the other hand (illuminated laser probe, 23G with Iridex adapter. DORC. 7510.IRI).

2.2.11 Endodiathermy Probe (Fig. 2.17)

An endodiathermy is useful for cauterizing bleeding retinal vessels such as in diabetic retinopathy or before large and more central retinectomies. Another indication is to mark a break in retinal detachment surgery or in preparation for a retinotomy. There are usually two different types of endodiathermy probes: "Active" endodiathermy probes are combined with a flute needle. This is very useful when treating an acute intraocular hemorrhage. The flute needle drains the hemorrhage, enabling localization of the bleeding site, which can then simultaneously be treated with endodiathermy. "Non-active" diathermy is a straightforward endodiathermy probe with a pointed tip. Appropriate use of the endodiathermy probe requires some training. If the settings are too strong or the tip is held too close to the retina, an iatrogenic retinal break can easily be created.

2.2.12 *Exodiathermy Probe*

The exodiathermy is used to cauterize (bloody) episcleral vessels.

2.2.13 *Instruments for Macular Surgery*

2.2.14 *Alcon Scraper* (Fig. 2.18a, b)

2.2.15 *Atkinson Cannula* (Fig. 2.19)

2.2.16 *Tano Diamond Dusted Membrane Scraper*

The instrument has a flexible diamond dusted silicone tip (Fig. 2.15). It is used for the peeling of the internal limiting membrane (ILM) or ERM by gently stroking the ILM until it tears. The ILM edge can then be removed with the Eckardt forceps.

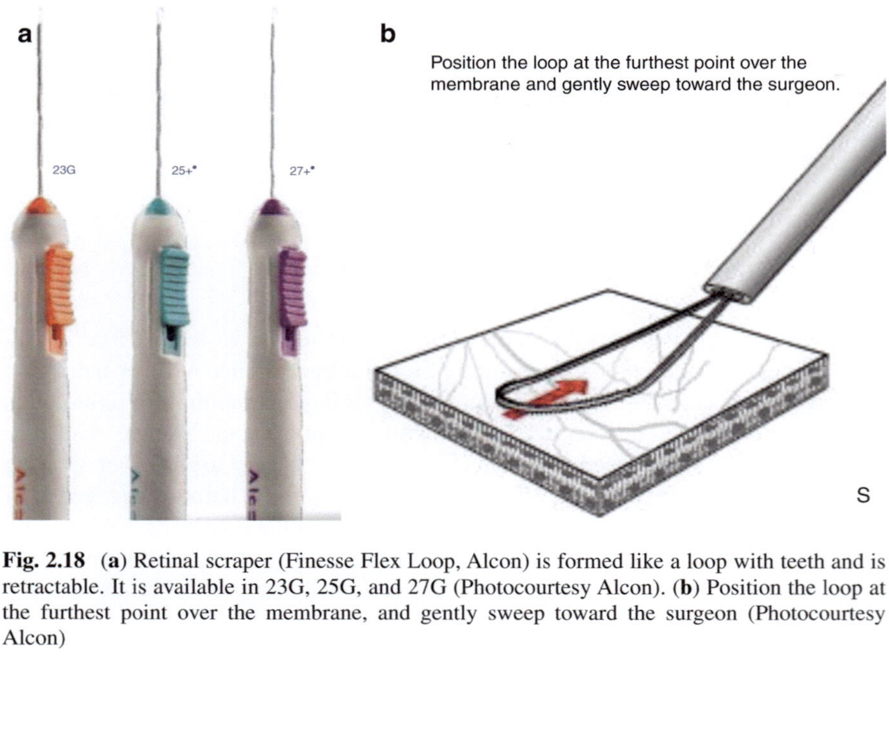

Fig. 2.18 (**a**) Retinal scraper (Finesse Flex Loop, Alcon) is formed like a loop with teeth and is retractable. It is available in 23G, 25G, and 27G (Photocourtesy Alcon). (**b**) Position the loop at the furthest point over the membrane, and gently sweep toward the surgeon (Photocourtesy Alcon)

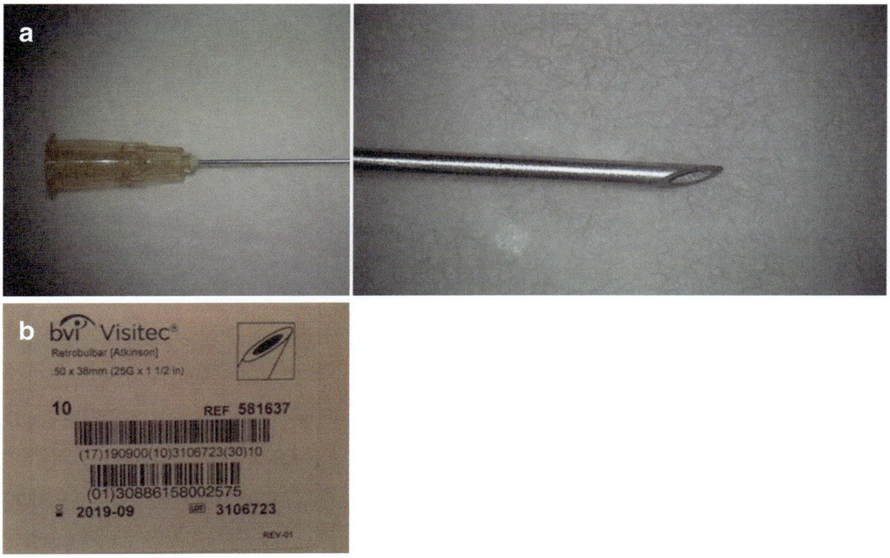

Fig. 2.19 The Atkinson retrobulbar cannula is a useful tool for manipulation of epiretinal membranes. (**a**) It is a good and cheap alternative to the Alcon retinal scraper. You carefully stroke the membrane or ILM with the Atkinson cannula until the membrane is loose or the ILM tears. The membrane edge can then be removed with the Eckardt forceps. Blunt 27G retrobulbar cannula (Atkinson, Beaver-Visitec, USA) (**b**)

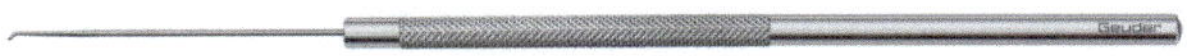

Fig. 2.20 The membrane pic is angled at the end. It is very useful for the lifting of membrane edges. A lifted membrane (edge) can then be removed with Eckardt forceps

Fig. 2.21 The Eckardt forceps has two jaws and is an instrument frequently used for the manipulation of membranes, removal of the internal limiting membrane (ILM), or the epiretinal membrane. The endgripping forceps is more powerful than the Eckardt forceps

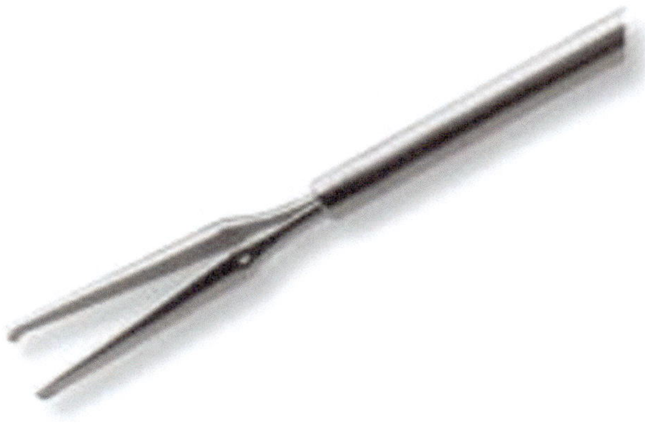

2.2.17 Membrane Pic (Fig. 2.20)

2.2.18 Eckardt Forceps and Endgripping Forceps (Fig. 2.21)

2.2.19 *Instruments for Peeling for Diabetic Retinopathy and Traction retinal Detachment with PVR*

2.2.19.1 **Serrated (Jaws) Forceps** (Fig. 2.22)

2.2.19.2 **Straight or Horizontal Scissors** (Fig. 2.23)

2.2.19.3 **Knob Spatula** (Fig. 2.24)

2.2.19.4 **Retinectomy Scissors (Vertical Scissors)** (Fig. 2.25)

2.2.19.5 **Instruments for Intraocular Foreign Body**

Foreign Body Forceps (Fig. 2.26)

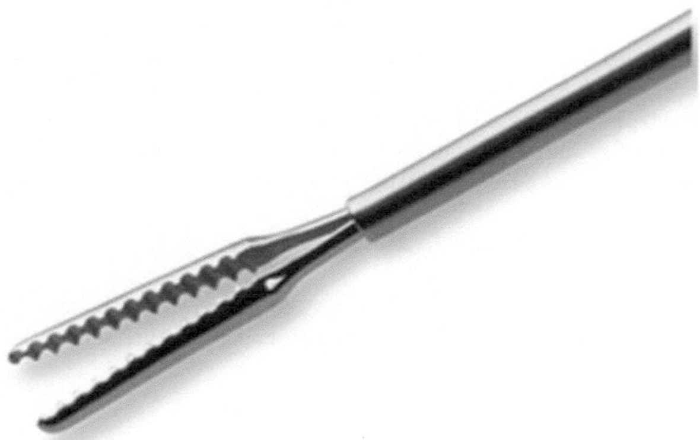

Fig. 2.22 These forceps have the shape of a crocodile jaw and exert more traction and grip than the Eckardt forceps. They are therefore more suitable for the removal of PVR membranes and grasping a dislocated IOL or intraocular foreign body. See also section Material

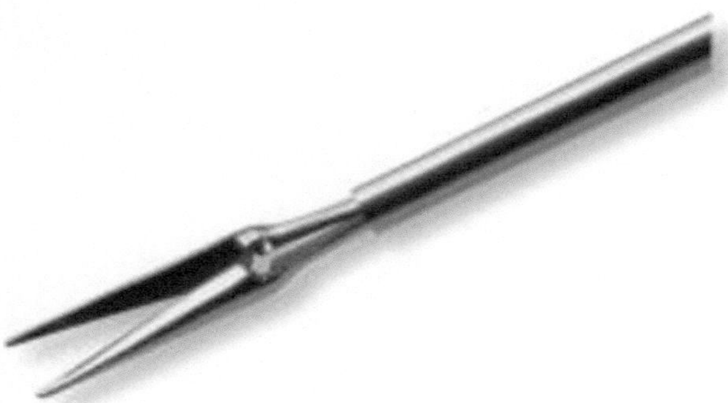

Fig. 2.23 The horizontal scissors have two straight blades. They are used for dissecting membranes from the retina, for example, in proliferative diabetic retinopathy or PVR retinal detachment

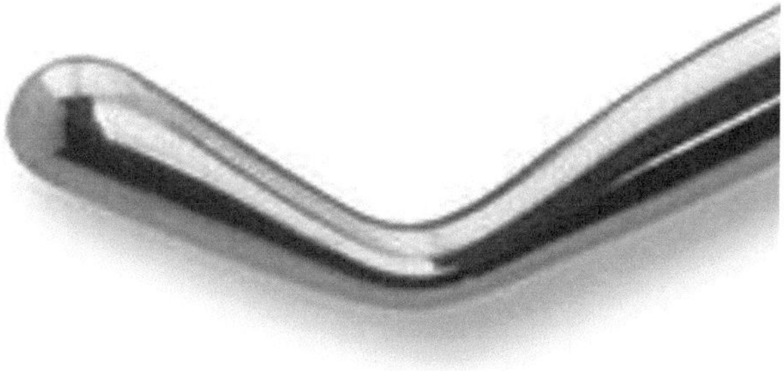

Fig. 2.24 The knob spatula has a thick knob at its tip. Indication for use is the manipulation of membranes or a retinal massage. A retinal massage is necessary if there are retinal folds

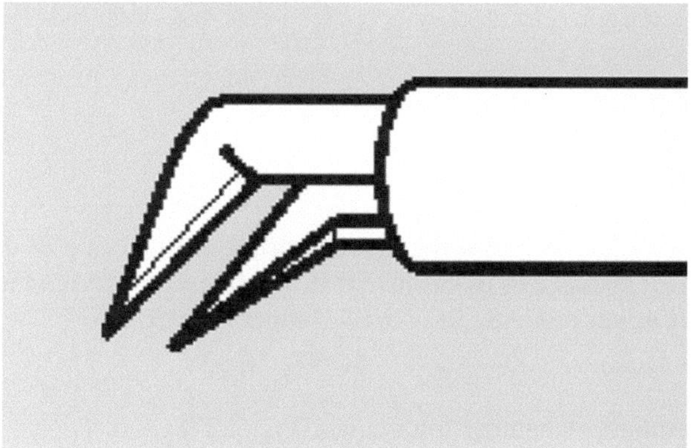

Fig. 2.25 These 23-gauge retinectomy scissors have two angled blades. They are used to create a retinectomy, for example, in PVR retinal detachment

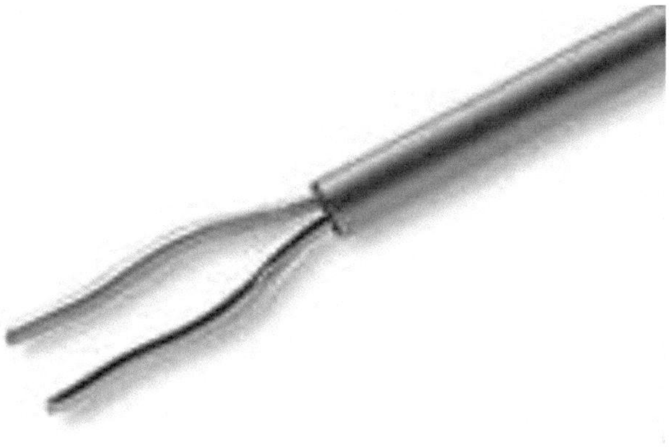

Fig. 2.26 The foreign body forceps are executed by a 20G sclerotomy (without trocar) in the eye. Available are 17G, 19G, and 20G foreign body forceps. The sclerotomy must of course be enlarged according to the size of intraocular foreign body. We recommend forceps with a roughened surface grip (diamond dusted)

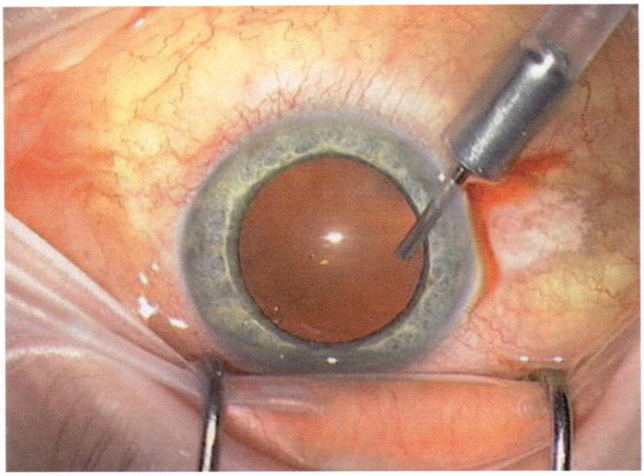

Fig. 2.27 An anterior chamber maintainer

2.2.19.6 Varia

Caliper

A caliper is useful for the measuring and marking of distances. Examples are correct distance of trocar insertion and scleral marking of a scleral buckle or a cerclage (Caliper of CASTROVIEJO Geuder No: 19135).

Anterior Chamber Maintainer (Fig. 2.27)

An anterior chamber maintainer can be used for a vitrectomy instead of a pars plana infusion, if there is sufficient flow between anterior and posterior chambers, e.g., aphakia. It cannot be used in a phakic eye because there is no sufficient flow from the anterior to the posterior chamber.

2.3 Gases and Liquids

In posterior segment surgery, various gases and liquids are used. It is therefore important to understand their characteristics and abilities. Four different intraocular gases are commonly used: air, sulfur hexafluoride (SF_6), hexafluoroethane (C_2F_6), and octafluoropropane (C_3F_8). In the vitreous cavity, these gases are colorless, odorless, and inert. When injected into the vitreous cavity, air does not expand, whereas pure SF_6, C_2F_6, and C_3F_8 gases do. All gases are, however, used in a non-expanding concentration (see Table 2.1).

Gases are temporary tamponades and are absorbed over several days (air) to months (C_3F_8). (Air < SF_6 < C_2F_6 < C_3F_8, see Table 2.1.) Silicone oil tamponades,

Table 2.1 Relative location of liquids, oils, and gases in the vitreous cavity. SG = specific gravity

Air/gas, SG = 0,0012	Vitreous space, SG = 1
Conventional silicone oils, SG = 0.97	
Water, SG = 1	
Heavy silicone oils, SG = 1.06	
Perfluorocarbon, SG = 1.75	

however, are permanent tamponades and are usually removed between 4 weeks and 6 months after the initial surgery. Perfluorcarbon (PFCL) is a temporary, preoperative tamponade used especially for detachment surgery.

Remark: If the term "water-filled eye" is used in this book, it means an eye filled with "balanced salt solution (BSS)." The BSS will be replaced postoperatively by aqueous humor.

In order to understand the function of the gases and liquids, one needs to know their physiologic abilities.

2.3.1 Physiologic Characteristics of Gases and Liquids: Specific Gravity

Substances with a specific gravity (SG) of 1 are neutrally buoyant, those with SG greater than 1 are denser than water, and will sink in it, and those with an SG of less than 1 are less dense than water, and so will float. The following diagram (see Table 2.1) gives the location of the fluids and gases depending on their relative weight within the vitreous cavity. Perfluorcarbon (PFCL) is the heaviest liquid and is always located on the bottom of the eye. Heavy silicone oils (Densiron 68®, Oxane Hd®) are heavier than water and tamponade therefore the inferior circumference. Conventional silicone oils are lighter than water and tamponade the superior circumference. The lightest tamponades used are gases; they are always located anteriorly.

In the eye, several gases or liquids may be present at the same time. In this context, the term phase is important. Phase is with regard to physical properties a spatially homogeneous field. One uses the term, for example, of a gaseous phase or liquid phase. A gas or liquid "bubble" refers to the spherical shape. Another important term is the meniscus: it refers to the curved surface of a liquid.

2.3.2 Physiologic Characteristics of Gases and Liquids: Surface Tension Pressure

The high surface tension between gas and fluid enables formation of an effective seal around a retinal break, thus allowing the retinal pigment epithelium (RPE) to absorb any remaining subretinal fluid to facilitate reattachment of the retina. The surface tension pressure of the gas/water interface is the greatest and therefore is the most effective in closing retinal breaks (70 mN/N). Because the specific gravity of any gas is lower than that of water, the intraocular gas bubble has buoyancy that presses the retina against the RPE, and this effect is greatest at the apex of the bubble. Buoyancy forces can be directed by careful positioning of the patient's head so that retinal break is placed at the apex of the bubble, until chorioretinal adhesions created by laser photocoagulation or cryotherapy can be established. Less effective are silicone oils because the surface tension pressure of silicone oil/water is only 50 mN/N.

2.3.3 All Gases and Liquids in Detail

2.3.3.1 Air

In the supine position, air exerts the most pressure on the anterior retina (ora serrata) and less on the posterior retina (Fig. 2.28). Because air is lighter than water or PFCL, the eye will be filled with air from the ora serrata and then down to the optic disk.

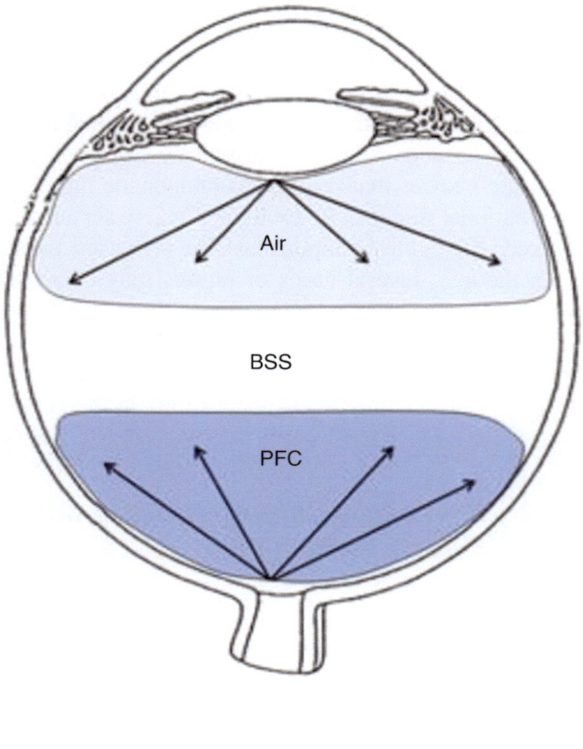

Fig. 2.28 Opposite effects of air and PFCL in the vitreous cavity. Air exerts pressure onto the retina from anterior to posterior, whereas PFCL exerts pressure from posterior to anterior

2.3.3.2 Expanding Gases

SF_6, C_2F_6, and C_3F_8 are expanding gases as dissolved nitrogen diffuses along the concentration gradient from the blood into the gas bubble and accumulates here. The postoperative extension may lead to strong increases in intraocular pressure when the gases are injected undiluted into the eye. To avoid this intraocular pressure rise, expanding gases are used in a concentration in which they do not expand. The non-expanding concentration of SF_6 is 20%, of C_2F_6 15%, and of C_3F_8 14% (see Table 2.1). Patients with a gas-filled eye should not undergo anesthesia with nitrous oxide, as it diffuses into gas-filled cavities and leads to an increase of volume. In addition, any air travel or trips to locations at greater heights (e.g., patients living in mountainous areas) are strictly prohibited. This should be part of any routine consent procedure before vitreoretinal surgery. We also advise on giving patients information leaflets with detailed instructions for themselves and referring physicians regarding these precautions.

Important: Air expands not at sea level. But patients with an air tamponade are not allowed to fly because air expands with increasing altitude. A plane flying at a height of 10.000 m above sea level has an air cabin pressure of 2400 m. The same also applies for a stay in the mountains.

SF_6 (Sulfur Hexafluoride)

The commonly used concentration of sulfur hexafluoride (SF_6) is 20%. It tamponades the eye for approximately 4 weeks. Indication includes macular holes, diabetic retinopathy, and retinal detachment surgery with superior breaks. SF_6 is not suitable for inferior breaks unless a specific posture can be maintained for prolonged periods of time (e.g., supine position or on one side opposite to the break). C_2F_6 (perfluoroethane).

C_2F_6 (Hexafluoroethane)

The usual concentration of C_2F_6 is 15%. It tamponades the eye for approximately 4–6 weeks. Indication includes difficult detachments with multiple breaks, inferior tears, or PVR detachment.

C_3F_8 (Octafluoropropane)

The usual concentration of C_3F_8 is 12–14%. It tamponades the eye for approximately 8 weeks. It causes ocular irritation. The indications are similar to C_2F_6.

Surgical Pearls No. 2

Injection of gas:

1. Errors in preparing the correct concentration of the air-gas mixture are potential sources of disasters, if different gases with varying concentrations are used regularly in one theater. Concentration levels, which are too high, can lead to a massive rise in the intraocular pressure, whereas lower concentrations may result in a shorter tamponade than desired. In every theater, a strict protocol for preparing the air-gas mixture must be followed. We recommend that every surgeon supervises the preparation of the mixture and checks on the gas used.

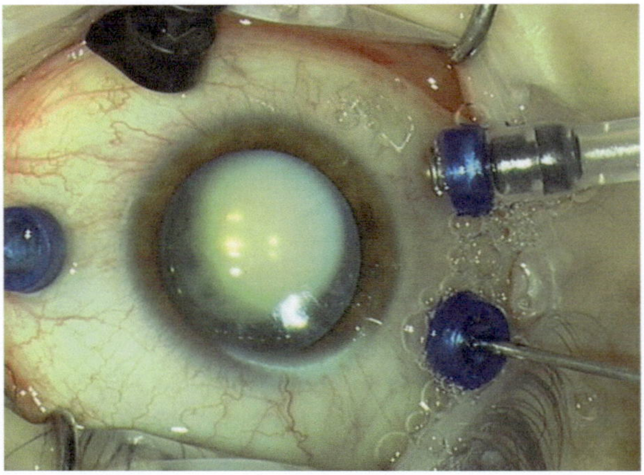

Fig. 2.29 An expanding gas is injected through the IV line to the top right into the eye. To the bottom right, a flute needle relieves intraocular air and reduces intraocular pressure

2. Gases are in 100% concentration in gas containers. They must be diluted with air before injection into the eye. For example, 20% of SF_6. 50 mL syringe: draw 10 mL 100% SF_6 in the syringe, and dilute to 50 mL with room air.
3. If you intend to inject a gas into the eye, first perform a fluid-air exchange. The gas-filled syringe is then connected to the three-way tap. The scrub nurse can inject the gas. At the same time, you hold a flute needle behind the lens to release pressure, so that the globe remains normotensive (Fig. 2.29). Always leave some 5–10 cc in the syringe. This gives you some extra volume to inject should the globe be hypotensive after removing the trocars.

2.4 Liquids

2.4.1 Perfluorocarbon

Perfluorocarbon (PFCL, "heavy water") has the highest density of all intraocular used liquids (see Table 2.1); the eye is filled up from the posterior pole to the ora serrata. In the supine position, PFCL exerts the most pressure on the posterior pole and less pressure anteriorly (Fig. 2.28); it flattens the retina from the posterior pole to the ora serrata. A big advantage is the good visibility under PFCL. One disadvantage is that it always needs to be completely removed, as it is retinotoxic if left within the eye for weeks to months, especially if it is dislocated into the subretinal space. PFCL is now an essential tool in retinal detachment surgery. It is used to flatten the detached retina and push subretinal fluid through the breaks into the vitreous. Additional advantages are an instant apposition of photoreceptors and retinal pigment epithelial cells in order to promote reattachment and facilitate laser treatment around the breaks. It also stabilizes the detached retina, thereby facilitating trimming of the vitreous base and decreasing the risk of iatrogenic breaks during surgery. Because it does not mix with vitreous, it clearly delineates vitreous remnants in the anterior periphery. One can fill PFCL without problems over the break itself; it will not spill through the break in the subretinal space due to its high surface tension. Finally, it can be used as a protectant of the posterior pole in cases of dislocated IOL or lens matter. Inject a small bubble of PFCL on the posterior pole in order to perform any necessary manipulations in these cases in some distance from the macula.

Dislocation of PFCL into the subretinal space can occur in two situations: if there is a large retinal break with significant residual traction on the retina or if one injects PFCL too briskly, thus splitting the PFCL stream into multiple small bubbles that can then be "blown" through the break into the subretinal space. Silicone oil tamponades are permanent tamponades and are usually removed between 4 weeks and 6 months after the initial surgery. Silicone oils with a lower viscosity (1000 csts conventional oil or heavy oils, which are a mixture of 1300 csts conventional oil and a heavy liquid) tend to emulsify earlier and are usually removed within 3 months. An advantage of these lower viscosity silicone oils is that they can easily be injected and removed with 25- and 23-gauge ports. Higher viscosity 5000 csts silicone oils tend to emulsify later and can usually be left in within the vitreous cavity for longer periods of time.

2.4.2 Light Silicone Oils

Conventional silicone oil is lighter than water and floats in the vitreous and in the anterior chamber. Indications for silicone oil tamponade are retinal detachments with multiple (superior and inferior) breaks, a giant tear, advanced proliferative diabetic retinopathy, PVR detachment, and a macular hole (if a prone position is not possible).

Light silicone oils are available with different viscosities of 1000 csts (centistokes), 1300 csts, 2000 csts, and 5000 csts. 1300 csts silicone oil is more and more replaced by 1000 csts silicone oil. 1000 csts silicone oil emulsifies more rapidly and is suitable for a tamponade of about 3 months. Occasionally, 5000 csts silicone oil should be left intraocularly as a permanent tamponade in cases with multiple redetachments after previously attempted oil removal or severe hypotony. All oils can easily be injected and withdrawn through 25- and 23-gauge trocars.

2.4.3 Heavy Silicone Oils (Densiron 68® and Oxane Hd®)

Densiron 68® and Oxane Hd® are a mixture of silicone oil and perfluorohexyloctane (F_6H_8) and are known as heavy silicone oils (Fig. 2.30a, b). They are heavier than water and therefore support the inferior periphery. Indications are multiple inferior breaks, PVR detachment, retinal detachment with giant tear, and a traumatic detachment.

Oxane Hd® and Densiron 68® should not come in contact with pure PFCL for longer periods of time because they would mix. However, a short contact (e.g., during direct PFCL-heavy silicone oil exchange) is possible. Oxane Hd® should be removed after 2 months and Densiron 68® after about 3–4 months as their tendency to emulsify is comparable to 1300 csts conventional silicone oil. The features of these tamponades are summarized in Table 2.2.

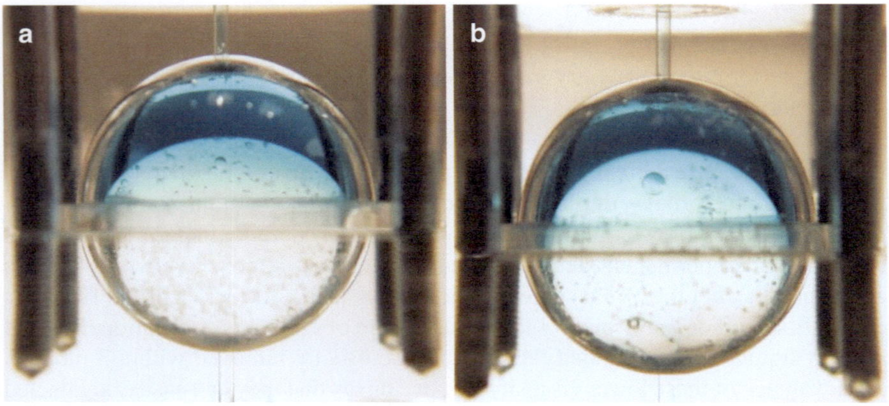

Fig. 2.30 (**a**) Tamponade with Densiron 68® in an eye model. The blue fluid is aqueous. Densiron 68® is less convex than Oxane Hd® and therefore tamponades the inferior retina better. Densiron 68® is widely accepted by vitreoretinal surgeons. With friendly permission of Dr. David Wong. (**b**) Tamponade with Oxane Hd® in an eye model. Oxane Hd® is much lighter than Densiron 68®. It is much more convex and tamponades the inferior retina less effectively than Densiron 68®. With friendly permission of Dr. David Wong

Table 2.2 Properties of gases and liquids for a tamponade (Densiron 68® is heavier than Oxane Hd® (see density) but almost as viscous as 1300 csts silicone oil (see viscosity) and therefore almost as easy to remove)

Gas	Tamponade duration (days)	Concentration in %	Indication
Air	7		Vitreous hemorrhage, diabetic retinopathy, epiretinal membrane
SF_6	14–21	20	Superior breaks from 8 to 4 o'clock, macular hole, diabetic retinopathy
C_2F_6	30	15	Inferior breaks, PVR detachment
C_3F_8	60	14	Inferior breaks, PVR detachment
Silicone oils (viscosity)	**Tamponade duration (months)**	**Density (g/cm³)**	
Silicone oil (1000 and 1300 csts)	appr. 3–6	0.97	Multiple breaks, PDR, PVR, trauma, choroidal detachment, endophthalmitis
Silicone oil (5000 csts)	> = 12	0.97	Multiple breaks, PDR, PVR, trauma, choroidal detachment
Oxane Hd® (3500 csts)	2	1.02	Inferior breaks, inferior PVR detachment
Densiron 68® (1400 csts)	2–3	1.06	Inferior breaks, inferior PVR detachment

Remark: There is no 100% tamponade, neither for gases nor for oils. This is because any tamponade will form the smallest possible surface, thereby forming a sphere within the eye that will never be able to cover all areas of the inner surface of the eye. This is also true for so-called double tamponades of silicone oil and PFCL. These two substances will mix well, but then they will form an hourglass-shaped tamponade within the eye with one part trying to folate upward and one part sinking down. Thus, a belt of fluid surrounds the tamponade in the middle of the eye. Finally, a "complete" vitrectomy is not possible. Remnant vitreous will always lead to an incomplete tamponade.

2.5 Dyes for Vitreous and Membranes

2.5.1 Staining of the Vitreous

Staining: triamcinolone acetonide, trypan blue (Monoblue®, Membrane Blue®)

Triamcinolone is a frequently used dye in vitreoretinal surgery. Many surgeons inject it at the beginning of the vitrectomy, because triamcinolone stains the vitreous well (comparable to asteroid hyaloid). In addition, triamcinolone is a popular staining agent for membranes but does not stain the ILM. Alternatively, trypan blue can be used to stain the vitreous (Table 2.3).

<u>Practical use:</u> For the injection of dyes, take a 3 mL syringe and a 23G backflush/extrusion needle. Inject before the vitrectomy 0.1–0.2 mL diluted triamcinolone, wait approximately 10 s,, and then continue the vitrectomy. You will now be able to recognize the vitreous well.

Surgical Pearls No. 3

Triamcinolone can be cumbersome to remove. If you inject too copiously, it will cover potentially important details of the retina and slow down the procedure. Use only diluted triamcinolone or minimal amounts of <u>triamcinolone for staining</u>; you can always reinject if necessary.

Table 2.3 Staining properties of different dyes

	Vitreous	Membranes	ILM
Triamcinolone	+	+	–
Trypan blue	+/–	++	+/–
Brilliant Blue G	–	+/–	++
MembraneBlue-Dual®	+/–	++	++

2.5.2 Staining of Epiretinal Membranes

Staining: triamcinolone acetonide, trypan blue (Monoblue®, Membrane Blue®, MembraneBlue-Dual®) Triamcinolone crystals stick onto the membranes, while trypan blue stains the entire membrane. Our best experience has been with MembraneBlue-Dual®. Practical modalities include slow injection (syringe with a blunt cannula) of dye onto the posterior pole (Monoblue® is heavier than water), waiting about 15 s, opening the infusion, and removing the dye again with the flute needle.

Practical use: For the injection of dyes, take a 3-mL syringe and a 23G backflush needle. Perform a PVD, inject dye slowly onto the posterior pole (Monoblue® is heavier than water), wait about 15 s, open the infusion, and remove the dye again with the flute needle.

2.5.3 Staining of the Inner Limiting Membrane (ILM)

Staining: Brilliant Blue G (Brilliant Peel®, ILM-Blue®, MembraneBlue-Dual®). Indocyanine green (ICG) is controversial as it is potentially neurotoxic and may cause visual field defects. Triamcinolone does not stain the ILM, and trypan blue stains the ILM only weakly.

Practical use: For the injection of dyes, take a 3 mL syringe and a 23G backflush needle (Fig. 2.24). Perform a PVD, inject dye slowly onto the posterior pole, wait about 60 s, open the infusion, and remove the dye again with the flute needle.

Remark: We use today only MembraneBlue-Dual® (DORC) since it contains both trypan blue and Brilliant Blue G and can therefore stain membranes and ILM at the same time.

Part III
Fundamentals of Pars Plana Vitrectomy

Chapter 3
Fundamentals to Pars Plana Vitrectomy

3.1 Introduction to Pars Plana Vitrectomy

As any surgical procedure, pars plana vitrectomy is learned in four steps: observation, performing sections of the procedure and then the entire surgery under supervision, performing the surgery without supervision but with an experienced surgeon as a backup close by, and finally performing the surgeries on your own. There is no shortcut to this process. However, with regard to pars plana vitrectomy, valuable knowledge and skills can be gained before starting to perform the surgery.

Surgical Pearls No. 4
Assist experienced surgeons as much as you can before you begin to perform vitrectomy. You will automatically acquire the basic "do's and don'ts" during these procedures. Get scrubbed to assist, this is the only way to get really involved and you will learn a lot more than by just looking at a TV screen.

Surgical Pearls No. 5
Examine all vitrectomy patients the day before the surgery. Overnight plan how you intend to operate on each patient (anesthesia, surgical procedure, instruments, dye, and tamponade). As a rule of thumb, assist in every type of surgery from silicone oil removal to retinal detachment ten times. Then you will have acquired specific knowledge on how a particular pathology is managed.

Surgical Pearls No. 6
You see only what you look for, you recognize only what you know. Acquire a broad knowledge of medical retina and develop your skills with binocular indirect ophthalmoscopy. If you master indirect ophthalmoscopy, you will be able to see things others will miss, in particular when there is a poor view of the fundus (e.g., vitreous hemorrhage with some areas of the peripheral retina still visible or a gas-filled eye). With a sound knowledge of medical retina, you will be able to establish the correct diagnosis before and during the surgery in certain cases. These skills will help you to plan your strategy for surgery, deal with unexpected findings during the surgery

U. Spandau, H. Heimann, *Practical Handbook for Small-Gauge Vitrectomy*,
https://doi.org/10.1007/978-3-319-89677-9_3

(e.g., unusual retinal changes after removing a vitreous hemorrhage), and, finally, avoid unnecessary interventions.

Surgical Pearls No. 7
If possible, try to learn and master cataract surgery before learning pars plana vitrectomy. This will not only teach you the ABC of ophthalmic surgery under an operating microscope but will also be very useful in cases of combined surgeries or anterior segment problems during the vitrectomy (e.g., silicone oil prolapse, dislocated IOL, or lens touch).

Surgical Pearls No. 8
Acquire a good knowledge of ultrasound echography and perform this examination yourself before your surgeries. This will enable you to construct a 3D image of the situation in front of you in cases of vitreous hemorrhage and poor view, help you to avoid unnecessary surgeries, and help you in developing the correct strategy for the surgery.

Surgical Pearls No. 9
Learn and practice scleral buckling surgery. This technique is still unsurpassed in localized retinal detachments, in particular in young and phakic patients with an attached vitreous. If you do not practice it, you will be unable to give the appropriate treatment to a child with a traumatic retinal detachment and an ora dialysis, for example.

3.2 Patient Selection

Before performing pars plana vitrectomies without supervision, the beginner should learn the techniques of pars plana vitrectomy (PPV) step by step. Most routine surgeries are suitable. Operate only pseudophakic eyes in the beginning. The best eyes to begin with are membrane peelings. The beginner can practice core vitrectomy, PVD, and a peripheral vitrectomy. Another good beginner eye is a diabetic vitreous hemorrhage without tractions. However, vitreous hemorrhage is an easy pathology, but visualization is poor, and this may be difficult for the beginner. **Important**: When operating a vitreous hemorrhage, pretreat the eye with Avastin, one injection every month for 3 months. One month after last injection, you can perform vitrectomy. Now vitrectomy is easy.

Recommended Learning Steps for Beginners

We recommend the beginner to train the following steps (the steps can be practiced separately):

1. Insertion and removal of trocars and suturing of sclerotomies. We recommend that the conjunctiva be opened before sewing up the sclerotomy.
2. Use of the light pipe and focus the image with the viewing system (BIOM, Eibos, Resight).
3. Staining of the vitreous (e.g., with triamcinolone) and core vitrectomy.

4. Induction of posterior vitreous detachment.
5. Trimming of the vitreous base with bimanual technique (chandelier light).
6. Peeling of an epiretinal membrane.

You can then perform the first surgeries from beginning to end. The following pathologies may be appropriate (with rising difficulty level).

Easy – More Advanced Surgeries:

1. Anterior vitrectomy from pars plana in posterior capsular rupture
2. ERM removal
3. PPV in diabetic retinopathy with mild vitreous hemorrhage and previously treated with laser photocoagulation
4. Silicone oil removal with passive and active aspiration with use of the BIOM
5. ILM peeling

Time perspective: If you perform 2–4 PPVs per week, one needs after our experience 3 months to operate an ILM peeling on your own and 6 months for a retinal detachment.

Complicated Surgeries for Advanced Surgeons

The following surgeries are hard nuts, which can be cracked with a little training. All surgeries demand a thorough and correct preoperative assessment. Draw up a plan on how you wish to proceed intraoperatively. An advanced proliferative diabetic retinopathy with tractional detachment can be very difficult to handle. A PVR detachment is technically challenging and demanding. Finally, the subchoroidal hemorrhage is an especially difficult surgery. You can be proud of yourself if you can manage this pathology.

Difficult Surgeries:

1. Retinal detachment
2. Endophthalmitis
3. Dislocated (hard) nucleus
4. Intraocular foreign body (IOFB)
5. Difficult proliferative diabetic retinopathy (PDVR)
6. PVR detachment
7. Subchoroidal hemorrhage

3.3 Do You Know What You Are Doing?

The A and O of a successful vitreoretinal surgery are optimal visualization, optimal instruments, and optimal technique. This is different to phacoemulsification surgery. Visualization is also very important in cataract surgery as well as a good phaco machine, but instruments and the technique are of minor importance. Regarding instruments, even for an experienced surgeon, there is a significant difference when using different peeling forceps. Test all available forceps and find the one which is most suitable for you. The vast pathological spectrum from PVR detachment to dislocated IOL requires different instruments, the optimal instrument for the specific indication. The same applies to technique. Every pathology requires an optimal technique. You can operate a dark-brown nucleus with phacoemulsification. But the likelihood that you will encounter a posterior capsular rupture, zonular lysis or decompensated cornea is high. This is not the case, if you use the SICS (modified ECCE) technique. If you operate a difficult diabetic retinopathy with tractive detachment with monomanual vitrectomy, you will likely run into problems such as retinal tears or incomplete removal of the membranes. Insert a chandelier light and things are easy. If you operate an ora dialysis with vitrectomy instead of episcleral buckling, then you made a risky choice because the success rate with buckling surgery is 100%.

3.4 Do You See What You Are Doing?

The most essential condition for successful surgery is optimal visualization. Do everything to optimize visualization. Even an excellent surgeon cannot unfold his skills, if he does not see well. The main factors for optimal visualization are the viewing system and the endoillumination.

Test all available viewing systems in order to find the best suitable viewing system for you. It will directly translate into better surgical quality. Of importance are also the lens and an easy lens change. Many surgeons operate with a 90D lens, which is an excellent compromise lens. But you cannot visualize the periphery well with a 90D lens, which makes it a bad candidate for retinal detachment surgery. We prefer therefore 120D lenses to visualize the complete retina. For macular peeling, we then change to a 60D lens. A suitable alternative to a 60D lens is a one-way contact lens.

The next crucial factor for optimal visualization is endoillumination. Three points here are essential:

1. The resterilization of light pipes reduces their quality. Use new light pipes.
2. The usage of an external light source. An external light source such as BrightStar (DORC) or Photon (Synergetics) provides more brightness than an internal light source. An alternative to an external light source is the internal light source of the newest generation of vitrectomy machines such as EVA (DORC), Stellaris PC (B&L), and Constellation (Alcon). The internal light source of the old generation vitrectomy machines such as Accurus (Alcon) is *not* sufficient for a chandelier light.
3. Choice of chandelier light. The brightness of chandelier lights varies a lot. Test many different chandelier lights until you have found a satisfying solution.

One author (US) uses a Zeiss microscope with a Resight viewing system (Zeiss). The Resight is simple to use, two different lenses can be rotated into the light beam and the view under air is excellent. Regarding endoillumination he uses an external light source (Photon, Synergetics) or the internal light source from the vitrectomy machine (Constellation and EVA). He uses predominantly the 25G chandelier light Awh from Synergetics for eyes with vitreous body and 25G chandelier lights from DORC and Synergetics for eyes without vitreous body. The latter light probes are inserted with a trocar and are therefore suitable for soft globes.

And again: It is worthwhile to set ambitious standards regarding visualization because it influences the surgical quality and outcome directly.

3.5 As Soon as You Enter the Eye, You Are in Jail

As soon as you enter the eye with the light pipe and vitreous cutter, you are in jail. Why? Because you decided to operate this eye and you cannot leave the eye any more without facing all negative consequences. So, you need to continue to the maybe bitter end and first then you can leave the jail again. An example: If you decide to perform a vitrectomy in an eye with retinal detachment but cannot treat the retinal breaks because your laser device is defective. Or if you operate an eye with transactional retinal detachment and don't have the intravitreal instruments to remove the membranes.

It is therefore essential to remember that the indication and right timing for vitrectomy is the key for success. This notion does not apply for cataract surgery. In cataract surgery, the indication remains the same and timing plays no role. In addition, the consequences of performing cataract surgery are not as negative as performing vitreoretinal surgery. The list of complications in vitreoretinal surgery is long: PVR detachment after vitrectomy of an attached retina, complete removal of the retina during detachment surgery, large retinal holes after diabetic vitrectomy, and an eye with 90% residual vitreous after a vitrectomy for endophthalmitis. Another example: If you decide to perform a phacoemulsification in an eye with rubeotic iris, you will encounter massive surgical intraoperative problems such as bleeding and massive postoperative problems such as increased iris rubeosis. So, why not treat first the iris rubeosis with an anti-VEF injection and perform phaco 1 month later?

3.6 Stepwise Surgery

Try to perform a stepwise surgery if possible. Stepwise surgery divides the complete surgery into small steps and reduces therefore the surgical trauma, facilitating the next step and resulting in an improved outcome. Stepwise surgery is especially advisable in inflamed and proliferative eyes. Avoid a combined phaco/vitrectomy in these eyes. Do instead first a phaco and later a vitrectomy. Doing surgery stepwise reduces inflammation and proliferation, and each step is surgically easier than a combined procedure.

Two examples: An eye with rubeotic iris and cataract is difficult to operate with phacoemulsification because intraocular bleeding will occur. Treat the eye first with intravitreal bevacizumab and perform 4 weeks later a phacoemulsification. An eye with diabetic tractional membranes and no laser treatment is difficult to operate because intraoperative bleeding will occur. Reduce the bleeding risk by treating the eye first with phacoemulsification and anti-VEGF and in a second step with vitrectomy.

This book will provide many examples for stepwise surgery. Stepwise surgery is intelligent and easy whereas complete surgery is difficult and has a higher complication spectrum.

3.7 Anesthesia

The choice of anesthesia is influenced by a variety of factors. It depends on the estimated duration and severity of the procedure as well as the preferences of the patient and the surgeon. Finally, organizational procedures also should be considered (e.g., out of hours, anesthetic cover, changeover times in theater, etc.). Ideally, beginners should learn the first steps while the patient is under general anesthesia. This greatly reduces stress levels for the surgeon, minimizes sudden head and eye movements, and allows for more discussion between the experienced and the student surgeon, and finally, as the surgical experience increases, more and more surgeries can be performed under local anesthesia. Experienced retinal surgeons perform almost all surgeries under local anesthesia. As a rough guideline, we usually perform macular surgeries and other vitreoretinal procedures up to 60 minutes estimated operating time under local anesthesia. The most painful surgical steps are indentation of the vitreous base, traction on rectus muscles, and cryotherapy. Procedures involving scleral buckling surgery are, therefore, commonly performed under general anesthesia, in particular in younger patients. Several colleagues have experienced good results with subtenon anesthesia. This usually needs to be topped up before starting the procedure to avoid excessive eye movements. One advantage of this technique is that it is classified as "blunt needle" anesthesia. In many departments, this avoids the need for the presence of an anesthetist in theater, which may facilitate out of hours' surgeries in units in which the anesthetic cover has to be shared with other surgical specialties.

For straightforward combined phaco/vitrectomy, we use a combination of short- and long-acting local anesthetic. The preferred techniques of the authors are:

US: Usually 3 mL solution (e.g., 50% bupivacaine (Marcaine®) and 50% mepivacaine (Carbocaine®)) inferotemporal and 2 mL superior at 12 o'clock next to the eyeball. For a PPV detachment, we recommend the following peribulbar anesthesia: 4-4–2.4 mL solution (50% bupivacaine and 50% mepivacaine) inferotemporal, 4 mL superonasal, and 2 mL through the caruncle (Fig. 3.1).

HH: Retrobulbar anesthesia with sharp 1 ½ inch retrobulbar needle, a mixture of 5 mL lignocaine 2%, 5 mL bupivacaine 0.5%, and Hylase (150 IU I 1 mL) are used and about 6–8 mL of this mixture are injected. Hylase is hyaluronidase, which is an

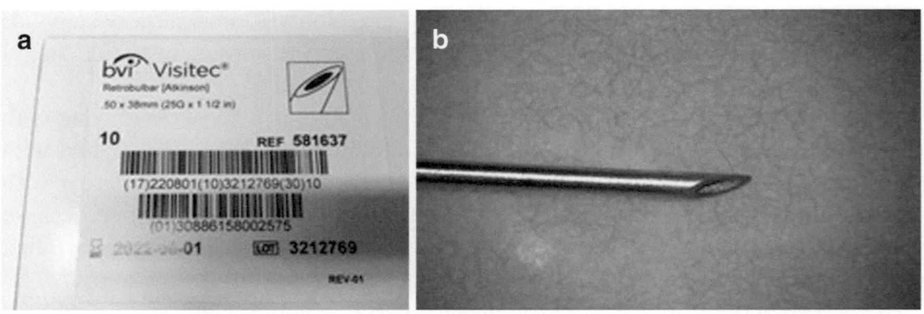

Fig. 3.1 A retrobulbar cannula from Atkinson. The blunt tip prevents a scleral perforation

enzyme that can be added to the local anesthetic solution when administering peri- or retrobulbar anesthesia. It promotes akinesia and is standard in some departments, whereas it is never used in others.

Surgical Pearls No. 10
Scleral perforation: If you use a 25G or 23G cannula, you may perforate the globe during retrobulbar anesthesia. Use a blunt 25G retrobulbar cannula from Atkinson instead. The blunt tip prevents a scleral perforation.

Surgical Pearls No. 11
If revisional surgery within several days of the initial surgery is necessary, consider general anesthesia, in particular after retinal detachment surgery with cryotherapy and extensive extraocular manipulations. The local anesthetic is less effective in inflamed tissue, and the procedure can be more painful under local anesthesia than anticipated.

Surgical Pearls No. 12
When performing potentially painful surgery under general anesthesia (cryotherapy, extensive extraocular manipulations), consider giving a small amount of sub-tenon anesthesia at the end of the surgery. This significantly reduces the pain in the immediate postoperative period when the patient is waking up and recovering from the general anesthesia.

Surgical Pearls No. 13
If you are using Hylase with retrobulbar anesthesia, one vial can be used for multiple cases during one surgical session. We routinely dilute one vial (1500 IU) with 10 mL saline for injection and then use 1 mL of this added to our local anesthetic mixture.

3.8 Lens-Sparing or Combined Phaco/Vitrectomy

There is an increasing trend toward combined surgery (phaco/IOL + vitrectomy) in patients over 60 years. This prevents the need for a second procedure (phaco/IOL) that will be required in almost every patient in this age group within 1–2 years postoperatively. Additionally, the disadvantages of cataract development (decreased vision, increasing myopization, and need for additional examinations) are avoided. Finally, manipulations at the vitreous base are significantly easier to perform in pseudophakic patients. This is of particular importance in retinal detachment cases. A lens touch is a serious complication. It will always result in rapid cataract development and creates a potential point of capsular damage during phaco/IOL. This again may cause prolapse of the posterior segment tamponade into the anterior chamber.

It must also be mentioned that several colleagues try to avoid combined surgery if possible, even in patients above the age of 60 years or patients with moderate cataracts. The reasons for this are that the lens also has a potential barrier function between the anterior and posterior segment. Increasing anterior chamber inflammation can sometimes be seen following combined surgery. In addition, more anterior segment problems can be seen compared to a two-step approach (e.g., posterior synechiae or lens capture). Finally, some authors argue that the additional anterior segment trauma together with the loss of barrier function may also increase posterior segment inflammation and may cause higher rates of cystoid macular edema. These hypotheses have never been examined in a prospective randomized trial. The authors usually combine vitrectomy with phaco/IOL in patients with moderate to advanced cataracts and in patients above the age of 60 years. In patients under 50 years with a clear lens, a lens-sparing vitrectomy should be performed.

In conclusion: The best solution is to perform first a cataract surgery and later a vitrectomy. In an acute case, such as a retinal detachment, however, a combined phaco/vitrectomy is necessary.

Surgical Pearls No. 14
If possible, try to establish biometry and IOL calculations as part of the routine preoperative assessment in all cases of phakic patients undergoing pars plana vitrectomy. This will enable you to perform unplanned phaco/IOL in cases of intraoperative lens touch if needed and provide you with the correct biometry should you need to use silicone oil as a tamponade (which greatly impairs the precision of biometry measurements).

There are two major surgical steps to understand and become skilled at if you wish to master pars plana vitrectomy: (1) To correctly assess the relationship of the posterior vitreous face and the retina, leading to completion of a posterior vitreous detachment (PVD) during surgery, and (2) to trim the vitreous base and to operate in this area without touching the lens in phakic eyes. Therefore, before the start of any pars plana vitrectomy, always ask yourself two questions: Is a PVD present and is the eye pseudophakic or phakic? A PVD should be induced in all posterior vitrectomies (some authors propose not to induce a PVD in asteroid hyalosis or floaters, as the vitreous cortex adheres firmly to the retina and a PVD can induce breaks; however, a PVD will eventually occur in most of these patients and this can either result in a "recurrence" of floaters or retinal breaks). The attached posterior vitreous is more important than most people think. It is involved in many retinal pathologies (maculopathy, diabetic retinopathy) and should therefore be removed by a PVD. For the beginner, the induction of PVD is often not easy. A PVD can be seen at the slit lamp or by ultrasound. Intraoperatively, you can stain the vitreous to determine if a PVD is present or not.

3.9 Monomanual and Bimanual Vitrectomy

A distinction is made between a three-port vitrectomy (Fig. 3.2) and a four-port vitrectomy (Fig. 3.3). The difference is that in a four-port vitrectomy, a fourth port is used for a chandelier light, which is best placed in an inferonasal position. Before

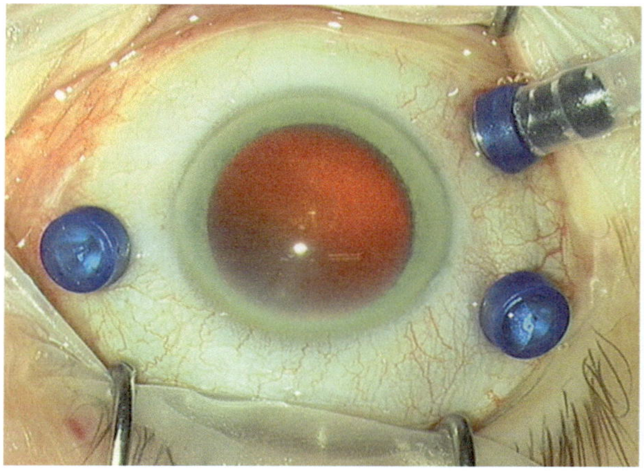

Fig. 3.2 An example of an operation with a three-port trocar system. One infusion trocar with infusion line and two instrument trocars

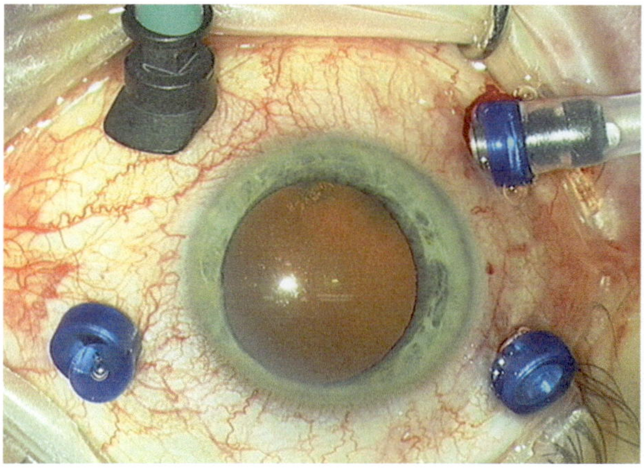

Fig. 3.3 An example of a surgery with a four-port trocar system. In the four-port trocar system, the fourth port is a chandelier light

starting a vitrectomy, you have to decide whether you want to perform a three-port or four-port vitrectomy and inform the theater staff accordingly. However, you can always add a fourth port during three-port PPV if needed.

3.9.1 Monomanual Vitrectomy

In monomanual vitrectomy (Fig. 3.2), one hand holds a light pipe and the other hand holds the vitreous cutter or a different active instrument. The three-port vitrectomy is sufficient for most surgical indications. A good help for detachment surgery consists of using an illuminated endolaser or an illuminated vitreous cutter (see instruments). These combined instruments can be used in combination with a scleral depressor.

3.9.2 Bimanual Vitrectomy with Chandelier Light

With the introduction of new chandelier lights (Fig. 3.3) and powerful external light sources (Photon, Xenon), more and more vitreoretinal surgeries are performed with two active hands (bimanual). Instead of a hand-held light pipe, a chandelier light is fixed in the sclera. The extent of bimanual surgery differs between the authors. US performs bimanual surgery for almost all pathologies except for macular surgery or silicone oil removal. HH uses four-port vitrectomy in cases of challenging membrane peeling (trauma, advanced cases of retinopathy of prematurity or von Hippel-Lindau disease, difficult proliferative diabetic retinopathy, or PVR retinal detachment). The surgeon then has two active hands to manipulate membranes. This is of particular advantage in very strong adhesions between retina and the posterior vitreous face or epiretinal membranes. Remember: No one can indent as good as your second hand.

Surgical Pearls No. 15
Try to use chandelier lights in your uncomplicated cases in order to practice their insertion and to trim the vitreous base bimanually with scleral depressor and vitreous cutter. This will give you greater control when you really need them in challenging cases.

3.10 Hybrid System

A hybrid system (Fig. 3.4) contains different gauges of trocars, for example, a 27G infusion trocar and two 25G instrument trocars. The advantage of 27G (small trocar= > small sclerotomy) is combined with 25G trocars which allows stiffer instruments. But you can also use 27G instruments for the 25G or 23G trocars. Prof. Eckardt, for example, performs his standard vitrectomy with a hybrid setup: One 27G infusion trocar and two 23G instrument trocars.

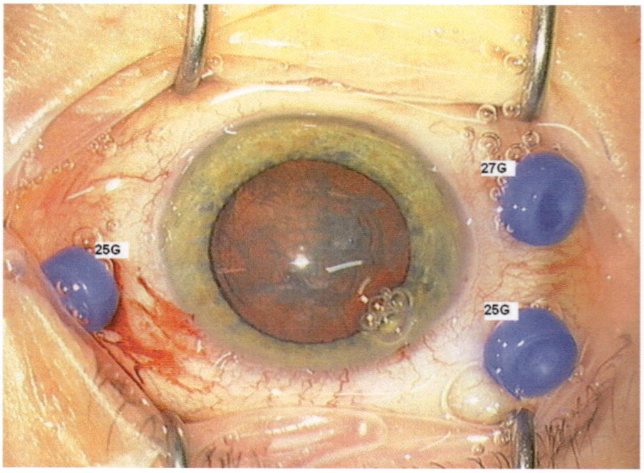

Fig. 3.4 An example of a surgery with a hybrid system. The infusion trocar is 27G and the two instrument trocars are 25G

Chapter 4
Pars Plana Vitrectomy for Beginners

Extras: Videos 4.1, 4.2, 4.3, 4.4, 4.5, and 4.6.

4.1 Topography in Vitrectomy (Figs. 4.1, 4.2, and 4.3)

The correct topography of the eye during surgery is more difficult than you might expect. The lens is located in front or anterior. The retina is located in the back or posterior. A peripheral break is equivalent to an anterior break and a central break

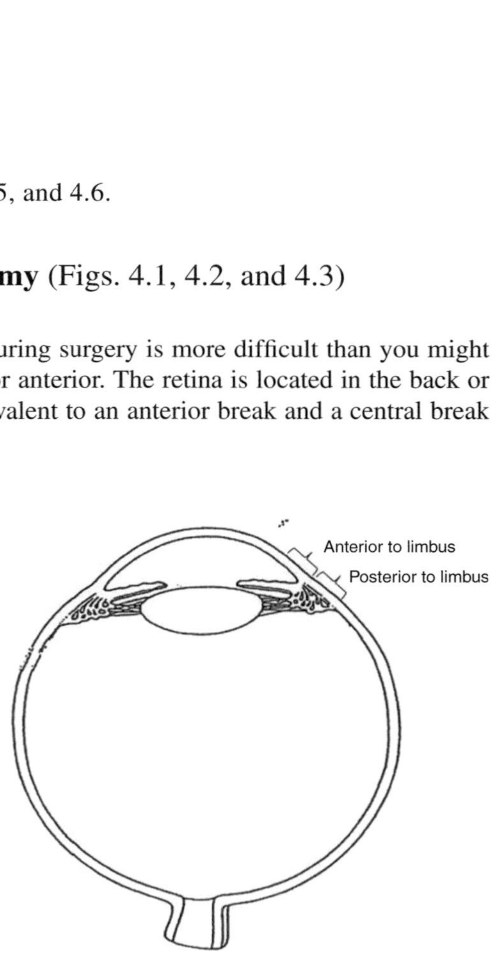

Fig. 4.1 The lens is located **anteriorly** and the macula is located **posteriorly**. The macula is located posterior in the center of the retina. The vitreous base is located peripherally

Electronic Supplementary Material The online version of this chapter (https://doi.org/10.1007/978-3-319-89677-9_4) contains supplementary material, which is available to authorized users.

U. Spandau, H. Heimann, *Practical Handbook for Small-Gauge Vitrectomy*,
https://doi.org/10.1007/978-3-319-89677-9_4

Fig. 4.2 A trocar is inserted **posteriorly (or behind)** to the limbus

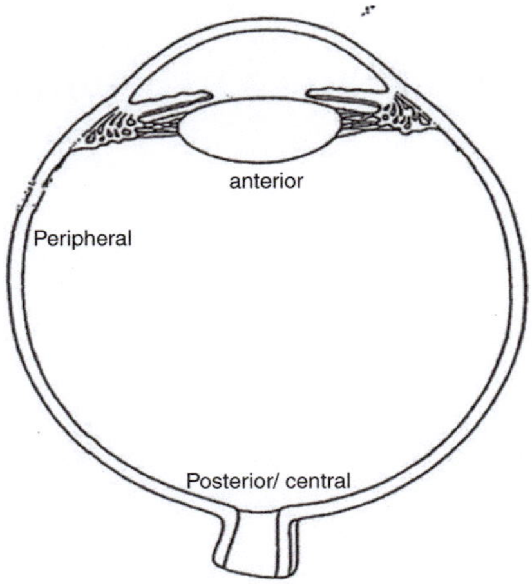

Fig. 4.3 The retinal break is located **anteriorly** to the encircling band. The retina is detached **anteriorly** to the encircling band **but** attached **posteriorly** to the encircling band

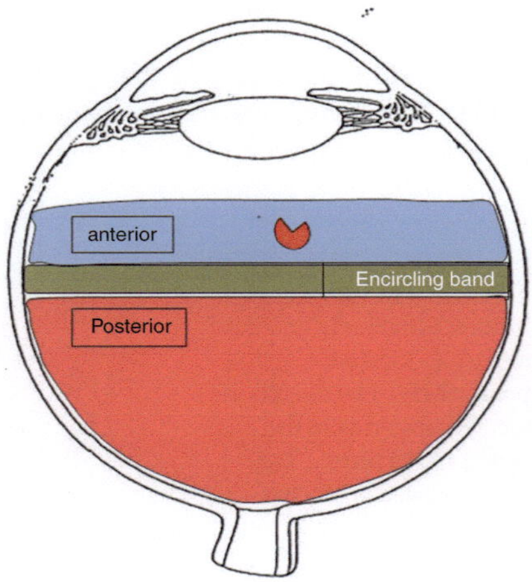

equivalent to a posterior break. You make a sclerotomy <u>not</u> below the limbus but behind or posterior to the limbus. You move the vitreous cutter from the back (retina) to the front (lens). Hold the Charles flute needle behind the lens (in the front of the eye).

4.2 Pars Plana Vitrectomy Step-by-Step

In the following section, a standard pars plana vitrectomy is explained. As in a cookbook, the ingredients (instruments, dyes, and tamponade) are listed first and then the practical approach is explained in detail step-by-step.

4.2.1 Instruments

1. Three-port trocar system
2. 120 or 90D magnifying glass
3. Light pipe
4. Vitreous cutter
5. Scleral depressor
6. Backflush instrument

4.2.2 Dye

Triamcinolone

4.2.3 Tamponade

Air, gas, silicone oil

4.3 The Surgery Step-by-Step

1. **Insertion of trocar cannulas**
2. **Phacoemulsification**
3. **Focusing**
4. **Anterior vitrectomy**
5. **Core vitrectomy**
6. **Induction of posterior vitreous detachment**

7. **Trimming of vitreous base**
8. **Internal search for retinal breaks**
9. **Laser photocoagulation of peripheral breaks**
10. **Cryotherapy of peripheral breaks**
11. **Intraoperative tamponade**
12. **Postoperative tamponade**
13. **Removal of trocar cannulas**
14. **Sclerotomy sutures**

1. **Insertion of Trocars**

The sclerotomies must be placed in the pars plana (here is no retina). The distance of the sclerotomies to the limbus is 3.5 mm in pseudophakic eyes and 4.0 mm in phakic eyes (Table 4.1). By using a scleral marker, you can measure and mark the sclerotomy. It is recommended that you always (even after the beginner phase) use this scleral marker to avoid unnecessary complications due to misplaced sclerotomies. There is no pars plana in newborns; refer to Table 4.1 for recommended placing of sclerotomies in children.

The insertion of the trocars is an important step. It may look frightening at the beginning, but it is actually easier than it looks. The standard position is 4 o'clock (left) or 8 o'clock (right) for the infusion and 9:30–10 and 2–2:30 o'clock for your working ports. See Figs. 4.4 and 4.5. The best position for the chandelier light is

Table 4.1 Site of sclerotomy in relation to the age [1]

Age	0	1–6 mts	6–12 mts	1–3 yrs	3–6 yrs	6–18 yrs	Adult phakic	Adult pseudophakic
Site of sclerotomy (mm)	1,0	1,5	2,0	2,5	3,0	3,5	4,0	3,5

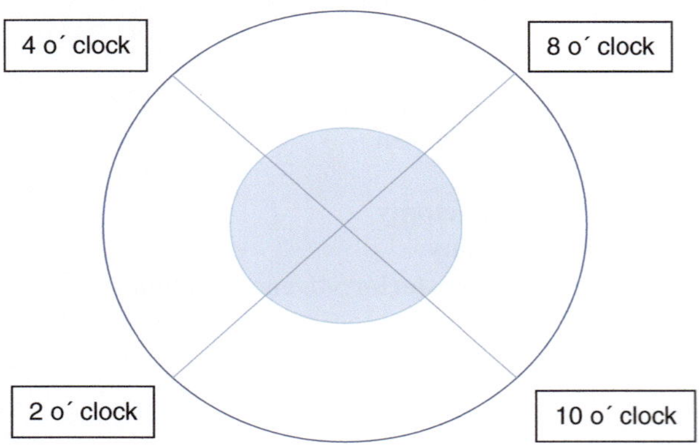

Fig. 4.4 Drawing of a four-port vitrectomy: two instrument ports, one infusion port, and one chandelier light

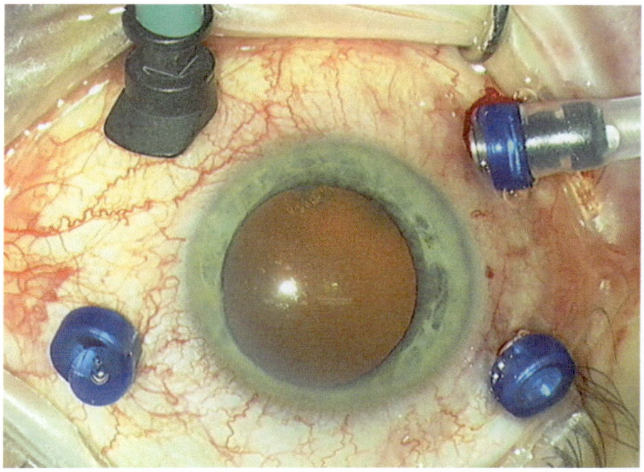

Fig. 4.5 Photo of a four-port vitrectomy: instrument ports, infusion port, and chandelier light

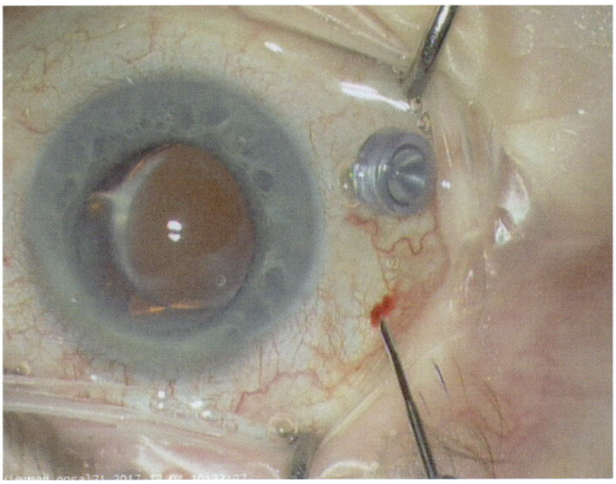

Fig. 4.6 A small bleeding highlights the sclerotomy site. Insert the trocar at an angle of about 15 ° parallel to the limbus

inferonasally because only in this position it does not interfere with the rotation of the globe. In phakic eyes, we recommend that you move your working ports closer to the 3–9 o'clock positions. This way, you have a better angle to trim the vitreous base at 12 and 6 o'clock with a lower risk for lens touch.

Practical procedure (Figs. 4.6, 4.7, 4.8, and 4.9): One always starts with the infusion port inferotemporally. Take a cotton swab in one hand, a 3.5 mm scleral marker (pseudophakic eye) in the other hand, and place the cotton swab posteriorly (behind) the limbus on the conjunctiva. Pull the conjunctiva a little to the side parallel to the limbus, mark the sclerotomy with the scleral marker, replace the scleral marker with the knife, and perform a transconjunctival sclerotomy at an angle of about 15 ° parallel to the limbus. Usually a minor bleeding highlights the sclerotomy site. Here, the trocar cannula is introduced. The first half of the insertion is 15 ° parallel

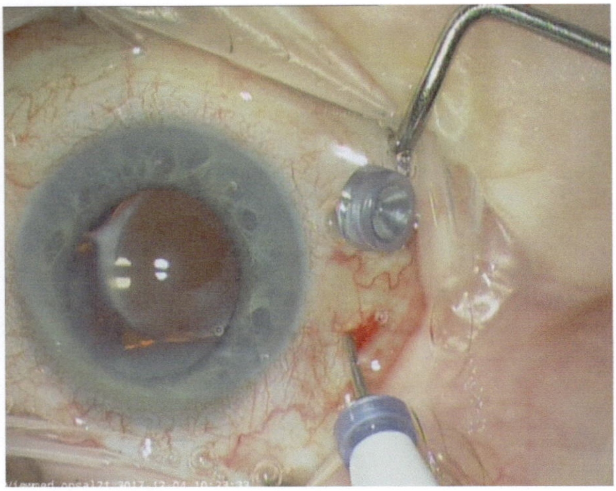

Fig. 4.7 The first half of the insertion is 15 ° parallel to the limbus

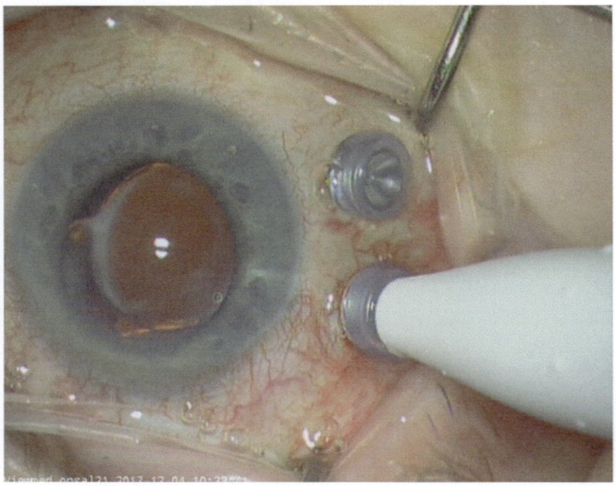

Fig. 4.8 The second half upright toward the middle of the eye (perpendicular)

to the limbus and the second half upright toward the middle of the eye (perpendicular). Finally, fixate the trocar cannula with the trocar forceps and remove the inserter.

Hold the infusion cannula with the trocar forceps (DORC, see materials) and insert the closed infusion line. Then ascertain whether the infusion cannula is located in the vitreous cavity: You turn the cannula with the trocar forceps in direction of the cornea until you can recognize with certainty the cannula's location in the vitreous cavity. The infusion is only opened at the beginning of the vitrectomy. Then the other trocar cannulas are inserted 2:30–2 o'clock and at 9:30–10 o'clock with the same procedure.

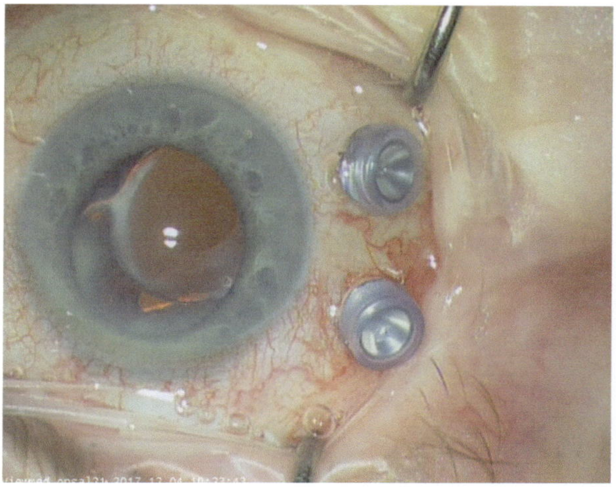

Fig. 4.9 Finally, fixate the trocar cannula with the trocar forceps and remove the insertor

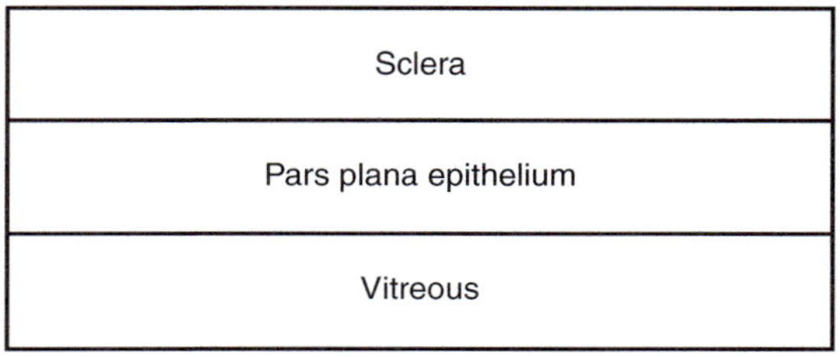

Diagram 4.1 Diagram of the anatomy of the pars plana (from outside to inside)

The procedure concerning the location of the infusion cannula in the vitreous cavity is very important as incorrect positioning of the infusion cannula can cause a number of complications, e.g., subchoroidal positioning can cause a choroidal detachment, subepithelial positioning can cause a detached pars plana, and a subretinal positioning can lead to a detached retina (Diagram 4.1).

Surgical Pearls No. 16
Conjunctival chemosis: If the conjunctiva has been ballooned through the local anesthetic or during previous phacoemulsification, then compress the conjunctiva at the sclerotomy site with a trocar forceps or a simple forceps.

Surgical Pearls No. 17
In patients with narrow lid margins (e.g., children or Asian patients), ports that are placed too superiorly may "disappear" under the upper eyelid. Constantly moving the eye inferiorly to expose the hidden ports and introduce your instruments can be extremely annoying during the surgery.

Surgical Pearls No. 18
Every surgeon will tell you that you have to avoid the 3–9 o'clock position because of the ciliary arteries and the risk for hemorrhage. We found this to be a surprisingly rare event.

Surgical Pearls No. 19

In revisional surgeries, try to identify the previous sclerotomy sites and avoid them. Reopening the previous sclerotomies may result in very irregular and leaking wounds.

Surgical Pearls No. 20

Infusion cannula:

1. Examination of the inner opening of the infusion cannula before starting the infusion is a must in each and every vitrectomy. Make sure that it is not blocked by ciliary epithelium or intraocular membranes. Opening the infusion while the opening is under the ciliary epithelium can within seconds turn a straightforward vitrectomy into a nightmare case.
2. When you can see that the opening is in the correct position but is blocked by blood or membranes, try to clear the opening with a sclerotomy knife, membrane pic, or the vitreous cutter. Be careful not to touch the lens during this maneuver in phakic patients. In the case of doubt, remove the infusion port and try a different site for your infusion.
3. If you are still unsure whether your infusion port is in the right place, introduce the light pipe through the port. You should be able to confirm the correct position even through hemorrhages in the vitreous base.
4. In very complicated cases when you cannot examine the infusion port (trauma, endophthalmitis), start the vitrectomy with infusion connected to an anterior chamber maintainer. Clear the vitreous immediately behind the lens with a vitreous cutter introduced through the pars plana to clear the view. Then insert the infusion trocar via the pars plana as soon as you can see the vitreous base. Even in such complicated cases, do not open the infusion without confirming that the infusion cannula is in the correct position.
5. One of the potential dangers of small-gauge vitrectomy systems is that the infusion cannula is more mobile than with 20-gauge system (with the 20-gauge systems, the infusion port is usually secured with a scleral suture). A mobile infusion port can easily be angled or displaced during small gauge vitrectomy. Secure a loop of the infusion tubing to the drape to avoid unintentional displacement of the infusion cannula.

2. **Phacoemulsification**

We recommend to insert the trocars before phacoemulsification because the globe is very soft after phacoemulsification which makes the insertion of trocars difficult. During phacoemulsification, the infusion is closed.

The phacoemulsification is performed as usual. Regarding the size of your rhexis, it is important to ensure that the edge of the rhexis circularly covers the intraocular lens, as the IOL optic can easily dislocate during vitrectomy in front of the anterior capsule. Therefore, perform a smaller capsulorhexis (4–5 mm). Furthermore, is it advisable to polish the anterior capsule (anterior capsule polishing) to enable a clear view into the periphery. The IOL is usually inserted at the end of the phaco and before the vitrectomy. In difficult cases, some surgeons prefer to insert the IOL at the end of the PPV, because the IOL edge disturbs the view into the periphery. After IOL implantation and irrigation and aspiration, hydrate the paracentesis and the tunnel well to ensure a stable anterior chamber during the vitrectomy. If the anterior chamber during vitrectomy is unstable, place a 10-0 nylon suture at the tunnel. This is particularly advisable if significant indentation is planned during the vitrectomy (e.g., retinal detachment cases), as indentation may open the corneoscleral wound and displace the IOL.

Important: In pseudophakic eyes, BSS is used as irrigation fluid and in phakic eyes BSS Plus®.

Surgical Pearls No. 21
Important remark: *Close* the infusion during an *anterior* segment procedure. *Open* the infusion during a *posterior* segment procedure.

Surgical Pearls No. 22
Perform phaco and vitrectomy only if you previously have gained considerable experience in performing phacos. This step of the surgery must be performed flawlessly. If you struggle with the phaco, the cornea is likely to opacify during surgery, making retinal manipulations later on extremely challenging. If you damage the bag or the zonules, you run the risk of tamponade prolapse into the anterior chamber.

Surgical Pearls No. 23
If you are really running into trouble during the phaco with corneal edema or damage to the lens in cases of elective surgery (macular hole, membrane peeling), think about delaying the vitrectomy part of the procedure until the situation has improved a couple of days later.

Surgical Pearls No. 24
Posterior capsular opacification: Should be removed if it reduces visibility. In addition, a YAG laser capsulotomy is significantly more difficult in vitrectomized eyes. A PCO can be removed from pars plana with the vitreous cutter. Settings: approx. 500 cuts/min and normal vacuum. Cut a circular hole in the posterior capsule. The IOL cannot be injured by this procedure. A small central capsulotomy is sufficient. A larger capsulotomy is associated with the dangers of IOL dislocation and tamponade prolapse into the anterior chamber.

Surgical Pearls No. 25
Blood in the anterior chamber: If you experience a bleeding during the PPV into the anterior chamber, you can either aspirate the blood with irrigation or aspiration instruments or inject a viscoelastics into the anterior chamber to push the blood to the edge of the anterior chamber and tamponade the bleeding. Ask the scrub nurse to remind you to remove the viscoelastic at the end of the vitrectomy. The removal has to be done before you instill the tamponade.

Surgical Pearls No. 26
Blood clots in the anterior chamber: If the bleeding has stopped, extract fibrous strands of blood with an Eckardt forceps through a paracentesis.

Surgical Pearls No. 27
Hypotony of the globe: If the globe is hypotone under phacoemulsification or any other situation, then inject BSS to normalize the IOP. Attach a flute needle (from backflush instrument) onto a syringe with BSS. Inject BSS via a trocar into the posterior vitreous room in order to normalize the intraocular pressure.

Surgical Pearls No. 28
Hypertony of the globe: If the globe is hypertone under phacoemulsification, then perform a dry vitrectomy. A dry vitrectomy is performed with a closed infusion. Place the vitreous cutter behind the lens and cut. Control constantly the pressure of the globe. If the pressure of the globe has become normal, retract the vitreous cutter and continue with phacoemulsification.

3. **Focusing**

The surgeon or the scrub nurse flicks in the BIOM (Oculus, Germany) (Fig. 4.10). Next, the light pipe is introduced in the temporal trocar toward the macula, until the pupil is bright. Then, the inverter is activated, the microscope light turned off, and the image is focused.

For beginners, it may be frustrating to adjust the focus at the beginning of vitrectomy. However, if you keep a few rules in mind, you will find focusing easy. There are three adjustable parameters: (1) focus wheel at the BIOM, (2) focus on foot pedal of the microscope, and (3) zoom on foot pedal of the microscope (Fig. 4.4). When focusing the image, you should only change the two parameters focus wheel BIOM and focus foot pedal and not the zoom. You should only change the zoom when you have a sharp image.

Remember the following steps:

1. Minimal zoom.
2. Turn the BIOM adjustment body with the focus wheel to the top position.
3. Move the microscope with the focus foot pedal so far down toward the cornea, until you get a fairly big image (red pupil).
4. Turn the focus wheel (BIOM) until you get a sharp retinal image.

If the image is sharp, move the microscope further down toward the cornea with the focus of the foot pedal (Cave: corneal touch!). Lastly, you can increase the zoom with the zoom pedal, but be aware that the resolution decreases the more zoom you have.

If the image is totally blurred and you eventually cannot continue or you changed the front lens, always return to the initial parameters (lowest zoom, BIOM adjustment body to the top).

If you are using the Resight viewing system (Zeiss, Germany), there is only one adjustable wheel at the viewing system. Minimize the zoom of the microscope with

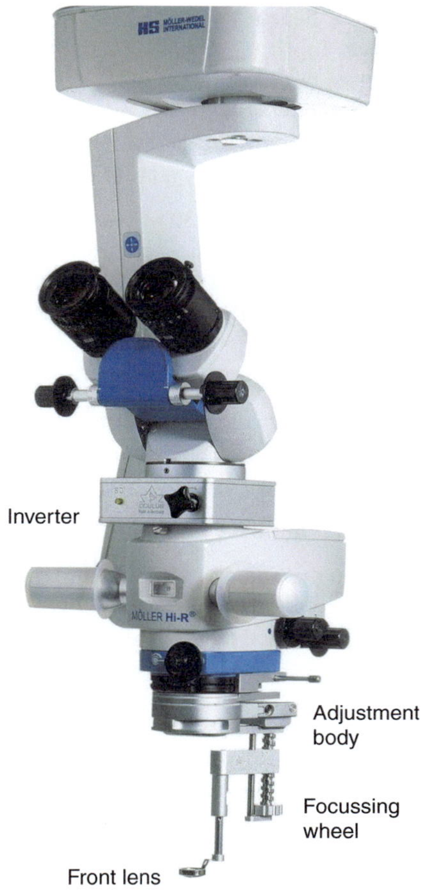

Fig. 4.10 A surgical microscope with attached BIOM. Integrated is an inverter, which may be operated manually or by foot pedal. At the front of the BIOM, the interchangeable front lenses are attached. The adjustment body can be adjusted with the focus wheel

the foot pedal, flick in the Resight viewing system (Zeiss, Germany), activate the inverter, and then turn the wheel at the viewing system until the image is sharp.

If you are using the Eibos system (Leica, Germany), try to reach the manual focus with your right index or middle finger. Once you have mastered this, it makes focusing a lot easier than advising the scrub nurse in focusing up or down.

Important: It may happen that the view to fundus is poor. The reason is media opacities. Hold the vitreous cutter behind the lens capsule. Is the vitreous cutter sharp and focused? If yes, then an opacity of the vitreous is present. If no, then a media opacity of the cornea, anterior chamber, or lens must be present. In latter case, you can perform a corneal abrasion, remove blood or fibrin from the anterior chamber and perform a phacoemulsification in case of a mature cataract.

Surgical Pearls No. 29
Corneal lubrication: A major problem during vitrectomy, especially in combined surgeries with a duration of over 1 h, is corneal epithelial edema. With the application of methylcellulose (Celoftal®, Alcon or Ocucoat®, Bausch & Lomb) on the cornea, the cornea can remain clear for many hours. A debridement of the epithelium is rarely necessary, but if needed use a broad blade (crescent knife).

Surgical Pearls No. 30
Small pupil: If the pupil contracts during surgery, inject 0.01% adrenaline into the anterior chamber. The pupil should enlarge within seconds. If the small pupil is caused by posterior synechiae, use stretching instruments such as a push-pull or insert iris hooks to enlarge the pupil.

Surgical Pearls No. 31
BIOM and air: If you perform water against air exchange, the image will become blurred. You can focus the image by turning the focus wheel of the BIOM so that the front lens moves up. The image will become focused again.

4. **Anterior Vitrectomy**

Remove the anterior vitreous without BIOM. Hold the vitreous cutter behind the posterior capsule and move the cutter in circular fashion while the opening of the cutter is directed downward in order not to injure the capsule.

As a beginner, it is amazing to learn how much vitreous is present in the eye (Fig. 4.8). This can be noticed intraoperatively when air bubbles are trapped in the vitreous behind the lens capsule. These air bubbles cannot be removed with the flute needle but only by removing the vitreous behind the lens capsule. An anterior vitrectomy is easy in pseudophakic patients; in phakic patients, it is dangerous because the location of the posterior capsule is difficult to determine. Therefore, injury to the posterior capsule is a common beginner's mistake. This happens less often when using trocar cannulas, as they limit your movements toward the capsule.

5. **Core Vitrectomy**

Here we start at last with the vitrectomy. You start with the core vitrectomy. In contrast to cataract surgery, you will be surprised by how much space you have in the vitreous cavity. In contrast to phacoemulsification where you hold the instruments almost horizontal, you hold the instruments during vitrectomy almost perpendicular (toward the optic nerve) (Figs. 4.11 and 4.12).

The main problem of vitrectomy is the poor visibility of the transparent vitreous. In eyes with synchisis scintillans or asteroid hyalosis, the vitreous can be seen very clearly. As a beginner, stain the vitreous body during your first surgeries with triamcinolone.

For visualization of the vitreous, hold the light pipe close to the vitreous cutter. You see the vitreous like holding a torch light into a smoke stack. This means that the light pipe and the vitreous cutter move in close vicinity while removing the vitreous body.

When performing vitrectomy, hold the instruments almost vertically toward the orbital apex. Make calm and slow movements, in contrast to irrigation/aspiration

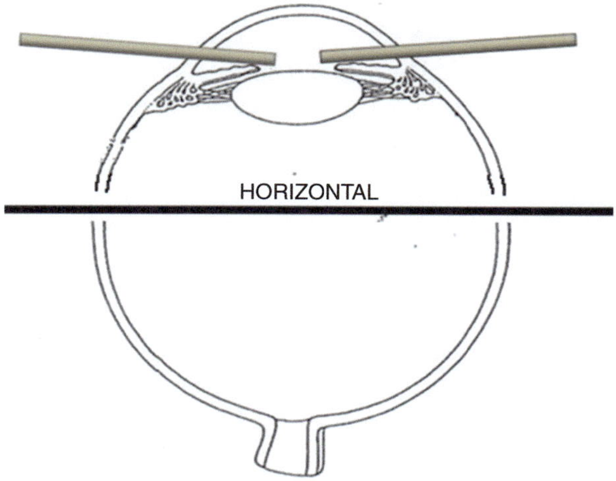

Fig. 4.11 In cataract surgery the instruments are held almost **horizontal**

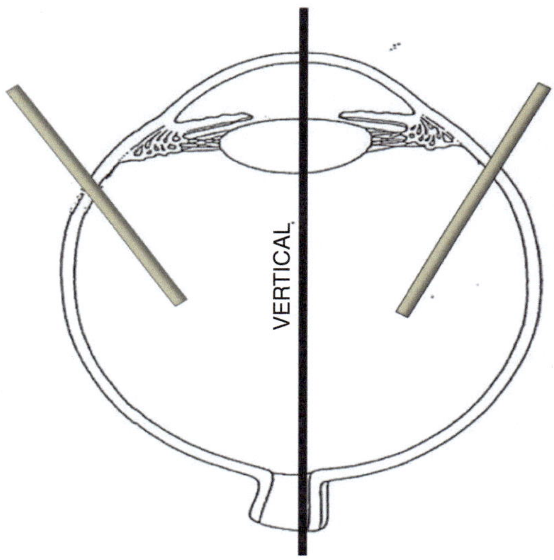

Fig. 4.12 In vitreoretinal surgery the instruments are held almost **vertical**

during phaco. Another important difference is that you hardly move the irrigation handpiece during phaco, but the light pipe in PPV is in constant motion. Light pipe and vitreous cutter move simultaneously, the light pipe illuminating the path of the vitreous cutter. You point the beam of the light pipe to the tip of the vitreous cutter. The vitreous is often difficult to detect. You recognize the vitreous best in the light cone. Move both instruments in a half circle in the vitreous cavity as if peeling an onion from inside to outside. In pseudophakic eyes, the nasal vitreous is cut with the vitrector from the temporal trocar and the temporal vitreous is removed from the nasal trocar.

One should always remember that the eye is a sphere. This means that you have little space behind the lens but plenty of room in the middle of the eye. Coming

Table 4.2 Approximate settings for small gauge with different vitrectomy machines

	Old-generation vitrectomy machines with 2500 cuts/min		New-generation vitrectomy machines with 8000 cuts/min	
	Cutting speed cuts/min	Vacuum mmHg	Cutting speed cuts/min	Vacuum mmHg
Core vitrectomy	1500	400	4000	300
PVD	0	400–600	0	400–600
Vitreous base shaving	2500	0–200	8000	200
Opening of posterior capsule	400	400	400	400
Retinotomy	200	100	300	100

closer to the posterior pole, you can estimate the vicinity to the retina by looking at the shadow of the vitreous cutter. Be aware: The retina forgives no mistakes, and retinal breaks are made quickly. Be cautious, if you come close to the retina with the vitreous cutter.

It is also important to clear the vitreous immediately in front of your ports. Otherwise, there is the danger of pushing the vitreous base forward when introducing your instruments, thereby causing retinal breaks in the vitreous base. This is of particular importance when introducing blunt instruments, for example, a flute needle or an injection cannula. The settings for the vitrectomy machine can be adjusted according to the individual preferences and the vitrectomy machine. For details, see Table 4.2.

Surgical Pearls No. 32

<u>Subepithelial location of infusion cannula:</u> Even an initially correctly placed trocar cannula may move subepithelially during a later stage of the operation. If you experience a retinal or choroidal detachment, stop the infusion, remove the infusion line, and insert it in a safe trocar cannula. Reopen the infusion and the retina or choroid will reattach. Now check the location of the infusion cannula. Is it 3.5 mm posterior the limbus? If not, replace the trocar cannula correctly. Is the trocar located subepithelial? If so, then free the trocar from the tissue with a membrane pic inserted in the opposite cannula.

6. **Induction of Posterior Vitreous Detachment** (Figs. 4.13 and 4.14)

For this step, we routinely use a 90D front lens. To induce a posterior vitreous detachment is a difficult procedure in the learning phase. We recommend beginners to stain the posterior pole at the beginning of vitrectomy with trypan blue. The vitreous is much easier to recognize, and especially the induction of a posterior vitreous detachment becomes considerably easier. Inject a small amount of trypan blue that will drop down onto the posterior pole. Do not inject too much trypan blue. The dye will very nicely stain the bursa premacularis of the vitreous. The bursa premacularis is a cavity anterior to the macula.

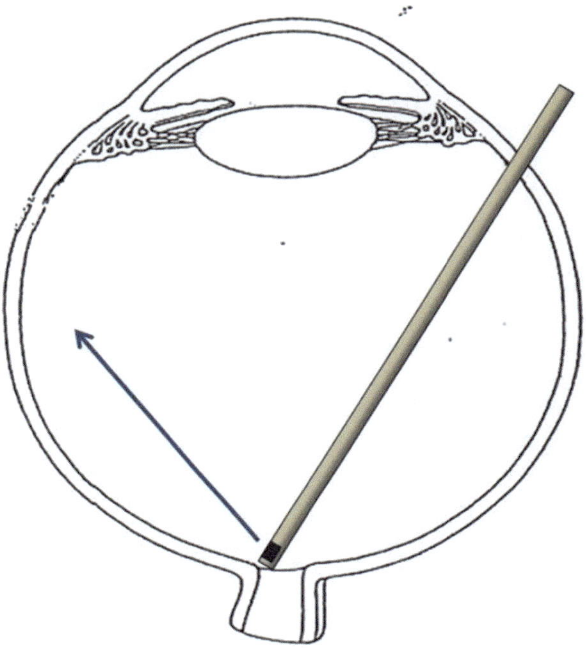

Fig. 4.13 Induction of PVD. Place the tip of the cutter at the nasal edge of the optic disc. Aspirate maximal, the vitreous cortex engages in the cutter opening and then pull the cutter slowly towards the ora serrata

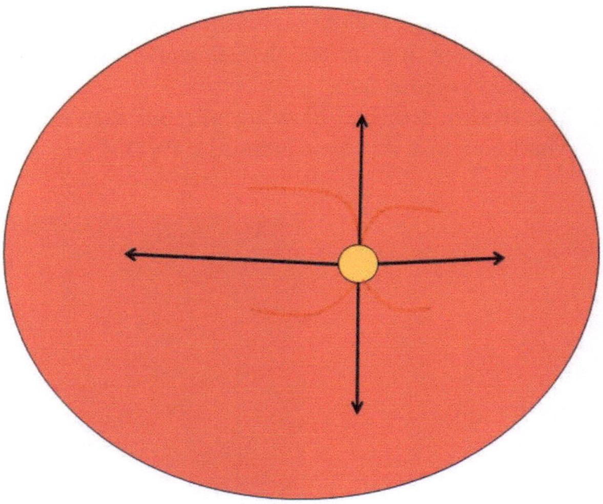

Fig. 4.14 Induction of PVD. Repeat this maneuver in all four directions but start always at the nasal pole

For induction of PVD, position the vitreous cutter at the nasal rim of the optic disc with the aspiration port pointing to the ora serrata. Then increase suction (foot pedal to bottom position) to maximum. In the suction phase, the cortex and especially the posterior hyaloid will be engaged in the aspiration port. Then draw the vitreous cutter slowly with maximal suction toward the lens. If the maneuver is successful, you will see a kind of fine silk screen that moves forward together with the vitreous cutter. Try to keep an eye on the advancing posterior vitreous face in the mid-periphery. This looks like a tidal wave. It is where breaks will develop during induction of a PVD. Sometimes, this whole maneuver must be repeated several times until it succeeds. Before you repeat the maneuver, cut the aspirated vitreous in the vitreous cutter to prevent traction and tractional tears and then place the vitreous cutter in front of the optic disc again.

Difficult PVD (Figs. 4.15, 4.16, and 4.17):

If you are not able to induce a PVD, try the following: (1) Increase the vacuum to 600 mmHg and try again. (2) Stain the vitreous with trypan blue or triamcinolone and try again. (3) Insert a 90D lens and mobilize the vitreous or even better, the posterior hyaloid membrane with an Eckardt forceps. If you have mobilized a larger piece or created a hole, try to aspirate this part with a vitreous cutter and provoke a PVD. If you cannot grasp the posterior hyaloid, you need to work with instruments. In these cases, the posterior hyaloid is a bit distant to the retina. You need to create a hole in the posterior hyaloid. Use a retrobulbar Atkinson cannula to create a hole. Then you can easily grasp the edges of the hole with an intravitreal forceps and enlarge the PVD (Figs. 4.15–4.17).

Surgical Pearls No. 33

PVD:

1. The correct assessment of the relationship between the posterior vitreous face and the retina/optic disc is one of the key steps to master pars plana vitrectomy. Always check if a PVD is present or not. Even in cases when you expect a PVD to be present (e.g., retinal detachments), you will sometimes be surprised by an attached vitreous face.
2. The freshly detached posterior vitreous face has a "beaten metal" appearance. You know that you have induced a PVD if you see this appear on the posterior

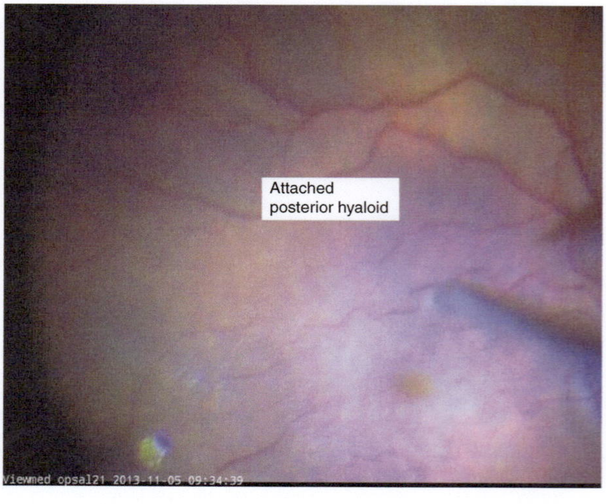

Fig. 4.15 Difficult PVD: the posterior hyaloid cannot be detached with the vitreous cutter

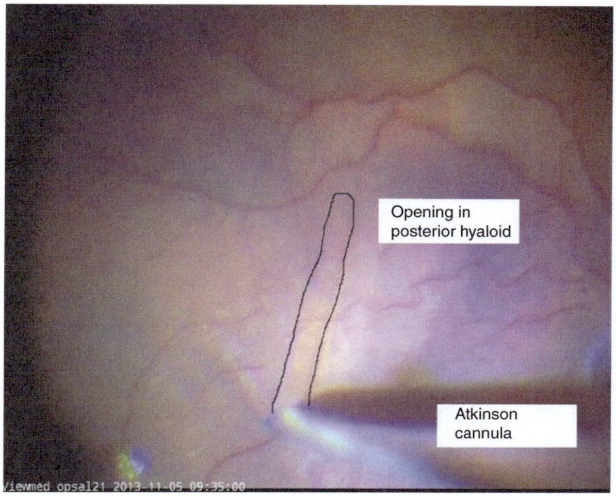

Fig. 4.16 Difficult PVD: open the posterior hyaloid with an Atkinson cannula

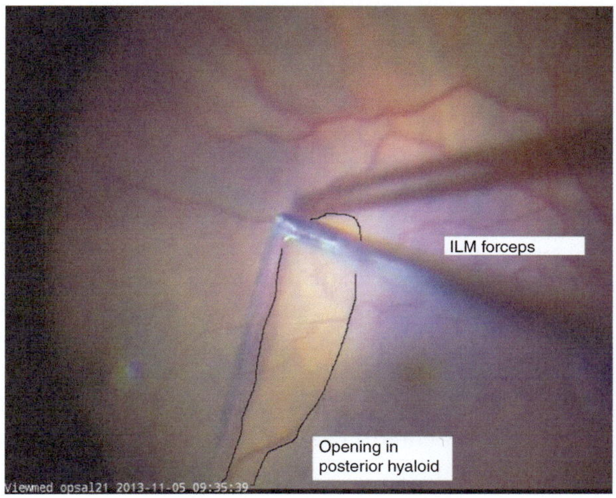

Fig. 4.17 Difficult PVD: grasp the edges of the posterior hyaloid with an intravitreal forceps

surface of the vitreous. When a PVD is induced, suddenly, a lot more vitreous, which must be removed, will appear in the vitreous cavity.

Surgical Pearls No. 34

<u>PVD and myopic eyes:</u> Beware of highly myopic eyes. They often have a "vitreoschisis." You may think that there is a complete PVD, yet, there only is a vitreoschisis with the posterior vitreous face still attached to the retina. In the case of doubt, stain with triamcinolone. The remnant vitreous face will appear as a thin membrane-like structure on the retina. Sometimes you can peel it off with the forceps, sometimes you have to use the flute needle to brush it off the retina.

7. **Trimming of Vitreous Base**

After successful PVD, continue with trimming of the vitreous base. We usually use a 120D or comparable wide-angle lens. Regarding the settings of the vitrectomy machine, decrease the vacuum and increase the cutting frequency the closer you work with the vitrector at the retina (Table 4.1).

In phakic eyes, you can cross the midline only when working at the posterior pole to mid-periphery. To reach the vitreous base, you are not allowed to cross the midline. The vitreous base can be removed from the opposite site by indenting the vitreous base or from the same side with the "backhand" and wide-angle viewing systems.

In detachment surgery, the vitreous base must be removed as completely as possible, because vitreous traction is causatively responsible for the retinal break and residual vitreous may continue to exert traction on the retina and cause post-operative new breaks. For surgeries, such as macular hole or macular epiretinal membranes, it is not necessary to remove the vitreous base completely, because the pathological changes are located here in the macula and not in the retinal periphery. In contrast, working too aggressively in this area may cause more harm by inducing retinal breaks or lens touch. The presence of the natural lens makes working in the area of the vitreous base challenging. Firstly, there is a risk of lens touch, and secondly, access to the vitreous base is more difficult as the lens is in the way, in particular in elderly patients with a thicker lens. Finally, a vitrectomy will induce cataract development in each and every case of phakic patients.

Surgical Pearls No. 35
Working in the area of the vitreous base and trimming the vitreous base is another key step to learn if you want to master vitrectomy. Numerous techniques can be used. Our favorite techniques are (US) using a chandelier light and indentation with a scleral depressor and (HH) scleral indentation with a light pipe or working with your "backhand" with the vitreous cutter facing the retina on the side of your vitreous cutter using wide-angle viewing systems. This avoids indentation and is used mainly for trimming the vitreous base during macular surgery.

Surgical Pearls No. 36
Scleral folds or soft globe during vitrectomy: If you view scleral folds during vitrectomy or if the globe is soft, then stop PPV at once. The most likely cause is a dislocated infusion line. Reinsert the infusion line and check if the globe is normotensive and if the scleral folds have vanished.

Surgical Pearls No. 37
Lens touch:

1. A lens touch is often caused by the light pipe (focusing the light beam on peripheral vitreous during trimming of the vitreous base) or the endolaser probe when

performing peripheral laser on the opposite site. One focuses on the opening of your vitreous cutter but "forgets" the other intraocular instrument. It has to become second nature to hold the second instrument in the correct position without thinking about it.

2. Another common cause of lens touch is pushing the infusion port into the lens during indentation. Avoid by taking extra care in this area and indent pushing the vitreous base toward the center of the eye, not anteriorly toward the lens.
3. If you notice a lens touch during or at the end of your surgery, clearly mark it in your surgical notes. It is important to know this if you are planning to perform the phaco at a later stage, as this weakens the posterior capsule. We have seen an entire lens dropping to the posterior pole during hydrodissection; the posterior capsule splits at the site of the previous lens touch and the lens dropped posteriorly.

8. **Internal Search For Retinal Breaks**

At the end of vitrectomy, breaks must be identified and treated accordingly. Inspect the entire peripheral retina with the aid of a scleral depressor. If a break is present, you must remove any residual vitreous adhesions, treat the break with laser or cryoretinopexy, and a gas tamponade needs to be installed, for example, with 20% SF_6. Otherwise a postoperative retinal detachment occurs.

Surgical Pearls No. 38
<u>Internal search for retinal breaks:</u>

1. Perform an internal search in each and every case of vitrectomy, even in low-risk cases. Perform the search at the very end of your procedure, as even minor intraocular manipulations may create breaks in the area of the vitreous base that may not be noticed if you have performed your inspection of the vitreous base beforehand.
2. Don't be complacent when performing the internal search. Identification of potential problems in the retinal periphery is one of the key steps to lowering your complication rate. Make sure that you visualize the entire retinal periphery 360° up to the ora serrata. Move your sclera depressor constantly when inspecting the vitreous base. This is a dynamic procedure. This way you will identify breaks opening up during your indentation that you may miss if the indentation is too "static."

9. **Laser photocoagulation of Peripheral Breaks**

If the break is so peripheral that you need a scleral depressor to see it, you must now either insert a chandelier light in order to have a free hand for the scleral depressor or you use a combined laser with optical fiber (see instruments) or indent the eye with your light pipe. Surround the break with one to three rows of laser burns (e.g., using the 532-nm diode laser OcuLight GL Company Iridex, we use the laser parameters: power 150 mW, duration 200 ms, interval 300 ms).

Surgical Pearls No. 39
Iatrogenic break: When a small break is located within the vascular arcades, a laser treatment is not necessary as the pigment epithelium in the central area has sufficient pumping function so that no detachment occurs. If the break is large, however, we recommend lasering the break with one row of laser burns. Even if you create a peripheral break, this is not a problem as long as you also recognize the break. Surround the tear with three rows of laser burns and perform a gas tamponade.

Surgical Pearls No. 40
Laser therapy:

1. A laser treatment can be carried out in a water (BSS)-filled, silicone oil-filled, and PFCL-filled eye. In an air-filled eye, it is difficult to laser due to a poor visibility.
2. It is easiest to laser breaks under heavy liquid, as you have a good apposition of retina and retinal pigment epithelium. One of the disadvantages of this technique is that the margins of the break are more difficult to see. Mark, therefore, the location of breaks with endodiathermy or laser spots before covering it with heavy liquid. This way it is easy to identify them under heavy liquid.
3. Beware of the "continuous" function of the laser. You can easily overtreat. This may result in mini-explosions, choroidal hemorrhage, retinal breaks, or predispose to postoperative tears. Pigmentation increases toward the periphery. Less energy is needed for peripheral laser spots.
4. The further you move the laser probe away from the retina, the larger the resulting spot size on the retina (and the more energy you need to create a burn). This can be quite useful if you want to treat larger areas as the resulting burns have softer edges and do not cut the retina like a knife.
5. Use 360° prophylactic laser with caution. It may not be necessary, may result in anterior segment ischemia and will make it very difficult to identify small breaks in cases of postoperative retinal detachments.

10. **Cryotherapy of Peripheral Break**

The cryotherapy of a peripheral break is a good alternative to laser photocoagulation, in particular in phakic eye where endolaser of breaks in the retinal periphery without touching the lens is challenging. You indent the retina with the cryoprobe and hold the light pipe in the other hand. Cryotherapy should be applied sparingly, preferably with one cryo effect in the middle of the break in order to reduce the risk for PVR. Cryotherapy induces more PVR than laser photocoagulation.

11. **Intraoperative Tamponade**

Sometimes during vitrectomy, an intraoperative tamponade with perfluorocarbon (PFCL) or air is performed. There are several indications. A fluid x air exchange is an important step in detachment surgery. A PFCL (heavy liquid) tamponade is important to remove subretinal fluid in detachment surgery and to attach the retina. PFCL must always be completely removed because it damages the retina. It is very important to know the physiologic properties of PFCL and air.

PFCL

Perfluorocarbon (PFCL, "heavy water") has the highest density of all intraocular used liquids; the eye is filled up from the posterior pole to the ora serrata. In the supine position, PFCL exerts the most pressure on the posterior pole and less pressure anteriorly (Fig. 4.18); it flattens the retina from the posterior pole to the ora serrata. A big advantage is the good visibility under PFCL. One disadvantage is that it always needs to be completely removed, as it is retinotoxic if left within the eye for weeks to months, especially if it is dislocated into the subretinal space. PFCL is now an essential tool in retinal detachment surgery. It is used to flatten the detached retina and push subretinal fluid through the breaks into the vitreous.

Air

In the supine position, air exerts the most pressure on the anterior retina (ora serrata) and less on the posterior retina (Fig. 4.18). Because air is lighter than water or PFCL, the eye will be filled with air from the ora serrata and then down to the optic disc. To fill the eye completely with air, the surgeon must aspirate the liquid behind the air bubble with a flute needle. This is most easily done by holding the flute needle just above the optic disc until the intraocular fluid is completely removed.

Air is important in detachment surgery for the fluid/air exchange maneuver, in which a detached retina can be flattened with air. This is possible due to the high surface tension pressure of air. In addition, in eyes with vitreous hemorrhage, air can be used as a tamponade to prevent a possible postoperative bleeding.

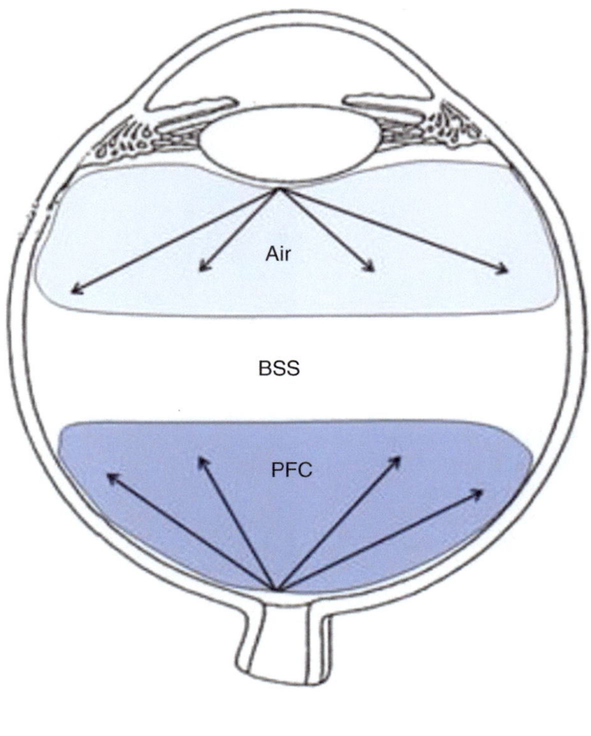

Fig. 4.18 Opposite effects of air and PFCL in the vitreous cavity. Air exerts pressure onto the retina from anterior to posterior whereas PFCL exerts pressure from posterior to anterior

Another indication for an air-filled eye is a better sealing of the sclerotomies. The air exerts pressure on the wedges of the tunnel sclerotomies and induces an improved closure of the sclerotomies.

A disadvantage of air and gases in general is the greater distortion of the optical image. One advantage is the wide-angle view up to the pars plana in an air-filled eye (Figs 4.19 and 4.20).

Surgical Pearls No. 41

BIOM and air: When filling air into the vitreous cavity, the image is out of focus due to the different refractive index. If you move the BIOM lens up a little, the image becomes focused again.

Fluid against air exchange (Figs. 4.21, 4.22, 4.23, 4.24, and 4.25)

Fluid x air exchange means fluid against air exchange. During this maneuver, the BSS inside the vitreous cavity is exchanged against air. This is a very common surgical maneuver during vitreoretinal surgery and at the end of vitreoretinal surgery. At the end of vitreoretinal surgery, the air may be used as tamponade or be exchanged against a longer-lasting gas such as Sf_6, C_2F_6, and C_2F_8. A fluid against air exchange is performed with a Charles flute needle (= backflush instrument).

Function of Charles flute needle:

Surgical procedure for fluid × air exchange: (Fig. 4.24)

Hold a Charles flute needle (backflush instrument) into the vitreous cavity. Switch from BSS to air infusion. Air enters the eye and the BSS is removed with the

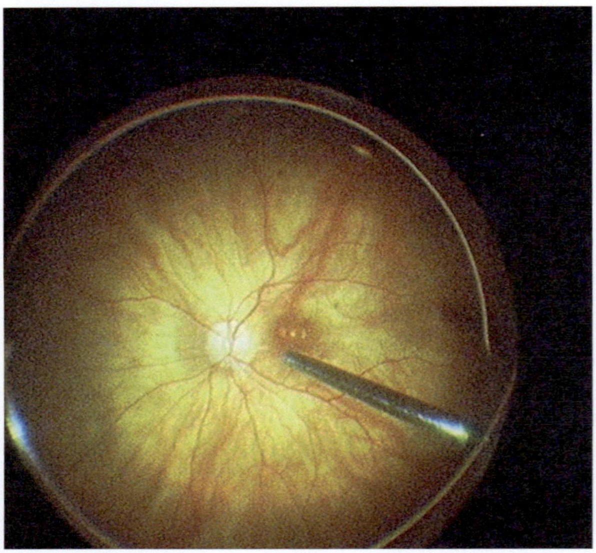

Fig. 4.19 View onto a fundus of a water-filled eye. The peripheral view is reduced by water, the advantage is a higher resolution

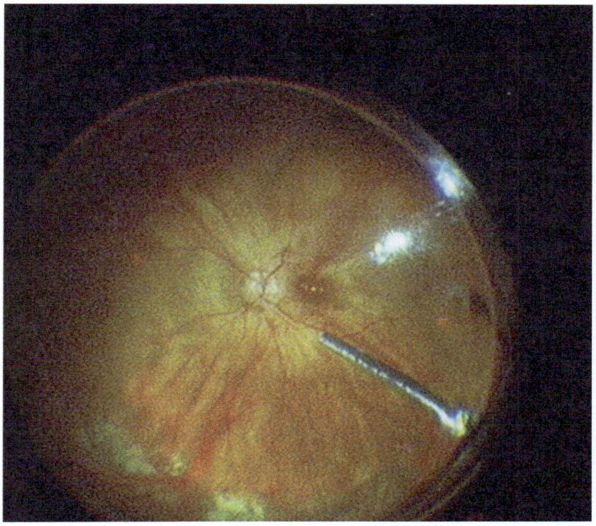

Fig. 4.20 View onto a fundus of an air-filled eye. The peripheral view is much enlarged up to the ora serrata, the disadvantage is a lower resolution

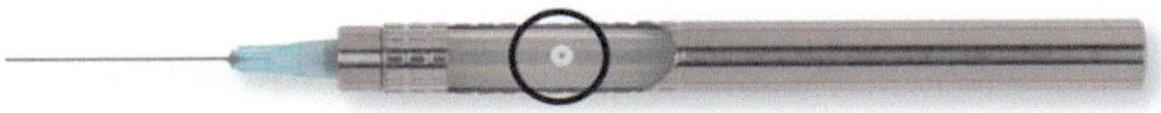

Fig. 4.21 The Charles flute needle aspirates fluid through the needle on the left side and the water flows out through the hole in the middle (circle). This is called **passive aspiration**

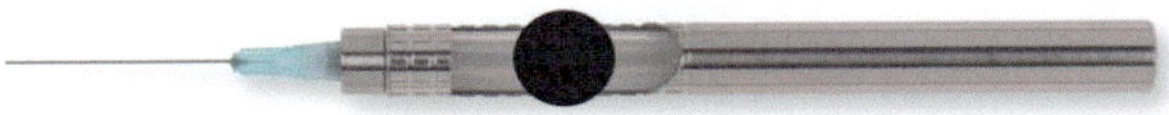

Fig. 4.22 If you close the hole at the side with your index finger, then the Charles flute needle does not aspirate. You do not need to press but only close the hole. During passive aspiration, you close the hole when you do not want to aspirate and open the hole when you want to aspirate

Charles flute needle. Refocus the viewing system, because the optical properties of air are different from BSS. Then place the Charles flute needle at the optic disc and aspirate the residual fluid.

Fluid tamponade (exchange of air against fluid) (Fig. 4.25)

Hold the flute needle directly behind the IOL. Then the scrub nurse switches from air to water and the eye fills up quickly with water. If small air bubbles remain at the end behind the IOL, then there is still (anterior) vitreous behind the IOL. If you plan to perform now macular surgery, you have to remove these irritating air bubbles. In order to do so, perform an anterior vitrectomy.

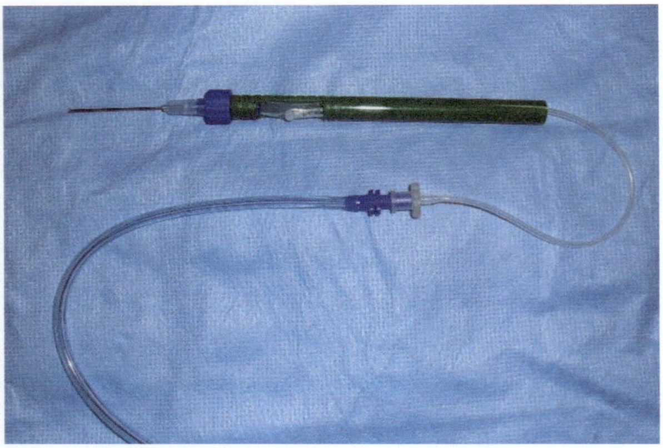

Fig. 4.23 **Active aspiration**: attach a suction pipe onto the Charles flute needle. For active aspiration, you must close the hole at the side **the whole time**. When pressing the foot pedal, you activate and steer the amount of active aspiration. The Charles flute handpiece is not needed during active aspiration. You can also attach the Charles flute needle directly to the suction pipe. Active aspiration is not necessary in 23 gauge, but necessary in 25 gauge and 27 gauge

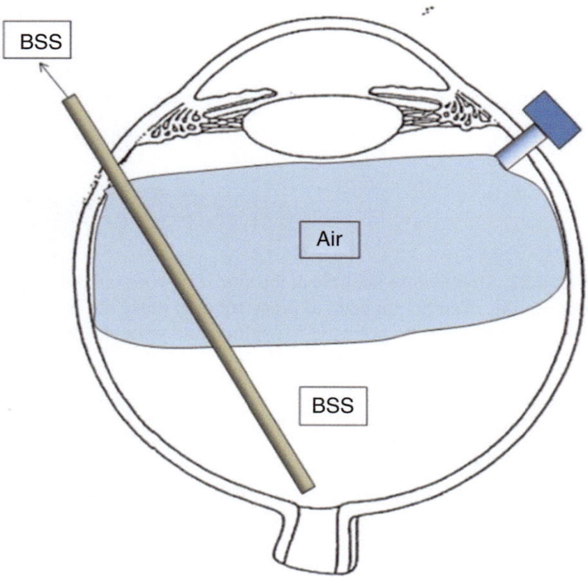

Fig. 4.24 Fluid against air exchange. Place the Charles flute needle before the optic disc. The air flows from the front (lens) to the back (posterior pole)

PFCL tamponade (exchange of fluid against PFCL) (Figs. 4.26, 4.27, 4.28, and 4.29)

Inject PFCL always in a fluid-filled eye and not in an air-filled eye. The PFCL must be injected slowly. PFCL injected too quickly can induce retinal damage. PFCL should never be injected in direction of the macula. You start with the injection nasal to the optic disc and then move the cannula slowly toward the lens leaving the tip of the cannula in the PFCL bubble. Leaving the tip of the cannula in the big

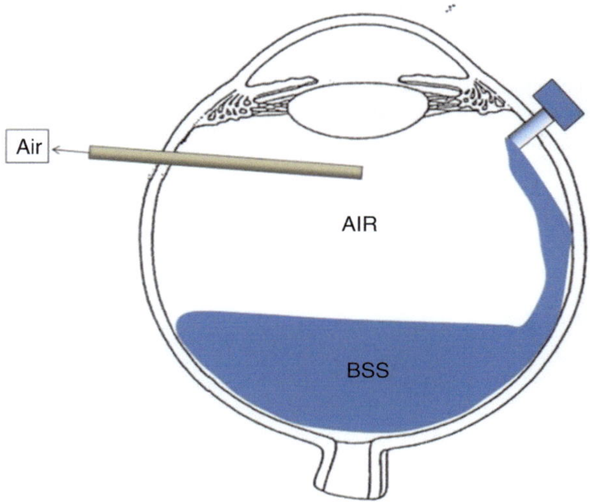

Fig. 4.25 Air against fluid exchange. Place the Charles flute needle behind the lens. The fluid flows from the back (posterior pole) to the front (lens)

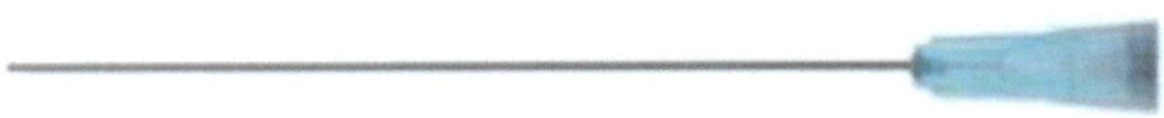

Fig. 4.26 A backflush needle. This cannula is used for the backflush instrument and for injection of fluids. DORC 1281.A5D06

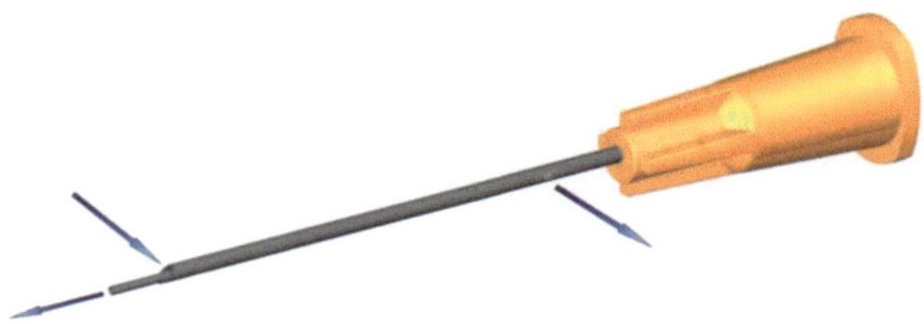

Fig. 4.27 Double-barreled cannula. This cannula is used for the injection of fluids. The cannula prevents an intraocular hypertension during injection. The injection is done monomanually. DORC: Double-bore cannula. EFD.06

bubble prevents the formation of small PFCL bubbles (fish eggs). PFCL can be injected (1) bimanual. At the same time, BSS is aspirated with a backflush instrument. A chandelier light is therefore needed (Figs. 4.26 and 4.28) (2) monomanual. You use a dual bore cannula (Fig. 4.27) which allows simultaneous injection and aspiration (Fig. 4.29).

Surgical Pearls No. 42

<u>PFCL injection</u>: Try to inject one bubble only. Start very slowly and then always keep the tip of your cannula in touch with the bubble. This avoids splitting the stream into multiple bubbles, which can then displace into the subretinal space.

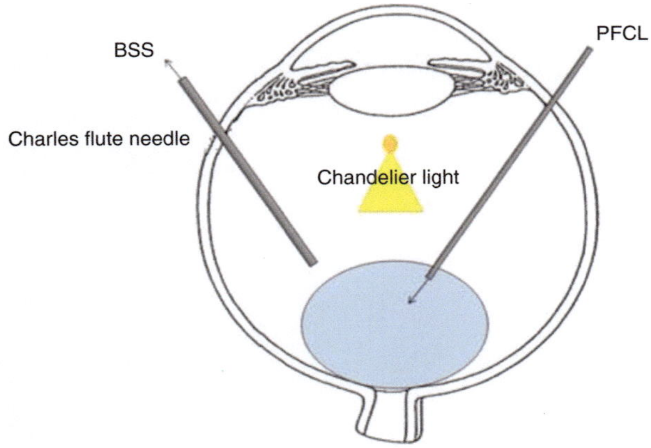

Fig. 4.28 Bimanual injection of PFCL with a normal extrusion cannula. At the same time, BSS is removed with a second extrusion cannula. A chandelier light is required

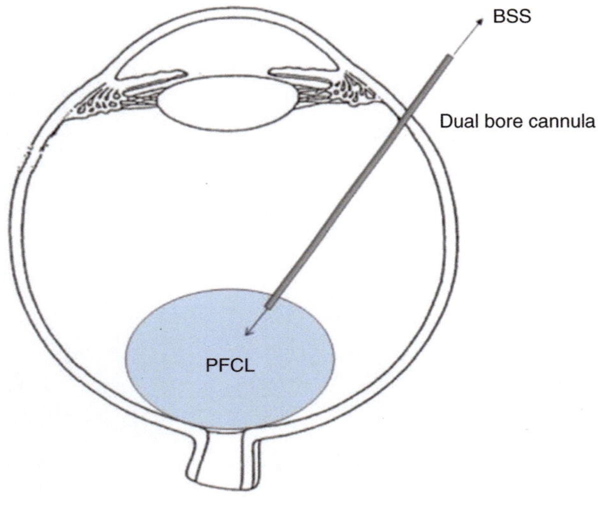

Fig. 4.29 Monomanual injection of PFCL with a dual bore cannula. The cannula injects PFCL as well as removes BSS at the same time. A chandelier light is not required

Removal of PFCL

Hold the flute needle in front of the optic disc and aspirate the complete PFCL bubble. If a small bubble remains and you do not succeed with the flute needle, then do not insist but aspirate the residual bubble with a silicone-tip flute needle in order not to damage the retina or the optic disc.

12. **Postoperative Tamponade (Gas and Silicone Oil)**

The choice of tamponade, gas, or silicone oil depends on the indication (Table 4.3). The main advantage of gas over silicone oil is that the surface tension pressure is higher. Gas presses the retina more against the underlying pigment epithelium than silicone oil. The main disadvantage of gas is that it causes ocular irritation and inflammation which makes it not suitable for vascular and inflammatory active eyes. Silicone oil is a good candidate for vascular and inflammatory active eyes. Silicone

Table 4.3 Gas or silicone oil tamponade for different pathologies

Pathology	Gas	Silicone oil
Easy retinal detachment	X	
PVR retinal detachment		X
Easy proliferative diabetic retinopathy	X	
Difficult proliferative diabetic retinopathy		X
Macular hole	X	
Silicone oil removal	Air	
Nondiabetic vitreous hemorrhage	Air	

oil is a good temporary tamponade. But silicone oil causes IOP increase and eventually a glaucomatous optic atrophy if left for several years inside the eye.

Practical Approach:

Make sure that all potential anterior segment problems are addressed before starting a tamponade. The air bubble will push the iris-lens diaphragm forward, making any manipulations in the anterior chamber extremely difficult. In addition, fluid injected into the anterior chamber will enter the posterior segment and displace the tamponade, potentially causing an "underfill."

In cases of large defects within the zonules or the lens capsule, inject miochol and an air bubble into the anterior chamber before fluid-air exchange. This prevents the iris-lens diaphragm from moving forward and avoids iris capture or displacement of the gas tamponade into the anterior chamber. With modern viewing systems and air in the anterior chamber, there usually is a sufficient view of the posterior pole to perform a safe fluid-air exchange.

Air Tamponade (Exchange of Fluid Against Air)

Remark: An air tamponade has several indications: (1) Air in the vitreous cavity presses against the wedges of the sclerotomy incision and thereby stabilizes the sclerotomies, which results in a reduced postoperative hypotony, (2) reduces postoperative bleeding (favorable for diabetic eyes), and (3) tamponade for macular holes.

The Surgery: Gas Tamponade (Exchange of Air Against Gas) (Figs. 4.30 and 4.31)

Gas has two great advantages over silicone oil. The surface tension pressure of gas is much higher than for silicone oil which enables a more effective sealing of retinal holes. Secondly, the gas is a temporary tamponade. Long-term damages of gas are therefore not existent compared to silicone oil.

Injection of gas: SF_6, C_2F_6, and C_3F_8 are due to the fluorine atoms heavier than air. The gases sink therefore to the ground whereas the lighter air stays above. Hold the Charles flute needle behind the lens to aspirate the air and the gases can fill the vitreous cavity from posterior to anterior (Figs. 4.30 and 4.31).

After the fluid to (against) air exchange, you can swing out the BIOM, activate the inverter, and switch on the light of the microscope. The surgical nurse attaches a 50 mL syringe with diluted gas to the three-way tap and injects the gas (about 45 mL) into the vitreous cavity. Instruct the scrub nurse to stop injecting immediately if he or she feels an increasing resistance to injection. To avoid an increased pressure in the eye, you must simultaneously decompress the eye. This can be

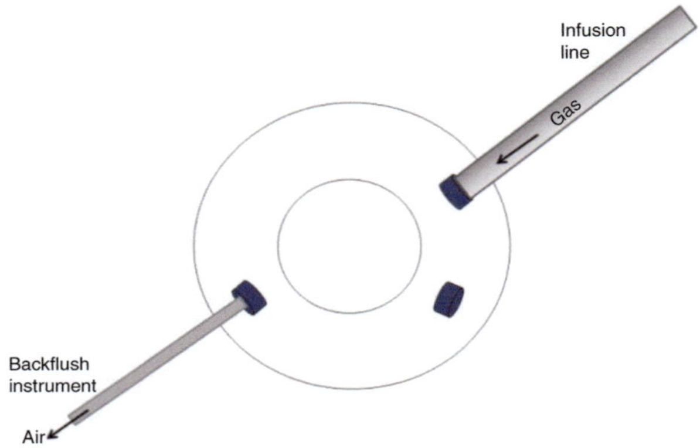

Fig. 4.30 The setup for a gas injection. The gas is injected through the infusion line and the flute needle evacuates the air

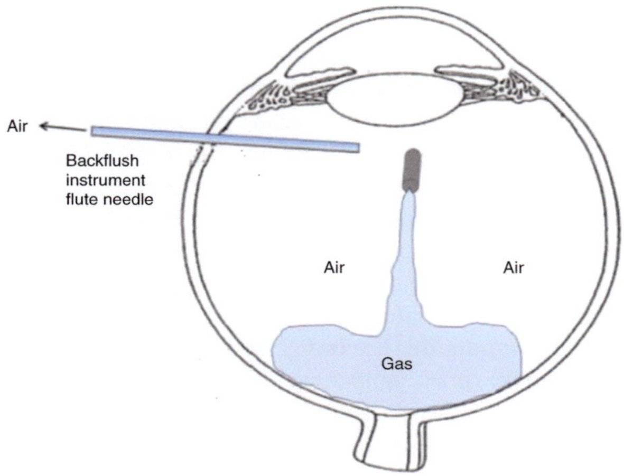

Fig. 4.31 The heavy gas fills the vitreous cavity from posterior to anterior and the flute needle aspirates the light air

achieved by holding the flute needle behind the lens and leaving the side opening half open (just enough that the eye remains normotensive). Leave approximately 5 mL of gas in the syringe. Now stop the gas insufflation, and remove both instrument trocar cannulas. Before removing the infusion cannula, check whether the eye is hypotensive. In this case, inject gas to achieve normotension and then remove the infusion cannula.

Silicone Oil Tamponade (Figs. 4.32 and 4.33)

Silicone oil is an excellent temporary tamponade but a very bad permanent tamponade. It causes high IOP and emulsifies and the final result is an optic atrophy. Silicone oil should be avoided in fresh and primary detachments. Silicone oil is indicated in recurrent detachments, in complicated PVR detachments, and in diabetic tractive detachments. But even in these cases, try to remove the silicone oil after 3 months.

Silicone oil tamponades can be used with 23-gauge and 25-gauge technology. It is straightforward to use 1000 csts and 5000 csts silicone oil. You can inject the oil

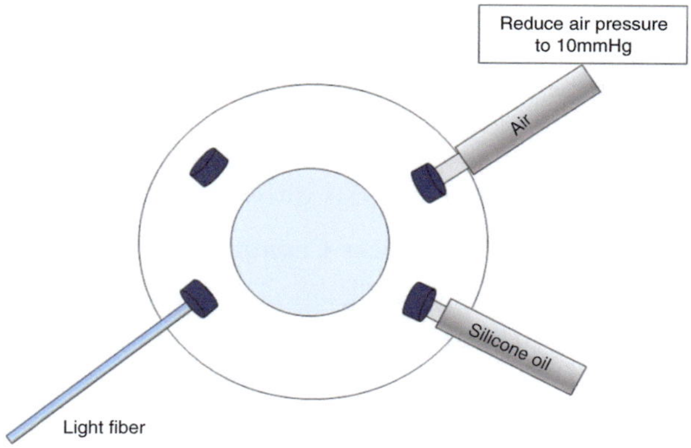

Fig. 4.32 Setup for silicone oil injection **without** chandelier light. **Remark**: Reduce the air pressure to 10 mmHg when injecting silicone oil

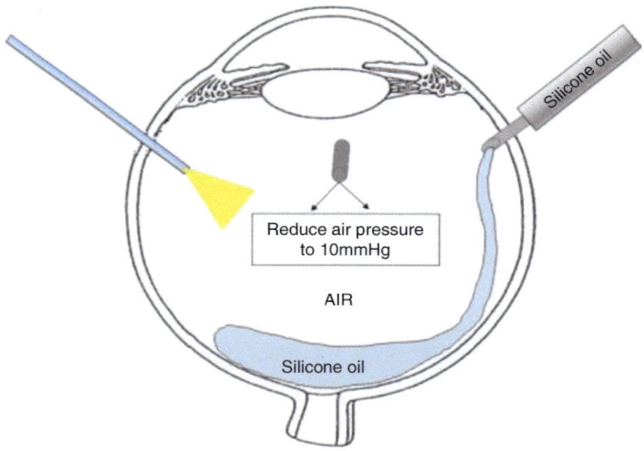

Fig. 4.33 If you use no chandelier light, then reduce the air pressure to 10 mmHg when injecting silicone oil

into a water-filled or an air-filled eye. But an injection into a water-filled eye is difficult because the two liquids are difficult to distinguish. We, therefore, recommend the exchange of air against silicone oil for most routine cases.

The Surgery: Exchange of Air Against Silicone Oil

The infusion line must remain in place because the air streaming in keeps the eye normotensive. We use a silicone oil 25-gauge metal cannula (Alcon) which works for all types of silicone oils. The oil falls from the anterior onto the posterior pole, i.e., the eye is filled from the back to the front with oil. At the same time, you must drain the air with a backflush instrument from a trocar. When the last bubble disappears behind the lens, stop the infusion of air and remove the residual air bubble. Then inject so much silicone oil until the globe is hypo- till normotensive. During this procedure, check for a positive venous pulse.

Perform a fluid × air exchange. Then reduce the infusion pressure of air to 10 mmHg. Then inject the oil. When the silicone oil almost reached the lens, stop the injection, exchange the light pipe against a backflush cannula, continue injection, and remove the residual air.

The sclerotomies should be sutured, because otherwise silicone oil can flow under the conjunctiva.

1000 csts or 5000 csts silicone oil: 5000 csts induces less IOP increase and less emulsification than 1000 csts. If you plan a long silicone oil tamponade (longer than 6 months), then use 5000 csts silicone oil. If you plan a short duration (shorter than 6 months), then use 1000 csts silicone oil.

13. **Removal of the Trocar Cannulas**

It is useful to remove the trocars in the following order: first the instrument trocars, then the chandelier light, and finally the infusion cannula. The infusion cannula remains in place until the end to avoid hypotension when removing the trocars. The infusion should therefore remain open until removal of the infusion cannulas.

To remove the trocars, pull out the trocar with the trocar forceps, and then press the edges of the sclerotomy together with a forceps, and massage the sclerotomy with a cotton swab. Lastly the infusion cannula is removed. Before you do this, check the intraocular pressure manually. If it is hypotensive, refill the eye with gas, until the eye is normotensive. Finally, the infusion cannula with running infusion (BSS, air or oil) is removed. The sclerotomies are usually not sutured. Exceptions are silicone oil tamponades, because the oil may cause subconjunctival cysts.

A major advantage of not suturing a gas-filled eye is that the eyes are rarely hypertensive, as the expanding gas can escape postoperatively through the non-sutured sclerotomies. If you observe uveal tissue or even a vitreous prolapse out of the sclerotomy, you should remove it with the vitreous cutter because otherwise there is a possible wicking and endophthalmitis risk. If the sclerotomy is still leaking, it should be closed with a suture. The sclerotomy should be covered by conjunctiva; otherwise it is recommended that the sclerotomy be sutured.

Surgical Pearls No. 43
<u>Sclerotomy:</u>

1. For beginners, we recommend opening the conjunctiva in the area of the sclerotomies in order to recognize the sclerotomies clearly. This is particularly important if you want to suture the sclerotomy at the end of the procedure.
2. In the case of doubt, suture the sclerotomy. The potential disadvantages of a leaking sclerotomy outweigh the discomfort of a single suture.

14. **Sclerotomy Sutures**

A suture is sometimes necessary in 23-gauge and seldom necessary in 27-gauge. In 23-gauge a suture is necessary in myopic eyes and after silicone oil removals. We suture 23-gauge, 25-gauge, and 27-gauge sclerotomies with silicone oil tamponade.

A 23-gauge and 25-gauge sclerotomy can be sutured with an 8-0 Vicryl simple interrupted stitch and a 20-gauge sclerotomy with a Vicryl 8-0 cross-stitch. To suture a sclerotomy is harder than you assume. Grasp one edge of the sclerotomy with surgical forceps, move the needle through the sclerotomy edge, and then grasp the opposite edge of the sclerotomy with the forceps and move the needle through the second edge. Test with the swab whether the sclerotomy is closed. If it still leaks, remove the suture and place a new suture.

Surgical Pearls No. 44

Leaking sclerotomies:

1. A leak can be identified by a chemotic conjunctiva above the sclerotomy in a flute-filled eye or by air bubbles in an air-filled eye. If the sclerotomies leak, then place a Vicryl 8-0 simple interrupted stitch on the sclerotomy (Figs. 4.34 and 4.35).
2. These can occur after multiple vitrectomies and a large opening, for example, for silicone oil removal or if multiple sclerotomies have been placed in the same location. It is not uncommon in high myopes with a thin sclera. To close these

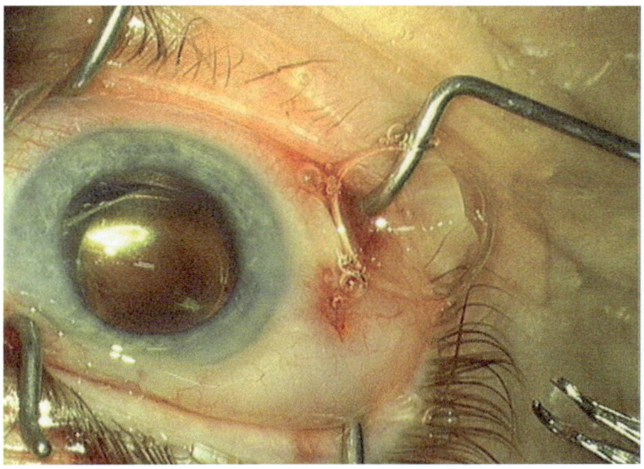

Fig. 4.34 Leakage of air from a 23G sclerotomy in an eye with air tamponade. In this case the sclerotomy should be sutured. This does not happen with 27G

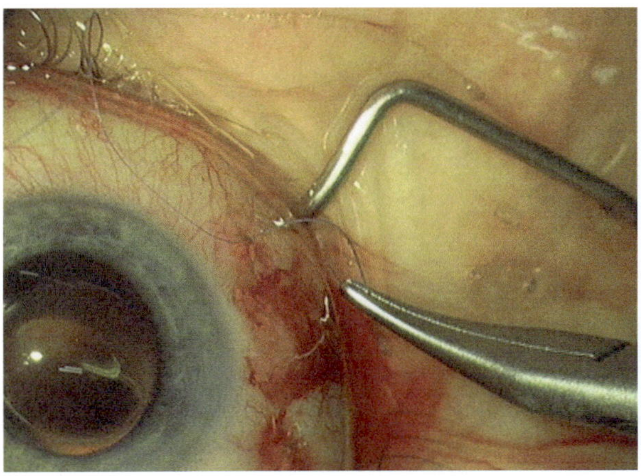

Fig. 4.35 After suturing the sclerotomy with a Vicryl 8-0 simple interrupted stitch, the sclerotomy is closed airtight

large sclerotomies, do not use multiple single sutures (they make it worse) or large sutures (the larger needles may cause additional holes in the sclera). Place a 7-0 or 8-0 Vicryl cross-stitch on the sclerotomy. Stay very superficially within the sclera and do not go "deep." Use a long intrascleral path. Finally, use four instead of three throws for your first knot and ask the scrub nurse to close the infusion temporarily while you tighten the knot.

Reference

1. Lemley CA, Han DP. An age-based method for planning sclerotomy placement during paediatric vitrectomy: a 12-year experience. Trans Am Ophthalmol Soc. 2007;105:86–9.

Part IV
Silicone Oil Injection and Removal

Chapter 5
Silicone Oil Tamponade

Extras: Videos 5.1 and 5.2.

Silicone oil is an excellent temporary tamponade but a very bad permanent tamponade. It causes high IOP and emulsifies and the final result is an optic atrophy. Silicone oil should be avoided in fresh and primary detachments. Silicone oil is indicated in recurrent detachments, in complicated PVR detachments, in diabetic tractive detachments, and in traumatic detachments. But even in these cases, try to remove the silicone oil after 3 months.

Silicone oil tamponades can be used with 23-gauge and 25-gauge technology. It is straightforward to use 1000–5000 csts silicone oil. You can inject the oil into a BSS-filled or an air-filled eye. But an injection into a BSS-filled eye is difficult because the two liquids are difficult to distinguish. We, therefore, recommend the exchange of air against silicone oil for most routine cases.

The infusion line must remain in place because the air streaming in keeps the eye normotensive. We use a 25-gauge metal cannula (Alcon) which works for all types of silicone oils. The oil falls from the anterior onto the posterior pole, i.e., the eye is filled from the back to the front with oil. At the same time, you must release air with a backflush instrument from a trocar. When the last bubble disappears behind the lens, stop the infusion of air and remove the residual air bubble. Then inject so much silicone oil until the globe is normotensive. During this procedure, check for a positive venous pulse.

We use predominantly 1000–1300 csts silicone oil. Earlier on, we used 5000 csts silicone oil but we switched almost completely to 1000/1300 csts silicone oil. We reserve 5000 csts silicone oil for cases which require silicone oil for a long time such as recurrent detachments or hypotony eyes. Apart from these rare cases, we use

---

Electronic Supplementary Material The online version of this chapter (https://doi.org/10.1007/978-3-319-89677-9_5) contains supplementary material, which is available to authorized users.

U. Spandau, H. Heimann, *Practical Handbook for Small-Gauge Vitrectomy*,
https://doi.org/10.1007/978-3-319-89677-9_5

1000/1300 csts silicone oil for all pathologies. We remove the oil after 6 weeks in detachments and after 3 months in diabetics. Within this time limit there are seldom problems with emulsification.

Duration of Silicone Oil Tamponade

Duration of **light** silicone oil tamponade:

Retinal detachment: 6 weeks

Diabetic retinopathy: 2–3 months

Macular hole: 4–6 weeks

Duration of **heavy** silicone oil tamponade:

Inferior detachment: 6 weeks

Macular hole: 4–6 weeks

5.1 Silicone Oil Tamponade

5.1.1 Introduction

The surgical method of choice regarding silicone oil exchange is the injection of silicone oil into an air-filled eye. This applies for light and heavy silicone oil. The injection of silicone oil into a PFCL-filled eye is also possible but technically more difficult. This applies for light and heavy silicone oil. Also heavy silicone oil (Densiron 68) can be exchanged with PFCL. The risk that heavy silicone oil and PFCL will blend during the short exchange time is low and both fluid phases can be well distinguished.

The 5.1 shows the location of the fluids in the vitreous chamber during an air x silicone oil exchange. Air is lighter than silicone oil. During surgery, the silicone oil is injected into the air-filled vitreous cavity. Depending on the amount of injected oil, more or less water will be localized at the inferior pole after surgery.

Regarding surgery: For injection of all types of silicone oil, we use the 23G and 25G cannula (Alcon) (Fig. 5.1). For injection in 27G we use the 27G metal cannula (Medilens). Silicone oil injection is easy with chandelier light and a bit tricky without chandelier light. With chandelier light the intraocular air is released with an extrusion cannula. See Sect. 5.2. Without chandelier light the air pressure must be reduced to 10 mmHg to avoid intraocular high pressure. See Sect. 5.3.

Intraoperatively	Postoperatively	
Air	Silicone oil	Vitreous cavity
Silicone oil	Water	

Diagram 5.1 Diagram of the location of liquids during an air × silicone oil exchange

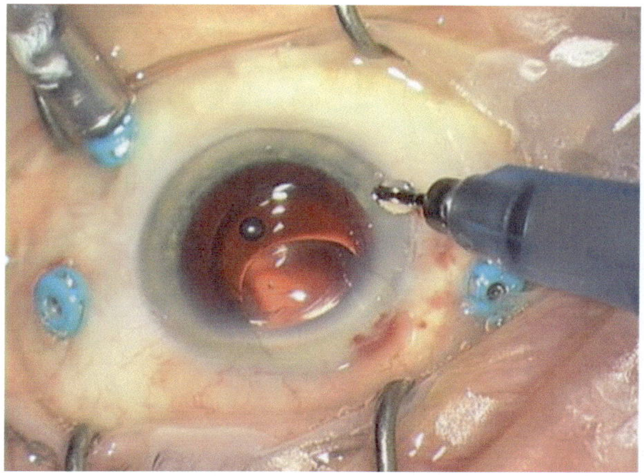

Fig. 5.1 We use a metal cannula (23G, 25G) for silicone oil and Densiron 68 injection (Alcon)

5.2 Silicone Oil Tamponade with Chandelier Light (Under BIOM View)

Instruments

23G or 25G metal cannula (Alcon)

The Surgery Step-by-Step

1. Prepare anterior chamber.
2. Fluid against air exchange.
3. Injection of silicone oil.

The Surgery Step-by-Step

1. Prepare anterior chamber.

Before you perform a fluid × air exchange, prepare the anterior chamber, stabilize the anterior chamber, perform an iridectomy, and inject methylcellulose if necessary (Fig. 5.2).

- 6 o'clock iridectomy for light silicone oils: If aphakia or zonular lysis is present, create an Ando iridectomy (6 o'clock) to prevent an increase in intraocular pressure. An Ando iridectomy prevents a secondary angle closure, because the aqueous can flow through the iridectomy at 6 o'clock into the anterior chamber and press the oil bubble back into the vitreous cavity. Work bimanually: Draw the pupillary edge at 6 o'clock with an intravitreal forceps. Place the vitreous cutter (low cut rate, about 200 cuts/min) with the opening forward behind the iris at 6 o'clock, aspirate the iris, and then cut a hole.

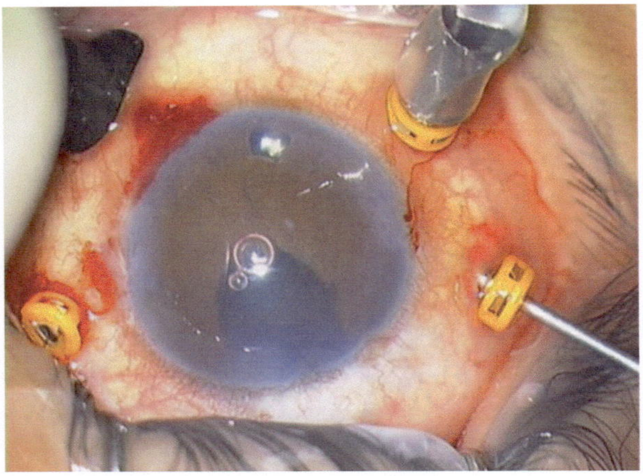

Fig. 5.2 A basal iridectomy. Place the vitreous cutter behind the iris and create an iridectomy with approximately 100 cuts/min. If the pupil is dilated, then stretch the pupil at 6 o'clock with a forceps

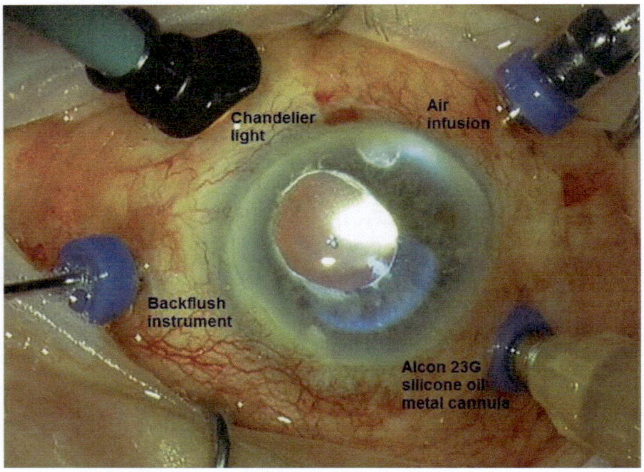

Fig. 5.3 Silicone oil injection **under** view to retina. Note that a chandelier light is required

- 12 o'clock iridectomy for heavy silicone oils: Densiron 68® (Geuder) is a heavy silicone oil and will tamponade the inferior retina. If an iridectomy is needed, it must be performed at 12 o'clock. Perform the iridectomy optimally in a perfluorocarbon liquid (PFCL) or water-filled eye, i.e., before silicone oil injection.
- Methylcellulose in anterior chamber: If a large zonular lysis is present, inject now methyl cellulose into the anterior chamber; it can be left there postoperatively. It holds the anterior chamber silicone oil free. There will be only a slight postoperative rise of IOP.

2. **Fluid against air exchange**.
3. **Injection of silicone oil**.

The infusion line must remain in place during the complete surgery because the air streaming in keeps the eye normotensive (Figs. 5.3–5.5). Attach a silicone oil 27-gauge metal cannula (Medilens) or a metal cannula (Alcon, all gauges) to a silicone oil syringe. The oil falls from the anterior onto the posterior pole, i.e., the eye

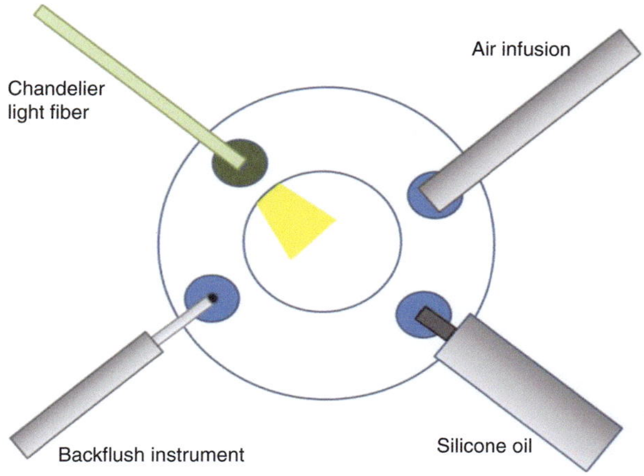

Fig. 5.4 Setup for oil injection **with** chandelier light

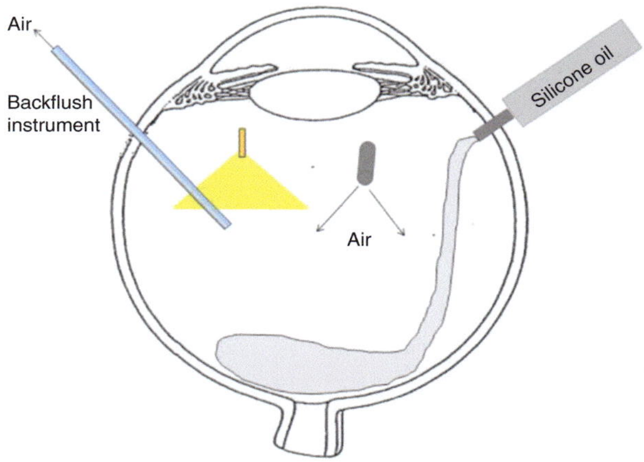

Fig. 5.5 You work bimanual in order to inject the silicone oil under view to retina

is filled from the back to the front. At the same time the surgeon must release the air with a backflush instrument from a trocar. When the last air bubble disappears behind the lens, stop the air infusion and remove the residual air bubble. Then inject silicone oil until the globe is hypo- to normotensive. During this procedure, check for a positive venous pulse. If the globe is hypertensive, then release oil by removing a valve or by simply cutting the infusion line.

5.3 Silicone Oil Tamponade Without Chandelier Light

Reduce the air pressure to 10 mmHg (Figs. 5.6 and 5.7). Inject the silicone oil. The second hand holds the light pipe. When the posterior segment is 90% filled with silicone oil, stop the injection. Flick out the BIOM, place an extrusion cannula behind the lens, and inject the final 10% silicone oil. Wait until the last air bubble disappears behind the lens.

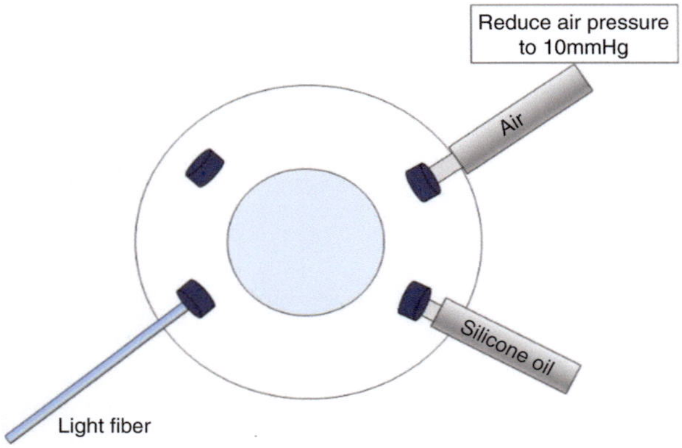

Fig. 5.6 Setup for silicone oil injection **without** chandelier light. **Remark**: Reduce the air pressure to 10 mmHg when injecting silicone oil

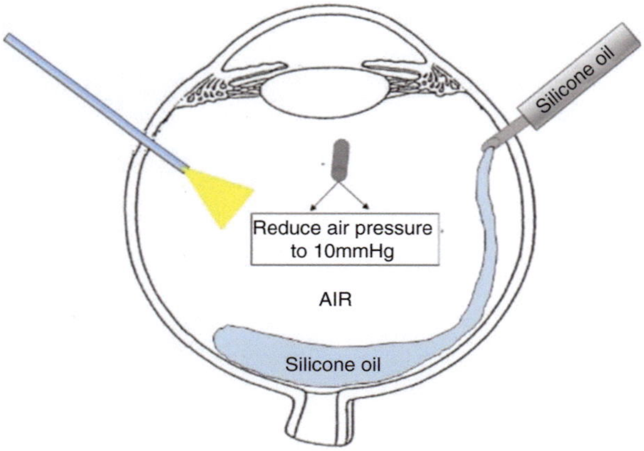

Fig. 5.7 If you use no chandelier light, then reduce the air pressure to 10 mmHg when injecting silicone oil

5.4 PFCL Against Silicone Oil Exchange (with DORC Infusion Line)

This situation is very different than the situation explained above. Why? The silicone oil is injected through the infusion line into the eye.

Surgery:

Instrument (Figs. 5.8 and 5.9)

1. 23G or 25G DORC infusion line with plastic cannula

Remark: An infusion line with metal cannula (Alcon) does not work.

The surgeon must work with the BIOM in order to remove the PFCL when injecting the silicone oil. There is only one method to inject the silicone oil:

Disconnect the infusion line from the BSS infusion and connect the infusion line to the silicone oil syringe. It is important to use a DORC infusion line (Fig. 5.9). An Alcon infusion line may fall off when injecting silicone oil (Fig. 5.8). Use instead a

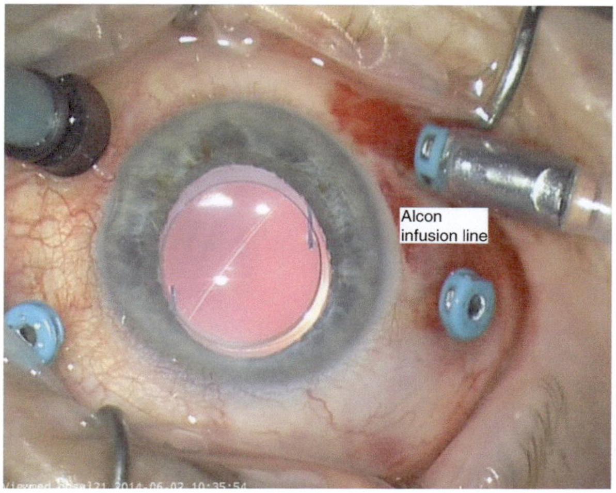

Fig. 5.8 PFCL × silicone oil exchange. An Alcon infusion line cannot be used for injection of silicone oil because the infusion cannula detaches

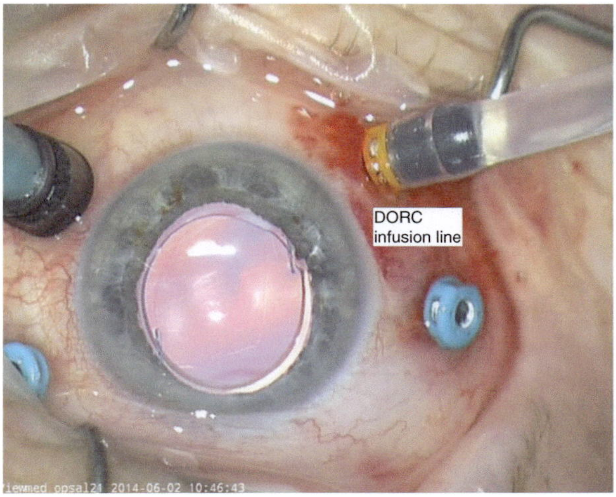

Fig. 5.9 PFCL × silicone oil exchange. Use instead a DORC infusion line with plastic cannula (not high-infusion line). The silicone oil is injected through the infusion line. The infusion line remains stable under injection of silicone oil

DORC infusion line which has a plastic cannula (Fig. 5.9). This infusion will remain stable in the infusion trocar when injecting silicone oil due to its special shape and different material of the DORC trocar cannula.

A chandelier light is not required. Hold the light probe in one hand and the back-flush instrument in the other hand. Inject the silicone oil with active injection modus into the vitreous cavity. Hold the flute needle in the beginning above the PFCL bubble in order to aspirate the residual water (BSS) (Fig. 5.10). Then hold the flute needle into the PFCL phase (Fig. 5.11). Check the pressure of the eye a few times with an index finger. If the pressure is too high, stop the injection of oil and aspirate more PFCL. If the globe is hard (no venous pulse), remove a valve at once and let excess silicone oil flow out.

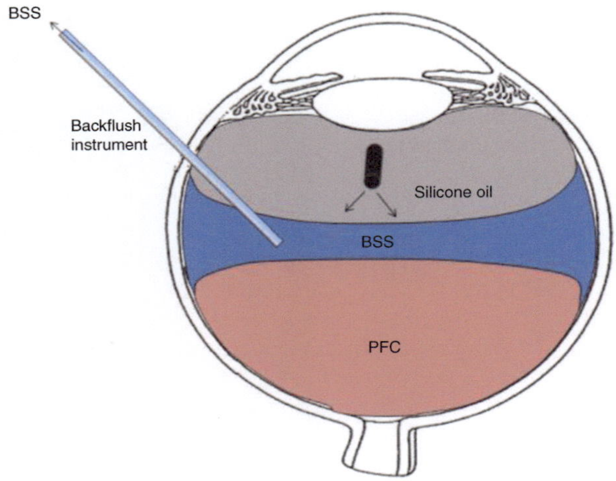

Fig. 5.10 PFCL × silicone oil exchange: Three fluid phases are present, PFCL on the posterior pole, silicone oil in the anterior pole, and BSS in between. Remove first BSS

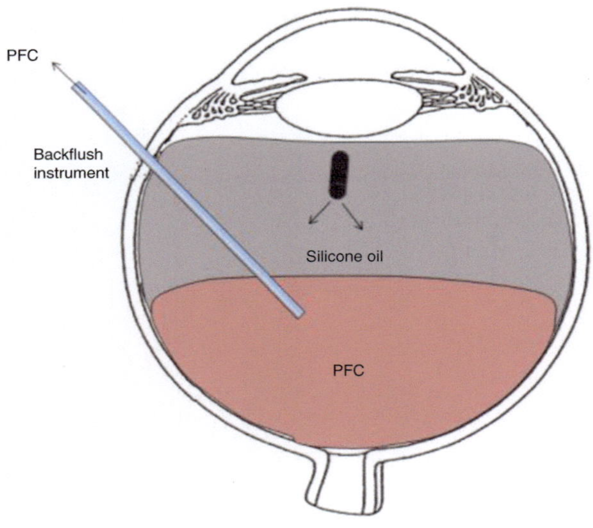

Fig. 5.11 Then remove the PFCL. The silicone oil is injected through the infusion line

If subretinal fluid is present, remove it by holding the tip of the flute needle in the break. Aspirate the subretinal fluid under the pressure of the incoming oil and increase the pressure in the eye by injecting more oil. If the break is fully attached, you can complete the photocoagulation.

At the end of the aspiration, you recognize clearly the PFCL meniscus and also the final PFCL puddle at the posterior pole. The final PFCL bubble may be tricky to remove. It requires sufficient intraocular pressure. This can be achieved by injecting more silicone oil. Or alternatively, compress the globe with one finger in order to increase the intraocular pressure.

FAQ

What is the difference between PFCL × silicone oil and air × silicone oil exchange?

Do not confuse this method with air against silicone oil exchange. If you disconnect the infusion line with air and connect it to the silicone oil syringe, then the eye will collapse. An air-filled eye needs constant air infusion in order not to collapse. This is not the case in a PFCL-filled eye. The eye is stable even if you disconnect the infusion line. In a PFCL × silicone oil exchange, the silicone oil is injected through the infusion line.

I have problems to remove the final PFCL puddle. Can you help?

1. If unsure whether there still is some heavy liquid left behind, pause and wait. The heavy liquid will collect and the interface will be clearly visible after approximately 20 s.
2. Removing the final puddle of heavy liquid is not an easy step. The danger is to aspirate retina into the flute needle at the posterior pole or to damage the optic disc. Either try to remove the final bubble "in one go" or let it collect over the optic disc. Then increase the pressure with the silicone oil injection, and touch the bubble with the opening of the backflush instrument. For small remnant bubbles, indent the eye with your ring finger. This will give you a much better pressure control than the injection of silicone oil with the foot pedal. Aspirate the heavy liquid bubble and immediately cover the opening of your backflush instrument before withdrawing it from the eye, otherwise the heavy liquid bubble will drop back onto the posterior pole.

Chapter 6
Silicone Oil, Densiron 68®, and Oxane Hd® Removal

Extras: Videos 6.1, 6.2, and 6.3.

6.1 Introduction

The removal of silicone oil preserves the late complications such as emulsification and secondary glaucoma and restores the binocular vision in operated patient. The silicone oil can be removed when the retina is completely attached, chorioretinal scars are formed, and the eye is not hypotensive. We remove the silicone oil 1,5–6 months after injection. We remove silicone oils as fast as possible in young patients (4–6 weeks). We are more tolerant with silicone oil in patients over 80 years and trauma eyes.

Traditionally, removal of silicone oil has been the first procedure to be performed independently when you make your first step into the field of vitreoretinal surgery. This is because in most cases, no major intraocular manipulations are performed, but a "proper" three-port setup is required and can be practiced. In addition, most patients will be pseudophakic, so you don't have to fear a lens touch. And finally, this procedure can be rather boring for advanced surgeons, so they are more than willing to let beginners do these cases. The result is that the importance and the difficulty of the procedure are often underestimated. Silicone oil removal is an ideal opportunity to learn and to deal with the trocar cannulas and get a feeling for the posterior segment of the eye. We always perform silicone oil removal with the BIOM because we remove emulsified oil bubbles through a fluid-air exchange and perform additional intraocular manipulations if necessary. The most common postoperative complication after silicone oil is a hypotony. For this reason, we prefer small sclerotomies and end surgery always with an air tamponade.

Electronic Supplementary Material The online version of this chapter (https://doi.org/10.1007/978-3-319-89677-9_6) contains supplementary material, which is available to authorized users.

U. Spandau, H. Heimann, *Practical Handbook for Small-Gauge Vitrectomy*,
https://doi.org/10.1007/978-3-319-89677-9_6

Remember that about 10–20% of patients undergoing silicone oil removal will need additional surgery at a later stage, e.g., for retinal redetachment or recurrent vitreous hemorrhage. The silicone oil removal procedure is an ideal opportunity to deal with any lesser or larger problems during the surgery. Therefore, perform a careful examination preoperatively for appropriate planning of the surgical steps. Exclude first a retinal detachment. Try to identify PVR membranes, which are a lot more difficult to see when silicone oil is still in situ. Be always prepared that additional vitreoretinal manipulations or even a "silicone oil exchange" may be necessary.

Before starting surgery, identify which type of silicone oil has been used. Light silicone oils are easy to remove as they float on water. Heavy silicone oils are rather more difficult to remove because they are heavier than water.

1000 csts silicone oil: We use in almost all cases 1000–1300 csts silicone oil. The duration is 2–6 months. The emulsification is acceptable, and an IOP increase can be treated with antiglaucomatous drops.

5000 csts silicone oil: 5000 csts silicone oil causes less ocular hypertension and less emulsification than 1000 csts silicone oil. It is therefore suitable for a permanent tamponade. We use 5000 csts silicone oil for eyes which require a permanent tamponade such as ocular hypotony, trauma cases, and PVR detachments.

Heavy silicone oil: The heavy silicone oil (Oxane HD, B&L) and Densiron 68 (Fluoron) are a bit tricky to remove, because the silicone oil sticks to the retina and the final oil bubble may fall onto the posterior pole. We remove Densiron 68 6–12 weeks after injection.

Which gauge? 25G and even more 27G are excellent choices for silicone oil removal because the risk of postoperative hypotony is significantly reduced. We use therefore a hybrid system with two 27G trocars and one 25G trocar. The 25G trocar is used for the removal of all types of silicone oil (1000 csts, 5000 csts, and Densiron 68).

Light Silicone Oil (1000, 1300, and 5000 csts) Removal

Silicone oil removal with a modern vitrectomy machine is simple and fast. Insert three trocars. Attach the high infusion (VFE, DORC) to the trocar and actively aspirate the silicone oil (Fig. 6.1). If you want a faster removal, then use the 25G trocar from Alcon (Fig. 6.2). The fastest removal is possible with a special adapter from Alcon (Fig. 6.3). When extracting the silicone oil, make sure that the tip of the aspiration cannula is always located in the silicone oil bubble and not in the BSS phase.

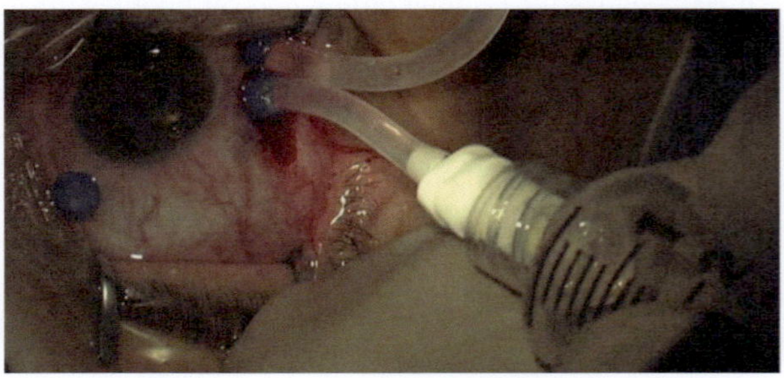

Fig. 6.1 Silicone oil removal with a silicone tube (VFE, DORC)

Fig. 6.2 Silicone oil or Densiron 68 removal with a 25G metal cannula (Alcon)

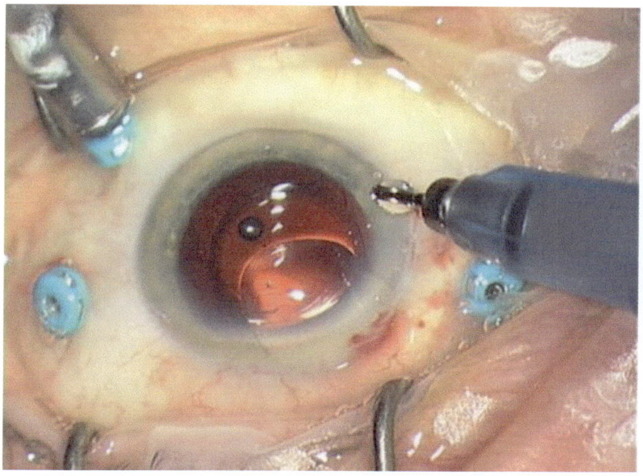

Fig. 6.3 This is the fastest silicone oil extraction cannula available. It fits to all gauges, and the valve is removed prior to use (Alcon)

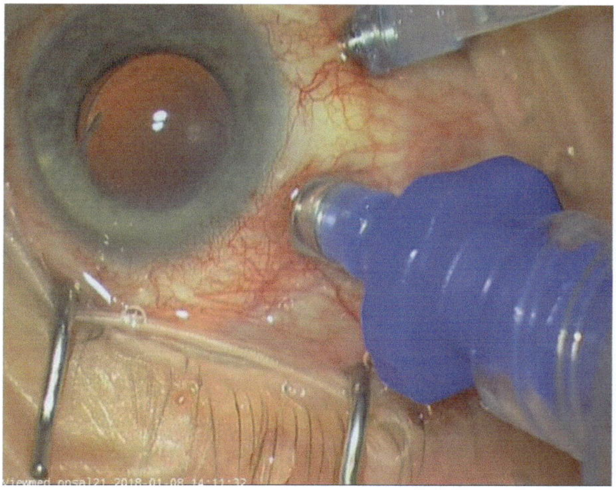

Heavy Silicone Oil (Densiron 68®) Removal

Heavy silicone oil removal cannot be performed with 27G. Heavy silicone oil removal can be performed with 23G and 25G. We prefer 25G because the eye has less hypotony after surgery due to the small sclerotomies. In any case perform a fluid × air exchange at the end. There are two extraction cannulas available:

1. Short 25G metal cannula (Fig. 6.2 Alcon): this cannula can be used with all modern vitrectomy machines (EVA, Constellation, or Stellaris).
2. 23G metal 10 mm cannula (Figs. 6.4 and 6.5, DORC): a good alternative is a longer 23G metal cannula from DORC. Especially recommended for long myopic eyes where you easily loose contact with the oil bubble this cannula is recommended.

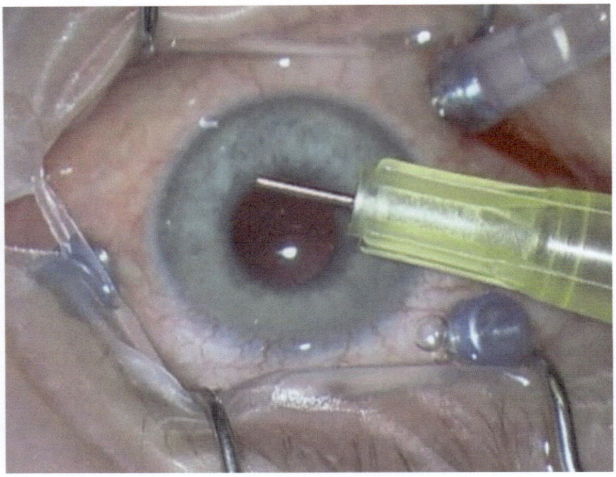

Fig. 6.4 Densiron 68 removal with a long 23G metal cannula (DORC), good for myopic eyes

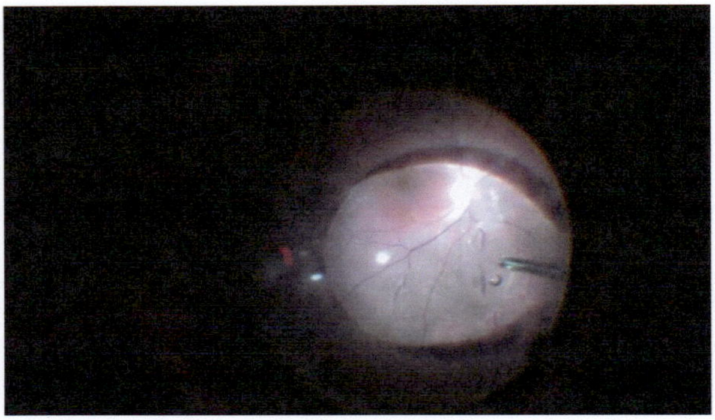

Fig. 6.5 Removal of Densiron 68 with a 10 mm long 23G metal cannula from DORC

6.2 The Surgery Step-by-Step

Instruments

1. Three-port trocar system (two 27G trocars and one 25G trocar), 120D lens
2. Silicone oil 1000 csts: active aspiration with 25 gauge metal cannula (Alcon)
3. Silicone oil 5000cts: active aspiration with 25 gauge metal cannula (Alcon)
4. Oxane Hd® and Densiron 68®: active aspiration with 25 gauge metal cannula (Alcon) OR 23G extrusion cannula (DORC)
5. 25G Charles flute instrument

Possible tamponade

Air or gas

Individual steps

1. **Three-port system**
2. **Active silicone oil removal**
3. **Fluid against air exchange**

4. **Air against fluid exchange**
5. **Flush anterior chamber with BSS**
6. **Internal search for retinal breaks**
7. **Air tamponade**
8. **Removal of trocars**
1. **Three-port system**
2. **Active silicone oil removal**

Insert the 25G metal cannula into the 25G trocar and aspirate the silicone oil. In the beginning of the procedure, the infusion line is often clogged: the reason of the clogged infusion line is silicone oil within the infusion because you compress the globe with the silicone oil cannula. Countermeasures are as follows: (1) Do not compress the globe during silicone oil removal. You will otherwise press the silicone oil into the infusion line. (2) Increase the IOP to 40–50 mmHg until the BSS comes. Then reduce back to 25 mmHg.

Remark for heavy silicone oil (Densiron 68 or Oxane) removal:

Remove the silicone oil bubble as one would with conventional silicone oil, always staying in touch with the bubble with active suction (Fig. 6.4). The residual bubble will stay connected to the short cannula through the "siphoning" effect, will move upward toward the cannula, and can easily be removed this way. Be aware that the cannula has constant contact to the Densiron 68 bubble. If you lose contact, then the residual bubble will fall on the posterior pole. In this case, fasten a 25G Charles flute cannula onto the silicone oil syringe and aspirate the residual bubble. Small remnant bubbles at the posterior pole can then be collected with the backflush instrument. The removal time is approximately 5 min.

3. **Fluid against air exchange**

Then perform a fluid × air exchange under view of the BIOM. Take the backflush instrument and try to "fish" residual oil from the water surface at the water/air interface (meniscus). In case of 23G, a passive suction is sufficient, but in case of 25G and 27G, an active suction is required. If there is a bigger residual oil bubble, it will be time-consuming to remove it with the flute needle. In this case, attach the backflush instrument to the silicone oil syringe or use a vitreous cutter to aspirate the residual bubble.

4. **Air against fluid exchange**

This maneuver may cause big complications, so be cautious. Hold the backflush cannula behind the lens. DO NOT use active aspiration. After you switched to BSS infusion, the globe will fill slowly with fluid. If scleral folds occur, close the opening of the backflush cannula until the scleral folds disappear and then release the opening again. The water × air exchange should be performed approximately three times.

5. **Flush anterior chamber with BSS**

If you see silicone oil bubbles in the anterior chamber, then flush the anterior chamber with BSS and remove the silicone oil bubbles.

6. **Internal search for retinal breaks**

Subsequently, check for peripheral tears or membranes, treat these pathologies and perform a tamponade if necessary. Perform an internal search for breaks and residual membranes, using endoillumination and indentation with a scleral depressor. Try to identify problems that may cause trouble at a later stage, for example, potential new retinal breaks, epiretinal membranes, or fibrovascular proliferations. These are best dealt with straightaway rather than during a later, potentially unnecessary additional procedure. The internal search will also identify larger remnant silicone oil bubbles that may hide in the vitreous base. If left behind, these larger residual bubbles can be extremely annoying for the patient.

7. **Air tamponade**

In order to prevent a postoperative hypotony, an air tamponade is strongly recommended.

8. **Removal of the trocars**

Remove the trocars as usual. In all cases, we instill a simple air tamponade in order to seal the sclerotomy sites. The air tamponade prevents or reduces the postoperative hypotony.

Surgical Pearls No. 45
A dreaded complication is a retinal and even sometimes choroidal injury from the infusion fluid. This happens in the beginning of an air × BSS exchange: the vitreous cavity is filled with air and you switch back to BSS. If you now aspirate actively with a Charles flute needle within the air phase, you will create an under-pressure, and the infusion fluid will stream with great force into the eye damaging the retina and choroid. In order to avoid this, aspirate only passively. You can control the intraocular pressure on your own by closing the side opening of the Charles flute needle with your index finger.

Surgical Pearls No. 46
Suprachoroidal hemorrhage (SCH). If a SCH develops, you should react quickly. First perform a fluid/air exchange, and in case of valveless trocars, close all ports with plugs to increase the intraocular pressure. This should stabilize the situation. Then inject silicone oil and terminate surgery.

Surgical Pearls No. 47
The removal time is of course much faster with 25G and especially 23G. With 23G the removal time for 1000 csts oil is 1–2 min and for 5000 csts oil 5–7 min. The disadvantage of 25G and especially 23G is the postoperative hypotony. In case of 23G and 25G, you need an air tamponade, and in myopic eyes you even need to suture the sclerotomies. The air tamponade and sutures are not necessary for 27G. It is therefore recommended to use a hybrid system: 27G trocars for infusion and light fiber and a 23G or 25G trocar for oil removal.

Surgical Pearls No. 48
Postoperative hypotony with choroidals occurs often after silicone oil removal. In order to avoid hypotony, take the following precautions:

23G: Close the sclerotomies with a suture and use an air tamponade.

25G: Use an air tamponade; a closure of sclerotomies is not necessary. Exception: Myopia.

27G: No sutures necessary even in myopia; in normal eyes an air tamponade is not required. In myopic eyes, an air tamponade is recommended.

Surgical Pearls No. 49

When removing Densiron 68® with a short cannula, it is important not to lose contact with the bubble before it starts "floating up" toward the cannula. If you lose contact with the bubble and it is too small to be reached with the short cannula, you need to proceed with a backflush cannula (which takes a long time) (Fig. 6.6).

Surgical Pearls No. 50

Passive removal of light silicone oil: This method is time-consuming but avoids strong aspiration, which might lead to a suprachoroidal hemorrhage. Insert three 23-gauge trocars. Remove the valves of both instrument trocar cannulas, open the infusion, and let the oil evacuate passively. The eye must be positioned so that the silicone oil flows in the direction of the open trocar cannulas.

Surgical Pearls No. 51

Always check the anterior chamber for residual oil bubbles. In particular, in cases with secondary glaucoma, it is advisable to flush the chamber angle to remove residual bubbles.

Surgical Pearls No. 52

In pseudophakic patients with an intact posterior capsule, perform a posterior capsulotomy with the vitreous cutter via the pars plana at the end of the procedure. These patients will otherwise almost always develop a thick posterior capsular fibrosis, and a YAG capsulotomy is more difficult in eyes in which the retrolental vitreous has been removed.

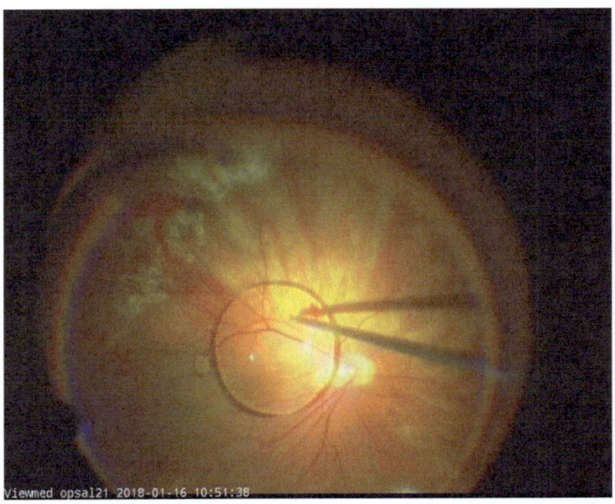

Fig. 6.6 If you lose contact with the Densiron bubble, then attach a 25G extrusion cannula to the silicone oil syringe, and remove the residual bubble

Surgical Pearls No. 53

"Sticky silicone oil" has sometimes been described after removing conventional or heavy silicone oils. This describes patches of silicone oil that are firmly attached to the retina and cannot be removed with suction alone. In our experience, this is most commonly caused by residual vitreous cortex in the area of adhesion, and the best prevention of sticky silicone oil is a complete removal of this layer during the primary surgery. If you are faced with "sticky" silicone oil, try to fill the eye with PFCL. This usually dissolves the sticky patches of oil that can then be removed with conventional suction.

Surgical Pearls No. 54

If a silicone IOL has previously been implanted, small remnant silicone oil bubbles can have remained stuck on the posterior IOL surface. They may cause severe visual disturbances if the center is affected. It may be difficult and sometimes impossible to remove these remnant bubbles. Again, prevention is better in such cases – never use a silicone IOL in cases of combined phaco and vitrectomy or cases that have a higher risk for retinal problems. If faced with such residual bubbles, you can try removing them by soaking a small piece of gauze or a cotton bud in heavy liquid and then wiping the posterior IOL surface with this solution. However, if you are unable to remove the remnant bubbles this way, it may be necessary to exchange the IOL. It is, therefore, best to know if a silicone IOL has previously been implanted. If, in addition, you know the optical power of the previously implanted silicone IOL, one can plan for an IOL exchange if needed, thus avoiding additional surgery at a later stage.

Part V
Macular Peeling

Chapter 7
Vitrectomy for Macular Peeling

Extras: Videos 7.1, 7.2, 7.3, 7.4, 7.5, 7.6, 7.7, and 7.8.

7.1 Introduction

A vitrectomy of a pseudophakic eye with a macular pucker is an ideal beginner eye. A combined phaco/vitrectomy is advisable in all patients above 60 years. Ideally the (non-acute) vitrectomy should be performed in a pseudophakic eye, i.e., the cataract surgery should be scheduled before the vitrectomy.

The first difficult surgical step (for a beginner) is the induction of a PVD. In almost all cases of macular puckers, a PVD is present. The contrary is the case in macular holes; here a PVD is seldom present. We therefore recommend to start with macular puckers and if you feel safe to proceed with macular holes.

7.1.1 Visualization

Before you start with the peeling, you need to change to a higher-resolution lens. You may take a macular lens (60D) or a plano-concave contact lens (DORC, 1284. DD), which is placed with contact gel on the cornea (Fig. 7.1).

Electronic Supplementary Material The online version of this chapter (https://doi.org/10.1007/978-3-319-89677-9_7) contains supplementary material, which is available to authorized users.

U. Spandau, H. Heimann, *Practical Handbook for Small-Gauge Vitrectomy*,
https://doi.org/10.1007/978-3-319-89677-9_7

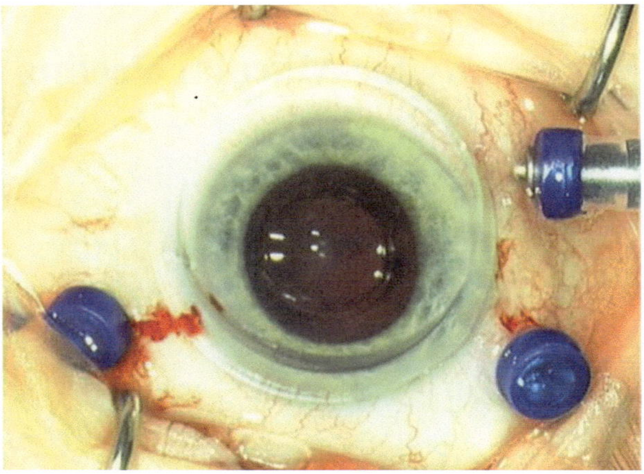

Fig. 7.1 A plano-concave contact lens has been placed on the cornea. DORC: 1284.DD

7.1.2 *Caution*

1. If you work with a contact lens, you only have a small visual field. And the risk of ramming an instrument into the retina is pretty high. Insert, therefore, an instrument only under minimal zoom.
2. The eye is a sphere. Follow during peeling the spherical shape of the eye, i.e., move the forceps obliquely upward. If you move the forceps at the posterior pole horizontally, you will ram the instrument into the retina.

7.1.3 *Peeling and Staining*

The next difficult step for a beginner is the peeling itself which is easier in membranes and more difficult for macular holes. The best case for a beginner is a thick macular pucker with uplifted edges. If you feel safe with peeling of puckers, then proceed with macular holes. The appropriate dye for macular puckers is trypan blue, and the appropriate dye for macular holes are Brilliant Blue G. Today a combined dye with trypan blue and Brilliant Blue G (Membrane Dual®, DORC) is available for staining both an epiretinal membrane and the ILM.

For peeling, only two instruments are required: a good forceps and a retinal scraper (27G retrobulbar cannula, Atkinson, Beaver-Visitec). Alternative scrapers are the Tano diamond duster and the loop scraper from Alcon (Vinesse®). The retinal scraper elevates an edge in membranes and creates a hole in the ILM in macular hole peeling. Many surgeons use only a forceps. One author (US) uses always a retinal scraper, and one author (MP) works only with forceps.

In macular pucker or idiopathic epiretinal membranes (ERM), the epiretinal membrane, which is usually stained with trypan blue, is peeled. Some surgeons recommend a subsequent peeling of the ILM, but there is currently no consensus on this. In a high proportion of cases, the ILM will already be removed together with the ERM. If you wish to peel the ILM after removal of an ERM, then use the dye Membrane Dual® (DORC) from the beginning. It stains the vitreous, the membranes, and the ILM.

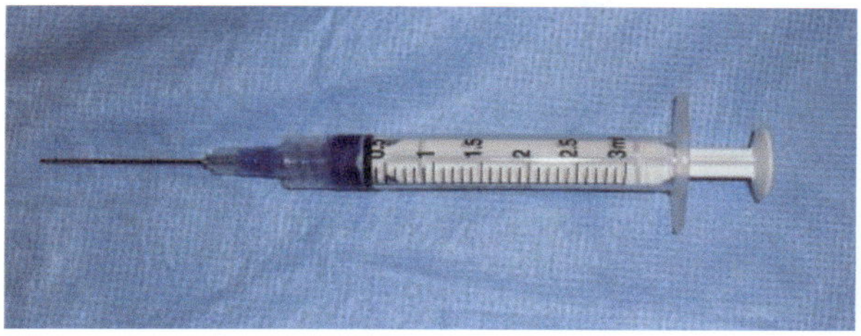

Fig. 7.2 A 3 mL syringe filled with trypan blue and a 23-gauge backflush needle (DORC 1281. A5D06). This syringe size is easy to handle

Staining may become difficult if you use the syringe of the company. If too much force is applied during injection, a sudden jet of dye can be injected into the eye which will obscure the view and is cumbersome to remove. We recommend therefore to change the syringes. We use a regular 3 cc syringe instead, which is predictable in its behavior (Fig. 7.2).

A gas tamponade is standard for macular holes. There is no standard present for membranes. We perform in the most cases an air tamponade to avoid hypotony and inject 0.1 mL triamcinolone if a macular edema is present. We use triamcinolone without benzalkonium chloride which is possibly toxic for the retina (Vitreal S®, Sooft Italy).

Which gauge?

All gauges are possible: 23G, 25G, and 27G. The advantage of 23G is the stiff peeling forceps. The 25G and 27G forceps are softer. For a beginner 23G is recommended.

7.2 Epiretinal Membranes

7.2.1 Introduction

The epiretinal membrane is a perfect beginner eye. The two most important tools for macular peeling are (1) the peeling lens – use a contact lens (e.g., plano-concave contact lens, DORC) or a 60D peeling lens on your BIOM, which suits you best – and (2) the peeling forceps. Test different variants of different companies until you found the forceps that suits you best.

7.2.2 Surgery

Instruments

1. 23G–27G three-port trocar
2. 120D lens, for peeling: 60D lens or plano-concave contact lens
3. Vitreous cutter
4. Backflush instrument
5. 27G ILM forceps (DORC)
6. 27G retrobulbar cannula (Atkinson)

Dye
Membrane: Triamcinolone acetonide, trypan blue.
For injection use a 3 mL syringe with 27-gauge backflush needle.

Tamponade
Possible air tamponade
Individual Steps

1. **23G–27G three-port system**
2. **Core and peripheral vitrectomy**
3. **Staining of the ERM**
4. **Peeling of epiretinal membrane**
5. **Inspection of periphery**
6. **Air tamponade with/without triamcinolone**
7. **Removal of the trocars**

The Surgery Step-by-Step (Figs. 7.3 and 7.4)

1. **23G–27G three-port system**
2. **Core and peripheral vitrectomy**

Insert the trocars. If the patient is older than 60 years, consider a combined phaco/IOL before the vitrectomy.

Perform a core vitrectomy and induce if necessary a PVD. If you are not sure, whether a posterior vitreous detachment is present, stain the vitreous with triamcinolone or trypan blue. If the posterior vitreous detachment has not been successful, you will now recognize the stained premacular vitreous cortex (bursa praemacularis). Continue with a peripheral vitrectomy but you can leave a vitreous skirt; this is in contrast to macular holes.

PVD: If you plan to stain with trypan blue, then use it also for PVD. It makes surgery so much easier. But if you stain the vitreous, you need to restain for the membrane.

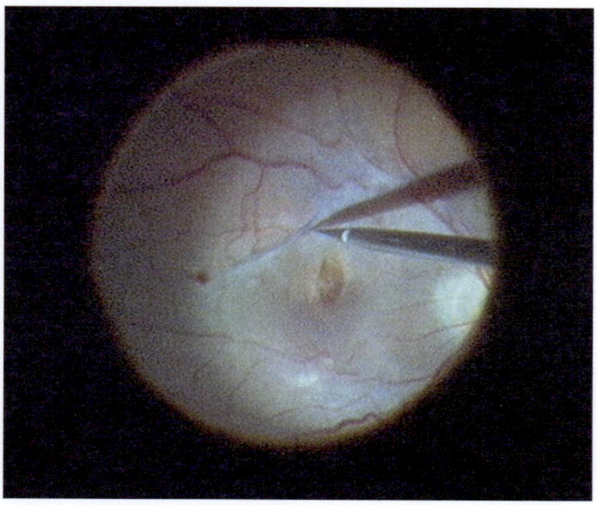

Fig. 7.3 A membrane, which has been stained with trypan blue, is mobilized with a CRVO knife. Use alternatively an Atkinson cannula

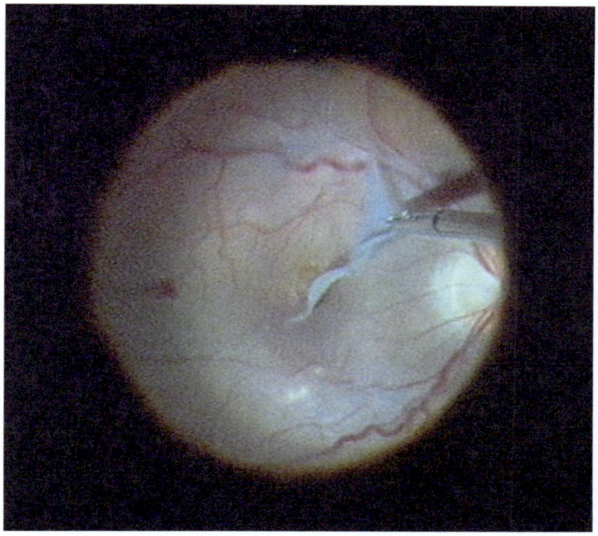

Fig. 7.4 The same membrane is now removed completely with the Eckardt forceps

3. **Staining of the ERM (epiretinal membrane)**

The next step is the staining of the ERM with triamcinolone or trypan blue. Stop the infusion. Then take the syringe with the dye in one hand and eject a few drops of the dye outside the eye in order to avoid blockage of the cannula and injection of air. Then insert the syringe until the tip is placed above the macula and slowly inject a little dye to fall on the macula. After a period of about 15–30 seconds, turn on the infusion and aspirate the dye with a flute needle or a vitreous cutter.

Surgical Pearls No. 55
<u>PVD:</u> If you plan to stain with trypan blue, then use it also for PVD instead of triamcinolone. It makes surgery so much easier. But if you stain the vitreous, you need to restain for the membrane.

4. **Peeling of epiretinal membrane**

Try to mobilize the membrane with a 27G membrane pic or scrape the membrane with the 27G Atkinson scraper (temporal, superior, or inferior to the macula), until a small defect is created. Once an edge is mobilized, it can be grasped with an Eckardt forceps (Figs. 7.3 and 7.4). Pull parallel to the retina until the complete membrane is removed. If the membrane is strongly attached to the retina, do not insist – you might create a retinal defect. If the edges of the membrane tear off and you no longer recognize them, stain again instead and avoid poking around in the retina with the forceps.

Surgical Pearls No. 56
<u>Membrane and dye:</u> Stain the membrane repeatedly, as there are often several membranes present. You can only exclude a residual membrane, if staining was negative. And the better the membrane is made visible, the easier it can be peeled.

Surgical Pearls No. 57
In cases of ERM, you can try a "two in one" peeling of ERM and ILM by starting your peeling more peripheral than usual (e.g., at the major vessel arcades). If you manage to grasp the ILM, continue your peeling toward the center. The ERM should sit on top of the ILM, and both layers can be removed with one peeling.

5. **Inspection of the periphery**
6. **Air tamponade and triamcinolone injection**
7. **Removal of the trocars**

Inspect the periphery for retinal tears and perform laser treatment if necessary. The best laser probe in this case is a combined laser probe with endoillumination. Alternatively, the scrub nurse or your assistant can indent.

Continue with a fluid against air exchange. If a macular edema is present, inject 0.1 mL washed triamcinolone (Vitreal S®, Sooft Italy) and close the case.

7.2.3 Complications

1. Retinal defect. A retinal defect temporal to the macula is less serious. It will appear as a retinal hole in OCT and does not need to be laser treated. A retinal defect in the papillomacular bundle is, however, serious because it causes a deep visual field defect.
2. Retinal vessel defect: A defect of an artery may cause occlusion of the vessel and appear as an arterial branch occlusion with visual field defect.

7.2.4 FAQ

Question: I removed the membrane completely. Do I need to restain?
Answer: Yes, restain. You will be surprised how much membrane or wrinkled ILM is left which you did not recognize before.
In case of epiretinal membrane, do you always remove the ILM at the same time?

No. If the ILM is wrinkled and deforms the macula, I remove it; if it is smoothly attached, I leave it. A recurrence of epiretinal membranes is very rare.

7.3 Macular Holes

7.3.1 Introduction

Macular holes are surgically more demanding than epiretinal membranes because a PVD has to be induced, and the ILM is more difficult to remove. The ILM is a thin layer and more difficult to elevate from the retina compared to a membrane.

We use to perform a combined vitrectomy with PVD, peeling, and gas. We use always 20% SF_6.

If the macular hole is long standing, consider 1000/1300 csts silicone oil. If the patient cannot sleep on the back, consider heavy silicone oil.

We position the patients the first night with face down posture and then 5 days with face down or to the opposite side. For example, if the right eye was operated, the patient shall position with face down or on the left cheek for 5 days.

7.3.2 Surgery

Instruments

1. 23G–27G three-port trocar
2. 120D lens, for peeling: 60D lens or plano-concave contact lens
3. Vitreous cutter
4. Backflush instrument
5. 27G ILM forceps (DORC)
6. Retinal scraper: 27G retrobulbar cannula (Atkinson) OR Tano diamond dusted scraper

Dye

Brilliant Blue G (several companies) or Membrane Dual® (DORC).

For injection use a 3 mL syringe with 27-gauge backflush needle.

Tamponade

20% SF_6, silicone oil (with macular holes in which no postoperative head positioning is possible)

Individual Steps

1. **23G–27G three-port system**
2. **Core vitrectomy**
3. **Induction of PVD**
4. **Staining of ILM**
5. **Peeling of ILM**
6. **Gas tamponade**
7. **Removal of trocars**

The Surgery Step-By-Step (Figs. 7.5, 7.6, 7.7, and 7.8)

1. **23G-27G Three-Port System**
2. **Core Vitrectomy**
3. **PVD**

Insert the trocars. If the patient is older than 60 years, consider a combined phaco/IOL before the vitrectomy.

Perform a core vitrectomy and induce a PVD. Position the vitreous cutter in front of the optic disc, the aspiration port almost touching the optic disc – induce maximal suction. Meanwhile, cortex and posterior hyaloid will be engaged in the aspiration port, and pull the vitreous cutter slowly toward the lens. Perform this maneuver in all directions.

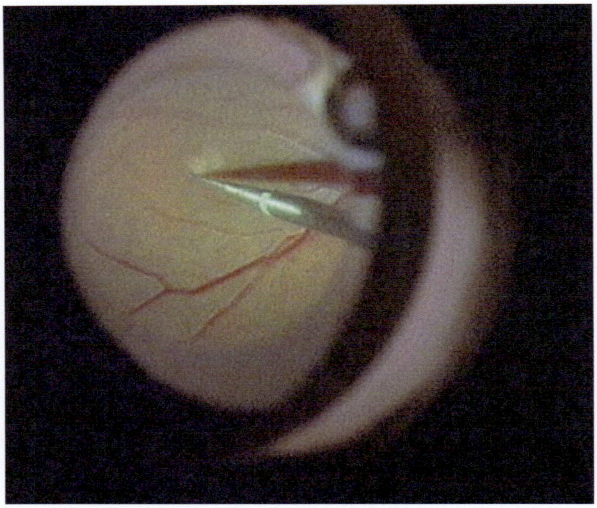

Fig. 7.5 A slight incision of the ILM is performed with a CRVO knife. Alternatively, you can also use a Tano diamond dusted membrane scraper or an Atkinson cannula

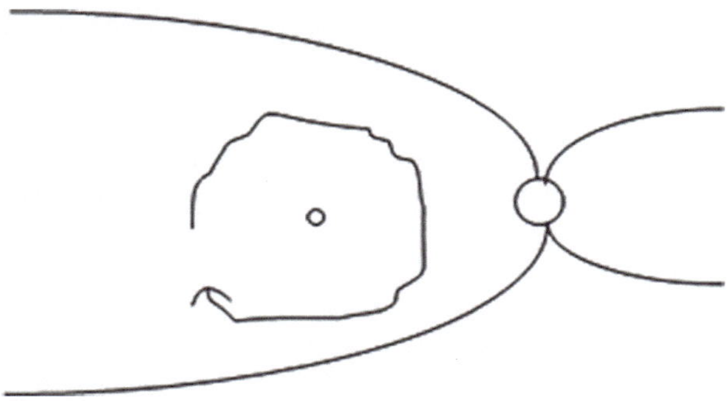

Fig. 7.6 Drawing for peeling maneuver. Start temporal to the macula, continue above or below the macula, and finish finally the circle. Be careful when peeling at the papillomacular bundle

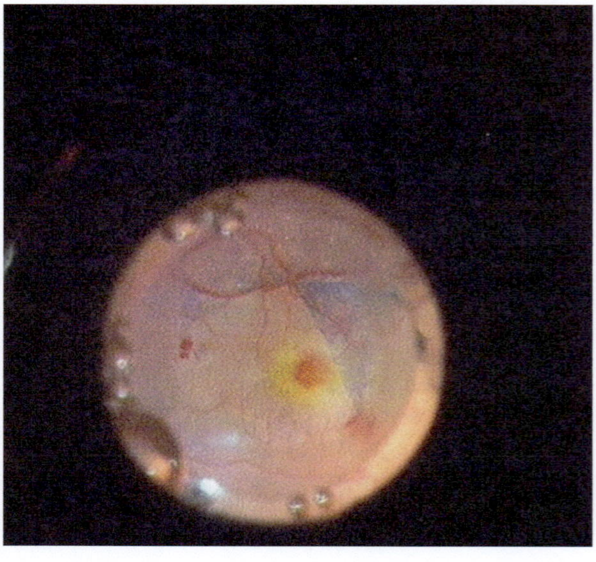

Fig. 7.7 An ILM rhexis. The ILM was stained with Brilliant Blue G. The circular removal of the ILM is comparable with the capsulorhexis. But it should be remembered that, in contrast to the convex capsulorhexis, the ILM rhexis runs concave. If you do not consider this, you can quickly drive the forceps into the retina

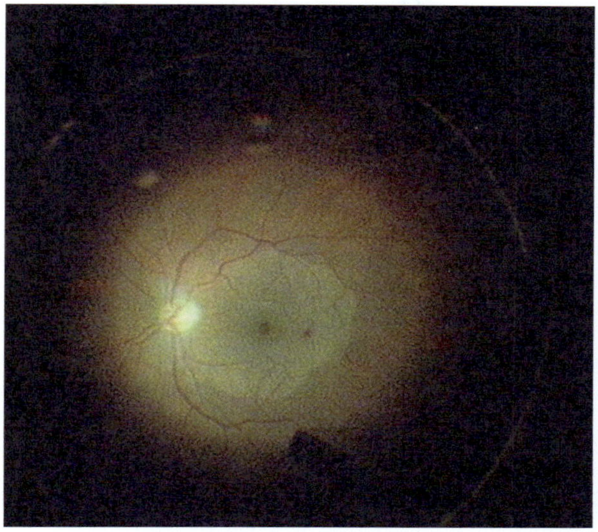

Fig. 7.8 The size of the ILM rhexis should reach approximately to the upper and lower temporal arcade

Surgical Pearls No. 58
PVD: If you plan to stain with Membrane Dual®, then use it also for PVD. It makes surgery so much easier. But if you stain the vitreous, you need to restain for the membrane.

4. **Staining of the ILM**

The internal limiting membrane (ILM) stains with Brilliant Blue G particularly well. The new dyes are heavier than BSS. They can therefore be injected in a BSS-filled vitreous cavity.

Surgical Pearls No. 59
Staining in air-filled eye: This method achieves a much higher concentration of the dye; you need less dye and staining is faster. Perform a water-air exchange and leave a small puddle of water on the central pole. Use a 3 cc syringe with a backflush needle for injection. Inject 2–3 drops of Brilliant Blue G into the puddle, wait 15 s, position the flute tip in the puddle, and remove the dye. Then perform an air-water exchange. The advantage here is the dye acts only in the water puddle, and the surgeon can remove it more quickly than if the dye is distributed throughout the vitreous cavity.

5. **Peeling of ILM**

Before you start with the peeling, you need to change to a higher-resolution lens. You may take a macular lens (60D) or a plano-concave contact lens, which is placed with contact gel on the cornea (Fig. 7.1).

To mobilize the ILM brush the retinal surface with the Tano diamond dusted membrane scraper or scrape it with the 27G Atkinson blunt cannula attached to a backflush hand piece (temporal, superior, or inferior to the macula), until a small defect is created (Fig. 7.5). You can also pinch the ILM with the ILM forceps, but the risk of retinal bleeding is higher with this technique. Grasp the edge with Eckardt forceps and pull the ILM parallel to the retina. Perform a circular rhexis of the ILM

(Figs. 7.6 and 7.7). Always perform the ILM peeling in a circular fashion pulling around and toward the macular hole (just like a capsulorhexis in phaco). Do not just pull the ILM in one sheet across the macular hole. The pathology is that there are usually strong adhesions between the posterior vitreous face and the edge of the macular hole. Therefore, by simply pulling a sheet across, you may enlarge the macular hole. If you do not recognize the edges, stain again. Remove the complete ILM up the vascular arcade (Fig. 7.8).

You (as a beginner) should work very carefully within the papillomacular bundle. You might create irreversible visual field defects. Therefore, you should never start the ILM rhexis in the papillomacular bundle but in an area with a good staining superior, inferior, or temporal to the macula (Fig. 7.6). Small retinal bleedings may occur during peeling. They will cause no harm and vanish within 1 month.

When the removal of the ILM has succeeded, change to the 120D lens, and with the help of scleral indentation, examine the retinal periphery for breaks.

Surgical Pearls No. 60
ILM peeling and dot hemorrhages: Small dot hemorrhages occur only during ILM peeling and do not appear with ERM peeling (Figs. 7.7 and 7.8).

Surgical Pearls No. 61
Peeling with chandelier light: Insert a chandelier light. Assist the dominant hand under peeling, you will be surprised how calm your hand is and without tremor. If you have a hand without tremor, take a Charles flute needle in the non-dominant hand, and aspirate the pieces of membrane or ILM. If you use a vacuum cleaner, you even lift up the edges of the membrane and then remove them with the forceps.

6. **Tamponade for macular hole** (Fig. 7.9)

To carry out the gas tamponade, position the flute tip above the optic disc and then switch to fluid-air exchange. The air streaming in has a different refractive index than water; therefore, the image becomes blurred but more wide-angled. You can focus the image by turning the focus wheel of the BIOM so that the front lens moves up. The image will come into focus again. Since a complete aspiration of BSS is not necessary, avoid an optic disc touch (optic neuropathy). Inject 20% SF_6 into the vitreous cavity and decompress the eye by holding the flute needle in a trocar. Open and close the side opening of the backflush instrument with your index finger depending on the tension of the globe. The intraocular pressure is checked with the index finger of the other hand.

Surgical Pearls No. 62
Backflush instrument: When working with 27G you should perform an active fluid aspiration. Use the backflush instrument with active suction or alternatively the vitrector. Be cautious when coming close to the retina. It is not possible to aspirate the water completely with the vitrector due to the position of the opening.

Surgical Pearls No. 63
Most vitreoretinal clinics use 20% SF_6 as tamponade for macular hole. However, some clinics prefer 15% C_2F_6, 14% C_3F_8, or even 1000 csts silicone oil. Silicone oil is also a good choice for patients who are unable to position themselves in the prone position.

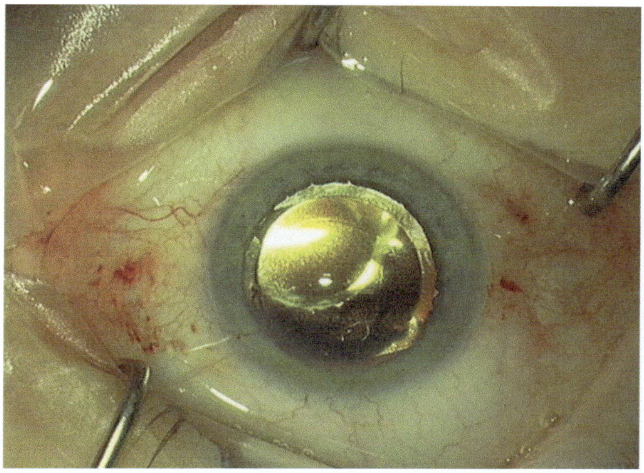

Fig. 7.9 Postoperative picture after combined 25-gauge phaco/vitrectomy secondary to an ERM. The characteristics are excellent sclerotomy closure, little tissue trauma, and subsequent fast postoperative and visual recovery

7. **Removal of the trocars**

   The sclerotomies need not be sutured. The big advantage of not suturing is that a postoperative hypertension due to the expanding gas, though rare, allows the gas to escape through the unsutured sclerotomies.

8. **Postoperative posture**

   We recommend face down when sitting and lying on the opposite cheek for 5 days. Some clinics do not posture their patients and have excellent results. There is unfortunately no randomized study published.

7.3.3 Complications

What complications may happen during peeling?
Retinal defects and even worse a defect of a retinal artery. Do not peel a membrane above a retinal vessel, and always observe the tip of the forceps during peeling (and not the membrane). The posterior pole is concave, and you may ram the forceps into the retina.

What do you do in case of recurrence?

If the macular hole is not closed after 4 weeks, we repeat the gas tamponade with 20% SF_6. If the macular remains open, we use silicone oil (1000 csts or Densiron 68). We achieve with this procedure almost 100% hole closure.

7.3.4 FAQ

Which magnification do you use for peeling?
I use a 60D plano-concave lens from DORC. It provides an excellent magnification and depth feeling. The disadvantage of contact lenses compared to 60D BIOM lenses is the small visual field. Be careful when inserting an instrument.

Which instruments are important for peeling?

A retinal scraper and a forceps. We use the blunt cannula from Atkinson as retinal scraper. It is available in 25G and 27G. It can be used for opening of the ILM and delamination of a membrane. Then we use a 25G or 27G ILM forceps from DORC.

How important is the forceps?

The peeling is very different with the different forceps. Test all available (ILM) forceps, and use the one you are comfortable with.

Is it possible to peel with the 90D or widefield lens?

Yes, it is. But it depends. If it is a membrane with elevated edges, you can use these lenses with a high zoom. But if you are a beginner and if you peel macular holes, then a 60D lens or contact lens is recommended.

How is the follow-up?

We have one regular follow-up after 1 day. After 1 week, we measure only IOP. After 1 month, we perform again a regular follow-up with OCT. In case of persistent open macular hole, we repeat a gas injection with SF_6. Approximately 95% of holes close after one surgery and the residual 5% after the second surgery.

What do you do in case of small holes?

We do not peel the ILM if small holes are present. After PVD we perform a fluid-air exchange, inject gas, and close the case. In our experience, almost all small holes close with this procedure without peeling.

7.4 Macular Peeling with a Cataract Machine

A vitrectomy with a cataract machine is possible. We perform combined phaco/vitrectomies and macular peeling with an Infinity machine and a Centurion machine from Alcon (Figs. 7.10 and 7.11). We used the 23G vitreous cutters which are used for anterior vitrectomy. As a light source, we used an external light source (Photon, Synergetics). In case of a dropped nucleus, you can also use a cataract machine.

<u>Devices</u>

Infinity or Centurion cataract machine
External light source (Fig. 7.12)
Viewing system

<u>Instruments</u>

1. Three 23-gauge trocars
2. 23-gauge infusion line (Fig. 7.13)
3. Light pipe

The irrigation is connected to the infusion line (Fig. 7.13). Insert three trocars. The infusion line is connected to one pars plana trocar (Fig. 7.14). The infusion is set to “Continuous irrigation”. Now you can perform a stable and safe vitrectomy.

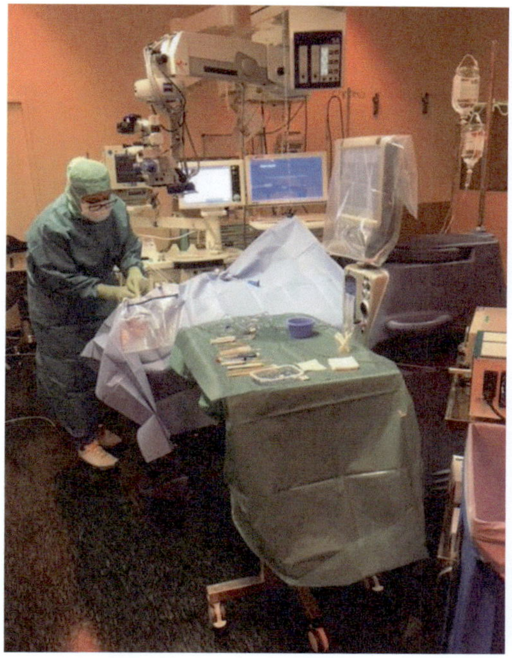

Fig. 7.10 Vitrectomy with an Infinity machine (Alcon). 23G cutter and 2500 cuts/min

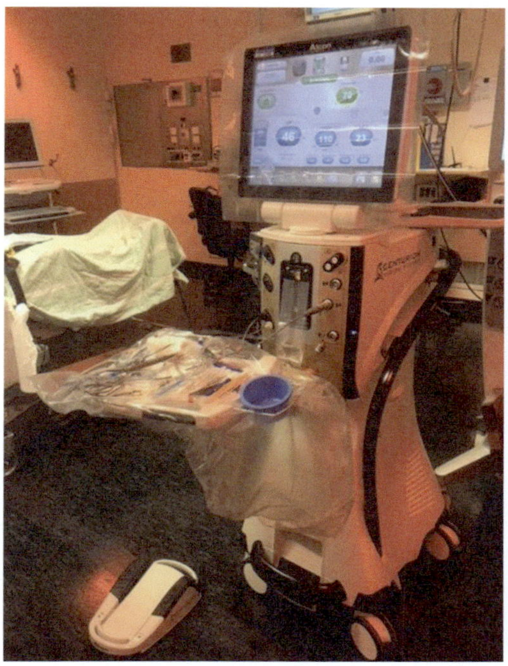

Fig. 7.11 Vitrectomy with a Centurion machine (Alcon). 23G cutter and 4000 cuts/min

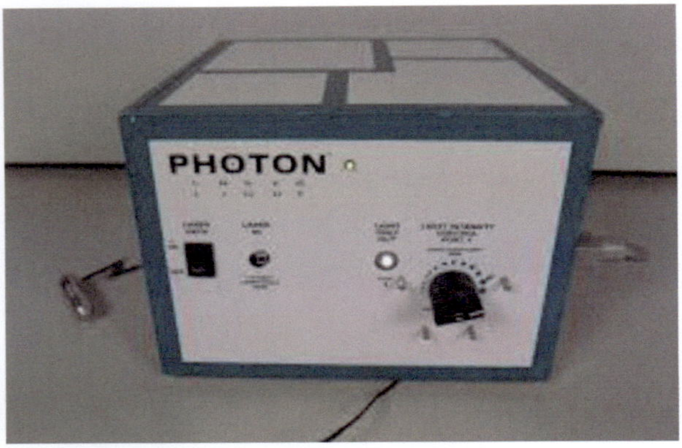

Fig. 7.12 An external light source (Photon from Synergetics, USA) provides light for the light pipe

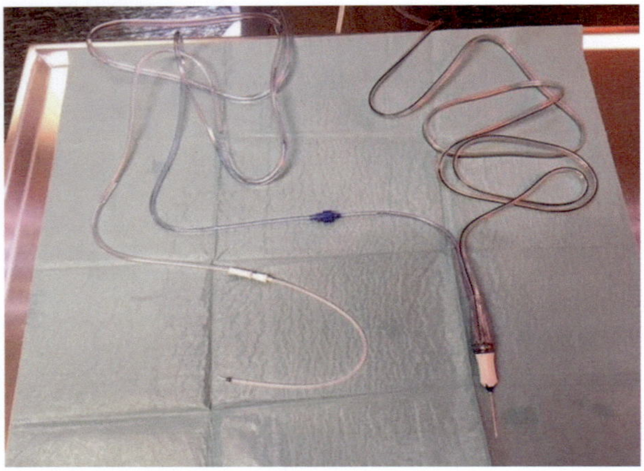

Fig. 7.13 The anterior vitreous cutter for Centurion or Infinity from Alcon. Attach a 23G infusion line (DORC or Alcon) to the irrigation

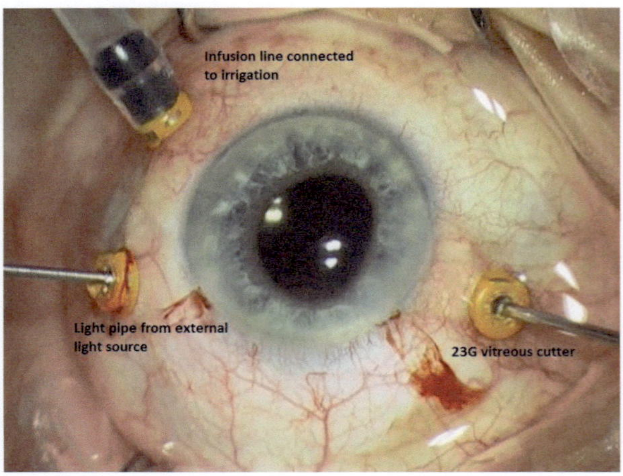

Fig. 7.14 Three 23G trocars are inserted. The vitreous cutter is the regular 23G vitreous cutter for anterior vitrectomy. The light pipe and the external light source must be purchased separately. The irrigation from the cataract machine is connected to a 23G infusion line (DORC, Alcon) and inserted into a trocar

7.5 Conclusion

I am convinced that anterior and posterior segment surgery will fusion in the future. The modern cataract machines have a very powerful vitrectomy function today and have reduced their gauge from 20G to 23G. In case of a dropped nucleus, the cataract surgeon can convert with the same machine to a vitrectomy and remove the nuclear fragments (Fig. 7.15).

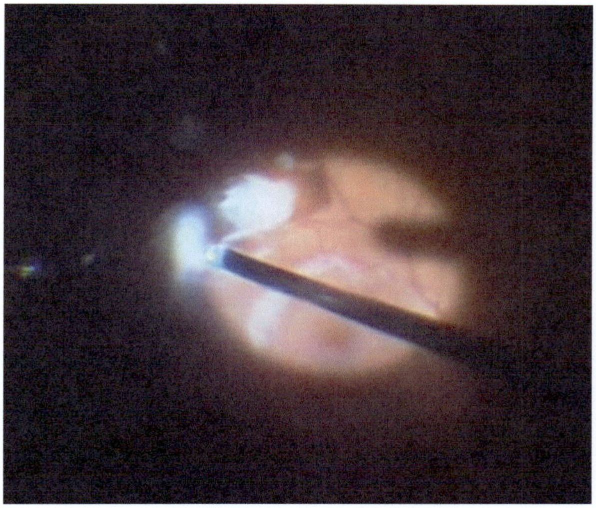

Fig. 7.15 You can also remove a dropped nucleus with a cataract machine and the 23G vitreous cutter. A fragmatome cannot be used with a cataract machine

Part VI
Secondary IOL Implantation

Chapter 8
Dislocated IOL Extraction and Secondary IOL Implantation

Extras: Videos 8.1, 8.2, 8.3, 8.4, and 8.5.

8.1 Introduction

The first part of the surgery is the extraction of the dislocated IOL. In most cases, the IOL is only subluxated because the vitreous body is present. The extraction is simple with serrated jaw forceps. In a few cases when the eye has been vitrectomized, the IOL is luxated to the posterior pole. In this case the extraction is trickier. The second part of the surgery is the IOL implantation. There are three main techniques for secondary IOL implantation.

1. Iris-fixated IOL (Artisan, Verisyse IOL)
2. Scleral fixation of IOL with suture
3. Intrascleral fixation of IOL (Scharioth, Agarwal, Yamane technique)

In the first technique, you remove the IOL with capsular bag and implant an iris-fixated IOL. In the second technique, a three-piece IOL is sutured to the sclera. In the third technique, the haptics are fixated inside the sclera. The first technique is fast; the disadvantage is the large, astigmatism inducing main incision. It is thus important to perform a sclerocorneal main incision. The second technique is time consuming, but it requires only a small main incision. The main disadvantage is that sometimes a lens tilt with a high astigmatism occurs. The third technique avoids this disadvantage because the haptics are fixated inside a scleral tunnel.

These surgeries may well be performed under local anesthesia. We prefer 27gauge instruments because aphakic eyes tend to have a postoperative hypotony.

Electronic Supplementary Material The online version of this chapter (https://doi.org/10.1007/978-3-319-89677-9_8) contains supplementary material, which is available to authorized users.

U. Spandau, H. Heimann, *Practical Handbook for Small-Gauge Vitrectomy*,
https://doi.org/10.1007/978-3-319-89677-9_8

8.2 Secondary Implantation of an Iris-Claw IOL

The benefits of an iris-claw IOL (Artisan) implantation are a short surgical time, a sutureless implantation, an excellent centration without risk of tilting, and a short learning curve (approx. five surgeries). The surgical time is approximately 15–20 min. A redislocation such as in scleral-fixated IOLs does not occur with iris-claw IOLs. The disadvantage is that the IOL is fixated into the iris tissue, and a too traumatic implantation may lead to an inflammation. This postoperative inflammation with cellular proliferation of the IOL is induced by macrophages. This occurs, however, only in the learning curve. If you combine the Artisan implantation with a complete PPV, then a pseudophakodonesis may occur. If the Artisan implantation, however, is only combined with an anterior vitrectomy, then the risk for a pseudophakodonesis is very low.

In addition, sufficient iris tissue is required for implantation, e.g., an implantation in case of aniridia is not possible.

We will demonstrate the implantation of an iris-claw IOL (Verisyse®, Abbott and Artisan®, Opthec) (Fig. 8.1). The iris-claw IOL can be implanted before the pupil or behind the pupil. If you implant the IOL retropupillary, then it has to be done "upside down" (on the back) because the haptics are bent upward.

We will demonstrate the retropupillary method, which is quite easy to learn. We recommend starting with an aphakic eye which underwent an anterior vitrectomy. The pupil should be constricted before surgery. We recommend retrobulbar anesthesia.

There are different A-constants for antepupillar and retropupillar IOL implantations; contact the companies.

The most difficult part of the surgery is the dissection of a scleral tunnel, which is the same as for the SICS technique (modified ECCE). We prefer a scleral tunnel

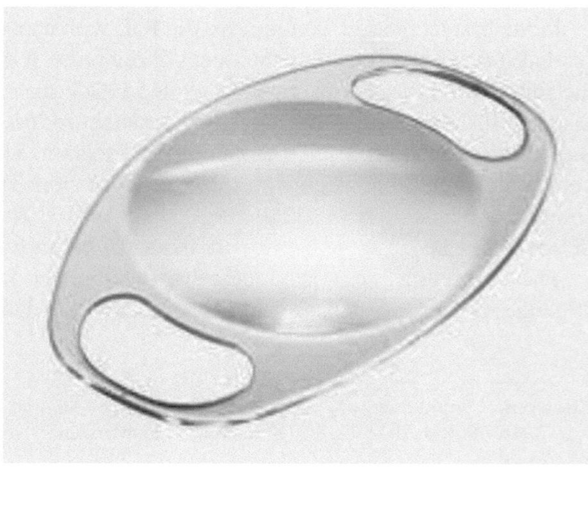

Fig. 8.1 An iris-claw IOL (Artisan®, Ophtec and Verisyse®, AMO)

to a corneal tunnel in order to reduce astigmatism; this tunnel is 6 mm wide. Why? Because the iris-claw IOL is 6 mm wide and because the extracted IOL is also 6 mm wide. What may happen if the tunnel is 8 mm wide? The wider the tunnel, the more you risk a choroidal detachment. In the beginning, we recommend to start with a 6 mm limbal tunnel. If you feel safe with the technique you can continue with a scleral tunnel.

Which gauge? We prefer 27G in order to avoid hypotony after surgery which may occur due to the 6 mm scleral tunnel.

How many trocars? We use usually only two trocars without a viewing system. We perform only an anterior vitrectomy and no core vitrectomy.

8.2.1 Special Instruments for Iris-Claw IOL Implantation

Instruments for Iris-Fixated IOL

The required instruments for the implantation of an iris-fixated IOL can be acquired from companies such as Verisyse®, Abbott and Artisan®, and Opthec:

IOL implantation forceps (Fig. 8.2).

Indication: holds the Artisan (Verisyse IOL) during implantation. A very important instrument.

Enclavation spatula (Fig. 8.2)

Indication: retropupillar fixation of IOL claws in iris tissue. This spatula is thin so that only a little iris tissue is enclavated. Sekundo enclavation spatula, Geuder-32,724.

Caliper (Fig. 8.3)

Indication: marking of main incision and sclerotomy. The main incision for the implantation of an iris-fixated PMMA IOL is 6 mm wide. Caliper by Castroviejo, Geuder 19,135.

Serrated jaw forceps (Fig. 8.4)

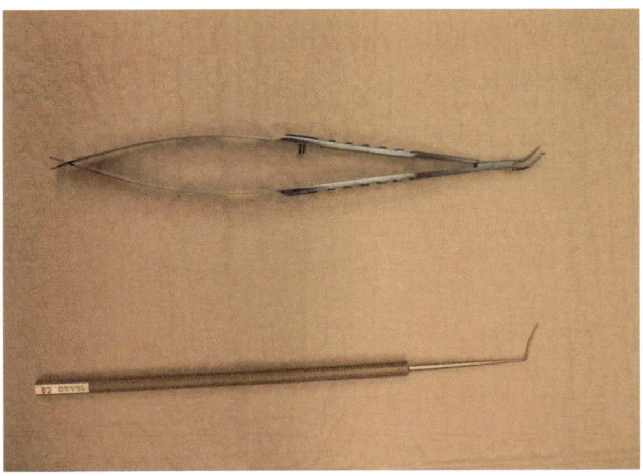

Fig. 8.2 Three instruments are required for the surgery of a subluxated IOL. (1) An IOL implantation forceps (AMO) and (2) an enclavation spatula from Sekundo (Geuder) for implantation of an iris-claw IOL

Fig. 8.3 A caliper to mark the frown incision (Geuder)

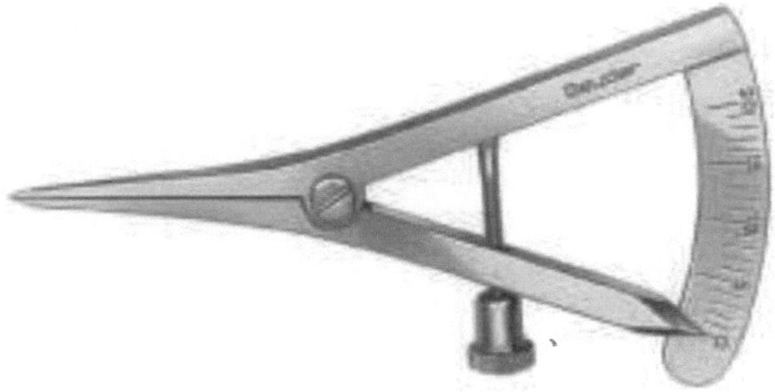

Fig. 8.4 A 23G intravitreal serrated jaw forceps (DORC). Indication: Extraction of the subluxated IOL from the anterior chamber

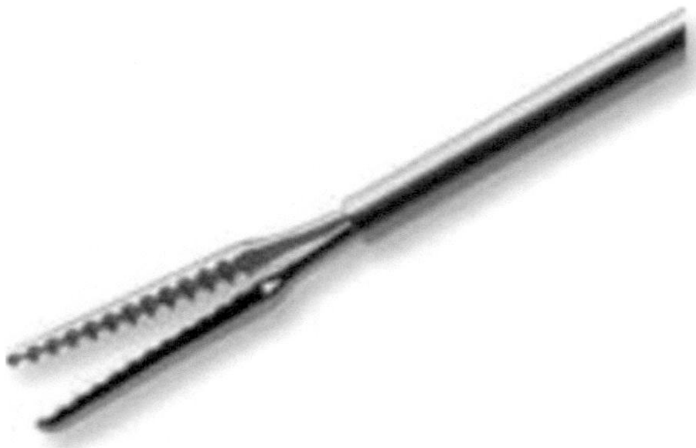

Indication: extraction of IOL with lens capsule. 20G or 23G. DORC. 1286.C06.

Endgripping forceps

Indication: luxation of IOL from posterior pole to anterior chamber. 27G. DORC 1286.WD04 Alternative: A 27G endgripping forceps (DORC).

8.2.2 Iris-Claw IOL Implantation Surgery

8.2.3 Instruments

1. Crescent bevel-up knife
2. 15° knife
3. 2.4 mm tunnel knife
4. Caliper
5. IOL implantation forceps (AMO)
6. Enclavation spatula
7. 20G or 23G Serrated jaw forceps
8. In case of IOL luxation: 27G ILM forceps

8.2.4 Material

Acetylcholine (Miochol).

Iris claw IOL (Artisan®, Verisyse®).

Maybe: Triamcinolone.

Individual Steps

1. **27G three-port trocar system**
2. **Paracentesis at 3–9 o'clock**
3. **Limbal main incision/scleral frown incision**
4. **Extraction of an anterior dislocated IOL**
5. **Extraction of a posterior dislocated IOL**
6. **Anterior vitrectomy**
7. **Injection of Miochol**
8. **Implantation of iris-fixated IOL (upside down)**
9. **Closure of the frown incision and conjunctiva**

8.2.5 The Surgery Step-by-Step (*Figs. 8.5–8.24*)

1. **25G or 27G three-port trocar system**
2. **Paracentesis at 3–9 o'clock**
3. **Limbal main incision/Scleral frown incision**

Insert two trocars at the temporal side. If you want to perform a core vitrectomy, then insert a third trocar and work with a viewing system (BIOM). Continue with a short paracentesis at 3 o'clock and 9 o'clock. The paracentesis is short so that you can reach the peripheral iris with the enclavation spatula.

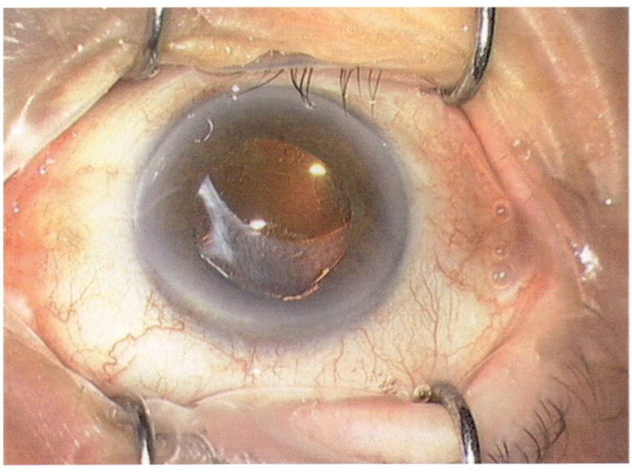

Fig. 8.5 An anterior dislocated bag-IOL complex secondary to zonular lysis

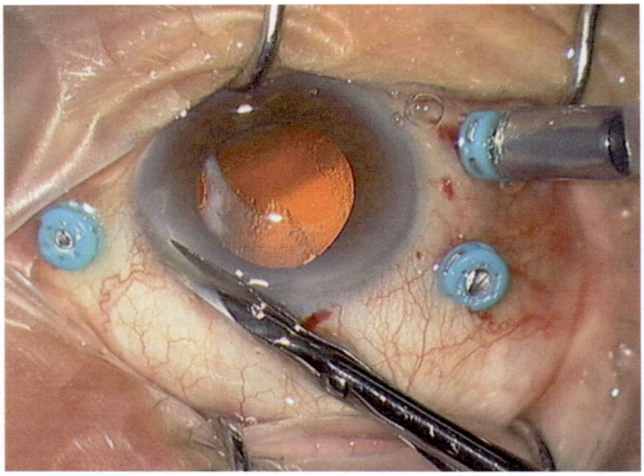

Fig. 8.6 Open the conjunctiva along the limbus from 11 o'clock to 1 o'clock with the Vannas scissors (limbal peritomy)

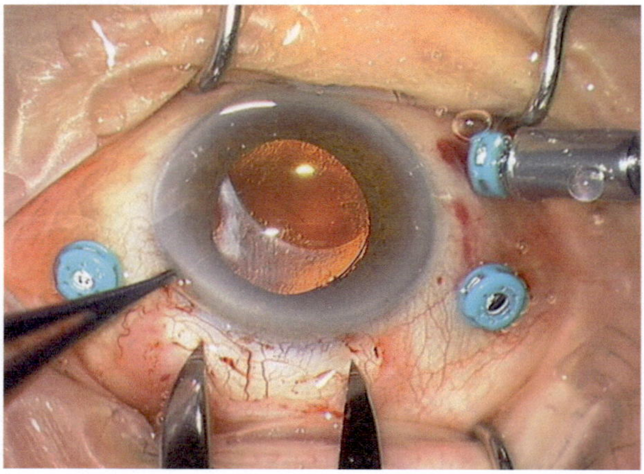

Fig. 8.7 Mark a 6-mm-broad scleral incision with the caliper

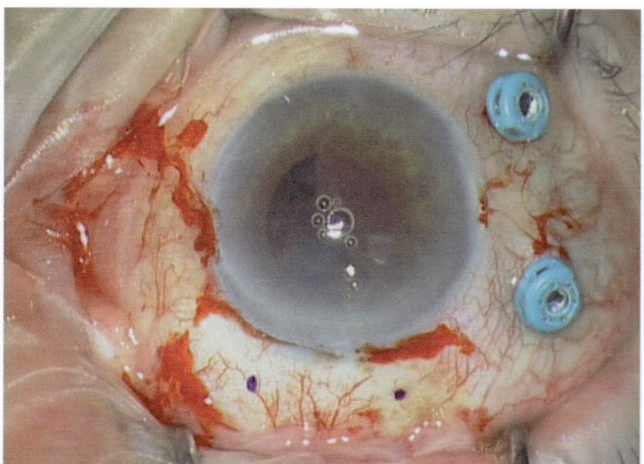

Fig. 8.8 The incision is approximately 1.5 mm behind the limbus

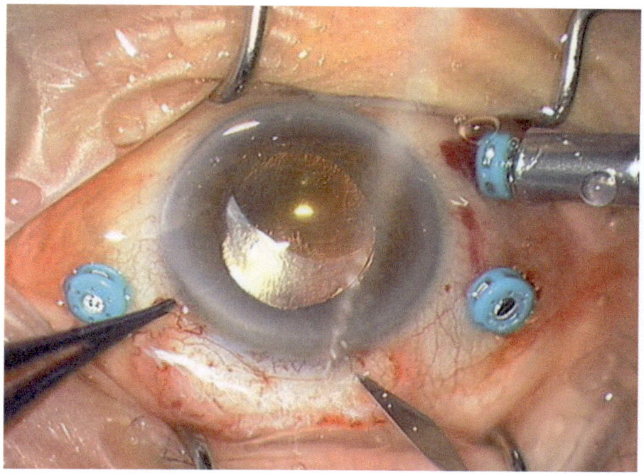

Fig. 8.9 A 50% scleral thickness incision with the 15° knife is performed

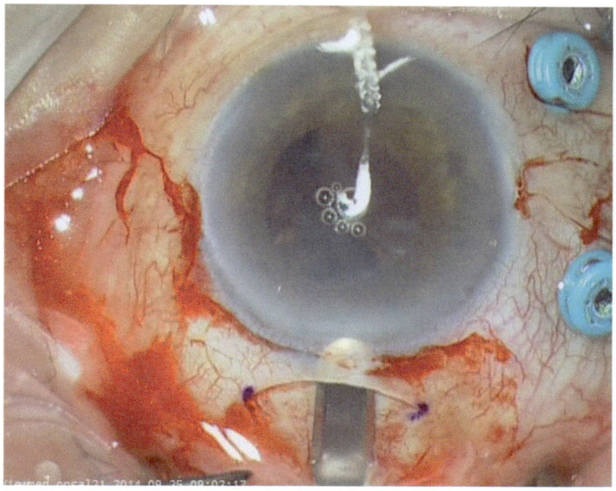

Fig. 8.10 Dissect a scleral flap with the bevel-up crescent knife. If the knife is visible through the sclera, then you have the correct depth

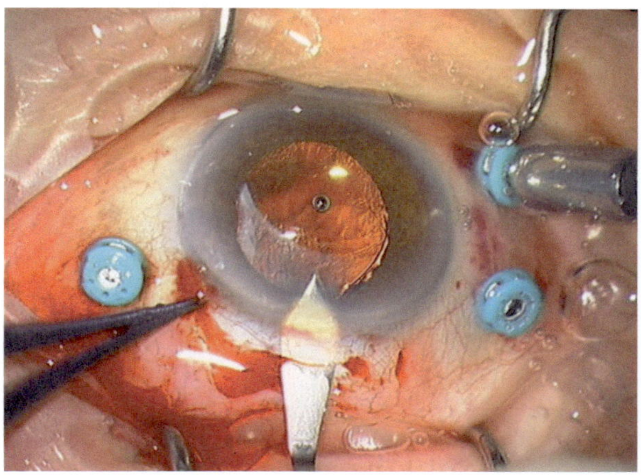

Fig. 8.11 Then open the anterior chamber with a 2.4 mm blade

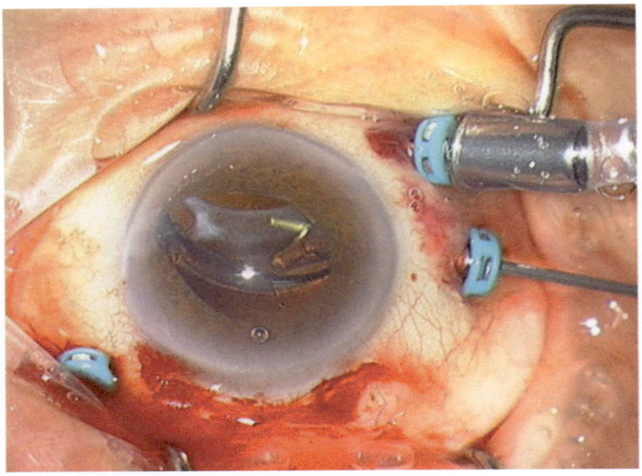

Fig. 8.12 Luxate the IOL at 12 o'clock up to the pupillary plane in order to access it with the forceps

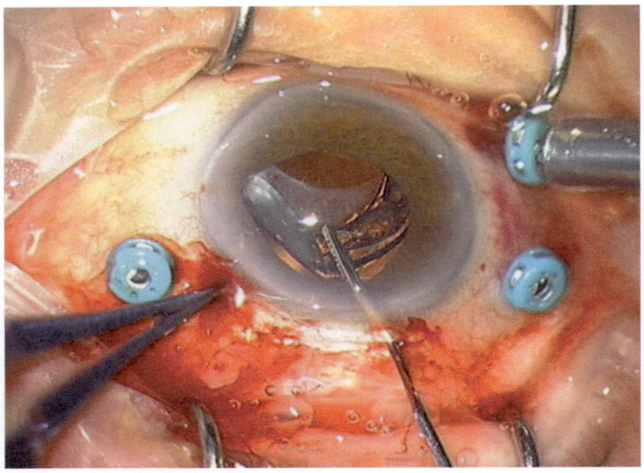

Fig. 8.13 Then remove the IOL with the serrated jaws forceps

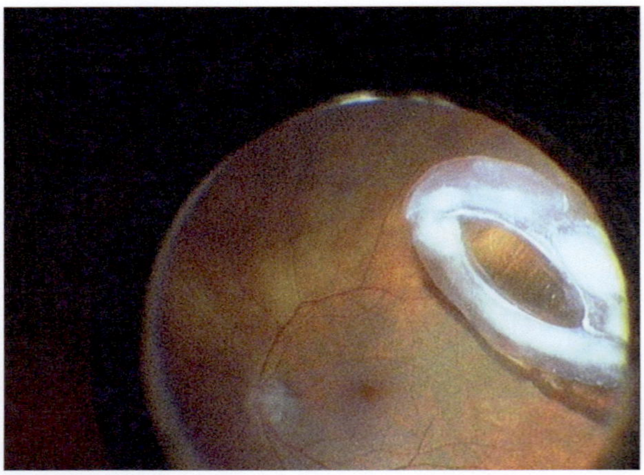

Fig. 8.14 A different approach is required in case of a posterior dislocated IOL

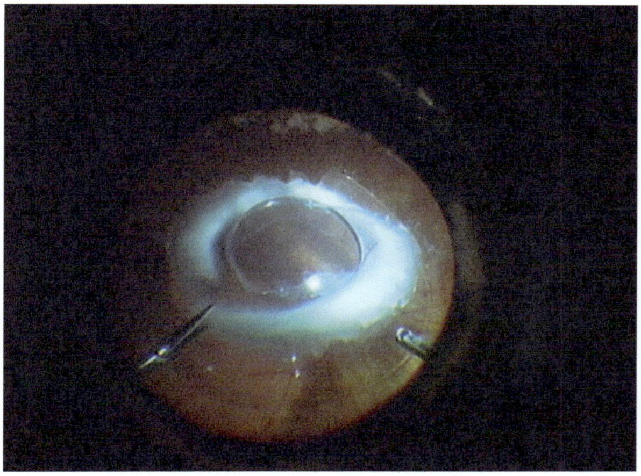

Fig. 8.15 Grasp the fibrotic capsular bag with an intravitreal forceps. In some cases the capsular bag gives no hold: Remove the capsule in order to free a haptic and grab it. It may be advisable to inject PFCL in order to protect the posterior pole

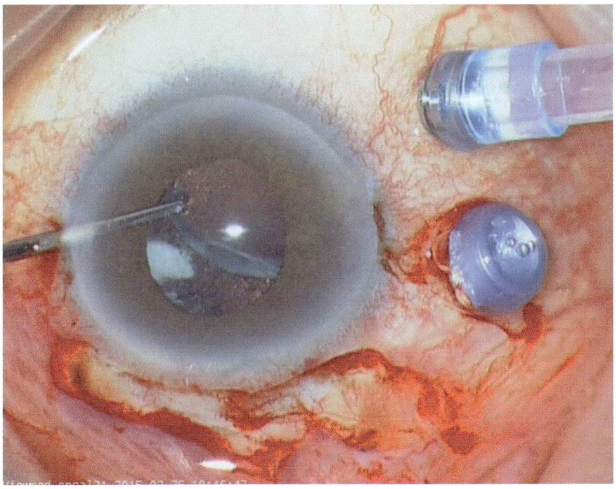

Fig. 8.16 Then lift the IOL forward to the pupil

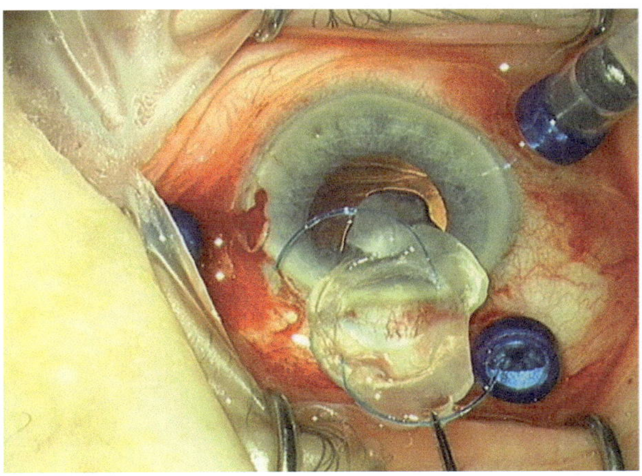

Fig. 8.17 And extract the IOL with an intravitreal forceps

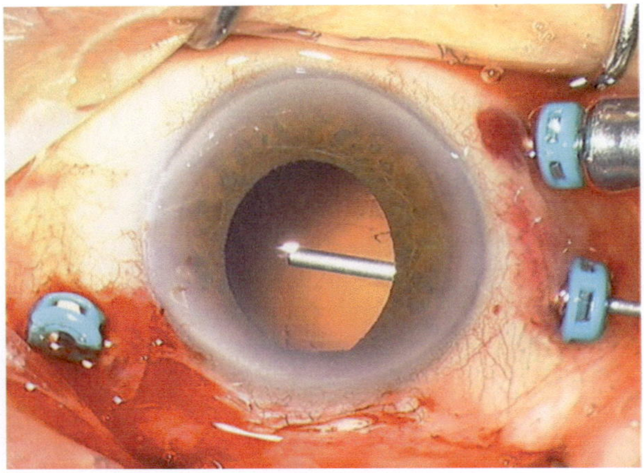

Fig. 8.18 Perform an anterior vitrectomy

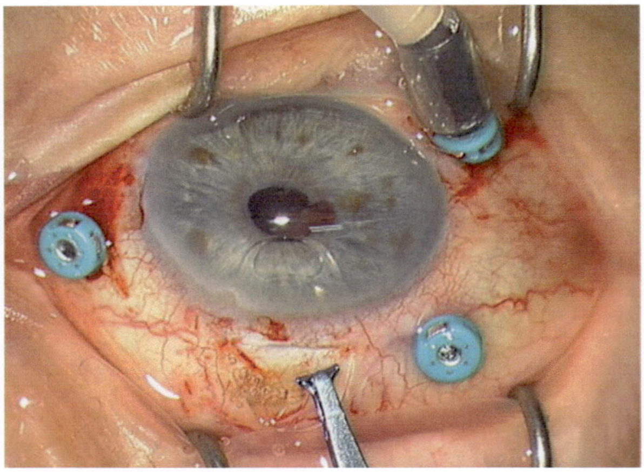

Fig. 8.19 Turn the iris-claw IOL upside down for implantation and place it on the iris with the IOL implantation forceps (AMO)

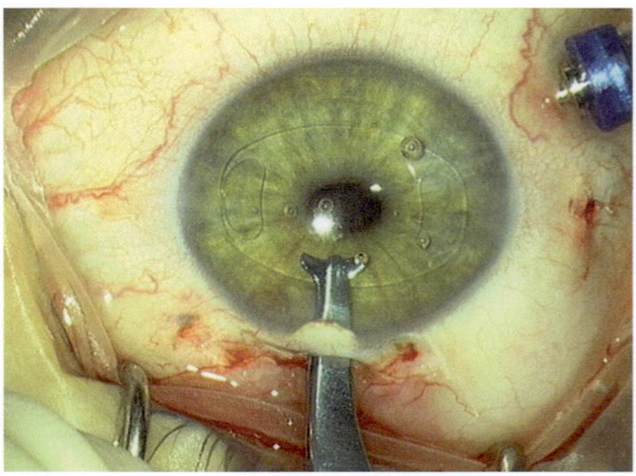

Fig. 8.20 Centrate the IOL, and fixate it with the IOL implantation forceps (AMO)

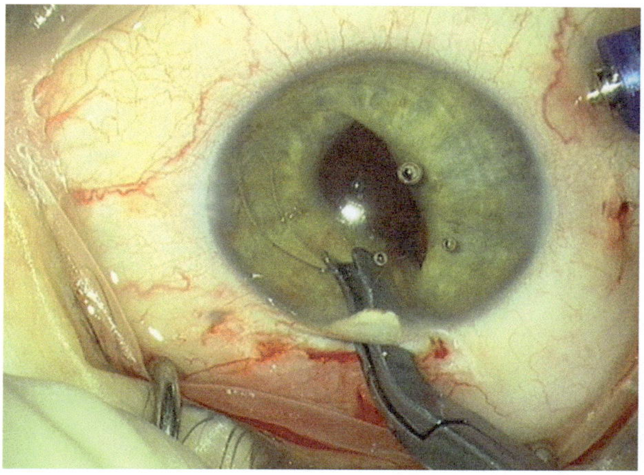

Fig. 8.21 Tilt the IOL behind the iris on one side

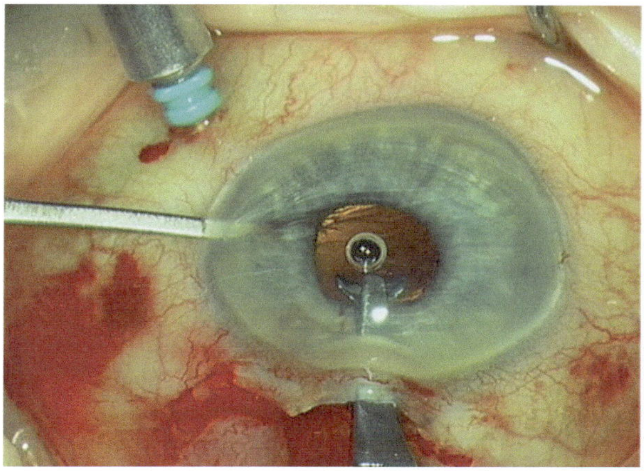

Fig. 8.22 Tilt the IOL behind the iris on the other side and then press the iris tissue with a Sekundo enclavation spatula (Geuder) (no push-pull instrument) behind the claws

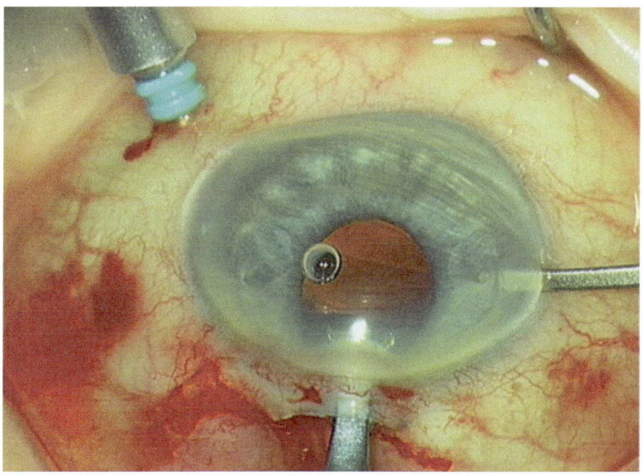

Fig. 8.23 Switch hands, and perform the same maneuver on the other side

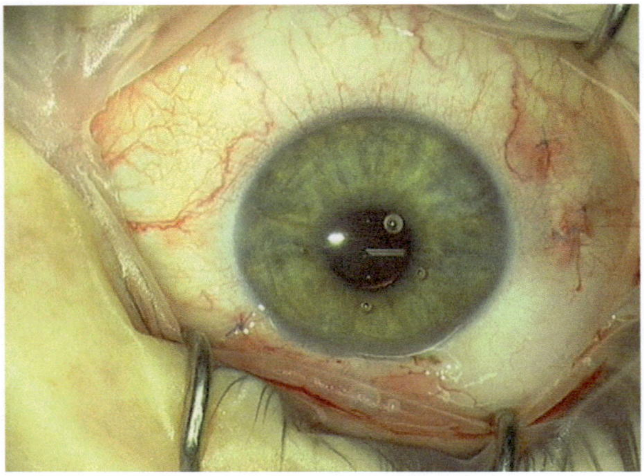

Fig. 8.24 Note the enclavated iris tissue at 3 and 9 o'clock

Note: The location of the IOL is determined by the position of the frown incision. If the claws are located at 3–9 o'clock, then the frown incision must be located at 12 o'clock. In case of an iris defect at 3 o'clock or a filtration bleb at 12 o'clock, you must choose the position of the IOL and frown incision accordingly.

Continue with the frown incision. Perform a limbal peritomy from 11 to 1 o'clock with Westcott scissors and cauterize the bleeding vessels (Figs. 8.5 and 8.6). Then mark a 6-mm-wide incision (not wider!) with a caliper (Figs. 8.7 and 8.8). The arc of the incision should be approximately 1–2 mm behind the limbus. Dissect a 50% scleral thickness deep limbus parallel incision with a 15° knife (Fig. 8.9). Then dissect a scleral tunnel with the crescent-angled bevel-up knife (Fig. 8.10), and open finally the anterior chamber with a 2.4 mm blade (Fig. 8.11). Note: Enter the anterior chamber with the 2.4 mm blade in the clear cornea in order to avoid an intracameral bleeding.

4. **Extraction of an anterior dislocated IOL**

The extraction is easier, if the eye is not vitrectomized and the IOL is located behind the iris. Close the infusion line during extraction. Inject viscoelastics into the anterior chamber and then behind the IOL and lift the IOL a little bit up at 12 o'clock so that the optic edge or a haptic is visible (Fig. 8.12). Grasp the IOL ideally at the haptic with the serrated jaw forceps, and extract the IOL with the lens capsule (Fig. 8.13). Often some fibrotic parts of the lens capsule remain in the anterior chamber. Remove them with viscoexpression, e.g., inject viscoelastics behind them into the anterior chamber and then press on the posterior scleral lip of the scleral tunnel.

Reopen the infusion line and continue with an anterior vitrectomy from pars plana.

5. **Extraction of a posterior dislocated IOL**

If the eye is vitrectomized and the IOL is located on the posterior pole, then you have to lift it up (Fig. 8.14). You need *two* intravitreal forceps, one 27G endgripping forceps and one 20G or 23G serrated jaws forceps. Grasp the edge of the optic or haptic with the first 27G endgripping forceps so that the IOL is standing up (Fig. 8.15). Fixate the upright IOL with the light pipe and then grasp the IOL again at the edge of the optic. Lift the IOL into the anterior chamber/pupillary plane, insert the serrated jaws forceps through a paracentesis, and grab the IOL (Fig. 8.16). Withdraw the first intravitreal forceps and reinsert it through the main incision. Grab the IOL with the endgripping forceps, withdraw the serrated jaws forceps (from the paracentesis), and extract the IOL (Fig. 8.17).

Surgical Pearls No 64
Difficult IOL in-the-bag extraction from posterior pole: Try the alternative maneuvers: (1) Work monomanual. Lift up the IOL with an endgripping forceps and place it against the light pipe. Now grab the haptic of the IOL. (2) Insert a chandelier light and work bimanual with one intravitreal forceps and one 27G membrane pic (DORC) to elevate the IOL. (3) Inject a small bubble of PFCL to elevate the IOL and to protect the macula. Grab the IOL. (4) It may be difficult to grasp the IOL due to the lens capsule. Remove the lens capsule around the haptic with the vitreous cutter (Fig. 8.15). If the haptic is freed from the lens capsule, it is easy to grasp with forceps.

6. **Anterior vitrectomy**
7. **Injection of Miochol**

Continue with an anterior vitrectomy (Fig. 8.18). Inspect then the periphery for retinal tears. The next step is pupil constriction. Before implantation of an iris-claw IOL, the pupil must be constricted. Inject first acetylcholine (Miochol®) and then viscoelastics into the anterior chamber. Using an IOL forceps (AMO), place the IOL upside down onto the iris.

8. **Implantation of iris-fixated IOL (upside down)**

Instrumentation
Dominant hand: IOL implantation forceps (Abbott)
Non-dominant hand: Enclavation spatula
Close the infusion line during IOL implantation (Fig. 8.19). Centrate the IOL with a manipulator (e.g., push-pull) inside the anterior chamber. Grasp the IOL at the edge with the IOL implantation forceps (Abbott) (Fig. 8.20). Flip the IOL to the right (Fig. 8.21) so that the IOL is behind the iris, and then flip it to the left so that the IOL is completely behind the iris. Hold the IOL now in the middle of the pupil. Do not move it to the left or right.

Take then the enclavation spatula in your left hand. Lift the IOL a little bit up, so that the iris claws are visible behind the iris tissue. Then insert the spatula in the 3 o'clock paracentesis, and clamp the iris tissue between the iris claws (Fig. 8.22). Then the hands for the implantation forceps have to be switched. This maneuver should be thoroughly practiced preoperatively. Then take the enclavation spatula in your right hand and perform the same maneuver at 9 o'clock (Fig. 8.23). Remove finally the implantation forceps, and open the infusion line to achieve normotension. A retropupillary implantation requires no iridectomy.

9. **Closure of the frown incision and conjunctiva**

Suture the frown incision with a Vicryl 8-0 cross-stitch and the conjunctiva with a Vicryl 8-0 interrupted stitch (Fig. 8.24).

8.2.6 Complications

Complete iris-claw IOL dislocation: The complete dislocation of an iris-claw IOL is very unusual. It may happen postoperatively secondary to a trauma.

Partial dislocation of an iris-claw IOL: Insert two iris hooks at 1–11 o'clock. Insert two trocars at 10:30–1:30 o'clock. Perform a corneal 2.4 mm main incision. Lift the IOL up from the trocars. Grasp the IOL with the IOL implantation forceps and then fixate the loose side.

Postoperative inflammation due to traumatic surgery, which occurs only in the learning phase. Do not enclavate too much iris tissue. It may cause ocular pain. In order to avoid this side effect, use the thin enclavation spatula from Sekundo from Geuder.

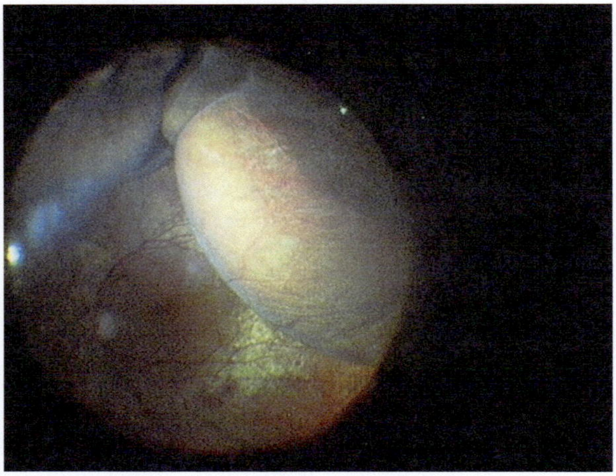

Fig. 8.25 A dreaded complication: Choroidal detachment. The reason is the big main incision and pressure fluctuations during manipulations at the main incision. It is therefore important to (1) perform a 6 mm incision (not wider) and (2) close the infusion and fill the anterior chamber with viscoelastics when working in the anterior chamber

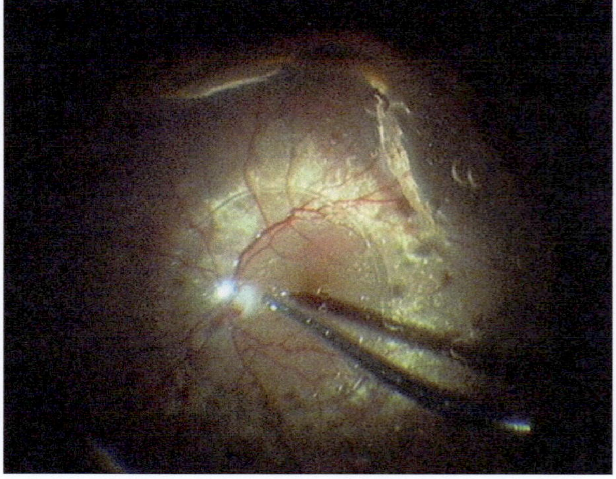

Fig. 8.26 In case of a shallow choroidal detachment, an air tamponade is sufficient. In case of a highly bullous choroidal detachment, it is advisable to inject PFCL and then perform a PFCL × 1000 csts silicone oil exchange

Choroidal detachment (Figs. 8.25 and 8.26)**:** The cause is the big main incision and pressure fluctuations during manipulations at the main incision. Make the main incision not wider than 6 mm, and perform an even cut so that the scleral lips are attached. A shallow choroidal detachment will resorb on its own after 2–3 months. In case of a highly bullous choroidal detachment, inject PFCL and then perform a PFCL × 1000 csts silicone oil exchange.

8.2.7 FAQ

Is an iris-claw implantation after trauma possible?

If the eye underwent a traumatic surgery due to a difficult cataract surgery with loss of the lens capsule, we would prefer a delayed implantation. We would implant the iris-claw IOL after approximately 1 month in order to obtain an uninflamed iris.

Why do you implant the Artisan IOL upside down?

The design of the Artisan IOL is convex; the haptics bend downward. This makes them difficult to enclavate into the iris tissue. If you implant the Artisan IOL upside down, then the haptics are bent upward and then the enclavation is much easier.

Is an iridectomy necessary?

No, not in case of an upside-down implantation.

Yes, in case of a non-upside-down implantation.

Is a core vitrectomy necessary?

A core vitrectomy increases the risk of a pseudophakodonesis. We perform therefore only an anterior vitrectomy.

Are three ports necessary?

In case of a subluxated IOL, two temporal ports are sufficient.

Is a BIOM necessary?

In the most cases, the IOL is only subluxated because the vitreous body is present. In this case, you may use only two trocars. An anterior vitrectomy is sufficient, and a BIOM is not required.

Pupil dilatation before surgery?

Only 1–2 drops tropicamide. Do not dilate maximally because you need a small pupil for implantation.

Is it possible to perform this surgery in two sessions?

Yes, of course. You may in one session extract the IOL and perform an anterior vitrectomy and then in a second session implant a Verisyse IOL. The advantage of two sessions is that the pupil can be constricted preoperatively with pilocarpine.

I am a beginner, what is the best eye to start with?

An aphakic eye with small pupil and removed anterior vitreous.

How do you treat a macular edema secondary to pseudophakia?

With topical eye drops or with intravitreal triamcinolone.

Is a treatment with Ozurdex possible?

No. The Ozurdex pellet will enter the anterior chamber and cause a corneal damage. An Ozurdex injection is contraindicated in eyes with aphakia and aphakic Verisyse IOL's.

8.3 Scleral Fixation of a 3-Piece IOL

Introduction

A fixation of an IOL with sutures is performed seldom nowadays. An intrascleral or iris fixation has become more common nowadays. The scleral fixation with sutures, however, is required with some IOL's such as a pigmented iris IOL (Opthec, NL; Morcher, Germany).

Materials

1. Polypropylene 10-0 suture with curved needle (i.e., Alcon. Polypropylene, blue monofilament, double armed. 8,065,307,601)
2. Three-piece IOL (Tecnis ZA 9003 or Alcon MA60AC)

Individual Steps

1. **Opening of the conjunctiva at 3–9 o'clock.**
2. **Two sclerotomies (1.5 mm posterior to the limbus) at 3–9 o'clock.**
3. **Extraction of a haptic at 3 o'clock; place a suture onto the haptic, and push it back into the eye. The same procedure at 9 o'clock.**
4. **Suture the haptic suture in a snake shape to the sclera.**
5. **Close the conjunctiva, removal of the trocars.**

1. **Opening of the conjunctiva at 3–9 o'clock**

Use a pars plana infusion or an anterior chamber maintainer. Open the conjunctiva at 3–9 o'clock to make space for one sclerotomy and a scleral suture, i.e., approximately from 2 to 4 o'clock and from 8 to 10 o'clock. Then cauterize the bleeding vessels.

2. **Two sclerotomies (1.5 mm posterior to the limbus) at 3–9 o'clock**
3. **Extraction of a haptic at 3 o'clock; place a suture onto the haptic, and push it back into the eye The same procedure at 9 o'clock.**

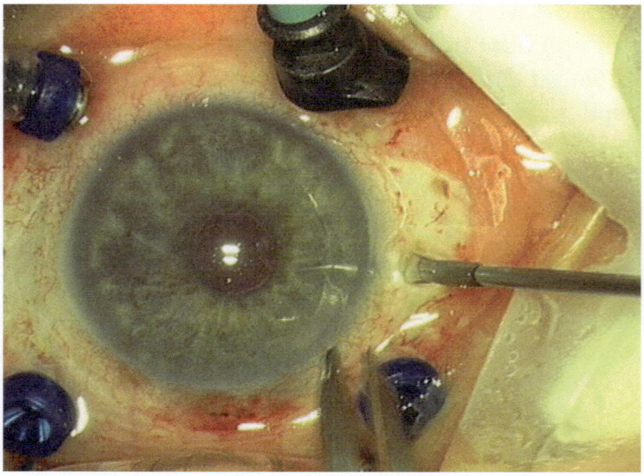

Fig. 8.27 A sclerotomy with a V-lance (Alcon) 1.5 mm behind the limbus

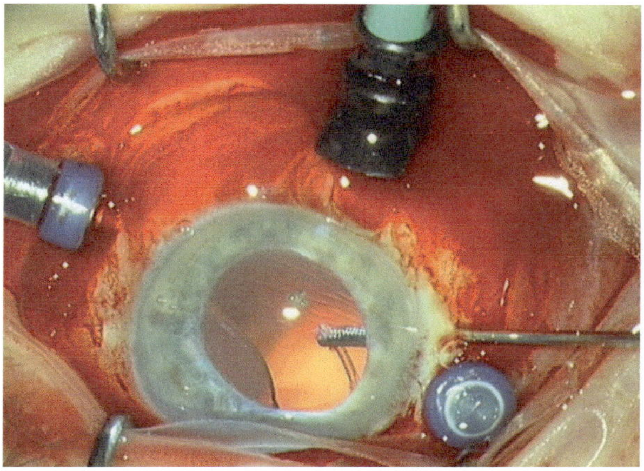

Fig. 8.28 Grab the end of the haptic and extract it through the sclerotomy

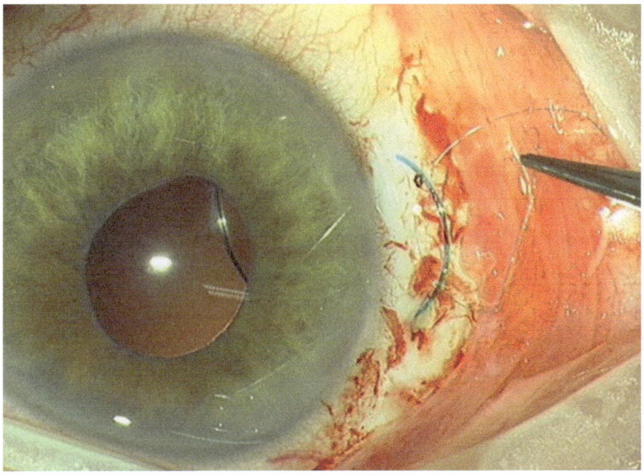

Fig. 8.29 Tie one end of a 10-0 Prolene 10.0 suture to one haptic. This suture has one straight needle. Then same maneuver on the other side

In case of a three-piece IOL, fasten the suture in the middle of the haptic and in case of an one-piece IOL at the end of the haptic.

In the area of the sulcus, 1.5 mm posterior to the limbus, perform an approx. 1.3 mm sclerotomy (Fig. 8.27). The sclerotomy must be perpendicular (i.e., approximately 90° to the sclera), in order not to harm the anterior chamber. Via the sclerotomy at 3 o'clock, grasp a haptic with an Eckardt forceps (Fig. 8.28) and pull it out of the eye. Cut a 10-0 polypropylene suture with two curved needles in two halves. Then place a 10-0 Prolene suture to the haptic (Fig. 8.29), and insert the haptic back into the eye. Perform the same maneuver at the 9 o'clock sclerotomy. After the haptic has been pushed back, center the IOL by pulling carefully on both sutures.

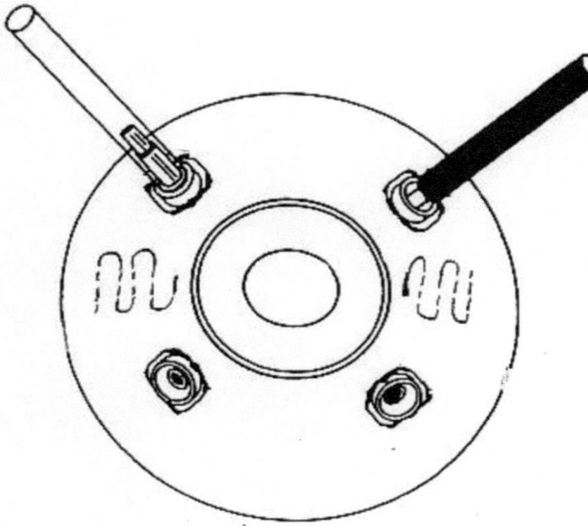

Fig. 8.30 5× snake-shaped suture. A knot is not necessary

4. **Suture the haptic suture in a snake shape to the sclera**

Different techniques are now possible. Move the suture in five U-shaped in a shape snake through the sclera and then cut off the suture without a knot. A knot can cause a disturbing foreign body sensation to the patient (Fig. 8.30). Alternatively, you can prepare a scleral flap, fasten the suture to the sclera and place the knot under the scleral flap.

5. **Close the conjunctiva, removal of the trocars**

The conjunctiva is closed with an 8-0 Vicryl stitch. The sclerotomies do not need to be sutured.

Part VII
Dropped Nucleus

Chapter 9
Dropped Nucleus (Posterior Dislocated Nucleus)

Extras: Videos 9.1, 9.2, 9.3, and 9.4.

9.1 Introduction

Surgical planning: two things should be assessed preoperatively:

1. How much of the nucleus is luxated? Or did only cortical fragments luxate?
2. Assess preoperatively whether the anterior capsule is intact. If the anterior capsule is intact, implant a three-piece IOL in the sulcus. If it is not intact, you can implant a sclera-fixated or even easier an iris-fixated IOL.

Necessity of surgery: If nuclear fragments drop, we always operate in order to prevent intraocular inflammation and hypertension. In case of dropped soft cortical fragments, it is possible to wait and not to operate so long as the eye remains quiet.

Timing of surgery: The surgery is not acute. Normally a dropped nucleus occurs under drop anesthesia. To proceed with vitrectomy under drop anesthesia will inflict much unnecessary pain to the patient. It is therefore advisable to stop surgery when a dropped nucleus occurs and to schedule a planned surgery within 1 week. During this time the eye can be treated against corneal edema and ocular hypertension.

Surgical Pearls No. 66
The most patients who underwent a complicated cataract surgery do not complain about the complication but about the painful procedure. Why? The cataract surgery was performed with drop anesthesia, and when the complication occurred, the surgery was continued with the same anesthesia. Our recommendation: If you experience a complication, decide if you continue or stop the surgery. If you decide to

---

Electronic Supplementary Material The online version of this chapter (https://doi.org/10.1007/978-3-319-89677-9_9) contains supplementary material, which is available to authorized users.

U. Spandau, H. Heimann, *Practical Handbook for Small-Gauge Vitrectomy*,
https://doi.org/10.1007/978-3-319-89677-9_9

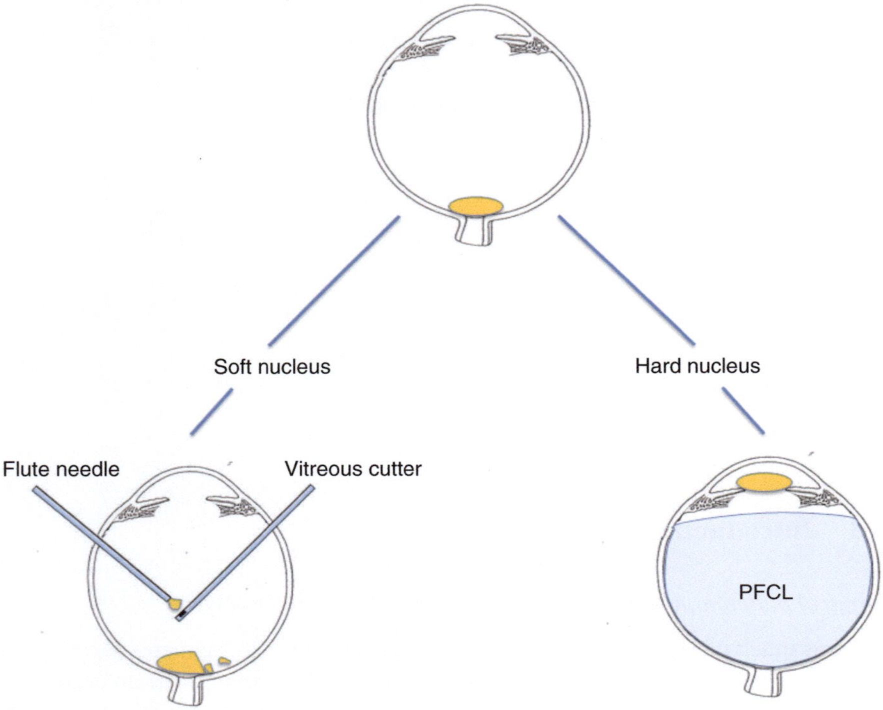

Fig. 9.1 Treatment algorithm for removal of soft or hard dropped nucleus

continue at once, then add a subtenonal or retrobulbar anesthesia. You will have a happy patient and an easier surgery.

The most difficult part of this surgery is the removal of the nucleus. There are two methods (Fig. 9.1):

1. You can remove the nucleus with a fragmatome inside the vitreous cavity. In case of soft to medium-hard nuclei, we recommend working with the fragmatome.
2. You can lift the nucleus with PFCL to the pupillary plane and remove it there with a conventional phaco hand piece or the SICS technique. The latter technique is very elegant and easy in case of a rock-hard nucleus. For details of SICS technique, see my book *Complications During and After Cataract Surgery* (Springer).

9.2 Extraction of a Posteriorly Dislocated Nucleus with Fragmatome

9.2.1 Introduction

The lens fragments are removed with the vitreous cutter and the fragmatome. Do you know which tissue you can remove with a vitreous cutter and the fragmatome? This is an important knowledge for this case. With the vitreous cutter, you can remove the cortex, the epinucleus, a soft nucleus, and the iris tissue. You cannot remove a dense nucleus or a thick capsular fibrosis. With the fragmatome you can remove a dense nucleus and a thick capsular fibrosis. A rock-hard nucleus is difficult to remove by a fragmatome. The fragmatome is less powerful than a normal phaco hand piece. To remove a rock-hard nucleus, it is advisable to perform phaco at the pupillary plane or a SICS.

9.2.2 Instruments

1. 23G, 25G, or 27G three-port trocar system with chandelier light fiber
2. 120D lens
3. Fragmatome
4. 1.3 mm V-lance for 20G sclerotomy

9.2.3 Surgery Step-by-Step

1. **23G, 25G, or 27G three-port system with chandelier light fiber**
2. **Anterior vitrectomy via pars plana**
3. **Removal of residual cortex from the lens capsule via paracentesis**
4. **Vitrectomy, if necessary PVD**
5. **20G sclerotomy at 9 o'clock**
6. **PFCL for macula protection**
7. **Emulsification of the nucleus with fragmatome and flute needle**
8. **Closure of 20G sclerotomy**
9. **Trimming of vitreous base**
10. **Implantation of an intraocular lens**
11. **Removal of trocar cannulas**

The Surgery Step-by-Step (Figs. 9.2, 9.3, 9.4, and 9.5)

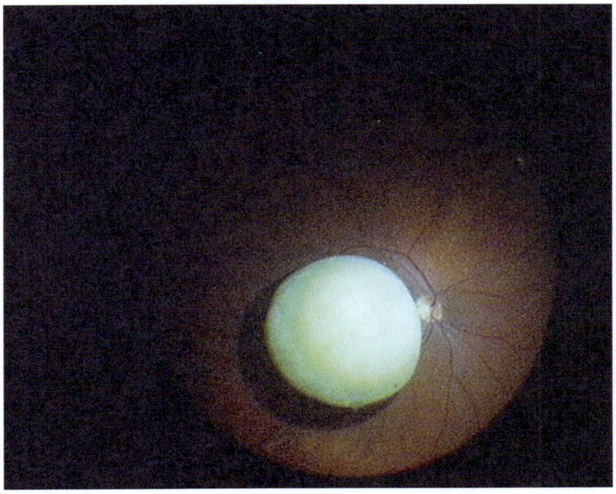

Fig. 9.2 A luxated white nucleus secondary to trauma for 20 years ago

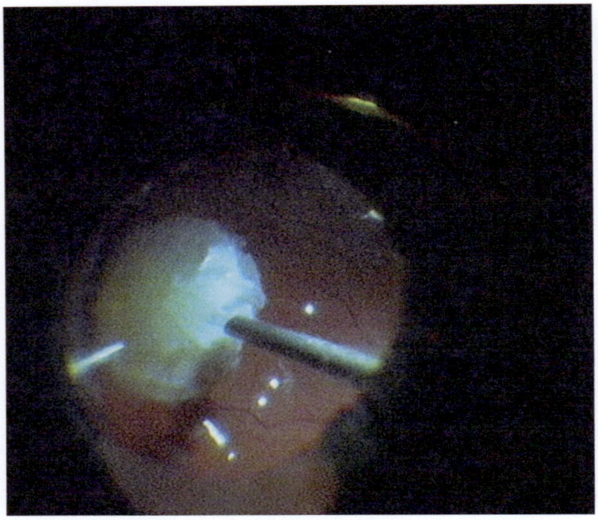

Fig. 9.3 Emulsification of a nucleus with fragmatome. A PFCL bubble was injected to protect the posterior pole

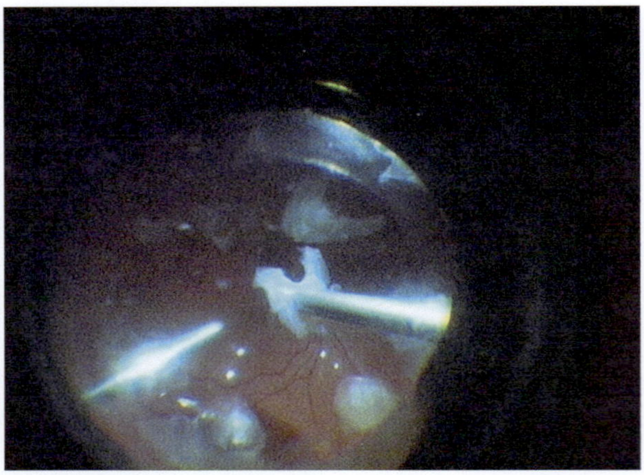

Fig. 9.4 Many small nuclear fragments. Every fragment has to be removed

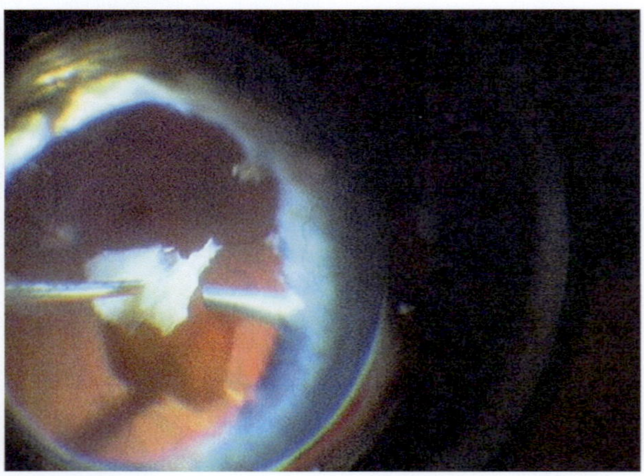

Fig. 9.5 The left hand fixates the fragment with a backflush instrument and the right hand removes it with the fragmatome. The fragmatome is a dangerous instrument which can cause severe retinal and choroidal damage

1. **Three-Port System with Chandelier Light Fiber**

After insertion of three trocars, we insert a chandelier light fiber, because we work bimanually in steps 7 and 9.

2. **Anterior Vitrectomy via Pars Plana**

3. **Removal of Residual Cortex from the Lens Capsule via Paracentesis**

4. **Vitrectomy, if Necessary PVD**

The anterior vitreous is cut with the vitreous cutter via pars plana. Make circular movements with the vitreous cutter. The vitreous cutter port points backward toward the posterior pole in order to avoid a damage of the lens capsule. Aspirate then the residual cortex with the vitreous cutter via a paracentesis. Alternatively, you can use two I/A hand pieces. It is important that you switch the vitreous cutter to aspiration and not to cutting. Otherwise you risk destroying the anterior capsule. If the lens capsule is free from the cortex, continue with a core vitrectomy from pars plana.

5. **20G Sclerotomy at 9 o'Clock**

6. **PFCL for Macula Protection**

7. **Emulsification of the Nucleus with Fragmatome and Flute Needle**

Then open the conjunctiva at 9 o'clock in the area of the sclerotomy and perform a non-lamellar (perpendicular) 20G sclerotomy with the V-lance. This sclerotomy is used for the fragmatome and closed as soon as the nucleus is removed, in order to avoid leakage from the sclerotomy. Inject next a small PFCL bubble to protect the macula.

Soft lens material can be removed first with the vitreous cutter (approximately 400 cuts /min). For hard lens fragments, you can use the flute needle in your left hand and the fragmatome in the right hand. Aspirate the lens fragments with the flute needle, move the needle to the central vitreous cavity, and emulsify them there safely with the fragmatome. This procedure is performed repeatedly until all the lens fragments are removed.

If you perform this procedure without flute needle (only with the fragmatome), there is a risk that during the frequent aspiration of the lens fragments with the fragmatome you may injure the retina (retinal break) or the choroid (choroidal hemorrhage). In addition, the frequent aspiration of the lens fragments clogs the vitreous cutter. If the suction is not working properly, the risk is increased to induce damage to the retina or choroid. In this case, it is advisable to inject a PFCL bubble in order to protect the posterior pole.

Surgical Pearls No. 67

Dropped nucleus: The difficulty of this step is that the nucleus is located on the posterior pole so that a damage of the retina is easily induced. Three advices: (1) Inject a PFCL bubble to (a) protect the macula and (b) elevate the nucleus. (2) Work bimanual so that one hand can fixate the nucleus and the other hand can remove it.

(3) If the posterior vitreous is attached, then the vitreous cortex is like a cushion for the nucleus making its removal difficult, in this case induce a PVD to free the access to the nucleus.

8. **Closure of 20G Sclerotomy**

The 20G sclerotomy must be sutured with a Vicryl 6-0 interrupted stitch or a Vicryl 8-0 cross-stitch.

9. **Trimming of Vitreous Base**

The fragmatome breaks the nucleus in many small pieces which are dispersed all over the posterior segment. These fragments must be removed meticulously, because every nucleus fragment which remains may cause a postoperative sterile uveitis. The most lens fragments are located in the vitreous base at 6 o'clock. In order to visualize and remove them you need to indent the vitreous with the scleral depressor. Use for this procedure a chandelier light.

Surgical Pearls No. 68
The trimming of the vitreous base is an important step because a residual nuclear fragment will cause a postoperative sterile uveitis. Conclusion: do not be satisfied after removal of the large nucleus but after complete removal of all small fragments.

10. **Implantation of the IOL**

11. **Removal of Trocar Cannulas**

If more than two third of the anterior capsule are intact, the lens can be implanted into the sulcus ("haptic out, optic in") (Figs. 9.11 and 9.12). If not, fixate a three-piece IOL to the sclera or implant an iris-fixated IOL (Verisyse®) (Fig. 9.12).

Surgical Pearls No. 69
One-piece IOL vs. three-piece IOL: Do not implant a one-piece IOL into the sulcus because the haptics cause a focal depigmentation of the iris resulting in a secondary pigment glaucoma. This does not happen with a three-piece IOL. The reason for this is that a one-piece haptic has sharp edges and a three-piece is round.

9.3 Extraction of a Posteriorly Dislocated Nucleus (Dropped Nucleus) with PFCL

9.3.1 Introduction

With this technique, the nucleus is luxated with PFCL into the anterior chamber and removed with a SICS technique or with phacoemulsification. The advantages of a SICS technique are a fast and complete removal of the dropped nucleus. The disadvantage is sometimes the destruction of the anterior lens capsule when luxating the nucleus into the anterior chamber. The advantage of phacoemulsification is that we are more used to this technique. The disadvantage is an injury of the endothelium with the phaco energy, which may result in a decompensated cornea.

9.3.2 Instruments

1. Hybrid three-port trocar system with chandelier light
2. 120D lens
3. 15° knife (Alcon)
4. Crescent-angled bevel-up knife
5. Tunnel knife, 2.4 mm
6. Double-barreled infusion cannula

9.3.3 Tamponade

Intraoperative: PFCL

Postoperative: none

9.3.4 Surgery Step-by-Step

1. **Three-port trocar system with chandelier light**
2. **Vitrectomy**
3. **Injection of PFCL and dislocation of the nucleus to the pupillary plane**
4. **Phacoemulsification of the nucleus**
5. **Extraction of the nucleus with the SICS method**
6. **Implantation of an intraocular lens**
7. **Removal of trocars**

Individual Steps (Figs. 9.6–9.12)

1. **Three-Port Trocar System with Chandelier Light**

2. **Vitrectomy**

3. **Injection of PFCL and Dislocation of the Nucleus to the Pupillary Plane**

The anterior vitreous is removed with the vitreous cutter via pars plana. Then the residual cortex is aspirated from the lens capsule with the vitreous cutter via a paracentesis. It is important that you switch the vitreous cutter to aspiration and not to cutting. Otherwise there is a risk of destroying the anterior capsule. If the lens capsule is free from the cortex, continue with vitrectomy from pars plana.Instill a PFCL bubble; if necessary luxate the nucleus with the flute instrument onto the PFCL

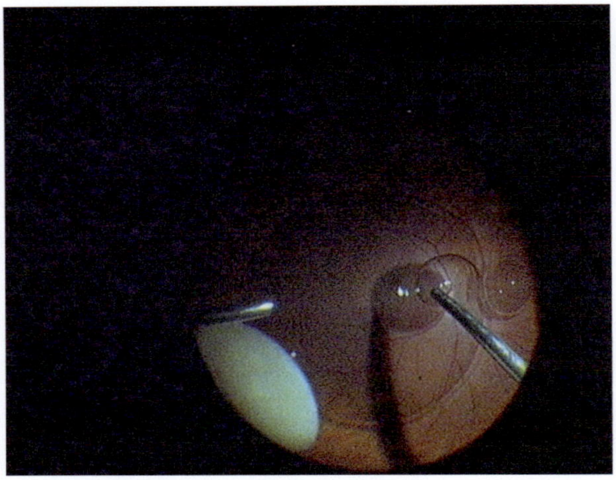

Fig. 9.6 A different nucleus removal method. PFCL is injected to lift up the nucleus

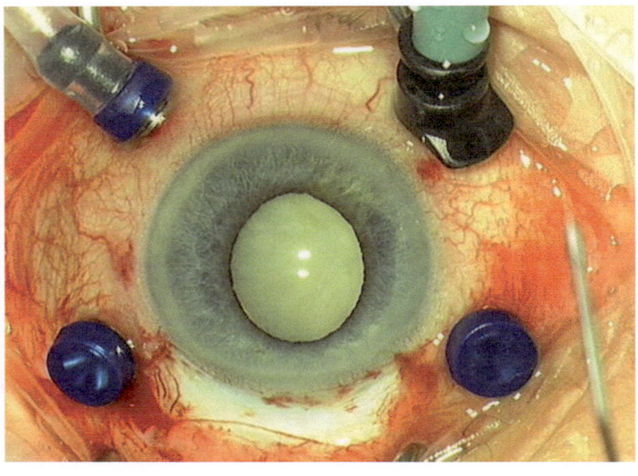

Fig. 9.7 The nucleus is now located behind the pupil

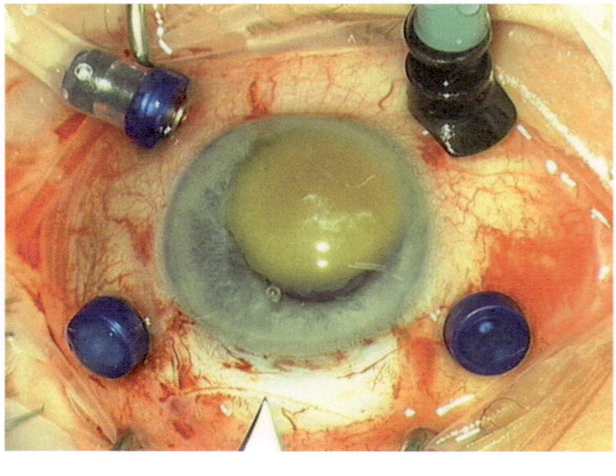

Fig. 9.8 Then the nucleus is luxated into the anterior chamber. This maneuver is not so easy because the lens capsule is slippery. Now a 8 mm frown incision is performed

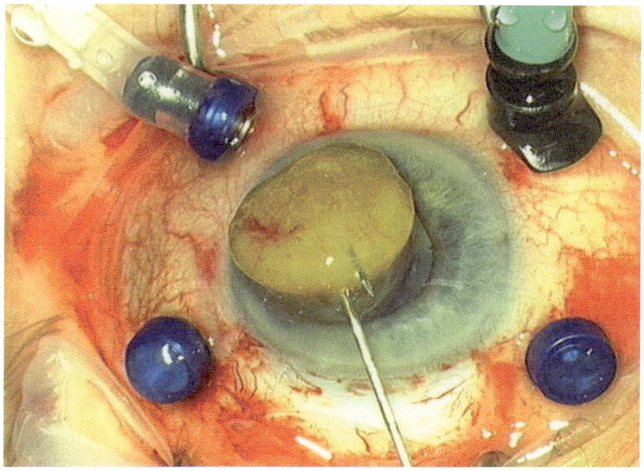

Fig. 9.9 The nucleus is removed with a so-called fish hook. Use alternatively a serrated lens loop

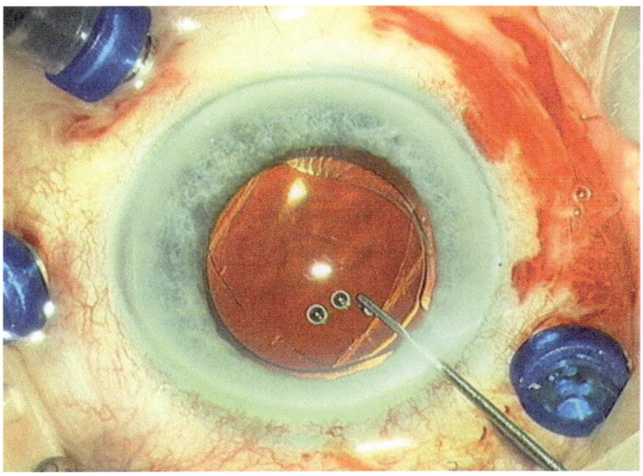

Fig. 9.10 Insert a three-piece IOL with haptics in the sulcus and the optic behind the rhexis

bubble (Fig. 9.6). Then inject PFCL up to the sclerotomies; the nucleus is then pushed up to the level of the pupil (Fig. 9.7).

4. **Phacoemulsification of the Nucleus**

Emulsify next the nucleus with a normal phaco hand piece. The phacoemulsification disintegrates the nucleus into small pieces which may slide away on the PFCL bubble in the retinal periphery and must be retrieved from there. Viscoelastics behind the nucleus can help to hold the lens fragments in the pupil.

OR

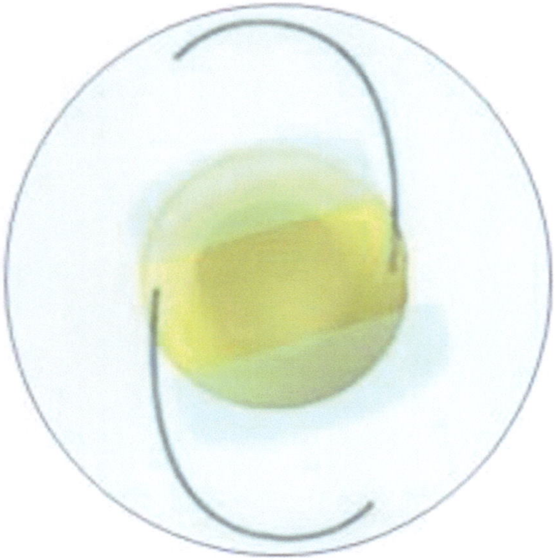

Fig. 9.11 An illustration of "haptic out, optic in." The IOL is centrated, and a barrier between posterior and anterior segment is created

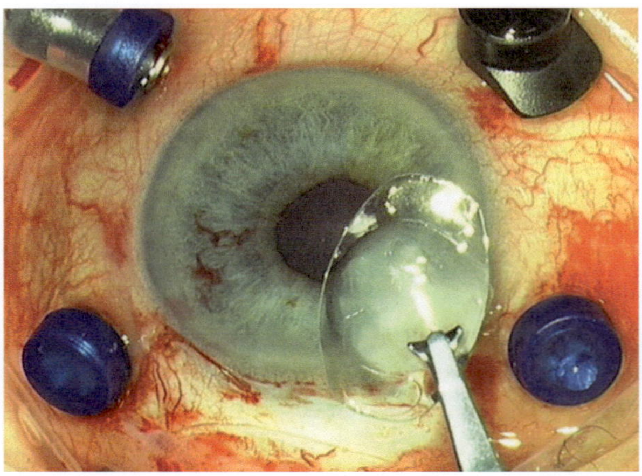

Fig. 9.12 If the lens capsule is absent, then implant scleral-fixated IOL or iris-fixated IOL (Artisan, Opthec, Verisyse, AMO)

5. **Extraction of the Nucleus with the SICS Method**

If the nucleus is too hard for the phaco, you can extract the nucleus faster and with a lower risk of complications in toto (Figs. 9.8 and 9.9). I recommend the so-called SICS technique (small incision cataract surgery), which is a modified form of ECCE. In short, limbal peritomy from 11 to 1 o'clock with Vannas scissors, mark then with the caliper an 8 mm wide frown incision, dissect the frown incision with a crescent bevel-up knife, and open the anterior chamber with a 2.4 mm tunnel knife. The next steps are the luxation of the nucleus into the anterior chamber, injection of viscoelastics below and above the nucleus, and finally extraction of the nucleus with loop, fish hook, or viscoelastics. The incision may be sutured with a Vicryl 8-0 cross-stitch.

6. **Implantation of the Intraocular Lens**

7. **Removal of Trocars**

If more than two thirds of the anterior capsule is intact, the lens is implanted into the sulcus ("haptic out, optic in") (Figs. 9.10 and 9.11). If not, fixate a lens to the sclera or to the iris (e.g., iris-fixated IOL) (Fig. 9.12).

9.3.5 Complications

Retinal break and choroidal hemorrhage are the most common complications and can be avoided, when you work bimanually or in other words, if you pick up the lens fragments with the Charles flute needle and not with the vitreous cutter.

9.3.6 FAQ

Which method do you prefer, SICS or fragmatome?
In case of a hard nucleus, I prefer SICS because this technique is faster and smoother and removes the complete nucleus. In case of a medium-hard nucleus, I would prefer the fragmatome.

I dislike about the fragmatome technique that it breaks the nucleus in many small pieces. And all pieces must be meticulously removed. Only one remaining nuclear fragment can cause a sterile endophthalmitis. This problem does not exist with the SICS technique.

Part VIII
Retinal Detachment

Chapter 10
Usage of a Chandelier Light

Extras: Video 10.1.

Surgery for retinal detachment means bimanual vitrectomy and the usage of a chandelier light. Bimanual vitrectomy is an essential part of modern minimal incision vitreoretinal surgery (MIVS). By inserting a stationary chandelier light in the sclera (four-port vitrectomy, Fig. 10.1), the surgeon has two active hands. To operate with two active hands is a new and exciting method of surgery. For example, in retinal detachment surgery you can indent the sclera with one hand and vitrectomize the vitreous base with the other hand. In diabetic retinopathy, you can apply laser photocoagulation up to the ora serrata with the help of a scleral depressor. You can remove membranes with two different instruments and also apply counteraction and so on.

For optimal use of a chandelier light, three requirements have to be met:

1. Inferonasal insertion enabling a good rotation of the globe
2. A rigid cable allowing aiming the light source in all directions in the vitreous cavity
3. Strong light source for optimal illumination

The chandelier light is best positioned inferonasally, because here its location does not affect the rotation of the eye. The 12 o'clock or 6 o'clock insertion sites disturb the rotation of the globe, and the light fiber is easily dislocated when the globe is rotated upward or downward. The rigid cable allows bending of the light fiber and henceforth the ability to maneuver the light to different directions in the vitreous cavity. The light source of modern vitrectomy machines (Constellation, Stellaris, Eva) is sufficient for optimal illumination of chandelier light. The light

Electronic Supplementary Material The online version of this chapter (https://doi.org/10.1007/978-3-319-89677-9_10) contains supplementary material, which is available to authorized users.

U. Spandau, H. Heimann, *Practical Handbook for Small-Gauge Vitrectomy*,
https://doi.org/10.1007/978-3-319-89677-9_10

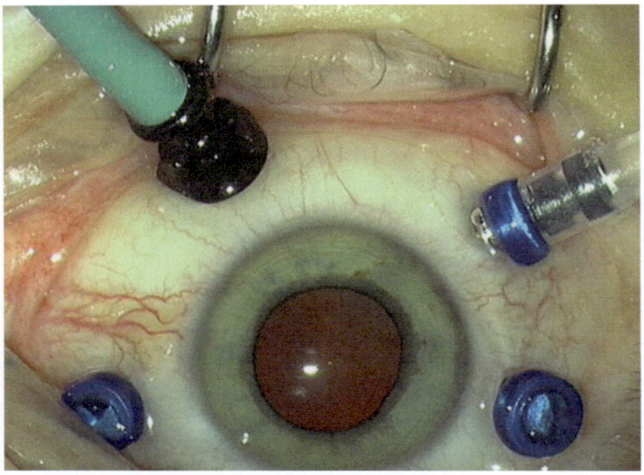

Fig. 10.1 An eye with four-port vitrectomy. In addition to the known three-port system, a chandelier light fiber (Awh chandelier, Synergetics) was firmly inserted into the sclera (top left)

Table 10.1 Features of different types of chandelier lights

Chandelier light	Alcon[a]	DORC[b]	Synergetics[c]
Light source	Photon	Xenon	Photon
Illumination	Good	Good	Very good
Rigid cable	Yes	No	Yes
Maneuverability	Average	Reduced	Good
Method of insertion	Trocar	Trocar	Sclera
Difficulty of insertion	Simple	Simple	Average

[a]Alcon: Chandelier Accurus 8,065,751,574
[b]DORC: 23-gauge chandelier light 3269.EB06
[c]Synergetics: 25-gauge Awh chandelier 56.20.25

source of old vitrectomy machines (Accurus) is <u>not</u> sufficient for optimal illumination of chandelier light. In the latter case, an external light source (Photon or Xenon) is required for a sufficient illumination of the vitreous cavity.

Insertion of Chandelier Light

If you have never used a chandelier light before, then start with one which can easily be inserted. The 25-gauge chandelier light from Alcon and the 23-gauge chandelier light from DORC are relatively unproblematic to use (see Table 10.1) as the light fiber can be placed inside a normal one-step trocar (Figs. 10.2 and 10.3).

The chandelier light from Synergetics is trickier to be put in place but on the other hand provides an excellent panoramic illumination of the vitreous cavity. Rotate the globe with a swab in a superotemporal direction so that there is space for the insertion of the chandelier light inferonasally. With the sclerotomy needle supplied by the manufacturer, one first performs a transconjunctival sclerotomy 3.5 mm posterior to the limbus with a perpendicular (not lamellar) path. The chandelier light is then inserted into the sclerotomy. This procedure requires some practice. The Synergetics chandelier light requires an external photon light source. By bending the rigid cable of the chandelier light, you can manipulate the light source. Sometimes you need to tape the cable to the drape.

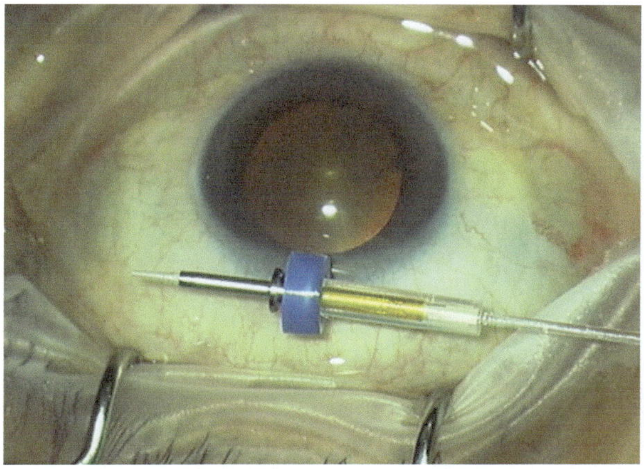

Fig. 10.2 A 23-gauge chandelier light from DORC, which is very easy to insert because it is placed in a trocar. Similar chandelier lights are available from Alcon and Synergetics

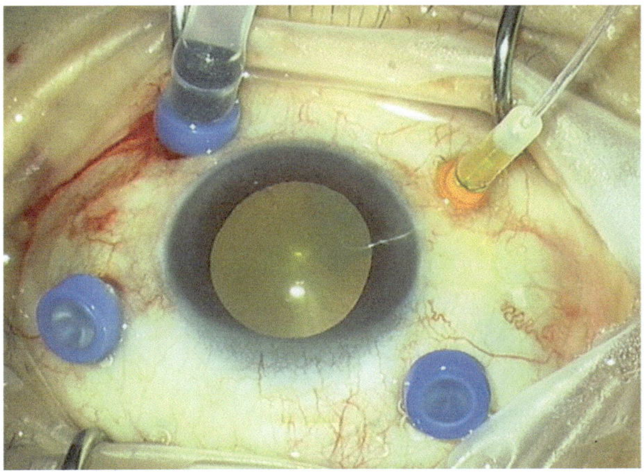

Fig. 10.3 Same 23-gauge chandelier light. Place inferonasally a 23-gauge trocar. Then insert the light fiber into an Alcon or DORC trocar (with or without valve). DORC: 23-gauge chandelier light 3269.EB06

Surgical Pearls No. 65
Chandelier light:

1. The insertion of the chandelier light is easier using your hands than with the trocar forceps. But you must exert a relatively strong pressure to insert the tip of the chandelier through the sclera. If you fail, you can expand the sclerotomy with a 23-gauge cannula/needle. The insertion is easier, but the chandelier sits a little loosely in the sclerotomy.
2. Conjunctival chemosis or hemorrhage may make it difficult to identify the sclerotomy. In such cases, open the conjunctiva focally with scissors and forceps in order to visualize the sclerotomy.

The following surgeries in bimanual technique are listed in increasing levels of difficulty. The most demanding surgeries are PVR detachment and proliferative diabetic retinopathy. In these pathologies, a bimanual peeling facilitates surgery immensely and is warmly recommended

Chapter 11
Episcleral Buckling for Detachment Surgery with BIOM

Extras: Videos 11.1, 11.2, 11.3, 11.4, and 11.5.

11.1 Introduction

The principle of buckle surgery can be explained very easily when comparing it with a puncture in a bicycle tire. The tire is the sclera and the tube is the retina. The first step in repairing a puncture is the search for a hole under water. Unfortunately, the same test is not available for the eye. Here we use an indirect ophthalmoscope and Lincoff rules. When the puncture in the tube is found, we mark it, and according to the size of the puncture, we place a patch on it. In the eye, we mark the hole on the sclera, and according to the size of the hole, we suture a sponge on it. Then we pump the tire up with air. If the tube remains filled, we solved the problem. If the tube gets soft again, then either the old hole is not well patched or a second hole is present. This situation correlates completely to the eye. If the retina is attached the next day, then the problem is solved. If the retina remains detached, then either the first hole is not located on the buckle or a second break is present. Remark: Would you place an encircling band on a bicycle tire? No. Why do we place an encircling band around an eye?

11.1.1 Minimal Buckling Versus Maximal Buckling Technique

Episcleral buckling with encircling band or segmental sponges is possible in vitrectomized and not-vitrectomized eyes. Episcleral buckling is possible in phakic and pseudo phakic eyes and in eyes with PVD and without PVD. Nowadays two different

---

Electronic Supplementary Material The online version of this chapter (https://doi.org/10.1007/978-3-319-89677-9_11) contains supplementary material, which is available to authorized users.

U. Spandau, H. Heimann, *Practical Handbook for Small-Gauge Vitrectomy*,
https://doi.org/10.1007/978-3-319-89677-9_11

episcleral buckling techniques are employed (Fig. 11.1): (1) minimal buckling surgery with a segmental silicone sponge which seals only the hole and (2) maximal buckling surgery with encircling band/tire and a grooved strip which covers the hole.

Our Surgical Technique at the University of Uppsala for Episcleral Buckling Is

Minimal buckling surgery: the episcleral buckling technique we apply is the minimal buckling technique according to Kreissig/Lincoff (1).

In short: (1) Cryopexy of the tear. (2) Application of a segmental buckle. Drainage only if necessary. No encircling band necessary.

The complete surgery is performed with a microscope. We use the microscope with BIOM instead of a helmet with binocular ophthalmoscopy. For endoillumination a chandelier light is inserted.

Why? Today vitreoretinal surgeons are more used to the microscope. It is easier for a vitreoretinal surgeon to inspect the retina with a microscope than with binocular ophthalmoscopy. In addition, suturing of the silicone sponge is easier under a microscope than with a helmet. This is especially the case for long myopic eyes.

Choice of Buckle (Table 11.1)

The choice of buckle is dependent on the size of the retinal break. If the break is 1 mm in size, then the sponge must be at least 3 mm in size. We have only 5–7 mm

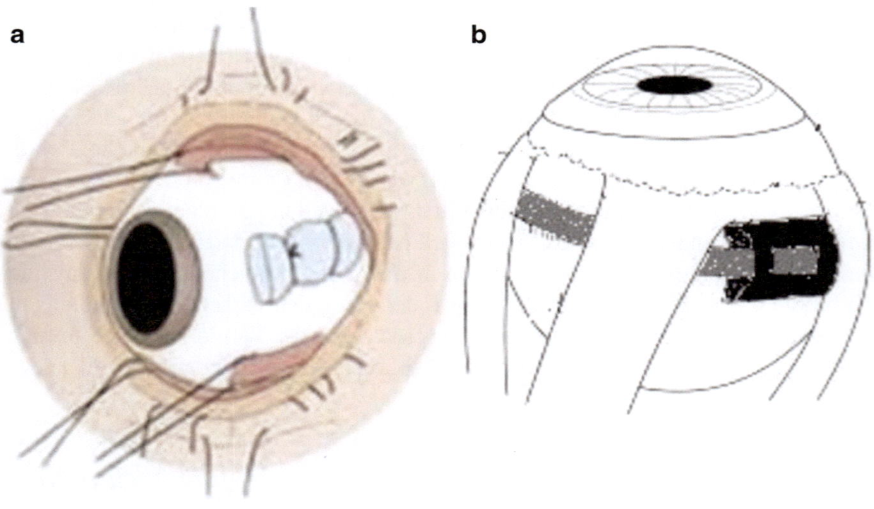

Fig. 11.1 Minimal buckling surgery with a radial sponge (**a**). Maximal buckling surgery with an encircling band and a grooved strip (**b**)

Table 11.1 Choice of silicone sponge depending on the size of the break

Break	Sponge	Suture
1 mm	5 mm radial	7 mm
2 mm	5 mm radial	7 mm
3 mm	5 mm radial	7 mm
4 mm	7 mm radial	9 mm
5 mm	7 mm radial	9 mm
6 mm	Circumferential	7 mm (in case of 5 mm sponge)

sponges and choose therefore in this case a 5 mm sponge. If the break is 4–5 mm in size, we choose a 7 mm sponge. If the break is larger than 5 mm, we place the 5–7 mm buckle circumferential. See Table 11.1.

11.2 Instruments

Here you will find all the details of our episcleral buckling instrument set, which we use at the University Hospital of Uppsala (Fig. 11.2). The instruments vary, of course, from hospital to hospital. The instruments in **bold** are absolutely necessary.

Blepharostat
1× Williams open adult
Cannulas
1× rough curved
Forceps
2× anatomical forceps
2× forceps claw 1 × 2
1× forceps Bonn
Scissors
1 scissors eyes straight sharp
1 scissors eyes bent sharp
1 scissors Westcott Geuder 19,750 (Fig. 11.3)
1 scissors straight Vannas **Geuder 19,760**
Clamping Scissors
2 clamping scissors bent Halstedt
2 clamping scissors Hartman straight
1 clamping scissors Crile straight 14 cm
Needle Holders
1 needle holder Barraquer without lock

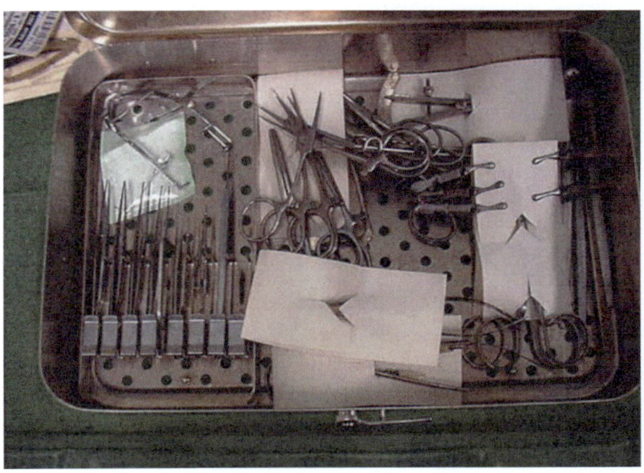

Fig. 11.2 Episcleral buckling instrument set

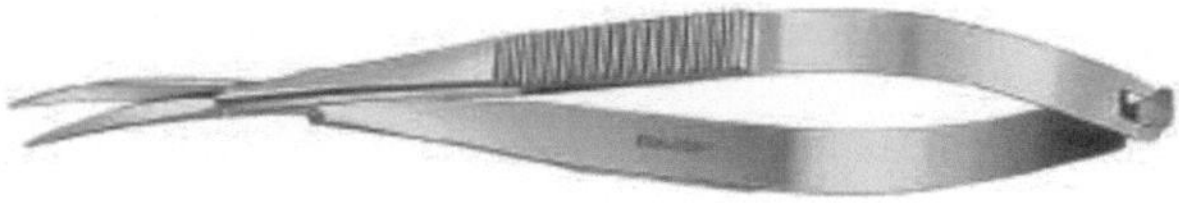

Fig. 11.3 Westcott scissors

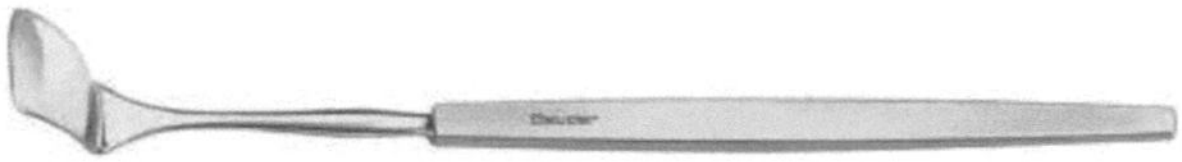

Fig. 11.4 Orbital spatula

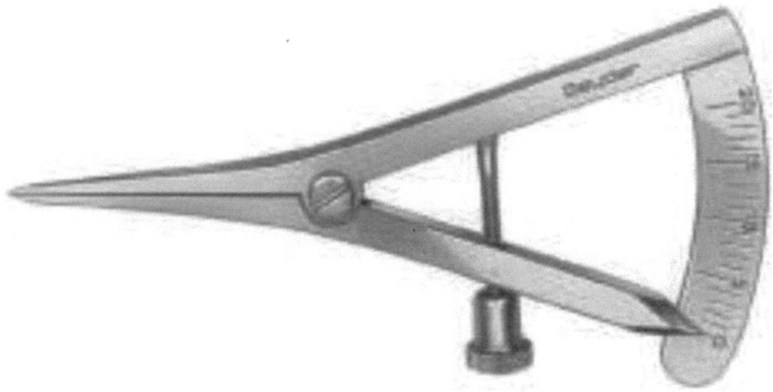

Fig. 11.5 Caliper

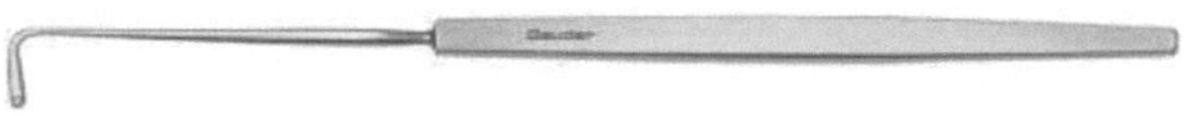

Fig. 11.6 Strabismus hook with hole

1 needle holder Snowden Pencer with lock
Orbital Spatula
1 orbital spatula Helvestone
1 orbital spatula Sautter Geuder 15,740 (Fig. 11.4)
Knot Holder
2 knot holder Rapp
Other
1 caliper Castroviejo straight 1–20 mm Geuder 19,135, (Fig. 11.5)
1 ruler.
4 clamp Diefenbach 2
1 depressor scleral with or without marker
1 strabismus hook Bonn 1 mm hole, Geuder 15,821, (Fig. 11.6)

11.3 Material

1. Silicone sponge (Fig. 11.7)

   • 5 × 3.77-mm-partial thickness sponge (Labtician, Canada) – our most commonly used silicone sponge. Indication: ora dialysis, all normal size breaks. This sponge requires a 7 mm marking.

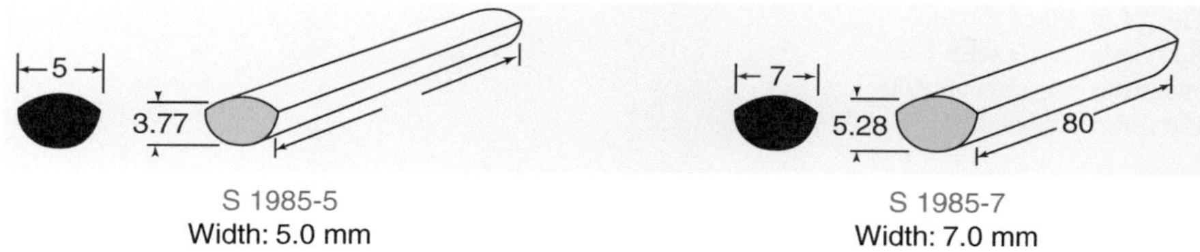

Fig. 11.7 Silicone sponge

- 7.0 × 5.28-mm-partial thickness sponge (Labtician, Canada) – less commonly used silicone sponge. Indication: big breaks. This sponge requires a 9.0 mm marking.

2. Surgical skin marker with ultra-fine tip (Many companies, e.g., 1456XL SR-100, Viscot Medical LLC, USA)
3. Supramid suture 4-0 (REF SP151399, Serag Wiessner, Germany); alternative: Polyester 5-0 (Alcon)
4. Silk suture 3-0 (Ethicon)

11.4 The Surgery

1. **180° limbal peritomy**
2. **2–3 traction sutures**
3. **Insertion of a chandelier light**
4. **Search for the retinal break with scleral depressor**
5. **Cryopexy of the break**
6. **Scleral marking of the break**
7. **Marking of sutures**
8. **Apply the sutures**
9. **Paracentesis, release aqueous from anterior chamber**
10. **Fasten the sponge**
11. **Inspect the retina**
12. **If sponge covers the break, fasten the sponge permanently. If sponge does not cover the break, then replace the sponge.**
13. **Remove the chandelier light and suture the sclerotomy with a Vicryl 8-0 suture.**
14. **Remove the traction sutures, and close the conjunctiva with Vicryl 6-0.**

The Surgery Step-by-Step (Figs. 11.8–11.25)

1. **180° limbal peritomy**
2. **Two or three traction sutures**

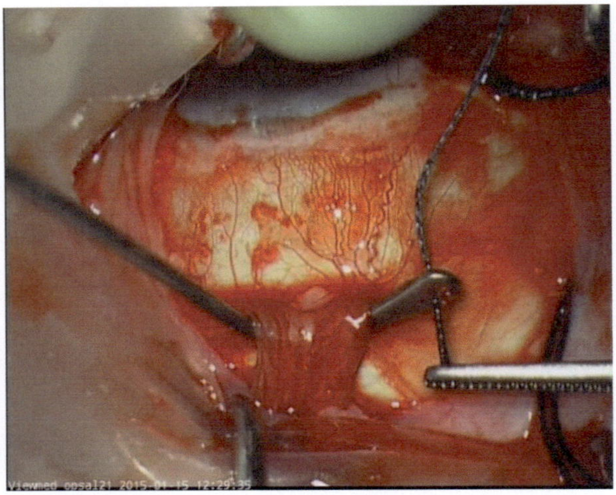

Fig. 11.8 Place a strabismus hook with hole under the complete muscle and insert a silk suture

The limbal peritomy and the three traction sutures are placed according to the location of the break. If the break is located at 12 o'clock, then the lateral rectus, medial rectus, and the superior rectus require traction sutures, and the limbal peritomy is located from 9 o'clock over 12 o'clock to 3 o'clock.

If the break is located at 1:30, then a limbal peritomy from 12:00 to 3:00 is performed, and two holding sutures are placed under the superior and lateral rectus muscle.

Perform a limbal peritomy, and place a strabismus hook with hole behind a straight muscle. Confirm that you grabbed the whole muscle because you may place a sponge beneath the muscle. Insert the silk suture into the hole, and retract the hook with the suture (Fig. 11.8). Tie a knot into the suture. Repeat this procedure with the two other straight muscles.

3. **Insertion of a chandelier light** (Fig. 11.9)

Continue with insertion of the chandelier light. The best location is opposite to the break. If the break is located superiorly, then insert the chandelier light inferiorly.

4. **Search for the break with scleral depressor** (Fig. 11.10)

Flick in the BIOM and search for the break. This maneuver is a bit more difficult compared to vitrectomy because the globe is more difficult to rotate. The search for a retinal hole goes like this: for example, with a retinal detachment from 6:00 to 10:00, place the scleral depressor at 10:00, and move it slowly in a straight line from the ora serrata toward the posterior pole. Look for a hole or a hole flap. Then continue placing the depressor at 9:30, move it in a straight line toward the posterior pole, and so on. It is like mowing a lawn.

5. **Cryopexy of the break** (Fig. 11.11)
6. **Scleral marking of the break** (Figs. 11.12 and 11.13)

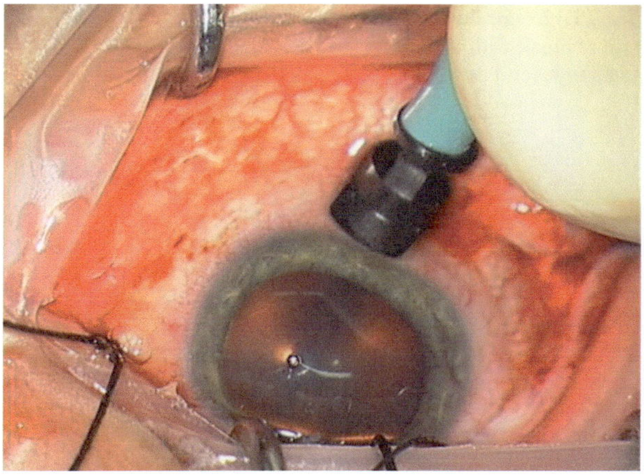

Fig. 11.9 Insert a chandelier light at 6 o'clock opposite to a break at 12 o'clock

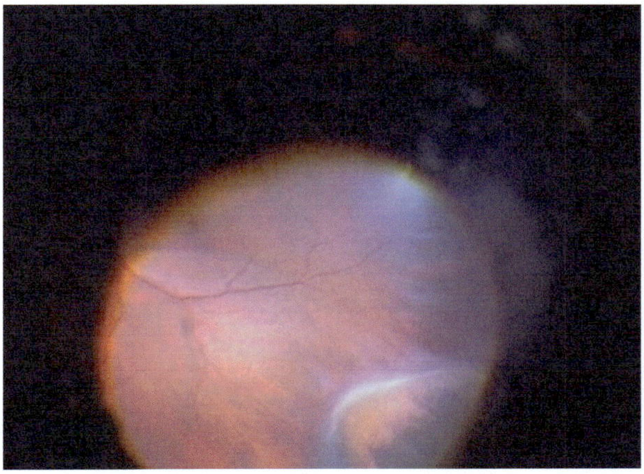

Fig. 11.10 It is easy to examine the retina with the microscope and a viewing system

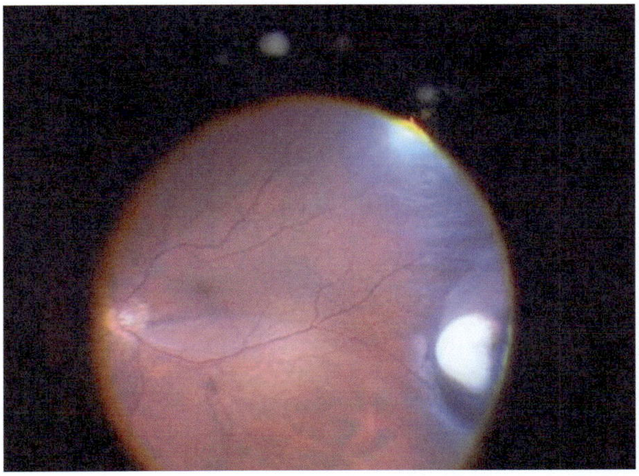

Fig. 11.11 Freeze the retinal break with the cryopexy hand piece

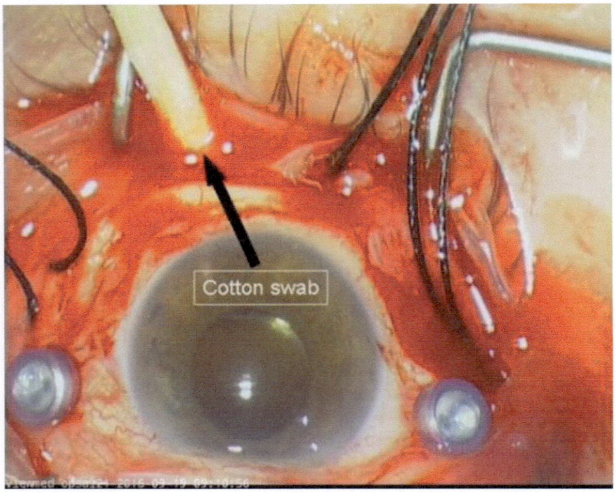

Fig. 11.12 Locate the retinal break with a cotton swab or scleral depressor

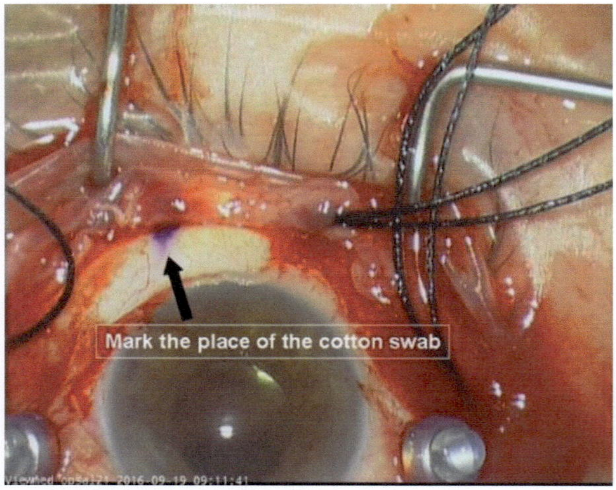

Fig. 11.13 Then mark the sclera or limbus at the position of the cotton swab

Freeze now the break (Fig. 11.11), keep the cryopexy hand piece in place, flick out the BIOM, rotate the globe, the assistant inserts an orbital spatula between tenon/conjunctiva and sclera to identify the freezing spot. Dry the freezing spot with a cotton swab and mark it with the surgical marker pen (Figs. 11.12 and 11.13). The sclera must be absolutely dry that you can mark it.

7. **Marking of sutures** (Figs. 11.14 and 11.15)

Decide now whether you want to apply a radial sponge or a limbus parallel (circumferential) sponge (Figs. 11.14 and 11.15). If the break is located under a muscle, an ora parallel (circumferential) approach is advisable because it is difficult to suture under the muscle. Paint the tips of the caliper with the surgical skin marker pen. Mark the sclera with the caliper (Geuder). How wide? Two millimeters more than the width of the sponge. If the sponge is 5 mm wide, then mark 7 mm.

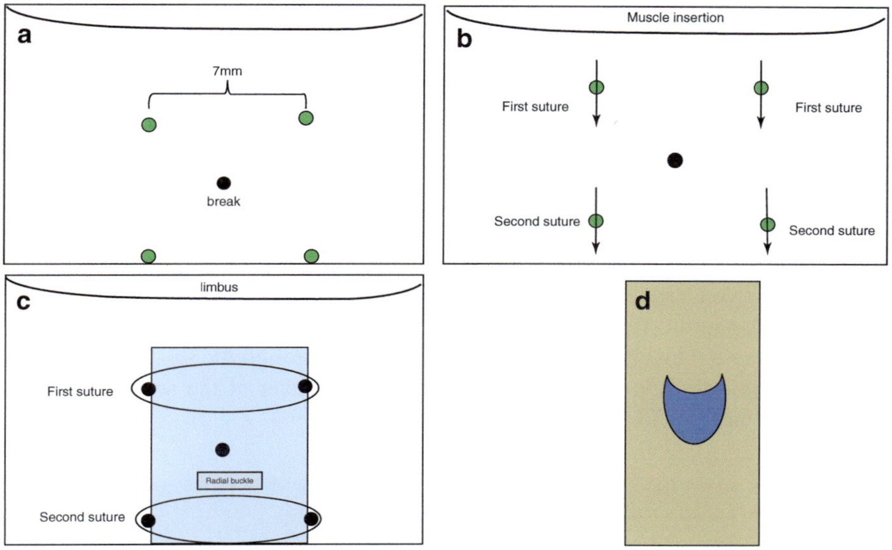

Fig. 11.14 A radial sponge. (**a**) Mark 7 mm anterior and posterior of the break. (**b**) Move the needle as depicted for the first and second suture. (**c**) After complete surgery. (**d**) The break is located in the middle of the radial sponge. No fish mouthing is possible

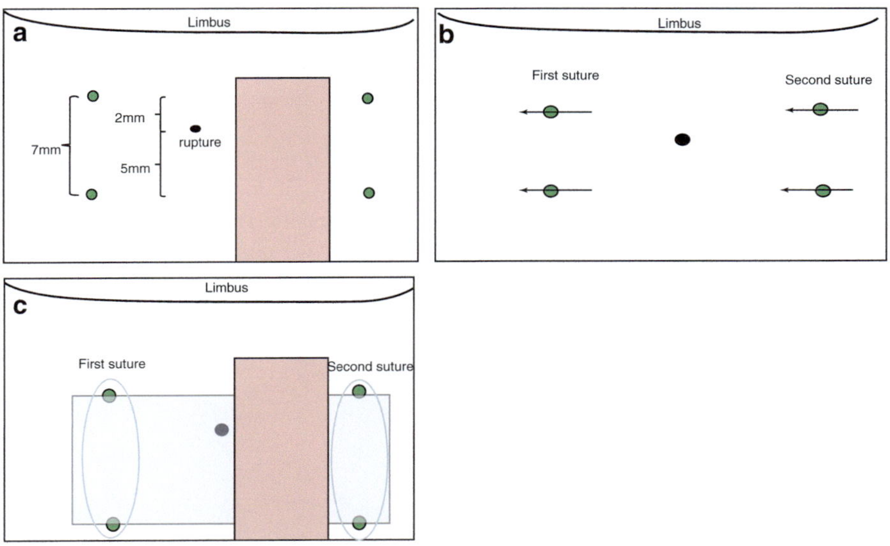

Fig. 11.15 A circumferential sponge. (**a**). Mark again 7 mm so that the retinal break is located in the upper half of the buckle. If the break is close to the muscle, then place the sponge under the muscle. (**b**) Place the first suture as depicted and then the second suture (**c**). Then place the sponge under the suture and tighten the knot with 2-1-1 throws (Supramid or Mersilene suture)

Where to mark? In case of a radial sponge, hold the caliper so that the hole is in the middle (Fig. 11.14) Make two markings approximately 2 millimeters anterior to the break and 2 millimeters' posterior to the break.

In case of an ora parallel (circumferential) sponge and a retinal break at 6:30 place two markings at 5:30 and two markings at 7:00 (Fig. 11.15). Place the silicone sponge under the inferior rectus muscle. The muscle force will help to indent the sponge.

8. **Apply the sutures** (Figs. 11.16–11.20)

You need one suture with one needle for two markings. Cut the suture in two halves so that you have two sutures with one needle each. How to suture? The suture is the most dangerous maneuver in the complete surgery because you can perforate the sclera. Move the needle less deep but a long way through the sclera. The needle must be visible through the sclera. Repeat this maneuver at the second marking (Figs. 11.19 and 11.20).

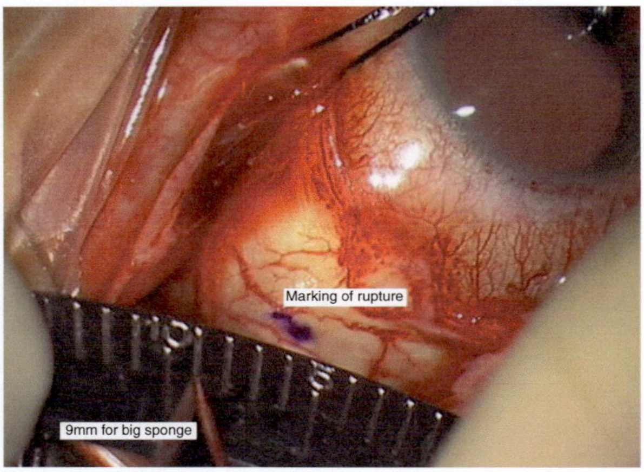

Fig. 11.16 Set the caliper to 9 mm for a big sponge and to 7 mm for a normal sponge

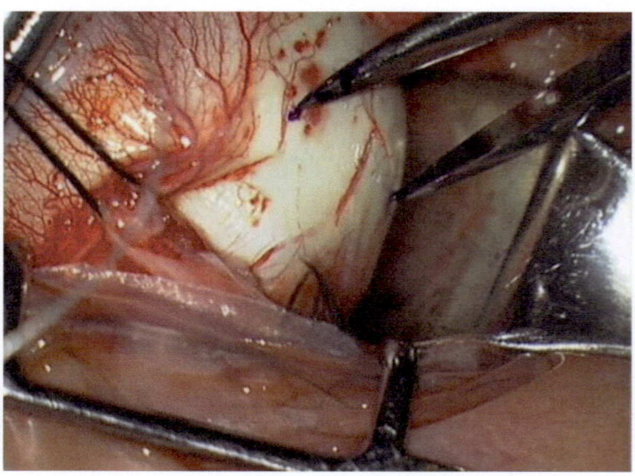

Fig. 11.17 Then mark the sclera with the caliper

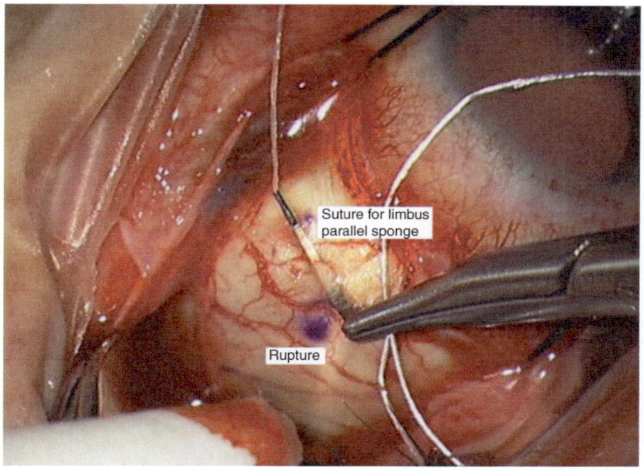

Fig. 11.18 Place the first scleral bite for limbus parallel (=circumferential) buckle

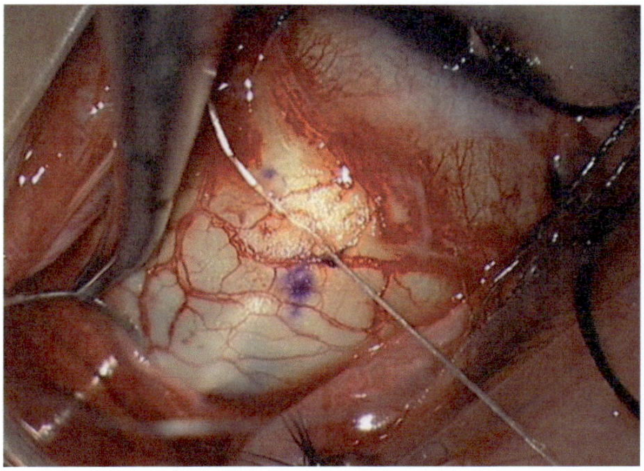

Fig. 11.19 Place the second scleral bite at the second marking

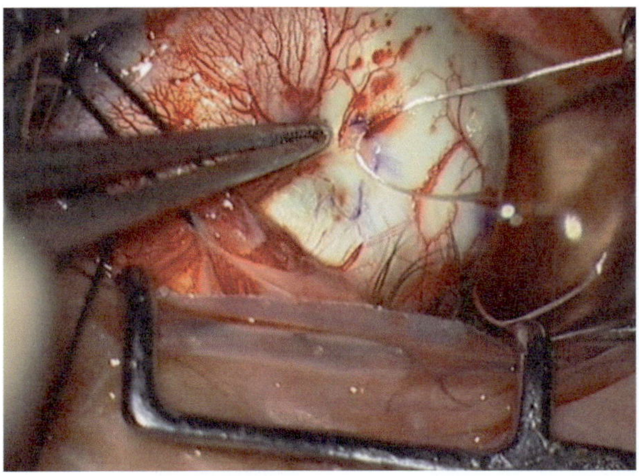

Fig. 11.20 The first suture is done

Surgical Pearls No. 70

Retinal tear under a muscle. Alternatively, to an ora parallel (=circumferential) sponge, you can apply a radial sponge. If you want to apply a radial sponge under the muscle, then remove the muscle, suture the sponge, and suture the muscle back to place or suture the sponge onto the muscle. If the patient experiences diplopia after surgery, you can remove the sponge after approximately 3–4 weeks.

9. **Paracentesis, release aqueous from anterior chamber**

You need a soft globe to achieve a proper indentation of the sponge. Perform a paracentesis and release aqueous from the anterior chamber.

10. **Fasten the sponge** (Figs. 11.21–11.23)

Place the silicone sponge under the sutures (Fig. 11.21), make two throws, tighten the suture a little bit, release tension on the traction sutures, and then tighten the suture again (Figs. 11.22, 11.23). The knot has 2-1-1 throws. Perform the same maneuver with the second suture. Important: do not pull the traction sutures while tying the sponge in order to achieve a good indentation.

11. **Inspect the retina**

Flick in the BIOM and inspect the retina. If the sponge does not cover the break, then reposition the sponge. The repositioning surgery goes usually faster than the first surgery.

12. **Remove the chandelier light**
13. **Remove the traction sutures and close the conjunctiva with Vicryl 6-0**

Remove the chandelier light and suture the sclerotomy with a Vicryl 8-0 suture. Continue with cutting the traction sutures and remove them. Replace the conjunctiva, and close it with Vicryl 6-0 or 8-0.

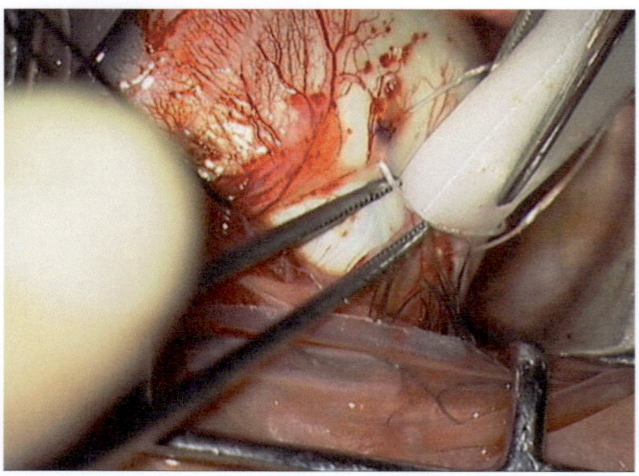

Fig. 11.21 Place the sponge under the suture

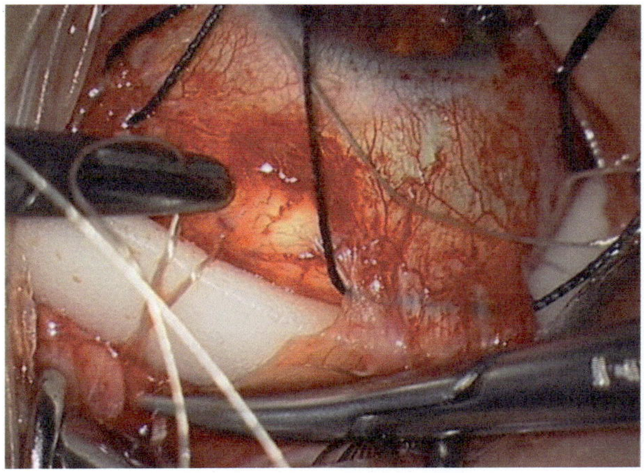

Fig. 11.22 Close the suture with 2-1-1 throws

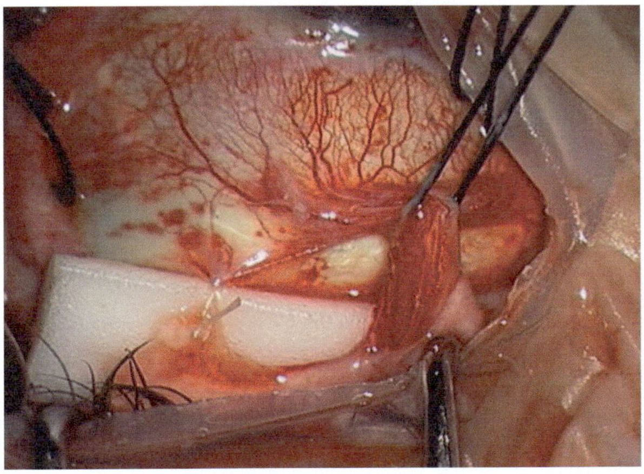

Fig. 11.23 Fasten the suture on both sides

11.5 Complications

Scleral Perforation (Video 11.4: **Complication During Episcleral Buckling**)

A scleral perforation can be seen by leakage of intraocular fluid. Redraw the needle, freeze the leakage site with cryopexy, and repeat the suture at a different location.

Repositioning a Buckle (Fig. 11.24 a–c)

It is no problem and in fact technically quite easy to reposition a wrongly placed buckle (Fig. 11.26a). In some cases, the perioperative visualization of the hole on the buckle is not easy. One day later at the slit lamp, the visualization is, however, in the most cases better. If the hole is located aside the buckle and not on the buckle, then try to estimate how many millimeters the hole is aside (Fig. 11.24b). Keep in mind that the silicone sponge is 5 mm wide. If, for example, the hole is located at 5:30 and the buckle at 6:00 (Fig. 11.24b), remove the old sponge, place new sutures 2.5 mm next to the old sutures, and refasten the same sponge (Fig. 11.24c).

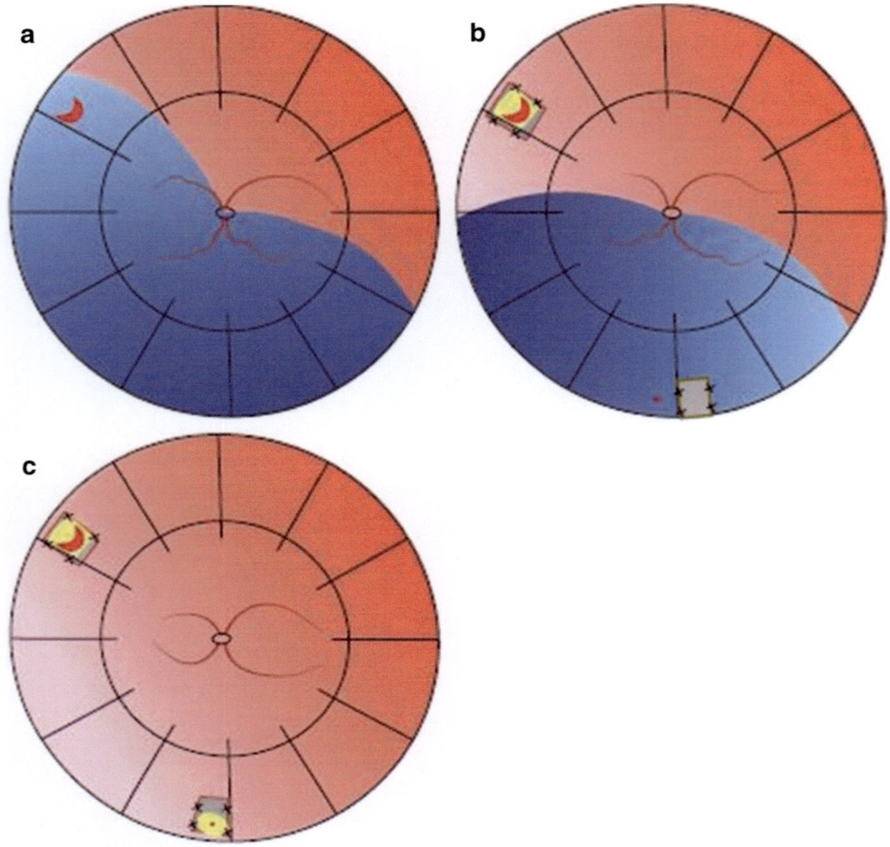

Fig. 11.24 (**a**) A superotemporal detachment with a rupture at 2 o'clock and at a second rupture at 6:15. (**b**) A residual detachment. The silicone sponge is placed on the break, and the break is dry. But the silicone sponge at 6 o'clock is wrongly placed, and the break at 6:15 is still detached. The buckle is 5 mm wide so you must replace the buckle 2.5 mm to the right side. (**c**) The sponge is correctly placed. 1 day later the retina is reattached, and the rupture is located now on the buckle

11.6 FAQ

Can I place a silicone sponge during vitrectomy?

Yes. If you want to buckle, for example, a break at 6 o'clock, then place a limbus parallel (=circumferential) silicone sponge under the inferior rectus.

What about episcleral buckling in a vitrectomized eye?

This is no problem. It is easier because the impression of the sponge is more pronounced due to the absent vitreous body. In case of a focal recurrent detachment, we often place a segmental buckle. Often the retinal break is difficult to find, and often it is a laser necrosis which causes a tiny break. Place a sponge on this laser-treated break, and the retina will be attached the next day.

Is it difficult to reposition a silicone sponge?

It is no problem and in fact technically easy to reposition a wrongly placed buckle, as well during the first surgery as during a second surgery. For more see chapter "Buckle with chandelier."

11.7 Brief Case Reports

1. 90 deg. circumferential buckle (Figs. 11.25 and 11.26)

Young myopic eyes with an inferior RD are a good indication for episcleral buckling surgery (Fig. 11.25 a, b). A 90 deg. circumferential buckle under one rectus muscle is required (Fig. 11.26). We employ always segmental buckles in these cases.

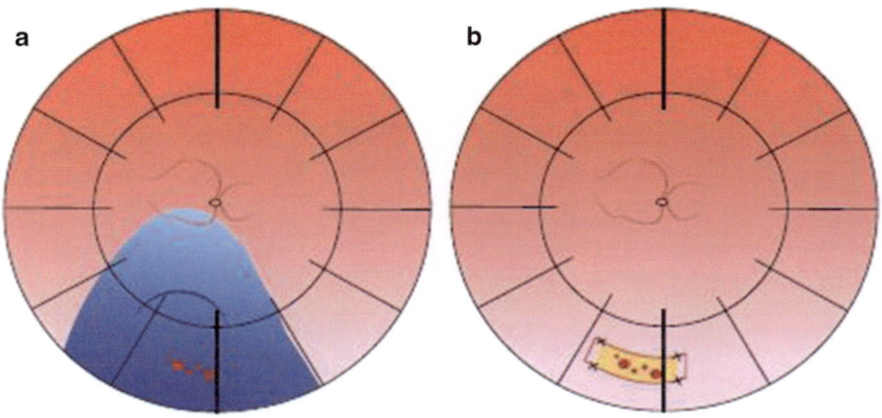

Fig. 11.25 (**a**) A young myopic patient with several retinal breaks at 6–7 o'clock. (**b**) A circumferential buckle is placed from 5:30 to 7:00, and the retina is reattached 1 day later

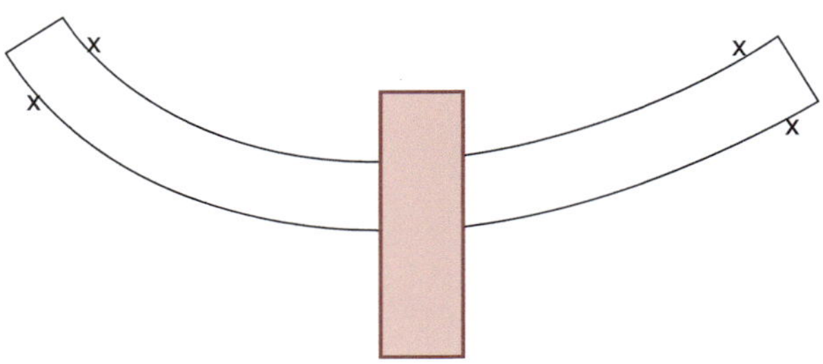

Fig. 11.26 A 90 deg. buckle is placed under one rectus muscle

Example: 27 y/o male patient with −3.5sph = 0.4 and an inferior detachment with six holes at 6–7 o'clock. Cryopexy and segmental buckle from 5 to 8 o'clock (under inferior rectus muscle).

2. Traumatic detachment: 90 deg. circumferential buckle (Figs. 11.27 and 11.28)

A traumatic detachment in a child's eye is a complicated retinal detachment (Fig. 11.29). But a reattachment is much easier to achieve with episcleral buckle than with vitrectomy. A vitrectomy is technically very difficult because you first need to perform most likely a phaco + IOL and then vitrectomize an inflamed eye resulting in increased PVR and recurrent detachment risk. If you choose episcleral buckling, things get much easier. The vitreous in children is clear and attached. The

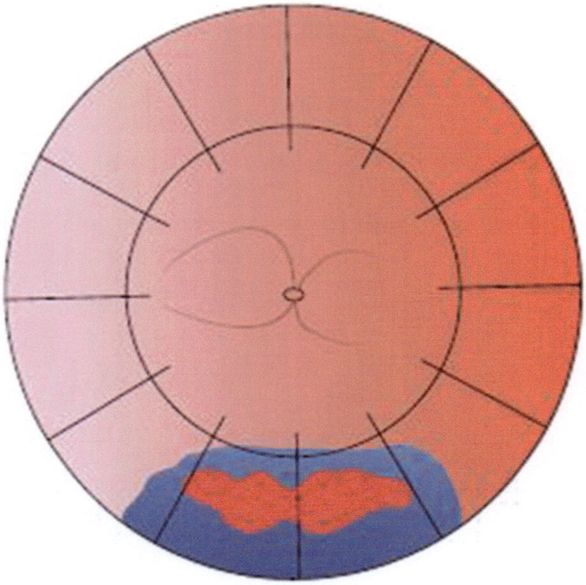

Fig. 11.27 A traumatic detachment from 5:00 to 7:00 and a focal detachment

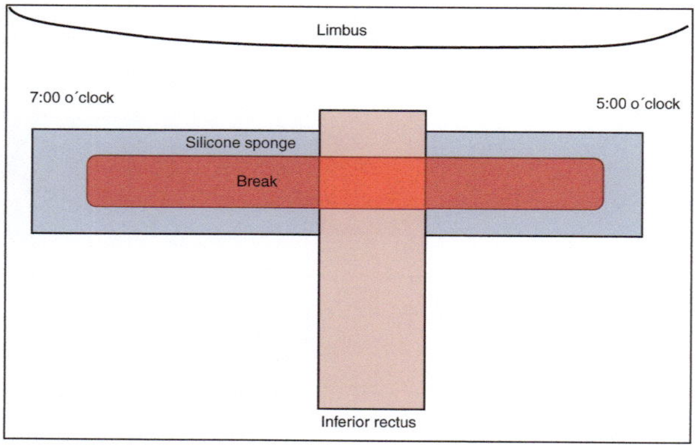

Fig. 11.28 A circumferential buckle is placed under the inferior rectus from 4:30 to 7:30

dense pediatric vitreous serves as a scaffold. These attributes facilitate working with a panophthalmoscope and the reattachment with a buckle. Example: 6 y/o boy with traumatic inferior detachment and a rupture from 5 to 7 o'clock. Cryopexy and segmental buckle from 4 to 8 o ´clock (under inferior rectus muscle) (Fig. 11.27).

3. Ora dialysis after trauma (Fig. 11.29)

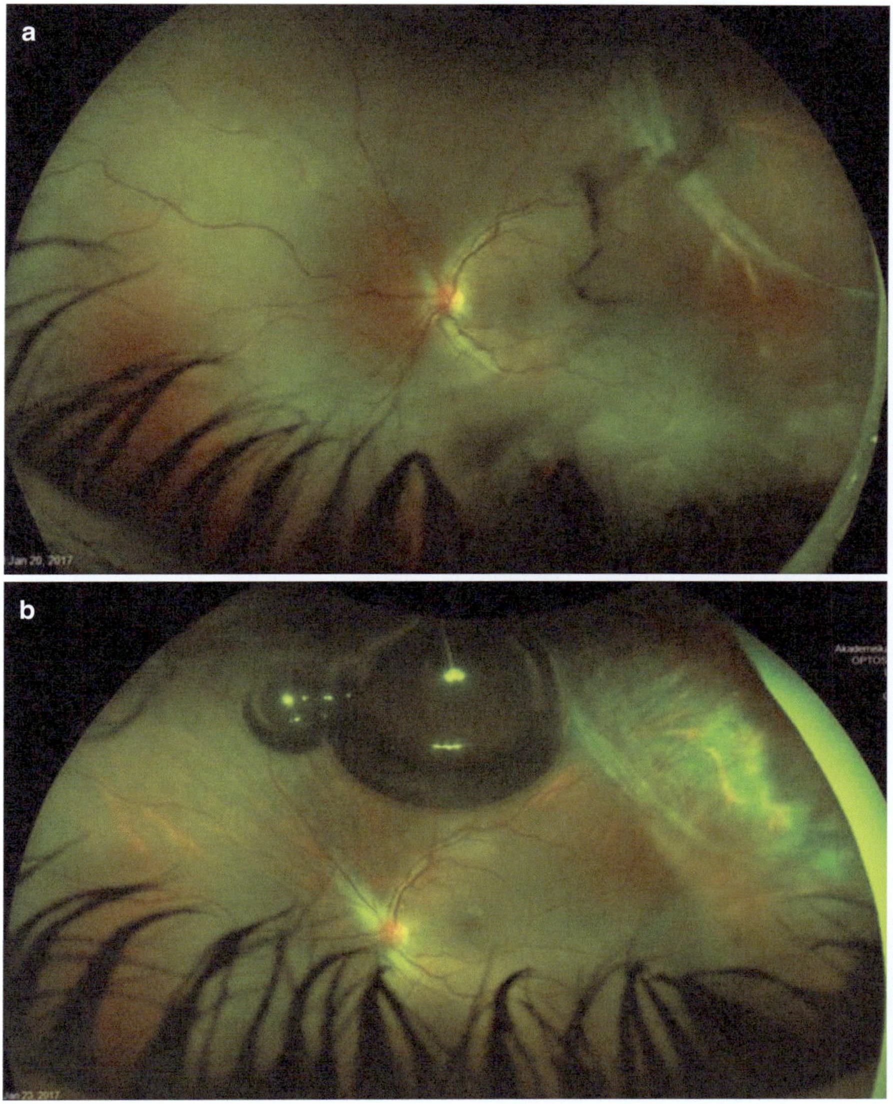

Fig. 11.29 A 7.0 × 5.28 mm partial thickness sponge (Labtician, Canada) was placed under the superior rectus at 12 o'clock and under the lateral rectus at 3 o'clock. In addition, 0.4 mL air was injected, and the patient was instructed to lie on the left cheek for 3 days. This pathology would be very difficult to fix with a vitrectomy

An 18 y/o male patient was hit in his left eye of a hockey stick. Due to visual acuity decrease, he visited an optician the following week. The optician stated a visual acuity decrease to 0.2 uncorrected and submitted him to the local eye clinic. Three weeks later he was examined at the local eye clinic, and a PVR detachment with a large ora dialysis was detected. The macula was shallowly detached, and the retinal edges at the ora dialysis were rolled in (Fig. 11.29). The visual acuity was +3.0sph = 0.1, and the IOP was 0 mmHg. He was consequently submitted to us for surgery.

I decided to perform an episcleral buckling. I always perform an episcleral buckling on young eyes because the optical media is excellent and the vitreous body is attached and intact and serves as an excellent scaffold when performing episcleral buckling. In my opinion a vitrectomy in these cases is extremely difficult and has a large complication spectrum. In contrast an episcleral buckling in traumatic detachment is fairly easy, and even if the surgery fails, you can convert to vitrectomy.

I operated with binocular indirect ophthalmoscope, cryopexy, and a 9 × 5,77 sponge from Labtician, Canada. The intraoperative retinal inspection showed a mini hole at 11:45, a large ora dialysis from 12 to 3 o'clock, and PVR from 3 to 6 o'clock. I placed the buckle under the superior and lateral rectus and placed a suture at 11:30, 1:30, and 3:30. The suture at 1:30 is necessary to achieve a sufficient impression. I injected 0.5 mL air to attach the enrolled retinal edge. I also injected triamcinolone subconjunctivally to reduce PVR risk and to increase the IOP.

The 3-day follow-up showed a completely attached retina, VA was 0.2 without correction, a 20% air bubble, and an IOP of 18 mmHg. The enrolled edges persist and the choroid is visible.

The 1 month follow-up showed a completely attached retina, VA was 0.2 with −3.0D an IOP of 16 mmHg. The retina is completely attached. The enrolled edges persist.

Further Reading

Kreissig I. A practical guide to minimal surgery for retinal detachment. Stuttgart: Thieme; 2000. isbn:9783131110619.

Chapter 12
Vitrectomy for Easy Retinal Detachment

Extras: Videos 12.1, 12.2, and 12.3.

12.1 Introduction

A rhegmatogenous retinal detachment (RRD) with multiple breaks is a surgery for experienced surgeons, as there is a significant complication profile. The beginner should start with a localized detachment (one to two quadrant detachment and a single break), as this is usually easier to manage.

Regarding surgery, we recommend two things, which simplify vitrectomy very much: phacoemulsification and usage of a chandelier light. First, we recommend performing a phacoemulsification in all patients older than 50 years because the anterior vitreous and the vitreous base can be removed completely (Fig. 12.1). Secondly, we recommend the usage of a chandelier light because it facilitates every step of the vitrectomy. Visualization and removal of the vitreous base are easier with a chandelier light. The retinal breaks are located in the periphery and need to be indented with the scleral depressor: nobody indents as well as your second hand.

PFCL or no PFCL?

Some vitreoretinal clinics use PFCL as a routine; others hate it. PFCL is an excellent tool for vitreoretinal surgery, and we recommend using it, if necessary. We use PFCL in large, macula-off detachments, and we work without PFCL in focal, macula-on detachments. In giant tears we always use PFCL due to the risk of slippage.

25G or 27G?

27G is superior to 25G in myopic eyes. 27G sclerotomies require no suture. Myopic eyes tend to leak, and 27G sclerotomies have only minimal leakage.

Electronic Supplementary Material The online version of this chapter (https://doi.org/10.1007/978-3-319-89677-9_12) contains supplementary material, which is available to authorized users.

U. Spandau, H. Heimann, *Practical Handbook for Small-Gauge Vitrectomy*,
https://doi.org/10.1007/978-3-319-89677-9_12

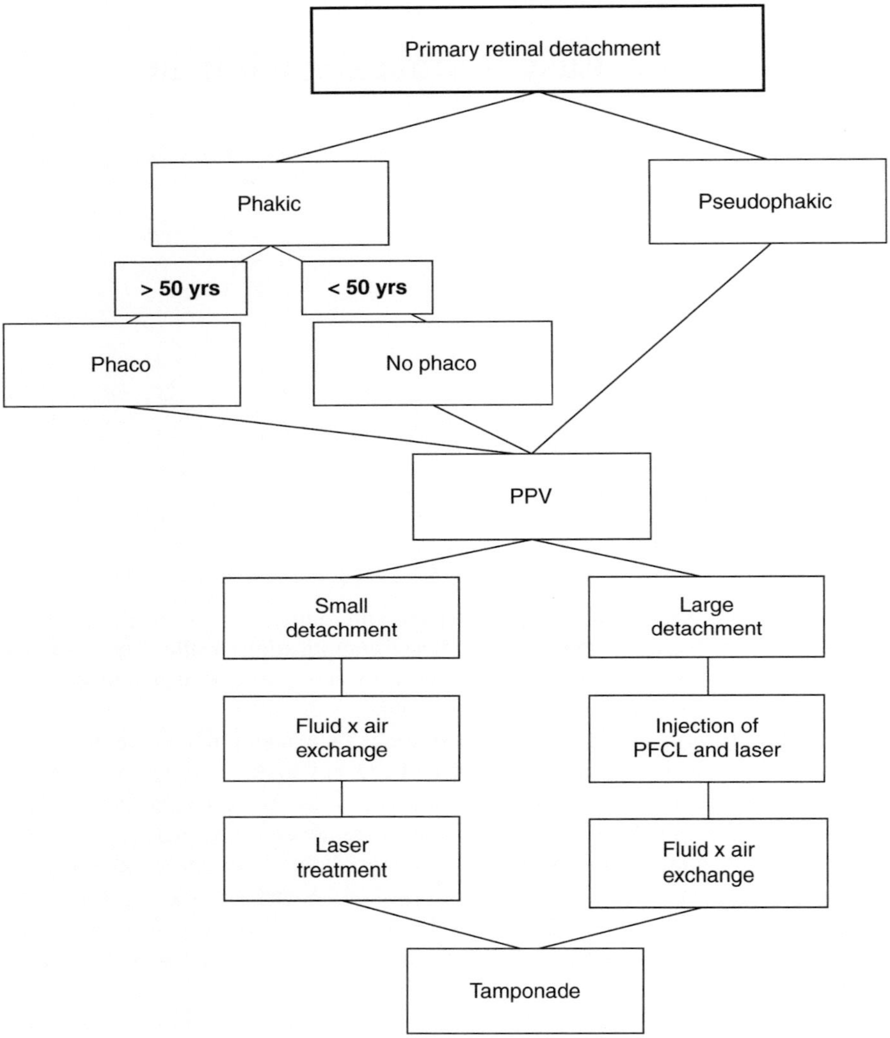

Fig. 12.1 Our treatment algorithm for retinal detachment surgery

Minimal leakage results also in improved gas tamponade. The disadvantage of 27G is the soft instruments. In normal eyes, a 25G cutter is therefore recommended.

12.2 The Surgery

12.2.1 Instruments

1. 25-/27-gauge three-port trocar system
2. Chandelier light

3. 120D lens
4. Endodiathermy
5. Endolaser
6. Backflush instrument
7. Scleral depressor

12.2.2 Dye

Possibly: Triamcinolone to stain the vitreous

12.2.3 Tamponade

Intraoperative: PFCL

Postoperative: 20% SF_6 and 15% C_2F_6

Individual Steps

1. **25G/27G three-port system with chandelier light**
2. **Phacoemulsification with IOL**
3. **Core vitrectomy and posterior vitreous detachment**
4. **Marking of breaks with endodiathermy**
5. **Injection of PFCL up to the posterior edge of the break and drainage of subretinal fluid**
6. **Vitrectomy of the break flap and the peripheral vitreous**
7. **PFCL injection up to ora serrata**
8. **Laser photocoagulation around breaks**
9. **Trimming of the vitreous base (shaving)**
10. **Fluid/air exchange**
11. **Drainage of subretinal fluid**
12. **Complete laser coagulation**
13. **Gas tamponade**
14. **Removal of trocars**
15. **Postoperative posture**

12.2.4 The Surgery Step-by-Step (Figs. 12.2–12.16)

1. **25G/27G three-port system with chandelier light** (Fig. 12.2)

Insert the trocars at the usual locations 3.5 mm behind the limbus. Visualize the location of the infusion cannula in order to avoid a choroidal detachment. Then insert the chandelier light inferonasally 3.5 mm behind the limbus.

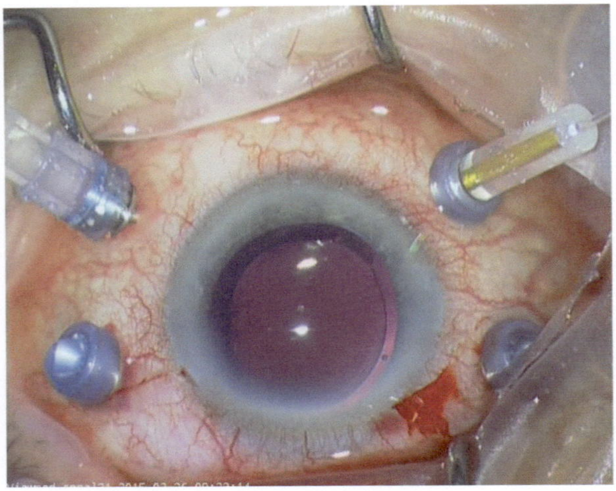

Fig. 12.2 Our regular setup for retinal detachment. Three-port vitrectomy and one chandelier light at the inferotemporal position

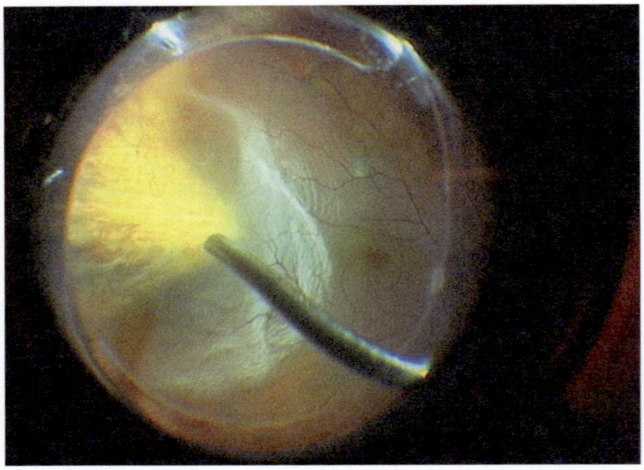

Fig. 12.3 The retinal break is hard to visualize

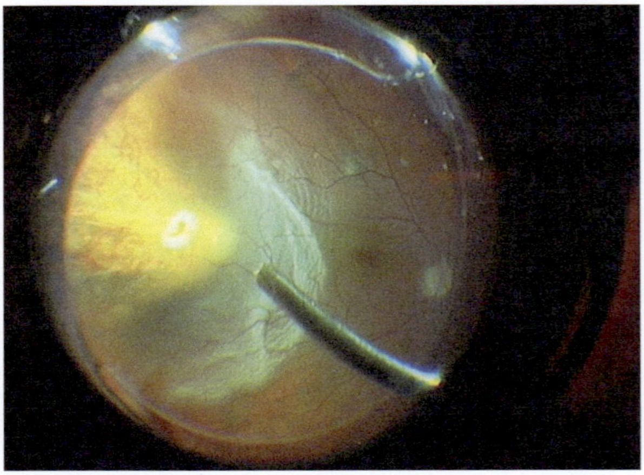

Fig. 12.4 After diathermy of the retinal edges, the retinal break is easy to visualize

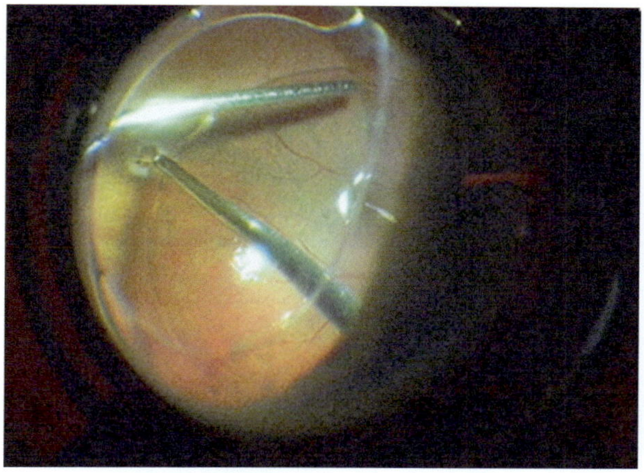

Fig. 12.5 Injection of PFCL and at the same time aspiration of subretinal fluid from the retinal break

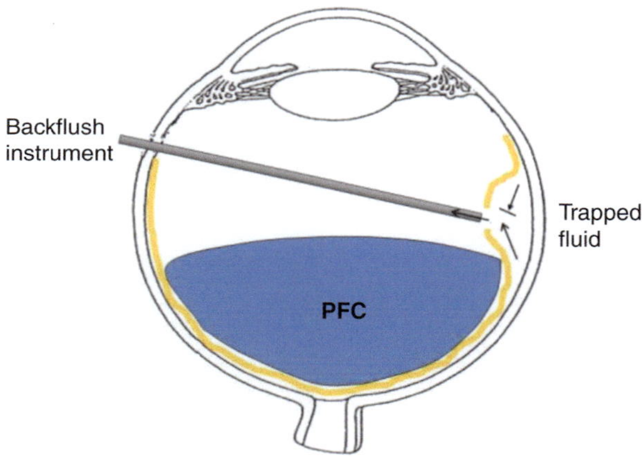

Fig. 12.6 Aspiration of subretinal fluid from retinal break. Note that only the posterior subretinal fluid can be removed and not the anterior located fluid. It will be removed later

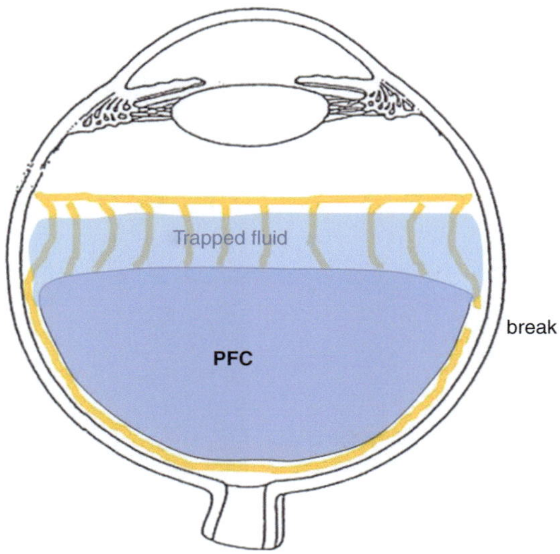

Fig. 12.7 Inject PFCL to the ora serrata. Note the trapped fluid anterior to the break

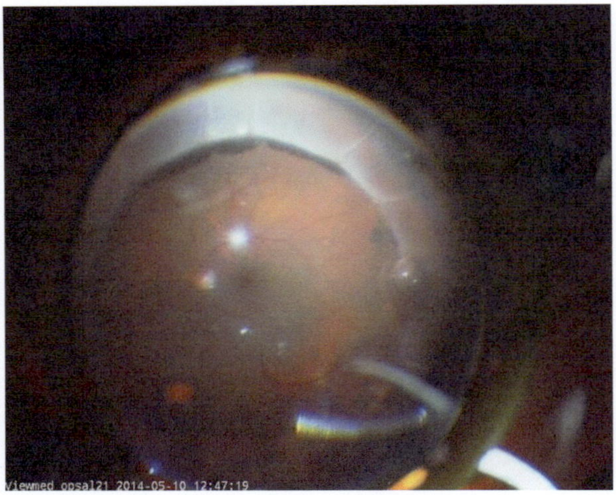

Fig. 12.8 Much trapped fluid anterior to the retinal break is visible

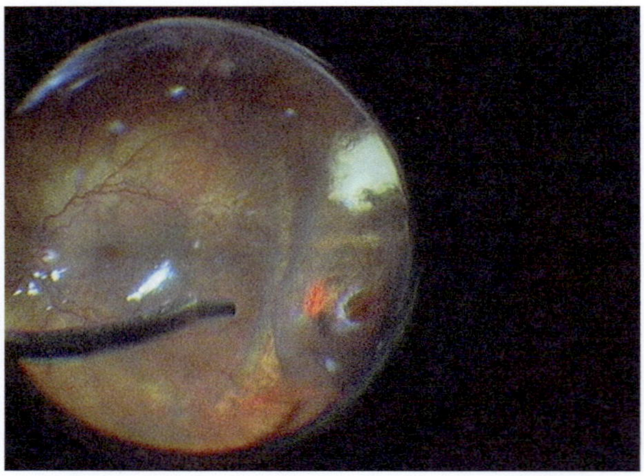

Fig. 12.9 Laser treat the complete hole after removal of subretinal fluid

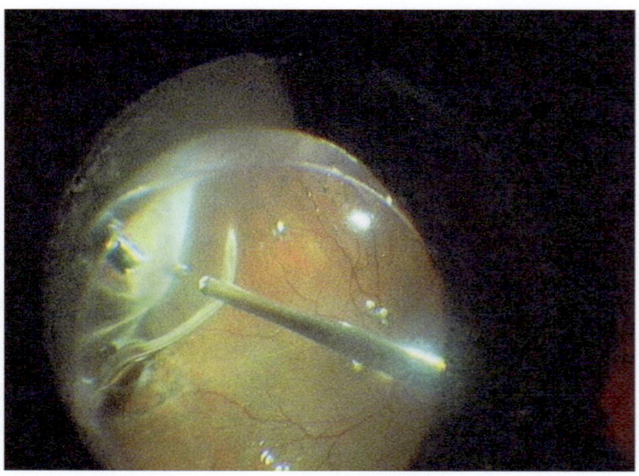

Fig. 12.10 Observe the "empty space" between the retina and PFCL. The empty space is vitreous

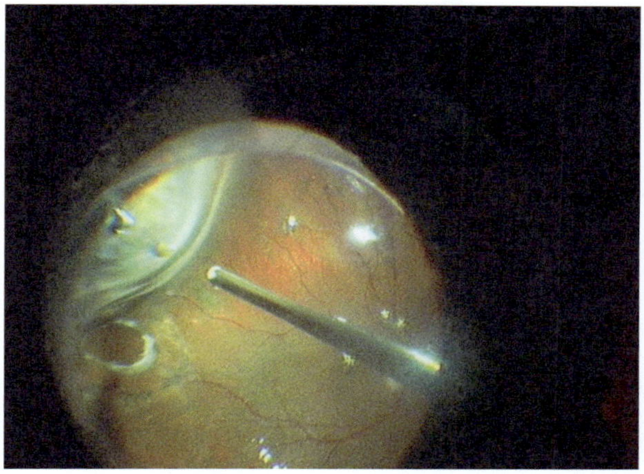

Fig. 12.11 Remove the peripheral vitreous and the PFCL will attach onto the retina

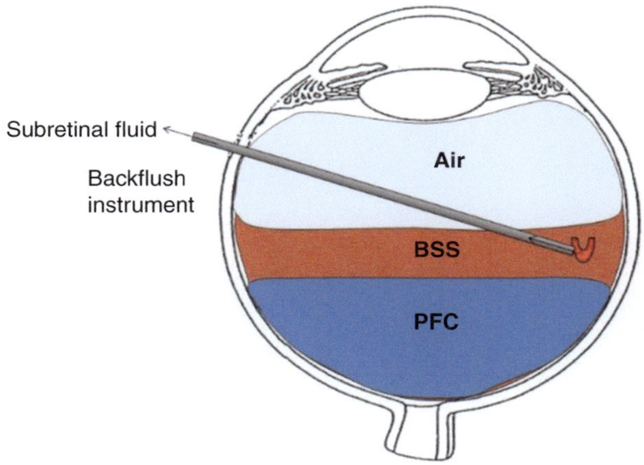

Fig. 12.12 Sandwich tamponade with air and PFCL. Aspirate first BSS and then PFCL until the PFCL meniscus reaches the posterior edge of the hole

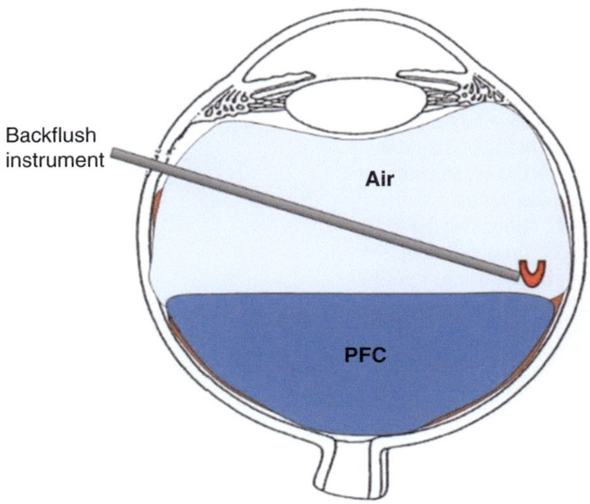

Fig. 12.13 If the PFCL has reached the posterior edge of the retinal break, then aspirate the subretinal fluid anterior to the retinal break. Then you can continue to remove the residual PFCL

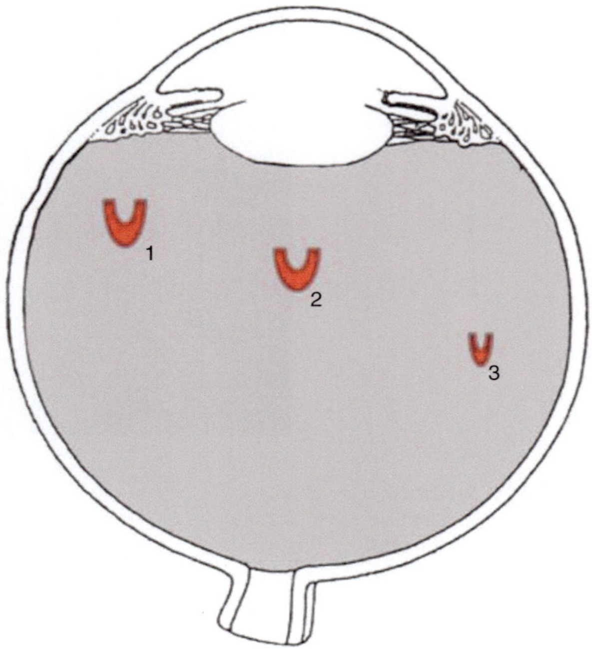

Fig. 12.14 If several holes are present, then start to remove subretinal fluid from hole 1 and continue with hole 2 and then 3

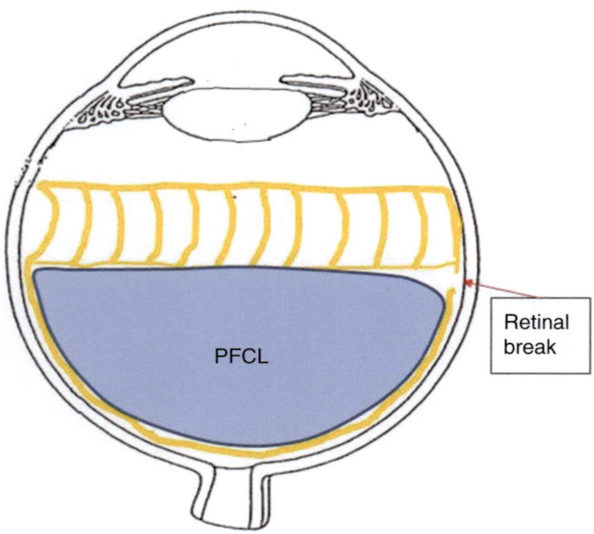

Fig. 12.15 Only if the complete trapped fluid is removed, you can continue with removal of PFCL. Otherwise the trapped fluid will flow toward the posterior pole and detach the macula

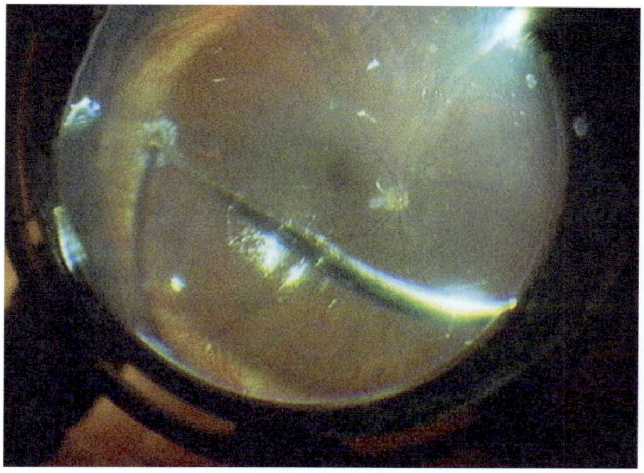

Fig. 12.16 Complete laser photo coagulation if necessary

2. **Phacoemulsification**

The IOL can be implanted in this step or later when all the breaks are treated (step 10). The advantage of early IOL implantation is that one works with a stable anterior segment and the IOL implantation is usually easier at this stage compared to the end of the surgery. The disadvantage is that the edge of the IOL may interfere with the view of the retinal periphery and the vitreous base. In detachment surgeries we prefer the implantation of a 3-piece IOL. Three-piece IOL's have stronger haptics than 1-piece IOL's resulting in an immediate stable fixation of the IOL in the lens capsule.

Surgical Pearls No. 71

Phaco or no phaco: If a cataract is present, then remove it during the same surgery. Why? The vitrectomy and the gas tamponade will increase the lens opacification resulting in a bad view to retina. The risk that you miss a recurrent detachment is high especially if it is inferior.

Surgical Pearls No. 72

Corneal suture: In case of an unstable anterior chamber, place a single 10-0 nylon suture at the end of the phaco and IOL. This avoids accidental opening of the corneal wound during indentation, which may lead to flattening of the anterior chamber and even dislocation of the IOL. The suture can be removed once the vitrectomy has been completed.

Surgical Pearls No. 73

Corneal lubrication: A major problem during vitrectomy, especially in combined surgeries with duration of over 1 h, is corneal epithelial edema. With generous application of methylcellulose (Celoftal, Alcon), the cornea remains clear for the complete surgery.

3. **Core vitrectomy and posterior vitreous detachment**

Perform a core vitrectomy and identify the posterior vitreous face to verify that a PVD is present. If the vitreous is still attached, perform induction of a PVD. Then continue with vitrectomy, and search for retinal breaks. Carefully remove the vitreous close to the retina in the area of detached, fluttering retina.

Surgical Pearls No. 74

PVD in RRD: In about 15% of patients with RRD, the vitreous is still attached at the posterior pole. One group at risk is myopic patients below the age of 50 years with multiple small round breaks. The vitreous may be very adherent to the retina in such cases, and trying to induce a PVD can lead to multiple iatrogenic breaks. These cases usually do very well with scleral buckling surgery. If in doubt, check the status of vitreous attachment/detachment with preoperative ultrasound before deciding to perform a vitrectomy.

Surgical Pearls No. 75

Triamcinolone and RRD: Many cases of RRD are caused by strong vitreoretinal adhesion. It may not be possible to separate the vitreous and retina simply by engaging the vitreous with the vitreous cutter and pulling it off the retina – you may enlarge pre-existing breaks or induce iatrogenic breaks in some cases. If you find very strong vitreoretinal adhesions, it is advisable to "stop pulling" and start "shaving" the vitreous of the retina. This is facilitated by staining the adherent vitreous with triamcinolone. When staining the vitreous with triamcinolone, use minimal amounts, and direct the injection to the area of interest. We dilute triamcinolone 1:3 with BSS. Injecting too much triamcinolone may interfere with your view, and it can be cumbersome to remove this later on in the procedure.

4. **Mark the breaks with endodiathermy** (Figs. 12.3 and 12.4)

The key concept of all retinal detachment surgeries is to identify and treat all retinal breaks. Perform a thorough internal search for breaks following Lincoff rules that point to the most likely areas of retinal breaks. If you fail to identify and treat a retinal break in detached retina, failure and retinal redetachment following vitrectomy are guaranteed. Mark the edges of the break with endodiathermy. A break, which is not marked, is hard to identify when it is attached to the underlying retinal pigment epithelium.

Surgical Pearls No. 76

Unseen breaks and Schlieren phenomenon: Inject PFCL slowly and watch for the "Schlieren phenomenon." In particular, in long-standing RRD, the subretinal fluid appears like a muddy stream when entering the vitreous cavity. This "Schlieren phenomenon" may point to the location of the retinal break at the entry site of the Schlieren in cases of "unseen breaks."

5. **Injection of PFCL to posterior edge of break and drainage of subretinal fluid**

The PFCL has three tasks in detachment surgery:

1. Stabilization of the mobile retina
2. Removal of the subretinal fluid
3. Elevation of the peripheral vitreous

The PFCL pushes the subretinal fluid from the central pole toward the periphery and presses it through the retinal break into the vitreous cavity. First, the PFCL is injected up to the posterior edge of the most central break, while we observe how the subretinal fluid is forced through the break into the vitreous cavity. You can accelerate this step by aspirating subretinal fluid actively with the Charles flute needle (Figs. 12.5 and 12.6). The PFCL also has the effect that the mobile retina is attached, and a vitrectomy in the vicinity of the detached retina is less dangerous (Fig. 12.7).

Surgical Pearls No. 77
PFCL is quite expensive. In more complicated cases, it may be necessary to perform multiple manipulations under PFCL, occasionally removing and then again adding PFCL at a later stage. If PFCL needs to be removed, you can easily aspirate it back into the injection syringe for re-injection at a later stage of the procedure.

6. **Vitrectomy of the tear flap and the peripheral vitreous**

After ensuring the presence and completion of a PVD, the next step is to perform a trimming of the vitreous base. Start within the area of the break(s) and also remove the flap, as the vitreous traction on the flap caused the detachment. The scleral depressor in the second hand is a great help when indenting the retina.

7. **PFCL injection up to ora serrata**

Depending on the anterior/posterior location of the break, there is more or less subretinal fluid anterior to the break (trapped fluid) (Figs. 12.7 and 12.8). If a break is located at the ora serrata, you can drain the residual subretinal fluid with a complete PFCL fill. However, if the break is located between the equator and ora serrata, then a complete drainage of subretinal fluid is not possible. The subretinal fluid is trapped between the break and the ora serrata (Figs. 12.7 and 12.8). In the first case, you can proceed with laser photocoagulation. In the latter case, a complete laser coagulation is not possible because the retinal break is partially detached. You can perform a partial laser photocoagulation and complete the laser after the fluid-air exchange in step 10.

Surgical Pearls No. 78
Iatrogenic break: If the retinal break and the bullous detachment are far apart from each other, it is difficult to drain the subretinal fluid from the break. In the first case, one can try to massage the subretinal fluid with a scleral depressor to the break or perform an iatrogenic break in the area of trapped fluid. Mark the inferior retina close to the ora serrata with endodiathermy. Then cut a hole with the vitreous cutter (setting, approx. 300 cuts/min) by suctioning the retina and then cutting it cautiously. Drain the subretinal fluid from this break. Another alternative is the aspiration of the subretinal fluid with a 41G cannula.

8. **Laser therapy of breaks** (Fig. 12.9)

Apply three rows of laser burns around the breaks. The settings depend on the laser device. It is possible that subretinal fluid has accumulated anterior to the break (so-called trapped fluid) which makes it difficult to apply a laser onto the anterior part of the break. Try to indent the break with the scleral depressor, so that the subretinal fluid is pushed away. Apply white laser burns. A good alternative is to freeze the break with a cryoprobe. If you do not succeed due to excess trapped fluid, then complete the laser treatment in a later step.

Surgical Pearls No. 79
Laser: Be careful with your laser energy. Only a mild whitening of the RPE is necessary. 200 msec duration is sufficient; 300 msec is too much, you may create a laser necrosis. Burns which are too strong will weaken the retina and are a predilection site for the formation of new retinal breaks. They may also cause contraction of the choroid or even choroidal hemorrhages. A typical beginner's mistake is to perform too much laser or cryotherapy as an extra safety measure that then may turn out to have exactly the opposite effect.

Surgical Pearls No. 80
Laser cerclage: A circumferential 360° laser is not recommended. It is essential to identify and treat all retinal breaks. A circumferential laser has the big disadvantage that in case of a redetachment, the breaks are difficult to find within the patches of chorioretinal atrophy.

Surgical Pearls No. 81
Laser necrosis: Another complication of laser is a retinal necrosis. Too high laser intensity may cause a necrosis of the retina and small, difficult-to-find holes. These tears occur often at the outer edge of the laser treatment. The same applies for cryopexy.

9. **Trimming of vitreous base (shaving)** (Figs. 12.10 and 12.11)

If it has not been performed before, a thorough vitrectomy of the vitreous base has to be performed at this stage using the scleral depressor. This procedure is also called "shaving." PFCL lifts the vitreous up and enables a secure and thorough trimming of the vitreous base. In those areas, where PFCL does not rest on the retina, there is vitreous which has to be removed. Indent the sclera and move the vitreous cutter along the meniscus of the PFCL. Hereby you can maneuver the vitreous cutter very close to the retina because the heavy liquid presses against the retina.

Surgical Pearls No. 82
Trimming of vitreous base: There are various ways to trim the vitreous base – (a) bimanual technique using a scleral indentor, (b) removal under coaxial light (only with microscope illumination) by using a cotton wool swab or a scleral depressor to indent the sclera, or (c) using the light fiber as an external scleral depressor (this gives you a focused beam of light transsclerally to illuminate the vitreous base).

10. **Fluid against air exchange**

If the shaving is finished, a PFCL × air exchange is performed. Before we perform this procedure, we have a look at Diagram 12.1, to get a better sense of the situation in the vitreous cavity. Before the PFCL x air exchange, the vitreous cavity

Intraoperatively			Postoperatively
PFCL x air exchange			
Before	During	After	
BSS	Air	Gas	Gas
	BSS		
PFCL	PFCL		Aqueous

Diagram 12.1 Diagram of the location of fluids during the PFCL × air exchange

is filled with PFCL, and on top of it is a layer of water. During the PFCL x air exchange, there is an anterior phase of air, a middle phase of water, and a posterior phase of PFCL. After the PFCL x air exchange, only air is in the eye, which is then replaced by gas. Postoperatively, water will accumulate again under the gas phase. Consequently, the gas does not effectively tamponade the lower pole.

The PFCL × air exchange is certainly the most difficult and most important maneuver in the whole detachment surgery, mainly because visibility under air is bad. Therefore, it is essential to understand the characteristics of PFCL and air. PFCL and air "work" as antagonists. Air exerts a pressure in the eye from peripheral (anterior) to central (posterior) but PFCL vice versa from posterior to anterior.

PFCL presses most of the subretinal fluid from the central pole to the periphery through the retinal break into the vitreous cavity, but a part of it flows beyond the break up to the ora serrata, where it cannot be aspirated ("trapped fluid") (Figs. 12.7 and 12.8). This "trapped fluid" can, however, be removed with air: the air attaches the retina beginning in the periphery and ending at the central pole and thereby pushes the "trapped fluid" in the direction of the break (Figs. 12.12 and 12.13).

11. **Drainage of subretinal fluid**

How do we proceed in practice? Before you switch to air, hold the flute tip in the middle of the break. If necessary, take the scleral depressor to help. If several breaks are present, start with the most peripherally located break and then move to the next more central break (Fig. 12.14). Now, the scrub nurse switches the three-way tap from BSS to air. In the beginning, disturbing air bubbles arise and the view deteriorates. Remain calm and turn the front lens with the BIOM-focus wheel up. The visibility will gradually improve.

In the beginning the break is covered with PFCL. After a short time, the PFCL is suctioned to the posterior edge of the break. Now the air presses the subretinal fluid in the direction of the break. The subretinal fluid is trapped between anterior located air and posterior located PFCL, so-called sandwich tamponade. Now you aspirate the subretinal fluid through the break and at the same time the BSS phase between air and PFCL (Figs. 12.12, 12.13, and 12.15).

Only when the "trapped fluid" and the BSS in the vitreous cavity are completely aspirated, can you continue to aspirate PFCL beyond the posterior edge of the break. This is very important because the subretinal fluid, which you do not aspirate, will continue to flow beyond the break in the direction of the optic disc.

If the "trapped fluid" is completely removed, you switch with the flute needle alternately between the PFCL bubble in order to reduce it and the break in order to aspirate fluid here. Try to aspirate without indenting the break. But sometimes you can only reach the break with the flute needle if you indent it with the scleral depressor. But you should not indent the break itself, but the retina on either side of the break. By indenting the break, you close it and prevent the aspiration of subretinal fluid. This procedure is usually not easy and requires patience.

The remaining PFCL is aspirated by holding the flute tip directly in front of the optic disc. Make sure that the PFCL is completely removed and that neither the retina nor the optic disc is affected.

If after complete removal of PFCL residual subretinal fluid remains in the central pole, then you may either inject PFCL again up to the break and aspirate the fluid or – if it is only a small amount – leave it. The subretinal fluid will be absorbed on the first postoperative day.

Surgical Pearls No. 83
Air test for detachment: When the retina is completely attached under air, you have drained the subretinal fluid completely. Air presses the entire subretinal fluid from the periphery to the optic disc, where it is easy to spot. This is only partly true for PFCL because PFCL pushes the subretinal fluid from the posterior pole to the periphery, where the "trapped fluid" is hard to detect.

Surgical Pearls No. 84
Active aspiration: In 25G/27G the aspiration of subretinal fluid is easier and more effective with active (than passive) aspiration. If you do not want to use PFCL, e.g., because only a focal retinal detachment is present, then you should absolutely aspirate subretinal fluid with active aspiration.

Surgical Pearls No. 85
Removal of PFCL: (1) When using a flute needle with silicone tip, the risk of retinal or optic disc touch is much lower. (2) If you are not sure whether you aspirated the entire PFCL, instill a little water into the air-filled vitreous cavity (with a brief water x air exchange), and then completely remove the residual PFCL/water puddle.

12. **Complete laser coagulation** (Fig. 12.16)

If necessary, complete now the laser therapy around the retinal break in the air-filled eye.

13. **Tamponade** (Diagram 12.2)

Concerning the use of tamponade, there are significant differences between vitreoretinal units at national and international level. The trend nowadays is to use SF_6 in a primary detachment and longer acting gases and silicone oils for redetachments.

We differentiate between detached breaks and attached breaks. The choice of tamponade depends only on the detached breaks. See Diagram 12.2. If all detached breaks are located above the 3–9 o'clock meridian, we use SF_6. If one detached hole is located below the 3–9 o'clock meridian, we use C_2F_6. If the detached break is

Diagram 12.2 Tamponade and posture for retinal detachment depending on the location of the break

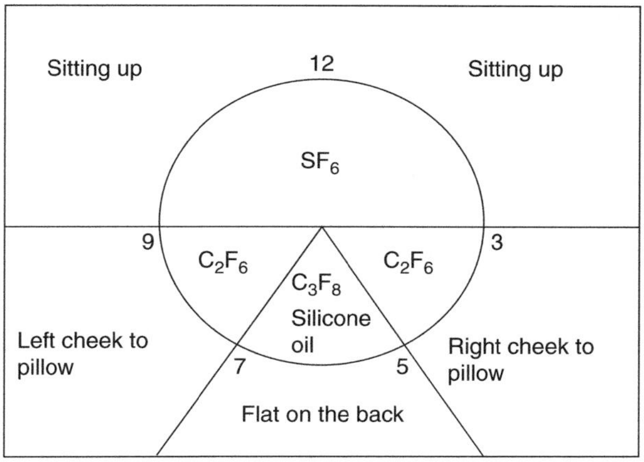

located at 6 o'clock, we would use Densiron 68 or perform episcleral buckling. An alternative is of course C_3F_8.

Surgical Pearls No. 86

1. 27G and air tamponade: 27G sclerotomies leak very little. In case of a superior detachment with a break between 11 o'clock and 1 o'clock, we use often only air as tamponade. There is an excellent tamponade present for 7–10 days, and laser treatment is effective after 3–4 days.

Why does it matter? Especially professionally active patients will appreciate to regain their visual acuity after 1 week. In comparison, C_3F_8 makes an eye blind and the patient earthbound for 2 months.

2. Gas tamponade: air against gas exchange: If the retina and the breaks are fully attached, you can flick the BIOM out and insufflate the diluted gas. The gas container is connected to the three-way tap, the scrub nurse injects the gas, and the surgeon decompresses the globe with use of a flute instrument. The globe should remain normotensive.

Surgical Pearls No. 87

Gas vs silicone oil: If the retina is attached under air in detachment surgery, then it will also be attached under gas but that's not necessarily the case for silicone oil. Why? The surface tension pressure of the gas/water interface is the greatest and therefore is the most effective in closing retinal breaks (70 mN/N). So, when the retina is attached under air, then it is also attached under gas. The same statement is not true for silicone oil. Why? Because the surface tension of silicone oil/water with 50 mN/N is less than that of air/water. So, when the retina is attached under air, it might not be attached under silicone oil.

14. **Removal of the trocar cannulas**

Finally, the trocars are removed. Remove first the instrument trocars and at the end the infusion trocar. In case of a gas tamponade, add some gas until the globe is normotensive. No suture is needed neither for gas nor for silicone oil.

15. **Postoperative posture** (Diagram 12.2)

For day 1 we recommend to keep a supine position (flat on the back) for the first hours after the surgery. Why? In some cases, you will not succeed in removing all subretinal fluid. If a substantial amount of subretinal fluid persists and cannot be removed, leave a puddle of preretinal fluid and instruct the patient to keep a supine position for the first hours after the surgery. In case of a prone position (face down) directly after surgery, a macular fold may occur. See Diagram 12.2.

From day 2 to day 7, we recommend "sitting up" if all breaks are above the horizontal meridian. If inferior breaks are present, the posture should support the breaks, for example, "left cheek to pillow" in a break in the nasal inferior quadrant of the left eye. If breaks in the superior and inferior periphery are present, a supine position "flat on the back" or "alternating sides, left and then right cheek to pillow" are recommended. Posture should be carried out for a week, day and night, for a minimum of 50 min on the hour.

12.3 Complications

1. Posterior capsular defect

This is a stupid complication during detachment surgery because the tamponade will press the IOL forward, and gas or silicone oil will flow into the anterior chamber. In case of a gas tamponade, we would inject air into the anterior chamber to counterpress, and in case of a silicone oil tamponade, we would perform an iridectomy and fill the anterior chamber with Healon GV.

2. Slippage

In cases of giant tears, the retina in the area of the break may slip/glide postoperatively toward the posterior pole (slippage). This is associated with the risk of developing retinal folds postoperatively which, in the worst of cases, may involve the macula. This phenomenon is caused by inadequate drainage of subretinal fluid during fluid-air exchange. To avoid slippage, perform a direct PFCL × silicone oil exchange.

3. Macular folds

Cause: Three factors are necessary to cause macular folds; (1) submacular fluid, (2) gas tamponade, and (3) face-down positioning.

Regarding 1: Macular hole patients have gas tamponade and face-down positioning and never have a macular fold. Why? The reason is that they do not have submacular fluid.

Regarding 2: Patients with silicone oil tamponade never have macular folds even in case of submacular fluid and face-down positioning. Why? The surface tension pressure of silicone oil is lower than that of gas.

Regarding 3: If an eye with submacular fluid and gas tamponade is positioned supine (on the back), then no macular fold will develop. Why? The gas presses against the IOL and not against the macula.

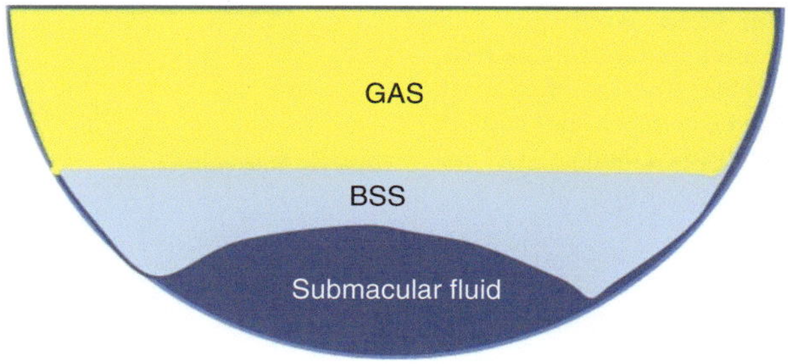

Fig. 12.17 In case of residual subretinal fluid, leave a puddle of BSS so that the retina is covered with BSS

What is the solution? (1) Leave so much BSS that the apex of the submacular fluid is covered with BSS (Fig. 12.17). Then position the patient the first postoperative hours on the back and then for the night on the opposite side of the retinal break. (2) Alternatively, use PFCL to remove the subretinal fluid.

12.4 FAQ

How do you deal with what type of detachment?

The general recommendations are that in phakic patients, one should perform a buckling surgery if possible. In pseudophakic patients, a PPV is recommended [2]. In pseudophakia with multiple breaks, we always perform a PPV; this is often named "primary vitrectomy for retinal detachment."

There is a strong tendency toward a combined phaco/vitrectomy for RRD in all phakic patients of 50 years or above. Phacoemulsification greatly facilitates the trimming of the vitreous base that is necessary in retinal detachment.

Must I change the position of the trocars according to the location of the detachment?

No. The trocars are always located at the same positions. You can however make small deviations according to the location of the break, i.e., to reach the break more easily. For example, if the retinal break is located at 12 o'clock, then place the trocars more toward 3–9 o'clock. This way you can reach the 12 o'clock break easier.

Can you give some tips for PFCL injection?

We inject PFCL bimanually; one hand holds the PFCL syringe and the other hand holds the Charles flute needle. Hold the tip of the PFCL cannula in the middle of the vitreous cavity and inject a little bit. If air bubbles escape, then aspirate them at once with the flute needle. Then start to inject the PFCL at the posterior pole and keep the tip of the cannula always in the PFCL bubble in order to prevent small bubbles (Fig. 12.18). These small bubbles will fusion after some time with the large bubble. Be cautious where the PFCL cannula is aiming to. Aim never toward the macula or a retinal break (Fig. 12.19). The PFCL bubble becomes bigger and bigger; pull the PFCL cannula slowly backward, but the tip remains constantly inside the bubble (Fig. 12.20).

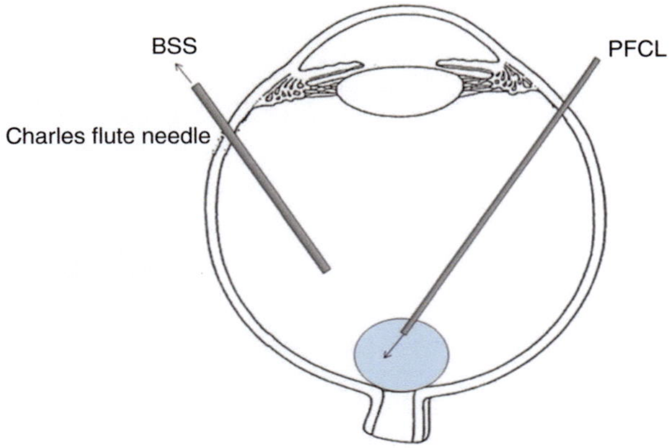

Fig. 12.18 Work bimanual. Aspirate first air bubbles from the PFCL needle and then start with a small PFCL bubble

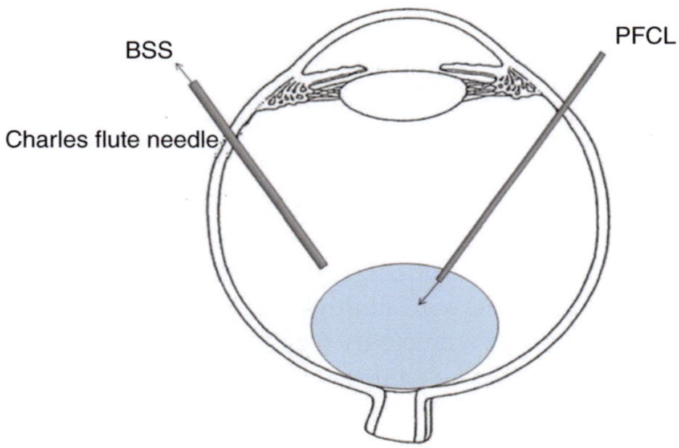

Fig. 12.19 Keep the Charles flute needle constantly in the PFCL bubble to prevent emulsification. Move the injection needle slowly forward to the lens

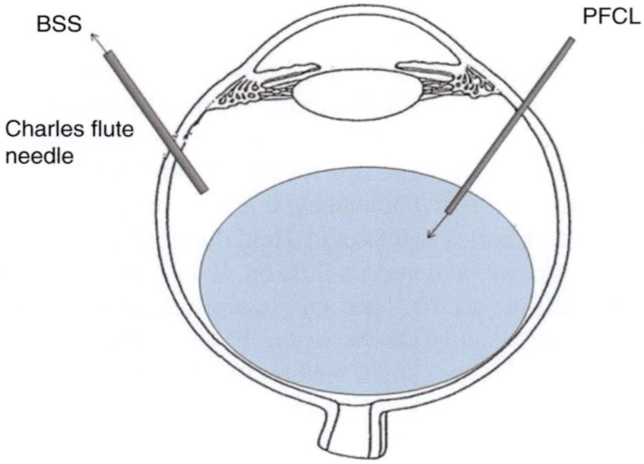

Fig. 12.20 Do not inject the PFCL toward the macula or a retinal break

What does fractionized injection of PFCL mean?

The PFCL is not injected at once but in fractions (Fig. 12.21). First you inject PFCL to the posterior edge of the retinal break. Then you inject PFCL up to the ora serrata. Fractionized PFCL injection helps to drain subretinal fluid, stabilize the retina, and remove the vitreous base.

What do you do if a macular hole is present?

Always check for the presence of a macular hole. This is present in 0.5% of all retinal detachments, and if you don't consider it, chances are that you will miss it. Check either during the preoperative examination or during the surgery. This is important for prognostication and your surgery, as you may be able to perform an ILM peeling during the vitrectomy in order to increase the chances of a postoperative hole closure. To correctly identify a macular hole in cases of macula-off RRD is difficult as the thinned retina at the fovea may be mistaken for a macular hole by the inexperienced examiner.

Should I perform an ILM peeling under PFCL?

If the retina at the posterior pole is attached, then perform an ILM peeling in a water-filled eye. If it is detached, then perform an ILM peeling under a PFCL bubble. Stain the ILM before you inject PFCL.

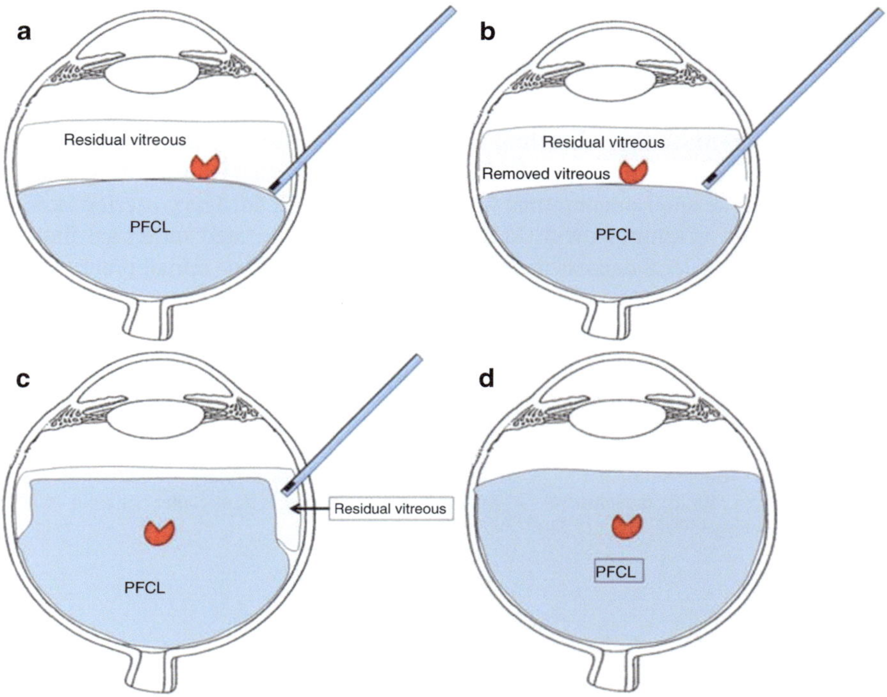

Fig. 12.21 (**a**) Inject PFCL to the inferior edge of the retinal break and remove the vitreous. (**b**) Remove the vitreous on height of the retinal break. (**c**) Inject now PFCL up to the ora serrata. Note the residual vitreous. (**d**) Remove the vitreous base (shaving)

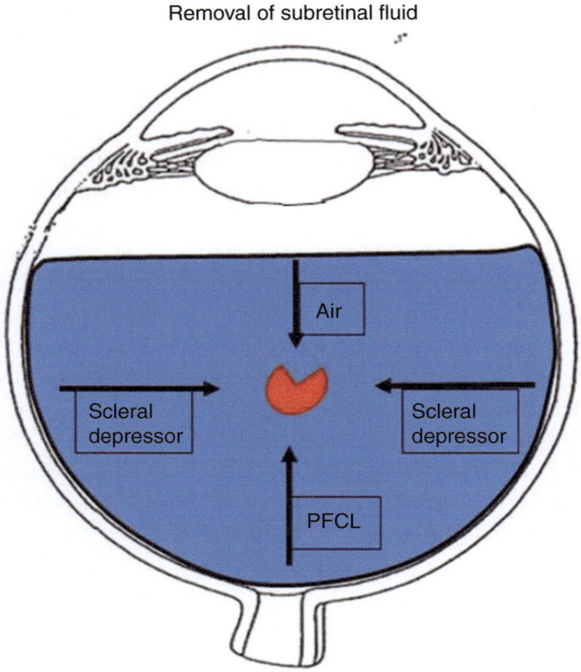

Fig. 12.22 A total retinal detachment with one retinal break. The anterior subretinal fluid is removed with air. The posterior located subretinal fluid is removed with PFCL. The horizontal located subretinal fluid is removed with a scleral depressor

How do I remove the subretinal fluid in case of a big retinal detachment?

You remove the complete fluid with air, PFCL, and a scleral depressor (Fig. 12.22). The anterior subretinal fluid is removed with air. The posterior located subretinal fluid is removed with PFCL. The horizontal located subretinal fluid is removed with a scleral depressor. Massage the fluid toward the retinal break.

References

1. Ingrid Kreissig. Minimal surgery for retinal detachment. Thieme ISBN 3131110619.
2. Heimann H, Bartz-Schmidt KU, et al. Scleral buckling versus primary vitrectomy in rhegmatogenous retinal detachment: a prospective randomized multicenter clinical study. Ophthalmology. 2007;114(12):2142–54.

Chapter 13
Vitrectomy for Difficult Retinal Detachment (PVR)

Extras: Videos 13.1, 13.2, 13.3, 13.4, 13.5, 13.6, 13.7, 13.8, 13.9, 13.10, 13.11, 13.12, and 13.13.

13.1 Introduction

The name *proliferative vitreoretinopathy* was provided in 1989 by the Silicone Oil Study Group [1]. The name is derived from *proliferation* of the retinal pigment epithelial and glial cells and *vitreoretinopathy* to include the tissues which are affected, namely, the vitreous and the retina (Fig. 13.1).

The **current management is t**he surgical relief of vitreal, preretinal, and subretinal tractions. The final aim is the reestablishment of retinal attachment and visual function.

The **principles of management** are (1) closure of all retinal breaks, (2) relief of traction, and (3) long-term retinal stabilization. The following Table 13.1 shows the principles and surgical procedures for PVR detachment.

Regarding the **timing of surgery** an early surgical treatment is favorable because it preserves the loss of photoreceptors and improves a favorable visual outcome. A delayed surgical treatment (after 6 weeks) is unfavorable for the visual function, but surgery is easier; the proliferative membranes become "mature" and are therefore surgically easier to remove.

Indication: Feasible pathologies for this surgery are the first surgery of PVR detachments grade C2, C3, and D.

Electronic Supplementary Material The online version of this chapter (https://doi.org/10.1007/978-3-319-89677-9_13) contains supplementary material, which is available to authorized users.

U. Spandau, H. Heimann, *Practical Handbook for Small-Gauge Vitrectomy*,
https://doi.org/10.1007/978-3-319-89677-9_13

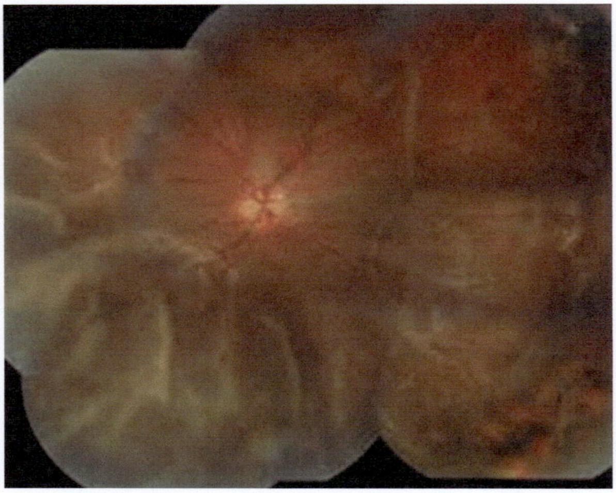

Fig. 13.1 PVR detachment stage C3

Table 13.1 Principles and surgical procedures for PVR detachment

Principle	Surgical procedure
Closure of all retinal breaks	• Identification • Closure
Relief of traction	• Membrane dissection • Retinotomy/retinectomy
Long-term retinal stabilization	• Laser photocoagulation • Scleral buckle • Intraocular tamponade

13.2 Surgery for PVR Detachment

Instruments for PVR detachment
Membrane Removal
Trypan blue
27G Endgripping forceps
27G DORC wide grip forceps (1286.WRD04)
Knob spatula
Membrane pic
Atkinson cannula
Straight scissors

The Surgery

1. Encircling band (cerclage)
2. Phacoemulsification and IOL implantation
3. Pars plana vitrectomy

4. Vitreous staining with triamcinolone
5. Vitreous base shaving
6. Staining of membranes with trypan blue
7. Removal of epiretinal membranes
8. Removal of subretinal membranes
9. 180 deg. retinotomy
10. Instillation of PFCL
11. Laser photocoagulation
12. Prepare the anterior chamber
13. Tamponade

Every Surgical Step in Detail

1. **Encircling band (cerclage)**

Introduction: An encircling band relieves traction at the vitreous base. It facilitates also the closure of peripheral retinal breaks. And finally, an encircling band supports the vitreous base during anterior dissection. An encircling band is used less and less nowadays. We place an encircling band in PVR stage C3 and in PVR redetachments.

The surgery of an encircling band is described in detail in **Chapter 13.3**.

2. **Phacoemulsification and IOL implantation**

For vitrectomy of PVR detachment, we recommend regardless of the age a phacoemulsification with IOL implantation in the bag. The lens removal allows the visualization of the vitreous base and assessment of anterior PVR, and it allows more importantly the surgical access to the vitreous base. We avoid a (pars plana) lensectomy because the lens capsule is absent which serves otherwise as a scaffold between the posterior and anterior chamber. For example, in case of a silicone oil tamponade, the oil may prolapse into the anterior chamber and cause anterior chamber complications.

Surgical Pearls No. 88

Management of miotic pupil: A miotic pupil may be a major obstacle for PVR surgery because the pathology is often located in the periphery. In many cases an intracameral injection of adrenaline (1:10) is sufficient. Adrenaline may also be given during surgery. If posterior synechiae are present, then a synechiolysis is recommended. This can be achieved through iris stretching. Insert two Sinskey hooks through the paracenteses and stretch the pupil (Fig. 13.2). Alternatively, iris retractors with four-point fixation or a Malyugin ring can be implanted (Figs. 13.3 and 13.4).

3. **Pars plana vitrectomy**

A main step in pars plana vitrectomy is the removal of the core vitreous resulting in relief of transvitreal traction.

We use a standard three-port PPV with 25G trocars. We use 25G and not 23G because smaller trocars require smaller instruments, and this results in less traumatic

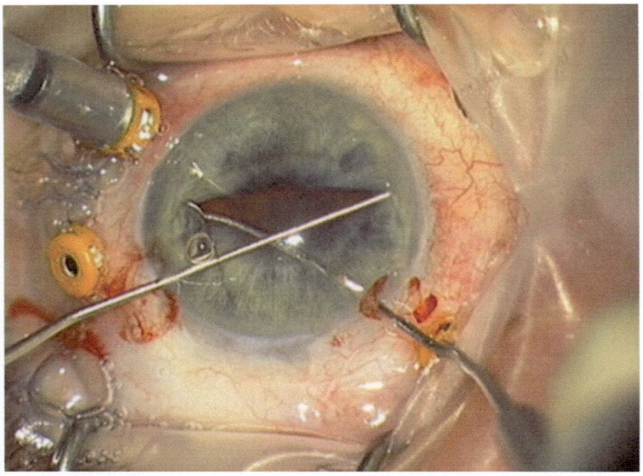

Fig. 13.2 Iris stretching with Sinskey hooks

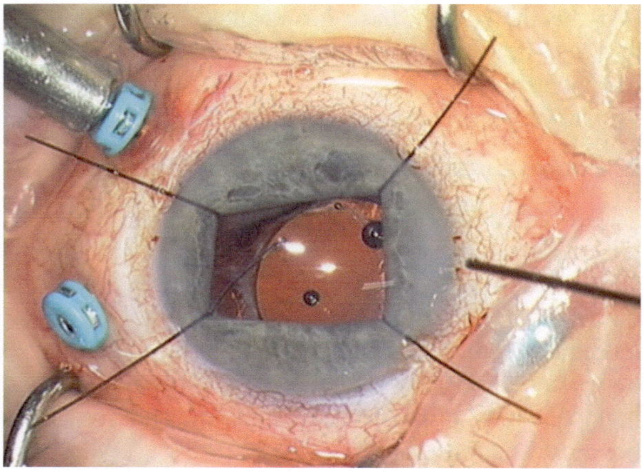

Fig. 13.3 Iris retractors

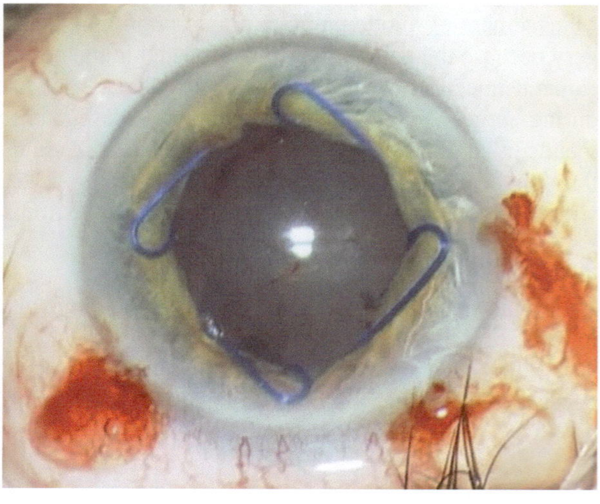

Fig. 13.4 Malyugin ring

surgery and less leakage from the trocars. In case of pseudophakia, the sclerotomies are placed 3.5 mm behind the limbus and in case of a natural lens 4.0 mm. Insert the infusion line in a quadrant without anterior traction. Otherwise the infusion will be located subretinally. In complicated vitrectomies, we insert always a chandelier light (four-port PPV) which allows for bimanual dissection of membranes, bimanual injection of PFCL, and injection of silicone oil under view to retina.

A vital point for successful and complication-free vitrectomy is a good visualization. Wide-angle viewing systems have a viewing field of 60 to 130°. They allow for anterior dissection and limit the need of scleral depression. The visualization in an air-filled eye is improved. The stereopsis is however reduced. The conventional contact lens system has a viewing field of only 20–30° and requires scleral depression. We use the RESIGHT Biom system from Zeiss together with a Zeiss Lumera microscope.

4. **Vitreous staining with triamcinolone**
5. **Vitreous base shaving**

A posterior vitreous detachment (PVD) is usually present in idiopathic PVR. In contrast, a PVD is not present in diabetic and traumatic PVR. Induce the PVD as far anteriorly to the vitreous base as possible. The vitreous in PVR is inflamed, and therefore a thorough removal is important. We recommend the staining of the vitreous with triamcinolone to assess if a PVD is present and to allow a meticulous shaving of the vitreous base. "Shaving" means that the vitreous cortex is removed to the surface of the peripheral retina. The settings of the vitreous cutter are a high clip rate (5000–7500 cuts/min) and a low aspiration rate (200 mmHg). Crucial for a successful shaving is a wide-angle viewing system and scleral depression. Ideally the scleral depression is performed bimanually under illumination of a chandelier light.

6. **Membrane dissection**

In general: The removal of preretinal membranes results in relief of preretinal traction. All **epi**retinal membranes must be removed. Even in case of retinotomy, remove all membranes up to the retinotomy edges. If you leave epiretinal membranes, then they will continue to proliferate and cause a tractive detachment. In contrast, remove **sub**retinal proliferation *only* if the posterior retina is not flattened under PFCL. Begin with removal of the membranes located at the posterior pole and continue with membrane dissection in the peripheral retina (Fig. 13.5).

Technique of membrane staining: We refill the dye into a regular 3 cc syringe because the dye can be ejected in more controlled manner (Figs. 13.6 and 13.7). In PVR detachments the membranes are located centrally and peripherally. It is easy to stain central membranes in a BSS-filled eye because the dye falls down on the posterior pole. This maneuver is, however, difficult for peripherally located membranes.

We stain, therefore, in an air-filled eye. In an air-filled eye, the contact between membrane and dye is longer and more concentrated before the dye falls down on the posterior pole. Perform a fluid x air exchange and drop a few drops of the dye directly on the membranes (Figs. 13.8 and 13.9). Wait for 30 sec, aspirate first the dye from the posterior pole, and then continue with an air x fluid exchange. With this method, a higher concentration of the dye is achieved and therefore a better staining of the membranes.

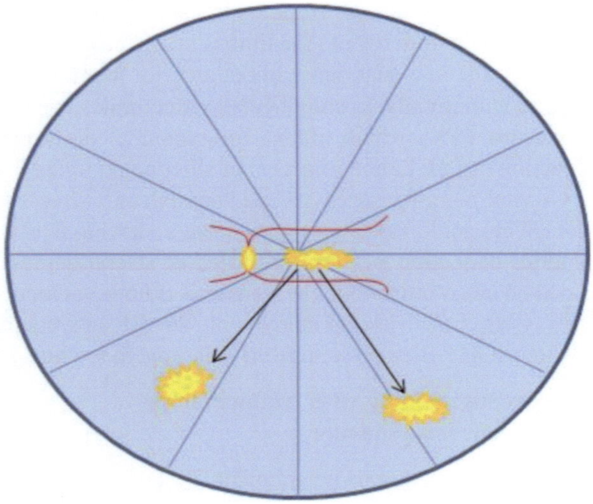

Fig. 13.5 In PVR detachment membrane dissection starts in the central posterior pole and continues in the periphery

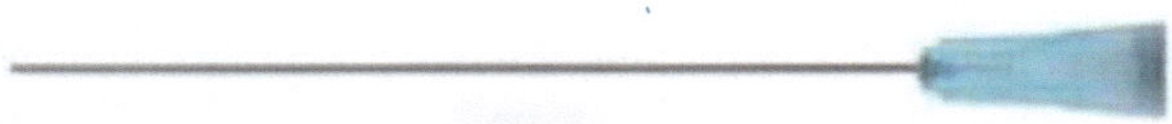

Fig. 13.6 A Charles flute needle

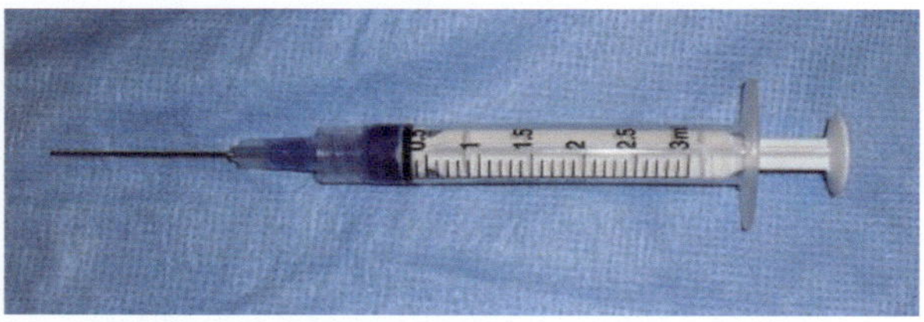

Fig. 13.7 A 3 cc syringe filled with trypan blue is easier to use than an original syringe

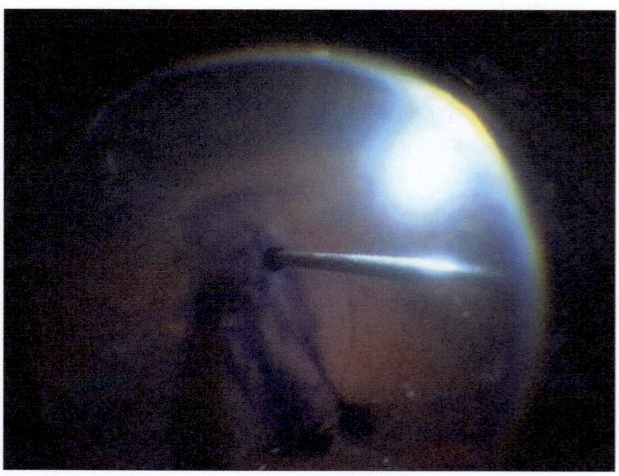

Fig. 13.8 The dye is dropped on the membrane

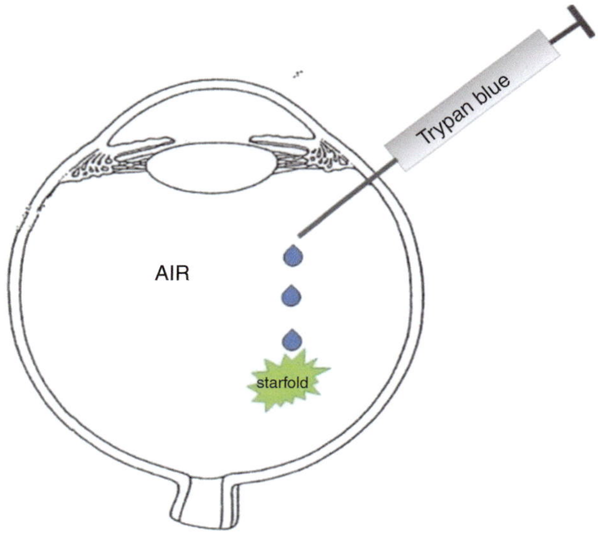

Fig. 13.9 The vitreous cavity is filled with air. This method increases the concentration of the dye and enables the staining of peripheral membranes

Technique of membrane removal: The peeling of PVR membranes is technically very difficult. It requires patience, good visualization, and good instruments. Centrally located membranes can be removed with one hand, but peripherally located membranes require bimanual peeling. Our setup is a four-port PPV with three trocars and one chandelier light.

7. **Removal of epiretinal membranes** (Fig. 13.10)

A successful membrane removal depends to a large amount on the instrument; even if you are an experienced vitreoretinal surgeon, you need good delamination instruments and good forceps. Test therefore many different peeling forceps to find the one which suits you best.

For delamination of the membrane, we use a 25G or 27G blunt retrobulbar cannula (Atkinson, Beaver Visitec); Alternatively, you can use a membrane pic (DORC). For dissection of membranes, three different forceps from DORC are available. In our experience the 27G endgripping forceps (DORC) is suitable for every tissue from ILM to thick membranes. Membranes with strong adhesions require stronger forceps such as the serrated jaws forceps or a strong endgripping forceps. Vitreoretinal tractions can be cut with straight 25G microscissors (Fig. 13.10) (DORC, NL and Eye Tech, UK) and curved 27G microscissors (DORC).

The most difficult surgical maneuver for removal of PVR membranes is the delamination of the membranes from the retina. This maneuver is even more difficult in eyes after a silicone oil tamponade. After a silicone oil tamponade, the membranes are even more adherent to the retina. Delaminate the membrane with an Atkinson cannula and create an opening between membrane and the retina. Then lift the membrane here with a forceps and move at the same time the delamination cannula or alternatively a 25G knob spatula (Eye Tech, UK) backward and forward through the opening.

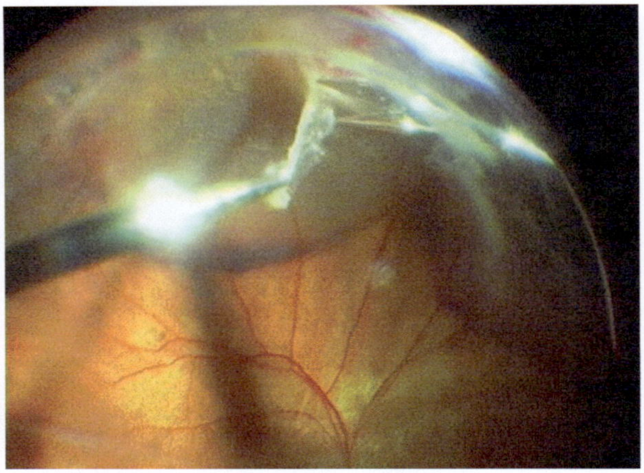

Fig. 13.10 Removal of peripheral membranes with endgripping forceps and straight scissors

The peripheral membranes are very difficult to remove because the retina is detached and because the membranes are difficult to reach with the instruments. Instill PFCL to stabilize the posterior retina and facilitate membrane removal. In addition, perfluorocarbon liquids (PFCLs) draw the vitreous base more posteriorly. This effect facilitates anterior dissection and reduces the chances of retina or vitreous incarceration in a sclerotomy site. Furthermore, it facilitates drainage of subretinal fluid through anterior retinal breaks. Important: all breaks must be *freed of traction* before they come in contact with the PFCL. Otherwise there is a risk that the PFCL tracks subretinally.

Subretinal proliferations are present in nearly half of the cases of PVR but rarely prevent retinal reattachment. Must all proliferations be removed? No, only the significant ones. A significant subretinal membrane is one that will preclude flattening of the retina unless it is removed. Their significance becomes obvious when PFCL is instilled. Remove a subretinal proliferation *only* if the posterior retina is not flattened under PFCL. A special case of a subretinal proliferation is a "napkin ring." A napkin ring is a tight annular band near the optic disc. Its removal requires a 360 deg. retinotomy. See chapter "Traumatic PVR."

8. **Removal of subretinal proliferations**

Before removing subretinal membranes, perform a complete posterior and anterior epiretinal dissection.

The complete surgery is shown step-by-step in **Chapter 13.4**.

9. **Retinotomy**

Introduction

If despite meticulous transvitreal, epiretinal, and subretinal dissection the retina remains foreshortened preventing an attachment of the retina with the retinal pigment epithelium, the surgeon should perform a retinotomy or retinectomy in order to relax the retina. **Retinotomy** involves incising the retina, whereas **retinectomy** involves excising the retina. The peripheral retina is cut parallel to the ora serrata

(180, 270, or 360 deg), and the retinotomy edges are treated with laser photocoagulation in order to reattach the retina.

Retinotomy could be performed in a **radial** fashion, but most commonly it is done **circumferentially**, parallel to the ora serrata. Most PVR cases can be managed without retinotomy/retinectomy. We almost never use it in the first surgery, except for the penetrating injuries with PVR and incarceration of the retina in the penetrating wound. **The circumferential retinotomy** in repeated surgery for idiopathic PVR detachment is performed in the area with persistent contraction of the retina usually affecting the two lower quadrants, due to the physical property of the 1000 csts silicone oil that is regularly used for the first surgery. This silicone oil is lighter than water and therefore is leaving some space filled with aqueous inferiorly, thus tamponing better the upper two quadrants where recurrent detachment almost never occurs.

The relaxing retinotomy consists of three main surgical steps:

1. Ora parallel diathermy
2. Retinotomy
3. Removal of anterior retina (retinectomy)

The most common problem with the retinotomy is underestimation of the necessary size of the tissue to be removed so that contraction persists. The most common size of retinotomy is 180° tapered to the two lower quadrants and extending from 3 over 6 to 9 o'clock. A 360° retinotomy is seldom and may be required in penetrating injuries with incarceration of the retina and PVR stage D. It is usually followed by some distortion of the retina after reattachment and requires relocation of the retina using the flute needle with silicone tip in order to reestablish its normal anatomical position. The complete surgery is shown step-by-step in **Chapter 13.5**.

10. **Instillation of PFCL**

As next step, we perform an **attachment test** (Fig. 13.11). For an attachment test, you can use PFCL or air. PFCL attaches the retina with its gravity. Air attaches the retina with its surface tension pressure. If the retina is attached under PFCL, then perform a PFCL against air exchange and check if the retina is also attached under air. If this is the case, then the retina will also be attached under a gas tamponade. BUT the retina is not necessarily attached under a silicone oil tamponade because the surface tension pressure of silicone oil is lower than the surface tension pressure of air.

Injection of PFCL: We inject PFCL bimanually; one hand holds the PFCL syringe, and the other hand holds the Charles flute needle. Hold the tip of the PFCL cannula in the middle of the vitreous cavity and inject a little bit. Then start to inject the PFCL at the posterior pole and keep the tip of the cannula always in the PFCL bubble in order to prevent small bubbles (Fig. 13.12). Aim never toward the macula or a retinal break. The PFCL bubble becomes bigger and bigger; pull the PFCL cannula slowly backward, but the tip remains constantly inside the bubble.

11. **Laser photocoagulation**

The aim of laser photocoagulation is a long-term stabilization of the reattached retina. Laser photocoagulation causes less RPE cell dispersion than cryotherapy and

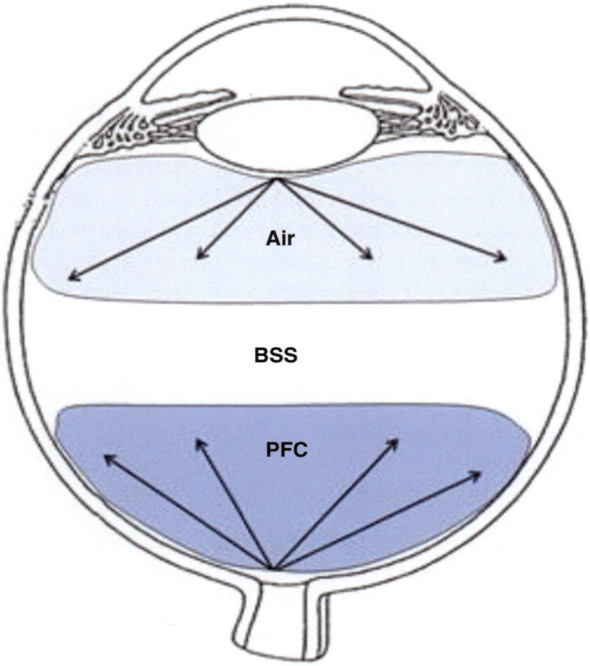

Fig. 13.11 Opposite mechanisms of action of PFCL and air in a BSS-filled eye. Air fills the globe from anterior to posterior. PFC fills the globe from posterior to anterior

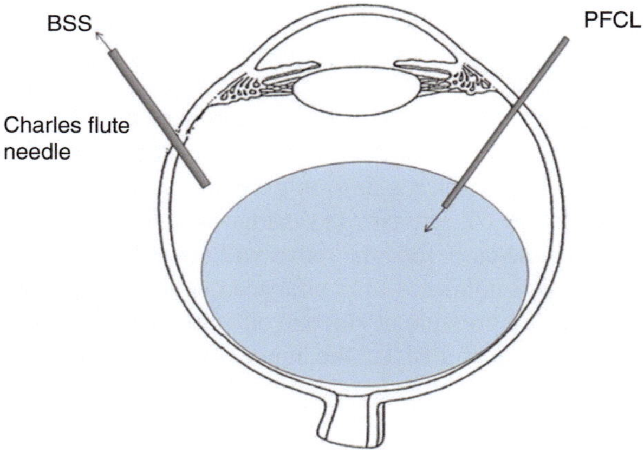

Fig. 13.12 Work bimanual. The left hand aspirates BSS with a backflush instrument and the right hand injects PFCL

consequently less PVR. In addition, laser photocoagulation induces no disruption of the blood-aqueous barrier.

Technique of laser photocoagulation

Laser photocoagulation can be performed in the PFCL-filled eye or in the air-filled eye. Apply the laser effects confluently surrounding all retinal breaks. Our laser power for retinal breaks with an argon laser (Iridex, CA) is as follows: power, 100–300 mW; duration, **200** msec; and interval, 300 msec.

Surgical Pearls No. 89

Laser cerclage ≠ encircling band (Fig. 13.13). Both, an encircling band and a laser cerclage, create a barrier for tears located anterior to the barrier. In addition, an encircling band creates an indentation of the retina which results in a relaxation of the shortened retina. A laser cerclage, however, does not create an indentation and can therefore not help in relaxing a shortened retina. This is important for PVR detachments with intraretinal PVR and a shortened retina.

Surgical Pearls No. 90

Cryopexy versus laser photocoagulation: Cryopexy creates PVR; this is especially the case if the posterior hyaloid is detached. In vitrectomy for retinal detachment surgery, laser photocoagulation is recommended because it induces less PVR.

12. **Prepare the anterior chamber**

Before finalizing surgery with the intraocular tamponade, **the anterior segment must be prepared** (Figs. 13.14 and 13.15). In case of 1000 or 5000 csts silicone oil,

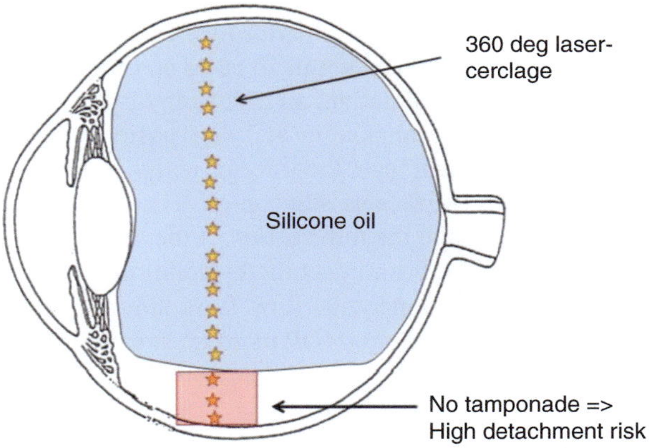

Fig. 13.13 In case of a 360 deg. laser cerclage, there is a risk of a laser necrosis at the inferior pole due to a lack of tamponade

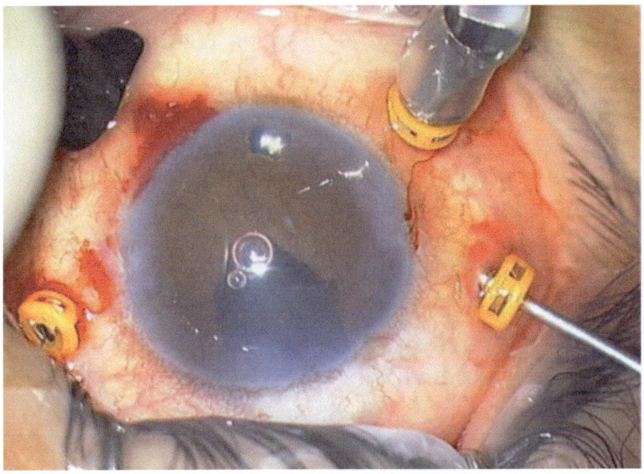

Fig. 13.14 Ando iridectomy with vitreous cutter

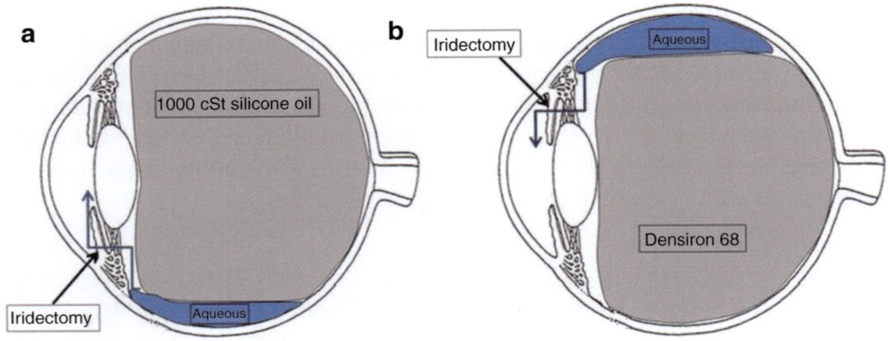

Fig. 13.15 An inferior (**a**) or superior (**b**) iridectomy depending on the silicone oil

an inferior Ando iridectomy is performed to enable a flow of aqueous from the inferiorly located aqueous phase in the posterior chamber to the anterior chamber. In case of a Densiron 68 tamponade, a superior iridectomy is performed to enable the flow of aqueous from the superior located aqueous phase in the posterior chamber to the anterior chamber. Not in all cases an iridectomy must be performed. In a normal pseudophakia situation, an iridectomy is not necessary. An iridectomy is however necessary in aphakia, in 360 deg. posterior synechiae, and in partial zonular lysis. In the aphakic eye, the inferior peripheral iridectomy prevents a pupil block by the anterior surface of silicone oil. Face-down positioning for the first 24 h is necessary to ensure the reformation of the anterior chamber.

In addition, you can inject methylcellulose into the anterior chamber to prevent an immediate postoperative flow from silicone oil to the anterior chamber. The methylcellulose causes no IOP increase in case of a silicone oil tamponade.

13. **Tamponade**

PFCL removal and tamponade

For gas tamponades, a PFCL × air exchange is routine. For silicone oil tamponades, two surgical techniques exist: (1) a PFCL against silicone oil exchange and (2) a PFCL against air and then an air against silicone oil exchange. We use a PFCL against silicone oil exchange in traumatic retinal detachments. Otherwise we use always a PFCL against air exchange.

Slippage is a complication which occurs in giant tears or retinotomies. If subretinal fluid is present at the posterior pole and the eye is filled with gas and the patient is located face down, then a slippage at the posterior pole with macular folds may occur. To avoid the slippage, use PFCL and perform a thorough aspiration of fluid at the giant tear edges and avoid face-down positioning directly after surgery. In silicone oil, slippage with macular folds does not occur. The reason for this is that the surface tension pressure of silicone oil is too low to press away the fluid at the posterior pole; the fluid is resorbed by the pigment epithelium and the retina slowly reattaches.

PFCL against silicone oil exchange (Fig. 13.16). For this step a chandelier light is not required. If you exchange PFCL against silicone oil, one hand aspirates the PFCL, and the other hand holds the light fiber, while the silicone oil is injected with the infusion line.

Intraocular tamponade

Gas or silicone oil: According to the silicone oil study, C_3F_8 is superior (higher reattachment rate and better visual outcome) to SF_6 in complicated detachments. The silicone oil study does not compare C_3F_8 with silicone oil. The advantages and disadvantages of C_3F_8 are listed in Table 13.2 and of silicone oil in Table 13.3. For complicated retinal detachments, we prefer silicone oil. The main reason is that the recurrent detachment risk in complicated RD's is higher than in easy detachments. And a recurrent detachment under silicone oil is better than a recurrent detachment under gas. Why? A recurrent detachment under gas develops fast into a PVR detachment. A recurrent detachment under silicone oil develops slowly. Under gas an immediate surgery is required. Under silicone oil you can postpone and plan surgery.

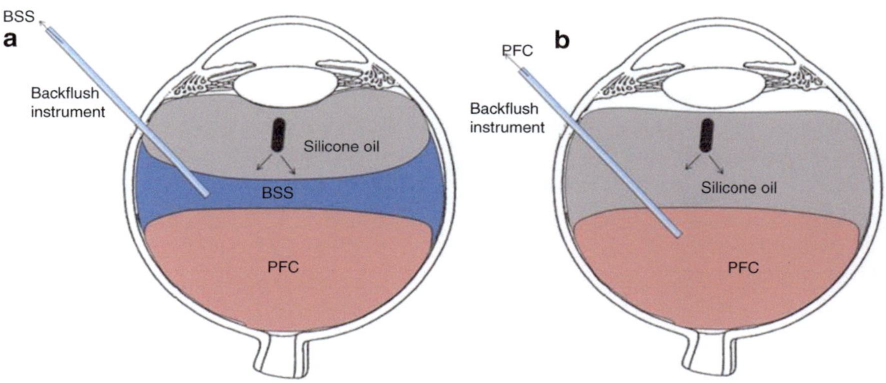

Fig. 13.16 PFCL against silicone oil exchange: In a first step (**a**) silicone oil is injected and fills the eye from anterior to posterior. Aspirate first the BSS phase. After removal of BSS (**b**), hold the flute needle into the PFCL phase and remove it

Table 13.2 The pros and cons of C_3F_8

Advantages of C_3F_8	Disadvantages of C_3F_8
Disappears spontaneously	Only temporary tamponade
High surface tension pressure	Specific head positioning (not for children, disabled)
	Air travel must be postponed (risk of expansion)
	Vision is restricted (not for monocular patients)
	Cataractogenic

Gas tamponade: Gas has two great advantages over silicone oil. The surface tension pressure of gas is much higher than for silicone oil which enables a more effective sealing of retinal holes. Secondly, the gas is a temporary tamponade. Long-term damages of gas are therefore not existent compared to silicone oil.

Injection of gas: SF_6, C_2F_6, and C_3F_8 are due to the fluorine atoms heavier than air. The gases sink therefore to the ground, whereas the lighter air stays above. Hold the Charles flute needle behind the lens to aspirate the air, and the gases can fill the vitreous cavity from posterior to anterior (Figs. 13.17 and 13.18).

Surgical Pearls No. 91

Shake the 50 cc gas syringe before injection because the gas sinks to the bottom of the syringe resulting in a wrong concentration of the gas in the eye.

Silicone oil tamponade:

Silicone oil is an excellent temporary tamponade but a very bad permanent tamponade. It causes high IOP and emulsifies, and the final result is an optic atrophy. Silicone oil should be avoided in fresh and primary detachments. Silicone oil is indicated in recurrent detachments, in complicated PVR detachments and in

Table 13.3 The pros and cons of silicone oil

Advantages of silicone oil	Disadvantages
"Non-temporary" longer tamponade	Need for a second operation
Does not require positioning	Scaffold for reproliferation (?)
Earlier visualization (option for monocular patients)	Cataractogenic
Air travel is possible	Low surface tension pressure
Lower risk of hypotony	

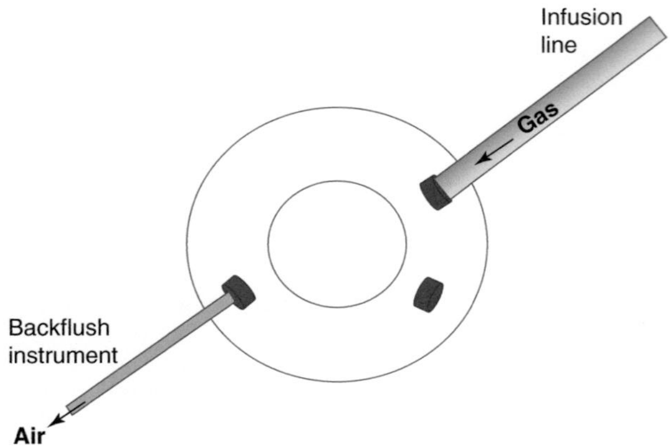

Fig. 13.17 The setup for a gas injection. The gas is injected through the infusion line and the flute needle evacuates the air

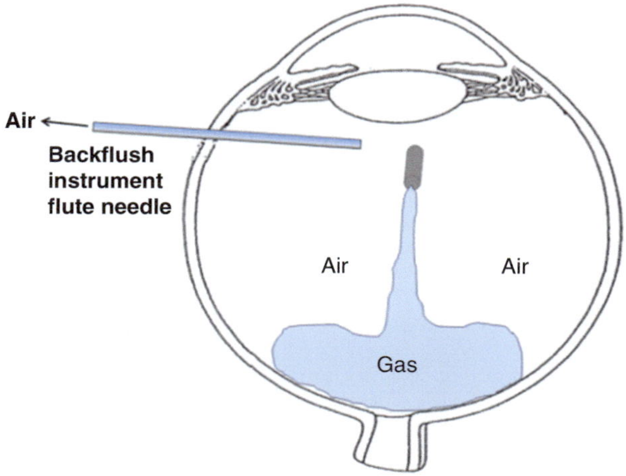

Fig. 13.18 The heavy gas fills the vitreous cavity from posterior to anterior and the flute needle air eracuates

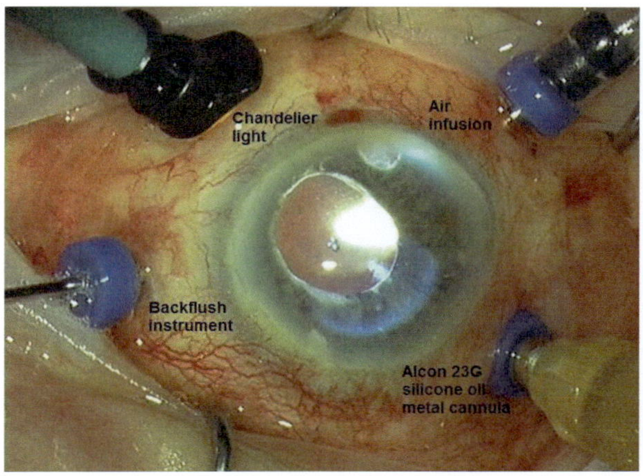

Fig. 13.19 Silicone oil injection **under** view to the retina. Note that a chandelier light is required

diabetic tractive detachments. But even in these cases, try to remove the silicone oil after 3 months.

Silicone oil injection (Figs. 13.19, 13.20, and 13.21)

1000 csts or 5000 csts silicone oil: 5000 csts induces less IOP increase and less emulsification. If you plan a long silicone oil tamponade (longer than 6 months), then use 5000 csts silicone oil. If you plan a short duration (shorter than 6 months), then use 1000 csts silicone oil. The duration of the silicone oil is listed in Table 13.4.

Surgical Pearls No. 92

Silicone oil overfill (Fig. 13.22): Cut the infusion line with a scissors so that the excessive silicone oil can escape. An IOP of approximately 10 mmHg is fine or wait so long until no more oil escapes from the infusion line.

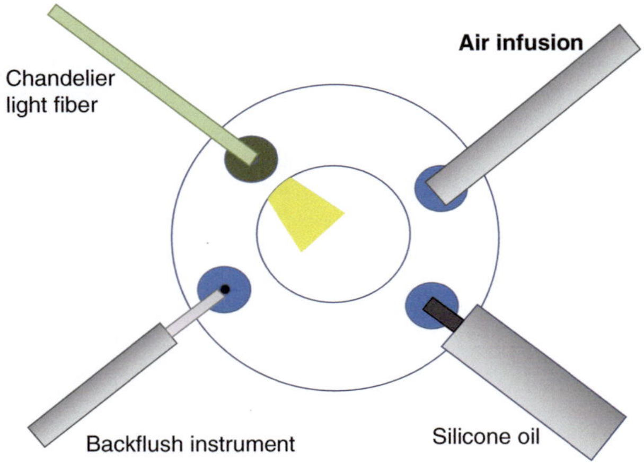

Fig. 13.20 Setup for oil injection with view to the retina

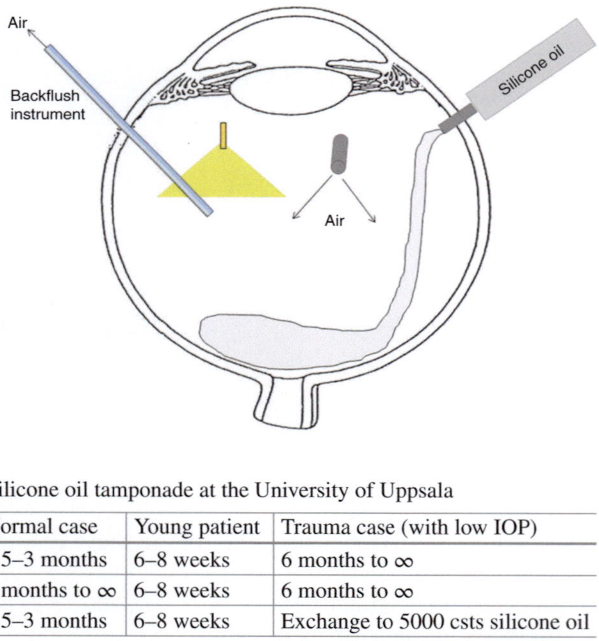

Fig. 13.21 You work bimanual in order to inject the silicone oil under view to the retina

Table 13.4 The duration of a silicone oil tamponade at the University of Uppsala

Duration of silicone oils	Normal case	Young patient	Trauma case (with low IOP)
1000/1300 csts silicone oil	1.5–3 months	6–8 weeks	6 months to ∞
5000 csts silicone oil	3 months to ∞	6–8 weeks	6 months to ∞
Densiron 68	1.5–3 months	6–8 weeks	Exchange to 5000 csts silicone oil

13.3 Surgery of an Encircling Band

Instruments

Mersilene 5-0

Silk 3-0

Encircling band (S2987, Labtician, Canada) (Fig. 13.23) and sleeve (S3083, Labtician, Canada) (Fig. 13.23)

Strabismus hook (of gas)

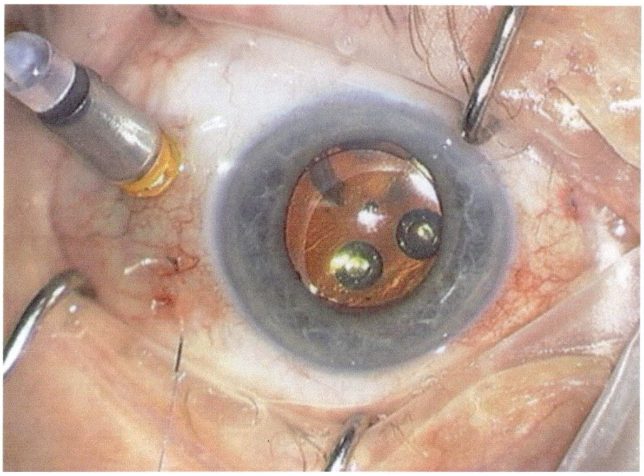

Fig. 13.22 Cut the infusion line after silicone oil injection so that excessive oil can flow out

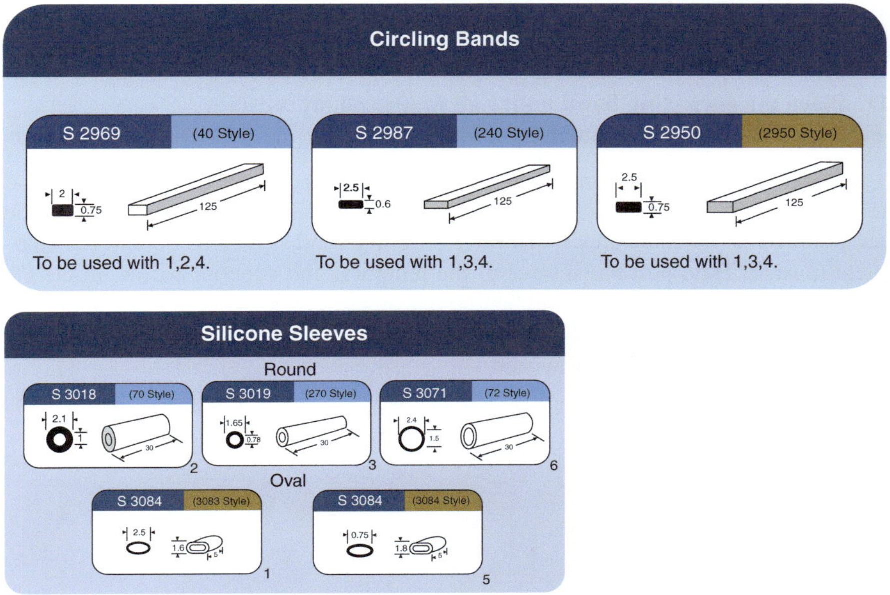

Fig. 13.23 Circling bands and silicone sleeves (Labtician, Canada)

Orbita spatula

The Surgery of an Encircling Band Step-by-Step

A. **Limbal peritomy 360 degrees.**
B. **Dissect Tenon from sclera.**
C. **Place four holding sutures (silk 3-0) on the straight muscles.**
D. **Place the encircling band under all four straight muscles.**
E. **Check that the band is not twisted.**
F. **Insert both ends of the band into the sleeve at the inferotemporal quadrant.**

G. **Mark the sclera with caliper at axial length/2 mm behind the limbus.**
H. **Place the first stitch (Mersilene 5-0) posterior to scleral marking, and hold the band at the same time anterior to the marking.**
I. **Place the second stitch anterior to scleral marking, and hold the band at the same time posterior to the marking.**
J. **Tie the suture and continue with the next three quadrants.**
K. **Tighten the band.**

The Surgery in Detail

A. **Limbal peritomy 360 degrees.**
B. **Dissect Tenon from sclera.**
C. **Place four holding sutures (silk 3-0) on the straight muscles.**

Open the conjunctiva 360 deg. at the limbus with a Westcott scissors and anatomic forceps. Then dissect the Tenon capsule from the sclera using a strabismus forceps. Dissect to the equator. Then place a strabismus hook with hole under a rectus muscle and insert a silk 3-0 suture. Pull back the hook with suture and place a knot on the suture. Repeat this step with all four rectus muscles.

D. **Place the encircling band under all four straight muscles.**
E. **Check that the band is not twisted.**

Start at the inferotemporal position. Pull the holding sutures of the inferior and temporal rectus, insert the orbital spatula, and insert the silicone band behind the temporal rectus. Double check that the encircling band is located behind the complete muscle. Then pull the sutures of the temporal and superior rectus, insert the orbital spatula, and place the band behind the superior rectus (Fig. 13.24); and so on until you are back to the inferotemporal position with both ends. Then check all four quadrants that the band is not twisted.

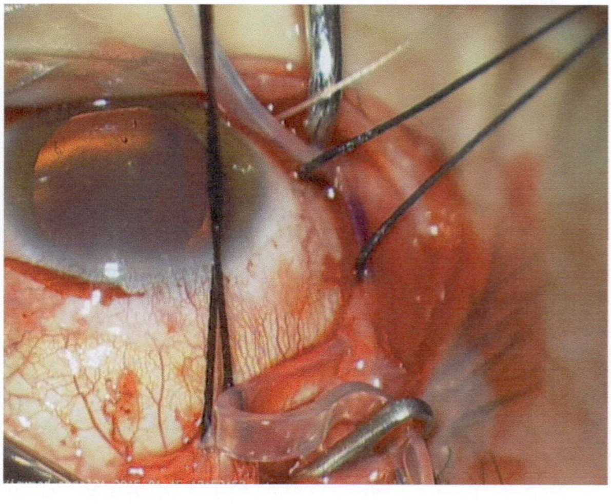

Fig. 13.24 With a strabismus hook with hole, the encircling band can be placed under all rectus muscles

F. **Insert both ends of the band into the sleeve at the inferotemporal quadrant.**

Now comes the most difficult step for this surgery: place the sleeve on the special forceps (Labtician, Canada), and insert first one end (this is easy) and then the second end (this is very tricky). If you succeeded, then tighten the band a little bit.

G. **Mark the sclera with caliper at axial length/2 mm behind the limbus.**
H. **Place the first stitch (Mersilene 5-0) posterior to scleral marking, and hold the band at the same time anterior to the marking.**
I. **Place the second stitch anterior to scleral marking, and hold the band at the same time posterior to the marking.**
J. **Tie the suture and continue with the next three quadrants.**

We continue now at the superotemporal quadrant. Pull the sutures and insert the orbital spatula. Then mark the sclera at AXL/2, i.e., the eye has an AXL = 23 mm, then mark the sclera at 11.5 mm. The marking is located in the middle of the band. Fixate then the band with a forceps anterior to the marking and place the first stitch (Mersilene 5-0) 1.5 mm posterior to the marking. Then fixate the band posterior to the first stitch and place a second stitch with the same suture 1.5 mm anterior to the marking. Then tie the suture and continue with the next three quadrants. The final suture is located at the sleeve.

K. **Tighten the band.**

Now tighten the band. The globe should be a little bit hypotensive, approximately 8 mmHg, to achieve a good impression. You can either tighten the band until the band lies tense on the sclera or tighten the band maximally 8 mm.

Surgical Pearls No. 93
A too tight encircling band may cause anterior segment necrosis and globe pain. If you cut the band, the pain disappears immediately. In addition, an encircling band reduces the ocular blood flow and ocular pulse. Cutting of the encircling band restores the ocular circulation [2].

13.4 Removal of Subretinal Membranes

Instruments

1. 20G subretinal spatula DORC 1295 1 0995
2. 20G subretinal forceps DORC 1286 01 1095
3. 20G or 23G serrated jaw forceps

The Surgery Step-by-Step

1. Identify the subretinal membranes which have to be removed and those which can be left: instill PFCL and identify those subretinal membranes which lift the retina.

2. Create two 20G sclerotomies. Remove either both instrument trocars and enlarge the sclerotomy with a V-lance (Alcon) or create two new sclerotomies (Fig. 13.25).
3. Insert a chandelier light.
4. Plan a retinotomy in the middle of the subretinal membrane.
5. Insert the subretinal spatula, pierce the retina, and dissect the subretinal membrane from the retina (Fig. 13.26).
6. Now work bimanual with serrated jaw forceps and subretinal forceps: place the subretinal forceps through the retinotomy, grasp the subretinal membrane with the subretinal forceps, and pull it through the retinotomy (Fig. 13.27). Then pull out the subretinal membrane with help of both forceps. If you do not work bimanual, then you will create a giant tear.
7. If the subretinal membrane breaks in small parts although it is not completely removed, then do not continue because the residual subretinal membrane creates no tension.
8. The maneuver 5–7 has to be performed from the nasal and temporal side for the same membrane.

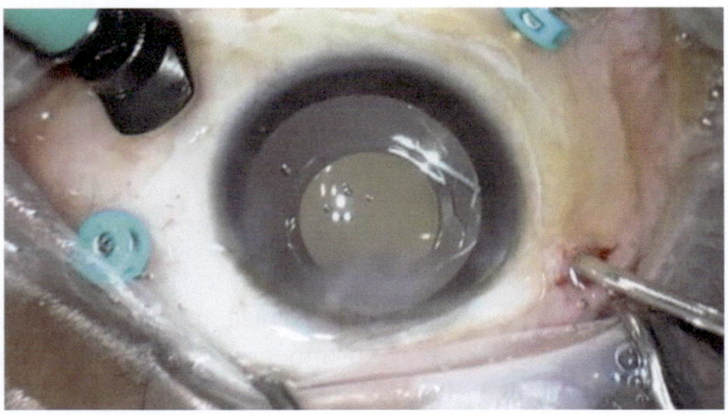

Fig. 13.25 Create first two 20G sclerotomies at 10 and 2 o'clock because the subretinal instruments are 20G

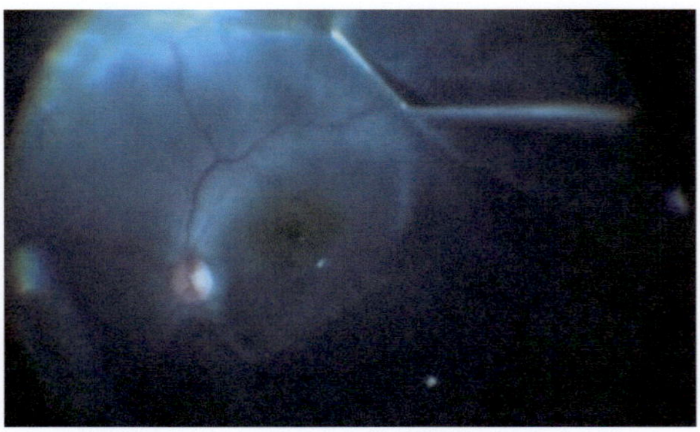

Fig. 13.26 Pierce the retina with the subretinal spatula and loosen the subretinal membranes

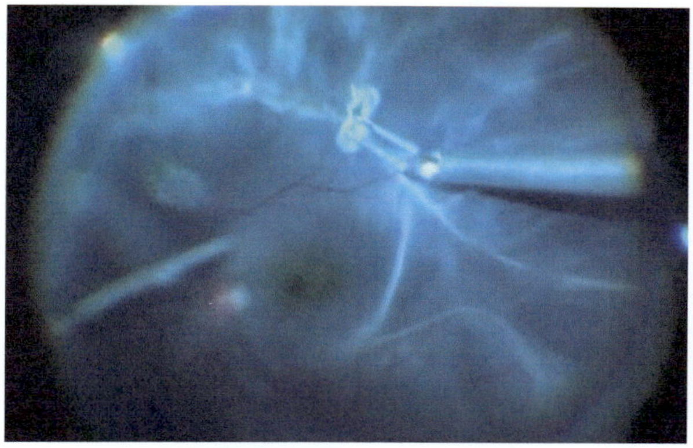

Fig. 13.27 Then grasp the membrane with the subretinal forceps and remove it together with a serrated jaws forceps

13.5 Retinotomy

Instruments

1. 25G or 27G Vitreous cutter **or** vertical scissors
2. 23G or 25G knob spatula (Eye Tech, UK) **or** flute needle with silicone tip
3. PFCL
4. 1000 csts or 5000 csts silicone oil

The Surgery Step-by-Step

1. **Row of diathermy as anteriorly as possible within the contracted retina**
2. **Retinotomy**
3. **Retinectomy (removal of remaining anterior retina)**
4. **Hemostasis of the retinotomy edge**
5. **Injection of PFCL**
6. **Flattening of retinotomy edges**
7. **Attachment test**
8. **Laser treatment**
9. **PFCL × air exchange**
10. **Air × silicone oil exchange**

Every Step in Detail

1. **Row of diathermy as anteriorly as possible within the contracted retina** (Figs. 13.28 and 13.29)

Retinotomy should be performed as anteriorly as possible in order to preserve the healthy retina. The area to be incised should be marked with a row of endodiathermy, and incision should be tapered into the normal retina at both ends of the contracted retina. If endodiathermy is not possible, i.e., the retina does not become white during endodiathermy, then vitreous is left. Remove the residual vitreous with the vitreous cutter and continue with diathermy (Figs. 13.2 and 13.3). If you find a membrane at the edge, remove it at once; otherwise it will continue to proliferate and cause a recurrent detachment.

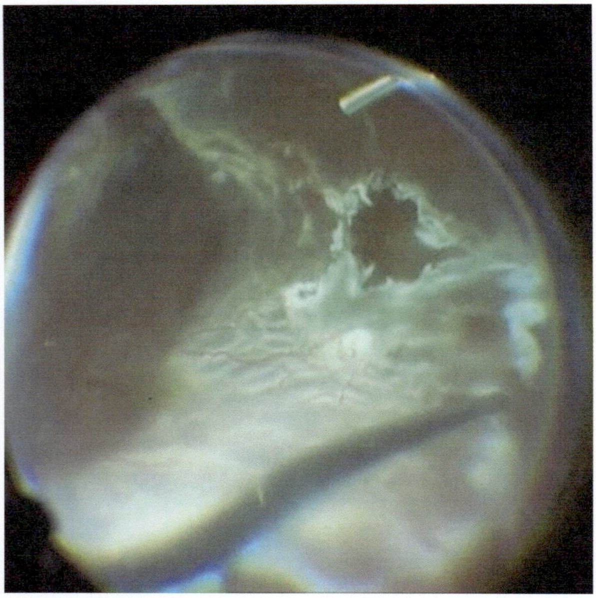

Fig. 13.28 A row of diathermy as anteriorly as possible

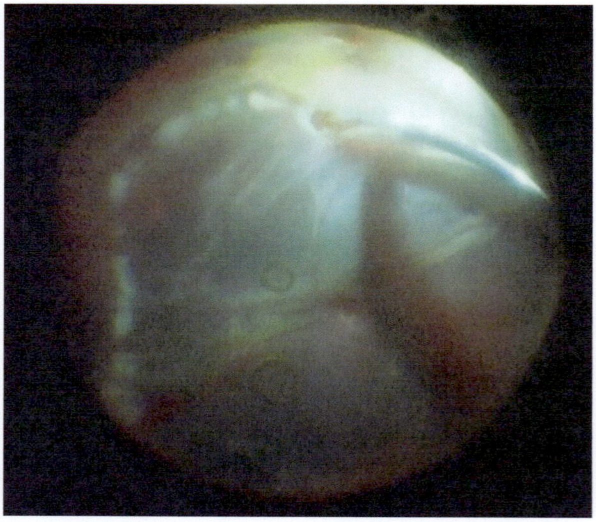

Fig. 13.29 Diathermy before retinotomy

2. **Retinotomy** (Fig. 13.30)
3. **Retinectomy (Removal of remaining anterior retina)** (Fig. 13.31)
4. **Hemostasis of the retinotomy edge**

The retinotomy is performed with the vitreous cutter at a low cut-rate of 100–150 cuts/min or vertical scissors (Fig. 13.4). A 27G vitreous cutter is due to its size very suitable for a retinotomy. The remaining anterior retina is then removed with the vitreous cutter at higher cut rate of 5000–7500 cuts/min and is called **anterior**

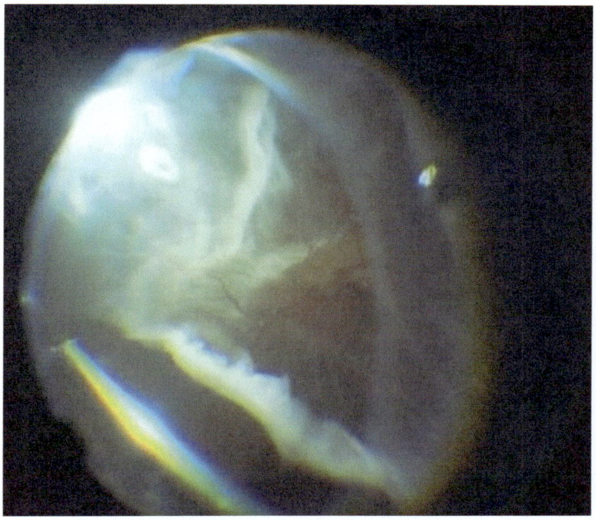

Fig. 13.30 A retinotomy anterior to the row of endodiathermy

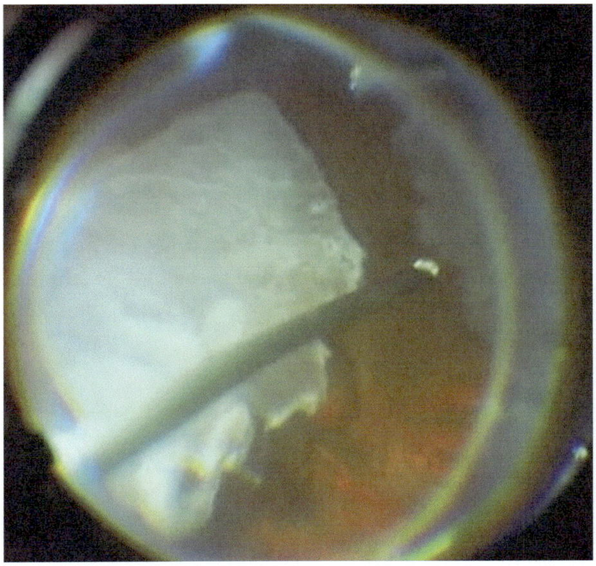

Fig. 13.31 A retinectomy of the anterior retina

retinectomy (Fig. 13.5). Meticulous hemostasis of the retinotomy edge is essential, as any bleeding may lead to recurrent PVR.

5. **Injection of PFCL**
6. **Flatten the retinotomy edges**

The retina is then reattached using perfluorocarbon liquid (PFCL). Instill PFCL up to the retinal edge. Folds or areas of retinal distortion are adjusted with a retinal manipulator (knob spatula) or a flute needle with silicone tip. In case of residual membranes, dissect the membrane with a membrane pic or CRVO knife. The PFCL is not removed for this maneuver; it creates counter tension. Grasp the membrane with a forceps and remove it. You may need to work bimanual with the forceps in one hand and the dissection instrument in the other hand. If you lift the retina carefully, then the PFCL will not spill over the edges and flow subretinal.

7. **Attachment test**
8. **Laser treatment** (Fig. 13.32)

Before continuing with laser photocoagulation, check whether the retinotomy edges are completely attached under PFCL. If not, then fix the problem: remove the membrane or enlarge the retinotomy. If the attachment test is positive, continue with laser treatment (Fig. 13.32).

For laser photocoagulation of retinal edges, we recommend a higher laser power than usual. A higher laser power induces an immediate congealing of outer retinal proteins by heat resulting in a more immediate adhesion. Our laser power for retinotomy edges with an argon laser device (Iridex, CA) is as follows: power, 100–300 mW; duration, **300** msec; and interval, 300 msec. This is especially the case for laser treatment of retinotomy edges. For retinal holes and for a laser cerclage, a reduced laser power is recommended.

Surgical Pearls No. 94
Laser photocoagulation for retinotomy: More laser power than usual – **300 msec** duration instead of 200 msec

9. **PFCL × air exchange**
10. **Air × silicone oil exchange**

For this step two methods are possible: (1) first a PFCL × air exchange and then a silicone oil injection and (2) a direct PFCL × silicone oil exchange. We prefer the first method because the retinotomy edges detach and enroll with the second

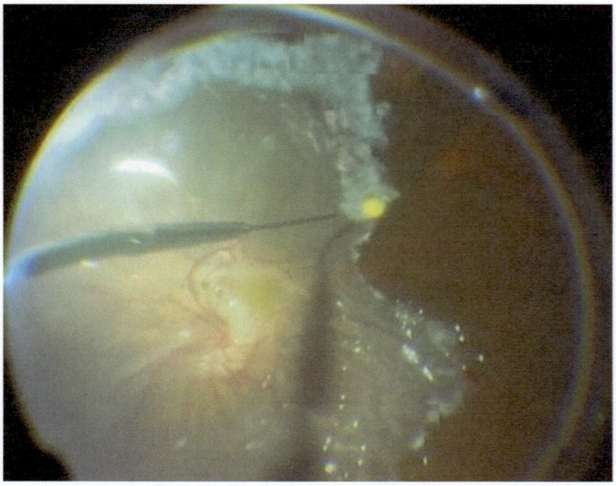

Fig. 13.32 Laser photocoagulation of the retinotomy edges

method.Start with a PFCL × air exchange until the air reaches the retinal edges. It is important to aspirate thoroughly the fluid at the edges of the retinotomy to avoid slippage. Then continue to remove the residual PFCL. The whole procedure is finished with an injection of 1000 csts silicone oil into the air-filled cavity. We never use gas in an eye with retinotomy because in case of recurrent detachment, there will be a fast progression to PVR. Heavy silicone oil such as Densiron 68 can be used but is not necessary. If the retina is relieved, then 1000 csts oil is sufficient.

References

1. Vitrectomy with silicone oil or sulfur hexafluoride gas in eyes with severe proliferative vitreoretinopathy: results of a randomized clinical trial. Silicone study report 1. Arch Ophthalmol. 1992;110(6):770–9.
2. Ingrid Kreissig. A Practical Guide to Minimal Surgery for Retinal Detachment. Thieme, Germany ISBN 9783131606914.

Part IX
Diabetic Retinopathy

Chapter 14
Easy Proliferative Diabetic Retinopathy

Extras: Videos 14.1, 14.2, and 14.3.

14.1 Introduction

The surgical planning of the diabetic eye is very important; this is especially the case in active proliferative diabetic retinopathies. What is the right timing for a vitrectomy? Do not operate too early; if the eye is not pretreated with PRP or anti-VEGF injections and the diabetes is badly regulated, then the vitrectomy becomes VERY difficult. Surgical trauma triggers the diabetic retinopathy and consequently the postoperative healing. It increases also the risk of recurrence of fibrovascular membranes. If you for example perform a phacoemulsification of an eye with active proliferative diabetic retinopathy, then the retinopathy will progress in the most cases and an iris rubeosis may occur. Therefore, combine a phacoemulsification always with an intravitreal anti-VEGF treatment in order to prevent a progression of the retinopathy and to quieten the retinopathy for the following vitrectomy.

We favor therefore a stepwise procedure, i.e., we operate the eye in several sessions: first phacoemulsification combined with an anti-VEGF injection and 4 weeks later a vitrectomy (see Fig. 14.1). The vitrectomy is much easier, if the eye is pretreated with phacoemulsification and Avastin. The posterior hyaloid is easier to open, less intraoperatively bleeding will occur, the membranes are easier to remove, and so forth. And the postoperative healing is of course faster.

Why a stepwise procedure? The difficulty of the vitrectomy depends on the severity of the PDR. A severe diabetic retinopathy requires a long traumatic surgery. The surgical trauma however aggravates the diabetic retinopathy, resulting in a vicious cycle. It is therefore vital to dry out the fibrovascular membranes BEFORE vitrectomy; i.e., remove the vascular component with laser and anti-VEGF.

Electronic Supplementary Material The online version of this chapter (https://doi.org/10.1007/978-3-319-89677-9_14) contains supplementary material, which is available to authorized users.

U. Spandau, H. Heimann, *Practical Handbook for Small-Gauge Vitrectomy*,
https://doi.org/10.1007/978-3-319-89677-9_14

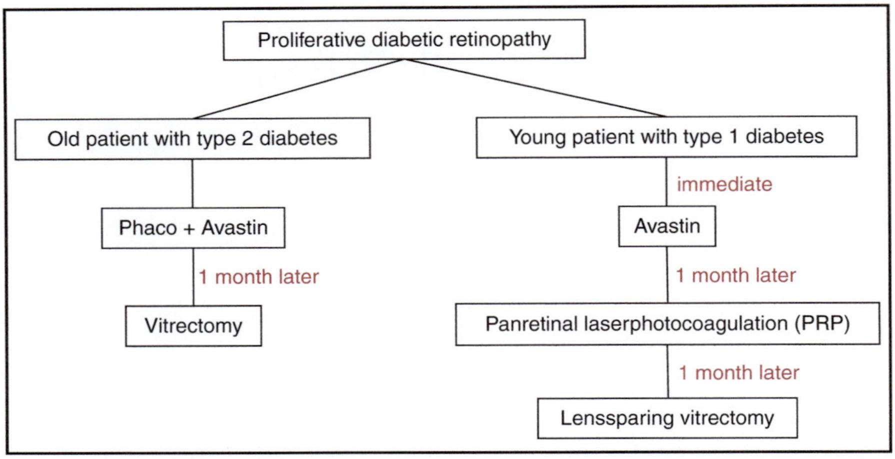

Fig. 14.1 Our treatment algorithm for surgical planning of a PDR for a young type 1 diabetic and an old type 2 diabetic

The main rule is not to perform a vitrectomy in an untreated eye. Pretreat the eye first with PRP and anti-VEGF, keep a tight follow-up until the retinopathy is inactive, and then schedule surgery. Secondly, avoid a combined phaco/vitrectomy. Operate instead first a phaco with Avastin and 1–4 weeks later a vitrectomy.

A cautionary note regarding the timing of phaco and Avastin treatment: The effect of Avastin lasts 6 weeks. After 4–6 weeks, a laser treatment with/without vitrectomy should be scheduled. Alternatively, repeat an Avastin injection. Otherwise the proliferative vessels will reopen, and the PDR will reoccur after 2–3 months.

In Conclusion: The grade of surgical difficulty depends on the severity of the diabetic retinopathy. We differentiate an easy and a difficult proliferative diabetic retinopathy:

Easy PDR: A complete PVD with vitreous hemorrhage is present. The retina is treated with scatter laser (Fig. 14.2).

Difficult PDR: Only a partial PVD is present. Fibrovascular membranes are located at the posterior pole. A tractional retinal detachment is present. No or insufficient laser treatment has been performed (Fig. 14.3).

The more active the retinopathy, the more stepwise we operate.

In an **easy PDR,** we operate in two sessions: (1) Phacoemulsification and intravitreal anti-VEGF and 4 weeks later (2) vitrectomy (Fig. 14.2).

In a **difficult PDR,** we operate in several sessions: In young type 1 diabetics, we inject within 1 week anti-VEGF in both eyes; 1 month later, if the vitreous is clear, we perform a laser photocoagulation. The laser photocoagulation is performed in general anesthesia with a laser helmet, so-called laser indirect ophthalmoscopy (LIO). If the vitreous is not clear, we repeat anti-VEGF. Then we perform a lens-sparing vitrectomy. In old patients, we start with phacoemulsification and intravitreal anti-VEGF and 3–4 weeks later vitrectomy (Fig. 14.1).

Caution: Do not forget the second eye while treating the first eye. We use to inject anti-VEGF in the second eye every time when operating the first eye. We have seen many times a second eye progress to a tractional PDR under a prolonged treatment of the first eye.

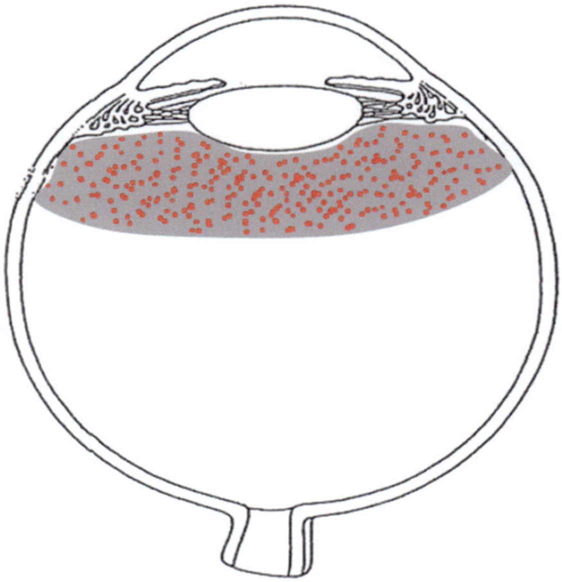

Fig. 14.2 A mild (surgically easy) PDR with vitreous hemorrhage. Note that a complete PVD is present. Fibrovascular membranes are usually not present because the posterior hyaloid is detached

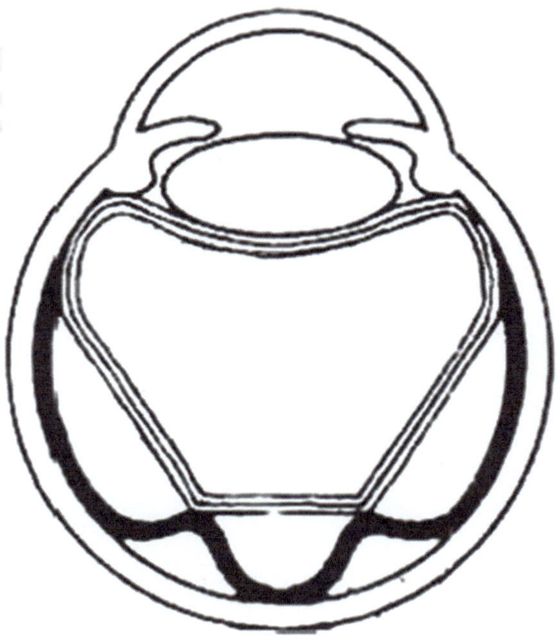

Fig. 14.3 Illustration of a difficult PDR. The retina is laser treated. Many retinal proliferations and vitreoretinal adhesions are present. The posterior hyaloid is attached in the posterior pole and partially detached in the periphery; the nasal posterior hyaloid is often attached

14.2 Combined Phacoemulsification and Anti-VEGF Treatment

A diabetic vitrectomy is easier if the eye is pretreated with anti-VEGF 1–4 weeks prior to the vitrectomy. If you have an opacified lens, and the patient is older than 50 years, then perform also a cataract operation before the vitrectomy. It only takes 10 min of extra surgical time. Especially in advanced diabetic retinopathy cases, avoid anterior segment inflammation with iris rubeosis. A diabetic eye, which is pretreated with anti-VEGF and cataract surgery, is much easier to vitrectomize.

Perform a phacoemulsification as usual. Inject the IOL and place it into the capsular bag. Before removing the viscoelastics, perform an intravitreal injection with an anti-VEGF medication. Inject 0.1–0.2 mL. Then remove the viscoelastics and hydrate the incisions (Figs. 14.4 and 14.5).

Surgical Pearls No. 95

If a patient has a bilateral PDR, and you decide to vitrectomize one eye, then do not forget the other eye. Treat the other eye in the same session (or shortly after) with phaco + IOL + Avastin or at least only Avastin. It easily happens that the clinical focus lies on the vitrectomized eye, and the other eye (often the better eye) gets worse.

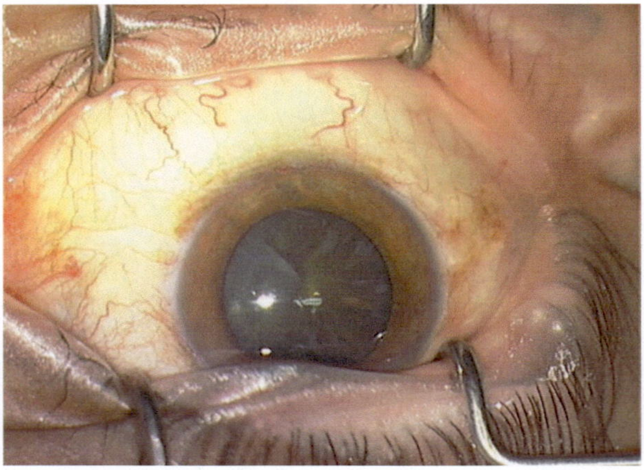

Fig. 14.4 A diabetic eye with vitreous hemorrhage. We apply a stepwise technique: first a combined phacoemulsification with intravitreal Avastin and 1 month later, if still necessary, a vitrectomy

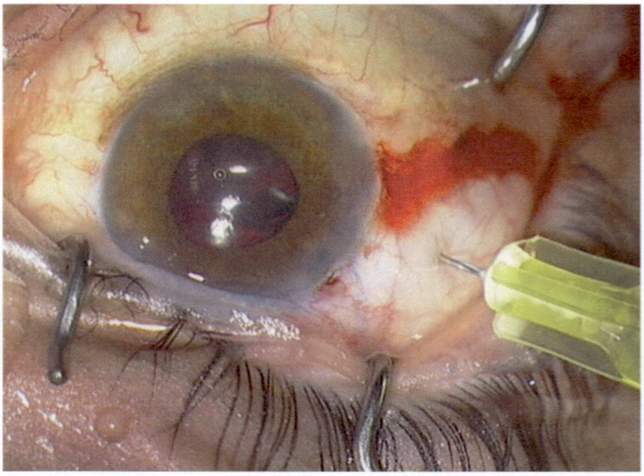

Fig. 14.5 After implantation of the IOL and before removal of the viscoelastics, an intravitreal injection of Avastin (0.1 mL) is performed

14.3 Vitrectomy

A vitreous hemorrhage with attached retina and no associated major vitreoretinal pathology is suitable for the beginner. In most cases, a PVD is present, and the hemorrhage fills out the vitreous gel behind the lens (Fig. 14.2). In the presence of vitreous hemorrhage, a previous history of panretinal photocoagulation usually facilitates the surgery, because it is associated with a higher rate of posterior vitreous detachment and promotes retinal adhesion to the RPE and choroid. He/she learns to work with the vitreous cutter and apply a PRP but does not need to perform any significant manipulations of the retina.

The main problem with this procedure is that there is no view of the fundus (Fig. 14.6). The procedure is even harder when the natural lens is still present, due to the risk of injuring the posterior capsule. In the learning phase, perform only PPVs in pseudophakic eyes.

Practice the application of panretinal laser photocoagulation (PRP) very well using a chandelier light. In one hand, hold the scleral depressor, and indent the sclera and retina, and in the other hand, hold the laser probe, and apply a PRP up to the ora serrata (Fig. 14.7). This surgery can be performed under local anesthesia. We use mostly 27G for these cases.

Surgical Pearls No. 96
B-scan: In cases with vitreous hemorrhage, always perform a detailed preoperative ultrasound examination. Try to determine the state of the posterior vitreous face (attached, partially attached or detached) and the retina.

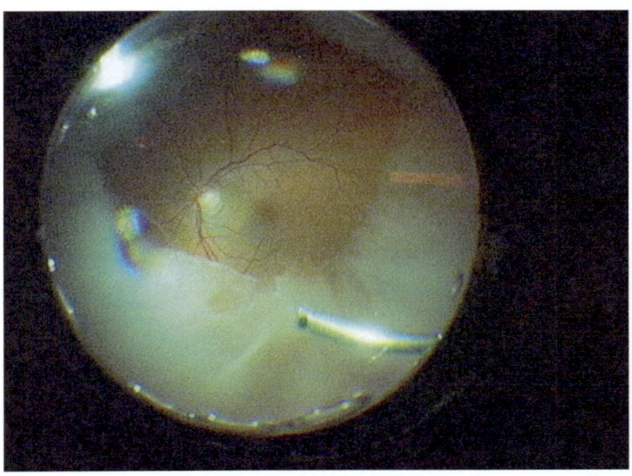

Fig. 14.6 A dense vitreous hemorrhage with attached retina behind the vitreous

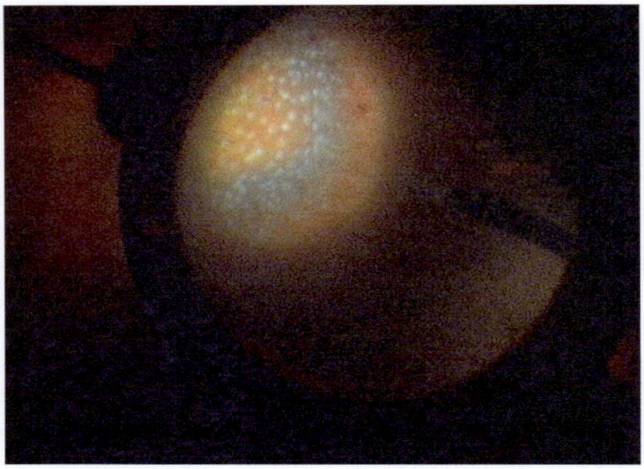

Fig. 14.7 Perform a PRP up to the ora serrata

14.3.1 Instruments

1. **23G–27G three-port trocar system with or without chandelier illumination**
2. **120D lens**
3. **Vitreous cutter**
4. **Backflush instrument**
5. **Scleral depressor**

14.3.2 Tamponade

Air, SF_6

14.3.3 Individual Steps

1. **Three-port trocar system with or without chandelier illumination**
2. **Core vitrectomy**
3. **Peripheral vitrectomy**
4. **PRP**
5. **Tamponade and intravitreal anti-VEGF treatment**
6. **Removal of the trocar cannulas**

The Surgery Step-by-Step: Figs. 14.6 and 14.7

1. **Three-port trocar system with or without chandelier illumination**
2. **Core vitrectomy**

The vitreous hemorrhage reduces the illumination of the light fiber, because the light cone is hidden by blood. Therefore, the surgeon should first make a core vitrectomy. Keep the vitreous cutter behind the IOL and remove all vitreous gel. It might be easier to work first without BIOM and use the microscope only as you would in cataract surgery. If the visibility is not improved, then try only to aspirate the liquefied blood. Try next to cut a break in the posterior hyaloid in order to obtain a view of the fundus (Fig. 14.6). It is important to identify the retinal vessels to make sure that the surgeon is in the right plane (and not in the subretinal space). If successful, continue the vitrectomy from the break into the posterior hyaloid.

Surgical Pearls No. 97
Blocked infusion: The hemorrhagic vitreous blocks sometimes the infusion. Check the infusion trocar before vitrectomy, and if in doubt, then cut the hemorrhagic vitreous around the infusion trocar.

Surgical Pearls No. 98
Removal of anterior hyaloid: In case of a hemorrhage directly behind the lens, it may be necessary to remove the anterior hyaloid. This is an easy procedure in pseudophakic patients but a lens-threatening procedure in phakic patients. We perform two techniques: work at the edge of the lens (i.e., behind the zonules) in order to avoid a lens touch. (1) With help of a serrated jaws forceps, grab the anterior hyaloid/vitreous, and pull it toward the center of the globe. Work from both sides. (2) With help of a vitreous cutter, suck the anterior hyaloid/vitreous (only aspiration), and pull the vitreous cutter toward the center of the globe. Cut the vitreous there. Work from both sides.

3. **Peripheral Vitrectomy**

Proceed to trim the vitreous base. Do not trim the vitreous base completely because the risk of causing damage to the retina is higher than the benefits. If the posterior vitreous body is not detached, then a PVD should be performed now. If the etiology of the bleeding is, for example, a bleeding vessel, treat it now with laser, diathermy, or cryo.

Surgical Pearls No. 99
How should epiretinal blood be removed? (1) Aspirate epiretinal blood by sweeping with a silicone tip flute needle over the retina. (2) By pressing several times on the side opening/tubing of the backflush instrument, water is ejected from the tip of the flute needle and blows the epiretinal blood upward. The blood can then be easily aspirated at the same time with the vitreous cutter. (3) Clotted blood can be grasped with an ILM forceps and be removed with the vitreous cutter.

4. **Panretinal Photocoagulation (PRP)**

We recommend completing a PRP intraoperatively in all cases of vitrectomy for proliferative diabetic retinopathy. This is the best opportunity to complete the PRP, as rebleeding into the vitreous cavity is a common problem following vitrectomy, which will have a negative influence on performing additional PRP after the vitrectomy. Use the scleral depressor and apply a dense PRP up to the ora serrata (Fig. 14.7). For PRP we recommend the following laser parameters: power, 100–150 mw; duration, 200 ms; and interval, 200–300 ms at an OcularLight GL Company Iridex. These values are dependent on the device and the pigmentation of the fundus.

After endolaser photocoagulation check if a new hemorrhage occurred at the central pole, and treat it before you move on to the tamponade.

Surgical Pearls No. 100
Small pupil: If the pupil constricts during surgery, inject 0.01% Adrenalin into the anterior chamber. The pupil enlarges within seconds. If the small pupil is caused by posterior synechiae, use stretching instruments such as a push-pull, or insert iris hooks to enlarge the pupil.

5. **Tamponade and Intravitreal Anti-VEGF Treatment**

An air or gas tamponade is recommended to avoid a rebleeding into the vitreous cavity. Inject 0,2 mL bevacizumab at the end of the procedure to inhibit proliferative vessels.

6. **Removal of Trocar Cannulas**

The trocars are removed, as described above. In cases of a 25G trocar and silicone oil tamponade, suture the sclerotomy.

14.4 Complications

Recurrent vitreous hemorrhage: After a vitrectomy for a vitreous hemorrhage, bleeding may reoccur after surgery. If the recurrence is associated with a hyphema, then check if the patient takes anticoagulants, i.e., aspirin. The patient should stop taking blood thinning medication for approximately 1 month. In most cases the hyphema resolves. Do not reoperate on the patient before the hyphema has resolved.

14.5 FAQ

Do you peel the ILM in diabetic retinopathy?
No, never. The only exception would be a very difficult case complicated by PVR. There are no double-blind studies published which justify the prophylactic removal of physiologic tissue such as ILM.
Anti-VEGF may increase tractions in diabetic eyes.
This is true. Anti-VEGF and laser increase preexisting tractions to a limited extent. The advantages of a bloodless surgical field, however, outweigh the disadvantage of an increased traction [1].

Reference

1. Arevalo JF, Maia M, Flynn HW, et al. Tractional retinal detachment following intravitreal bevacizumab (Avastin) in patients with severe proliferative diabetic retinopathy. Br J Ophthalmol. 2008;92:213–6.

Chapter 15
Difficult Proliferative Diabetic Retinopathy

Extras: Videos 15.1, 15.2, 15.3, 15.4, 15.5, and 15.6.

15.1 General Introduction

A vitrectomy for diabetic retinopathy is the most difficult and challenging vitreoretinal surgery nowadays and will become the most dominant surgery in the future. The two key features for a successful and complication-free surgery are two key elements:

1. Stepwise surgery
2. Bimanual vitrectomy

In proliferative diabetic retinopathy we apply the periphery to disc (outside-in) technique. You start with a posterior hyaloidal rhexis (outside) and continue with a removal of the membranes in the center (in). The surgical time is approximately 90–120 min.

The eye should be pseudophakic, an exception is the young type I diabetic patient. In the latter case, we perform a lens-sparing vitrectomy. We usually work with a 27G trocar system. The 27G vitreous cutter can work very close to the retina and be very helpful for dissection of membranes. If extensive membranes are present, we use a 25G system because the whole range of 25G peeling instruments is required.

Surgical Pearls No. 101
BSS damages the phakic lens: In pseudophakic eyes BSS is used as irrigation fluid and in phakic eyes BSS Plus® (Alcon). BSS Plus® also contains glutathione, glucose, and sodium bicarbonate.

Electronic Supplementary Material The online version of this chapter (https://doi.org/10.1007/978-3-319-89677-9_15) contains supplementary material, which is available to authorized users.

U. Spandau, H. Heimann, *Practical Handbook for Small-Gauge Vitrectomy*,
https://doi.org/10.1007/978-3-319-89677-9_15

15.2 Surgery

Instruments

1. **27G three-port trocar system with chandelier illumination**
2. **120D lens, for peeling: 60D lens**
3. **Vitreous cutter**
4. **Backflush instrument**
5. **27G endgripping forceps (DORC)**
6. **27G curved scissors (DORC)**
7. **Silicone tip Charles flute needle/vacuum cleaner**
8. **Endodiathermy (DORC, Alcon)**
9. **Laser probe**
10. **Scleral depressor**

Maybe

25G straight scissors
25G knob spatula

Dye
Triamcinolone or Trypan blue

Tamponade
20% SF_6, 1000 csts silicone oil

15.2.1 Individual Steps

1. **Three-port trocar system with chandelier illumination**
2. **Posterior hyaloid rhexis**
3. **Removal of tractional membranes**
4. **Instruments for removal of membranes**
   - Delamination of membranes with membrane pic, knob spatula, and vacuum cleaner
   - Dissection of membranes with curved scissors
   - Removal of dissected membranes with vitreous cutter
5. **Hemostasis**
   - Slight bleeding
   - Moderate bleeding
   - Strong bleeding
6. **Removal of attached posterior hyaloid in the periphery**
7. **PRP under BSS**
8. **Fluid against air exchange**
9. **Intravitreal Avastin**

10. **Internal tamponade**
    - Gas tamponade
    - Silicone oil tamponade
11. **Removal of trocars**

    The Surgery Step-by-Step: Figs. 15.1–15.29

1. **Three-Port Trocar System with Chandelier Illumination**

Insert first three trocars and then inferonasally the chandelier light. Continue with a core vitrectomy. We recommend 27G trocars (Fig. 15.1); an alternative is a hybrid system.

Surgical Pearls No. 102

Corneal lubrication: A major problem during vitrectomy, especially in combined surgeries with a duration of over 1 h, is corneal epithelial edema. With the application of methylcellulose (Celoftal®, Alcon or Ocucoat®, Bausch&Lomb) on the cornea, the cornea can remain clear for many hours. A debridement of the epithelium is rarely necessary; but if needed use a broad blade (crescent knife).

2. **Posterior hyaloid rhexis** (Figs. 15.2 and 15.3)

The posterior vitreous is usually attached in eyes with fibrovascular membranes. An important aim of surgery is the induction of PVD. The induction of PVD is extremely challenging in eyes with ischemic retina because the posterior hyaloid is firmly attached to the retina. When inducing a PVD, the surgeon can easily make tears in the retina.

To avoid this damage, the surgeon should begin with a peripheral vitreous detachment. In most cases of proliferative diabetic retinopathy, a partial vitreous detachment is present. This means that the vitreous is still attached centrally but partially detached in the mid-periphery. Try to find where the peripheral vitreous is detached. Create here an opening of the posterior hyaloid on the height of the equator. Then remove the vitreous along the posterior vitreous face (Figs. 15.2 and 15.3) on a

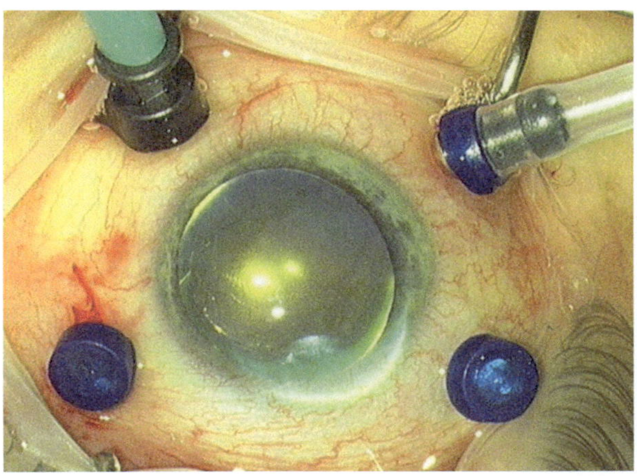

Fig. 15.1 A 3-port vitrectomy with chandelier light is the best surgical setup for a difficult PDR; a chandelier light allows bimanual surgery and bimanual removal of membranes

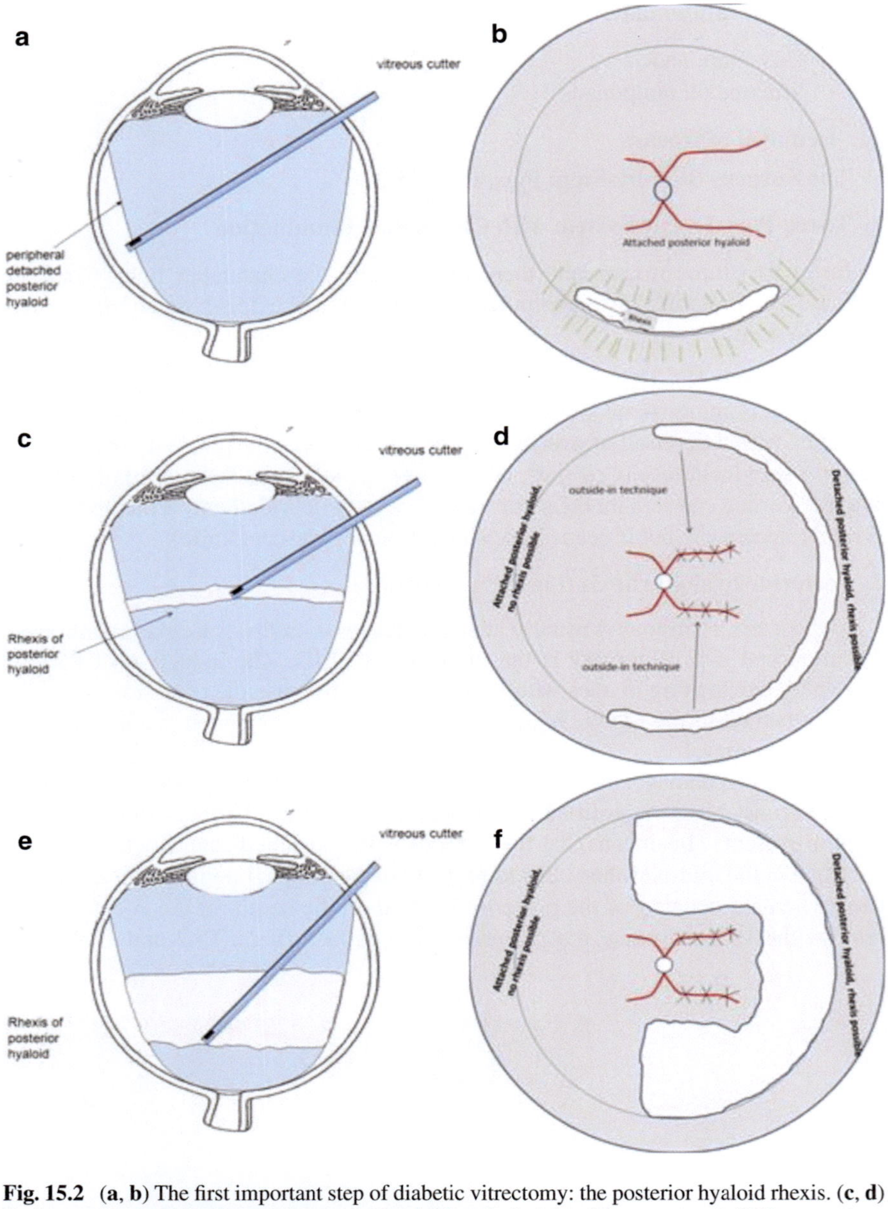

Fig. 15.2 (**a**, **b**) The first important step of diabetic vitrectomy: the posterior hyaloid rhexis. (**c**, **d**) Perform a rhexis of the detached posterior hyaloid on the height of the equator. (**e**, **f**) Then continue with the removal of the vitreous to the nasal and temporal arcades. The attached (nasal) hyaloid cannot be removed in this stage (f).

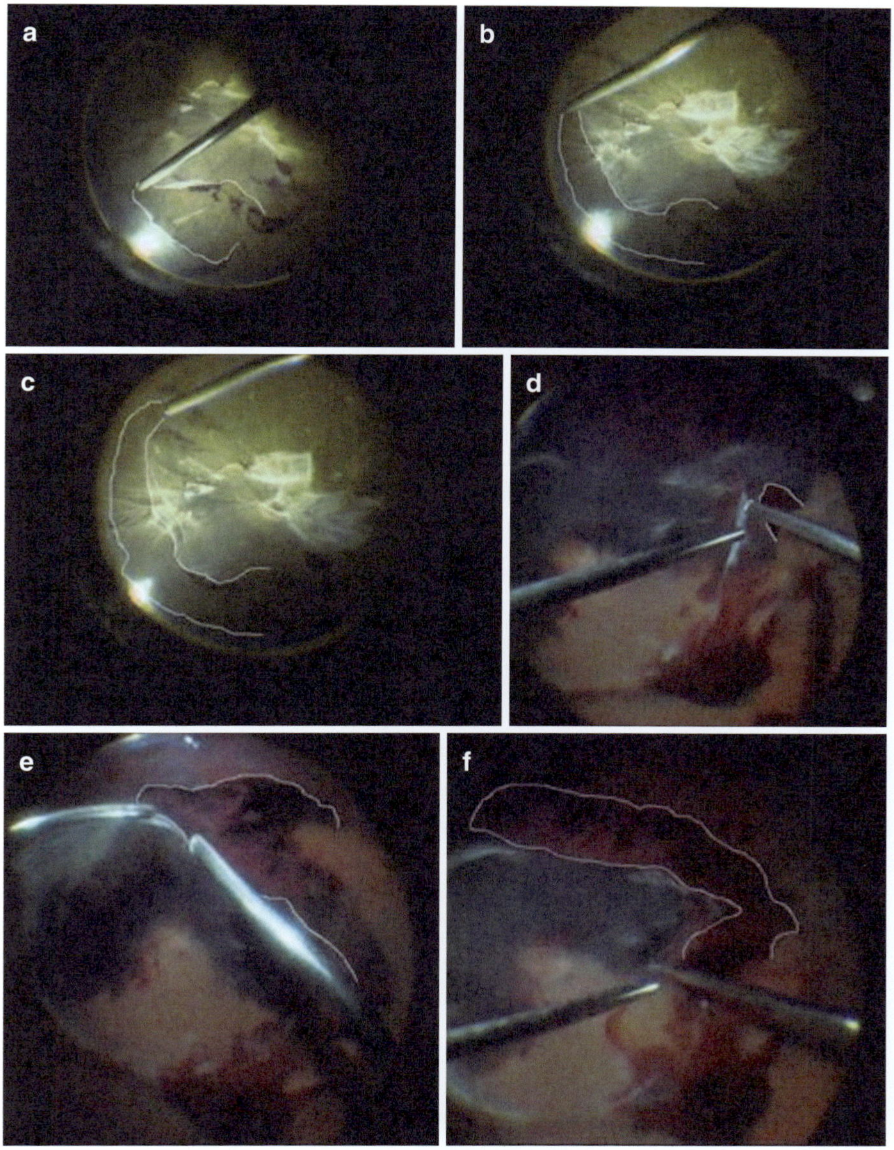

Fig. 15.3 (**a**) Posterior hyaloid rhexis without subhyaloidal hemorrhage. (**b**) Be careful not to damage the retina. (**c**) Perform a posterior hyaloid rhexis of the detached hyaloid. A rhexis of the attached hyaloid is not possible. (**d**) An opening of the posterior hyaloid with presence of subhyaloidal hemorrhage. (**e**) Use the vitreous cutter with a low cutting frequency such as 1000 cuts/min. (**f**) Open the posterior hyaloid as far as possible, i.e., try to perform a round rhexis as far as possible

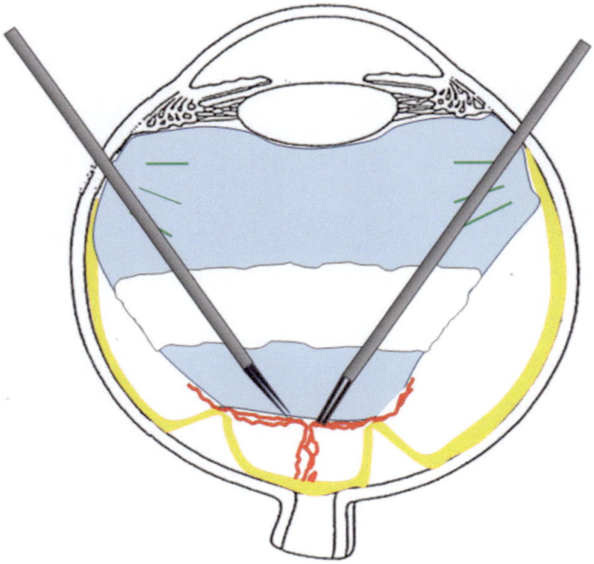

Fig. 15.4 The next and most difficult step is the bimanual removal of fibrovascular membranes

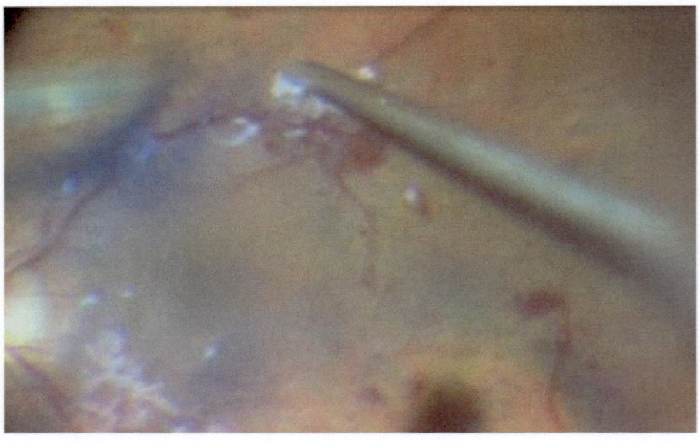

Fig. 15.5 Create an opening in the posterior hyaloid with the 27G blunt cannula (Atkinson, B&D)

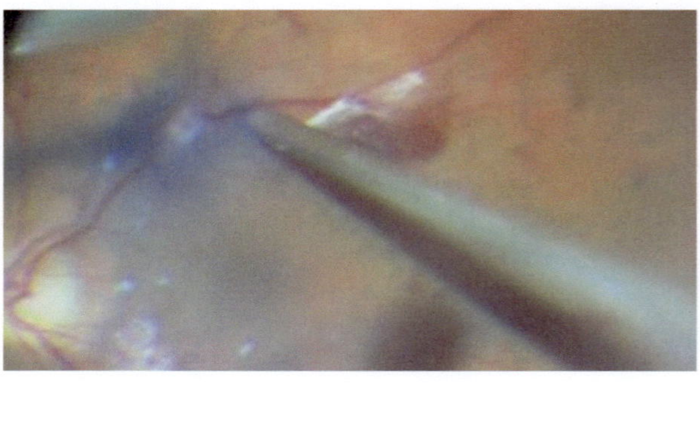

Fig. 15.6 Enlarge the opening in the posterior hyaloid

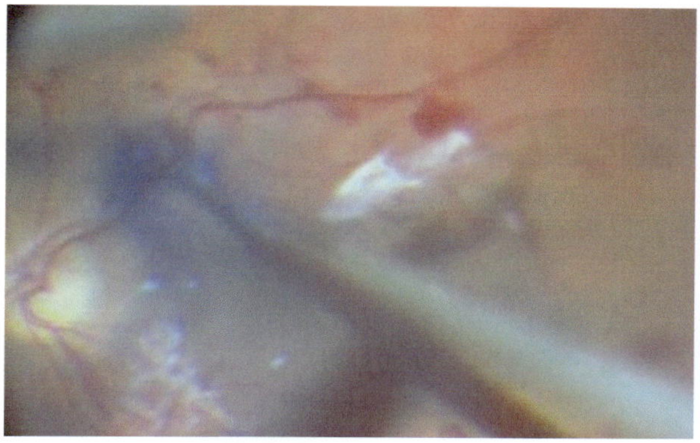

Fig. 15.7 The blunt cannula (25G and 27G) is a very convenient instrument for opening of the posterior hyaloid and for delamination of membranes

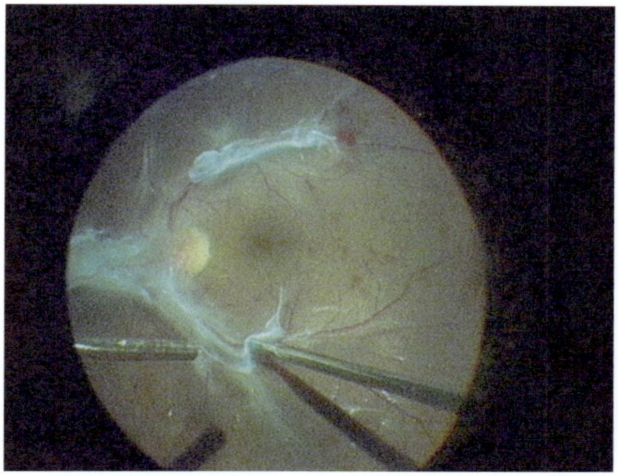

Fig. 15.8 Delaminate the membrane with a knob spatula or a vacuum cleaner

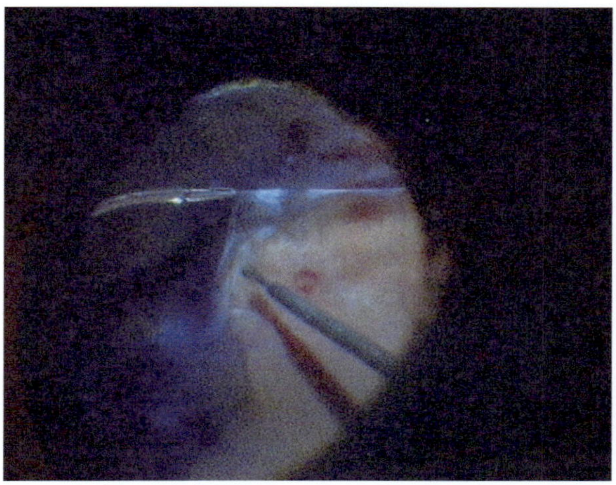

Fig. 15.9 If necessary stain the posterior hyaloid with trypan blue and delaminate it from the retina

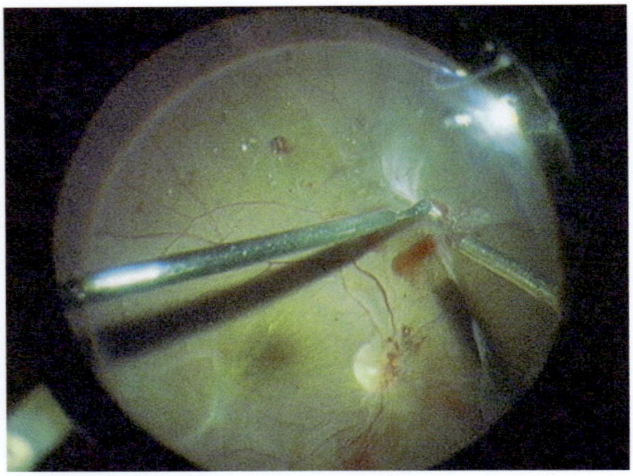

Fig. 15.10 Use a knob spatula or Charles flute needle with silicone tip or membrane pic for delamination

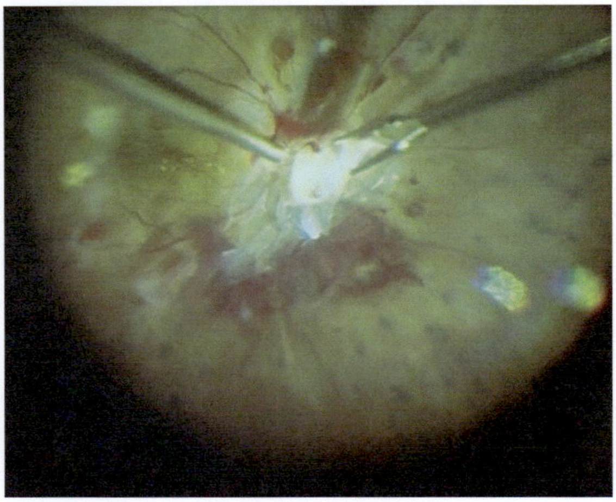

Fig. 15.11 You can also remove membranes with a silicone tip flute needle and a forceps

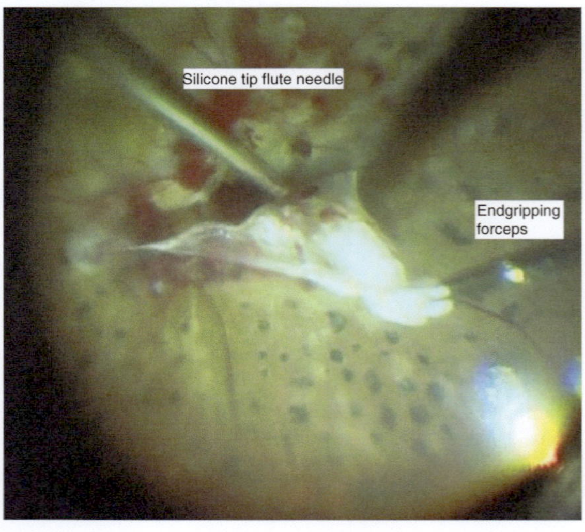

Fig. 15.12 Always pull the membrane parallel to the retina. Pulling vertically may cause a choroidal bleeding

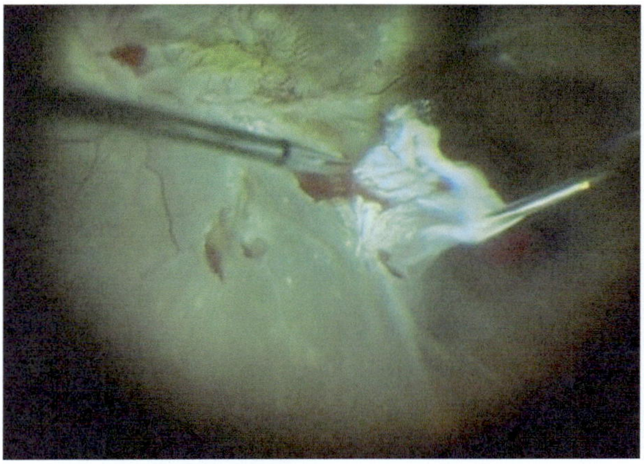

Fig. 15.13 For delamination of membranes, the knob spatula and the silicone tip flute needle are superior to the membrane pic

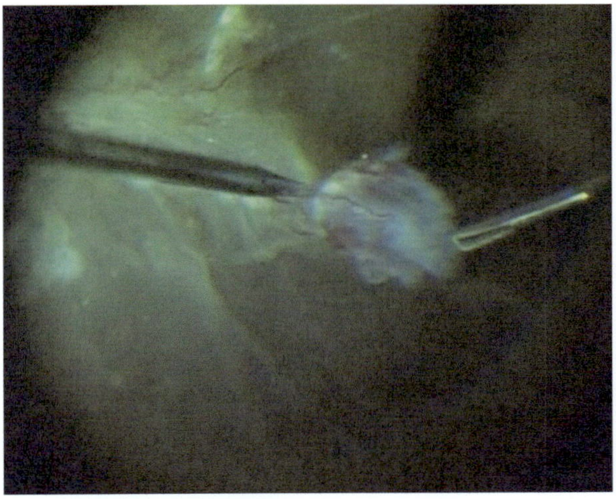

Fig. 15.14 The surgeon's right hand pulls the membrane parallel to the retina, and the left hand cuts the tissue bridges with the straight scissors

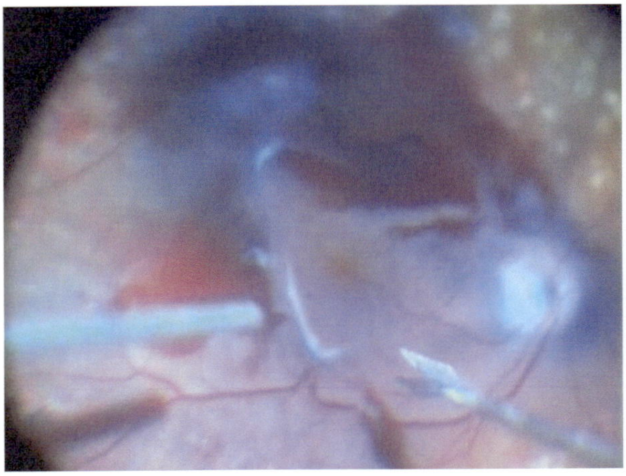

Fig. 15.15 The 27G curved microscissors allows precise cutting of vitreoretinal adhesions

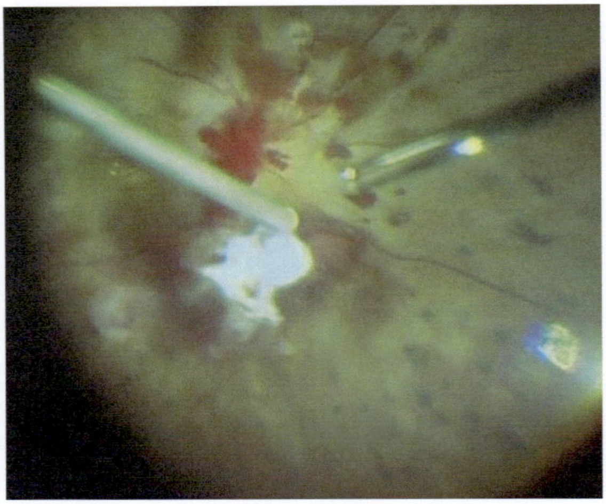

Fig. 15.16 Hold the membrane in the middle of the vitreous cavity and cut the membrane

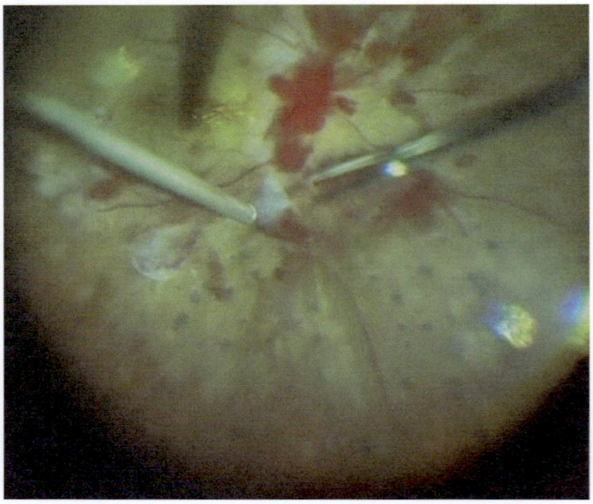

Fig. 15.17 The membrane is completely removed

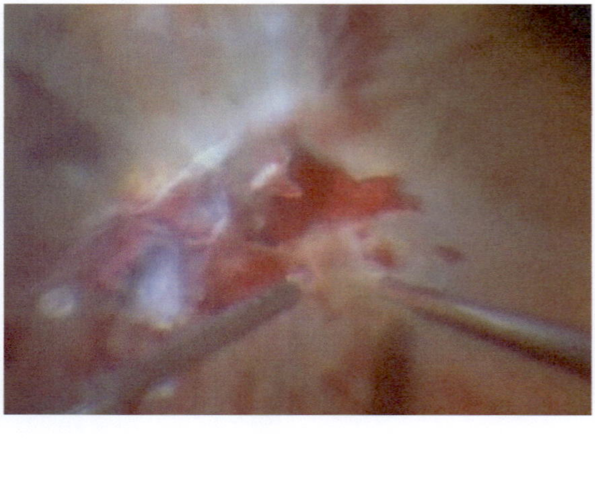

Fig. 15.18 Perform a meticulous hemostasis. We use endodiathermy outside the temporal arcades and laser inside the temporal arcades

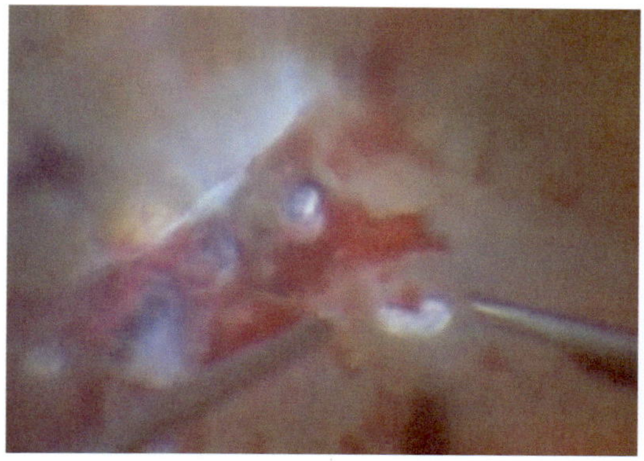

Fig. 15.19 Also hemostasis is performed bimanually. The surgeon's left hand holds the Charles flute needle and aspirates the blood. The right hand cauterizes the bleeding source

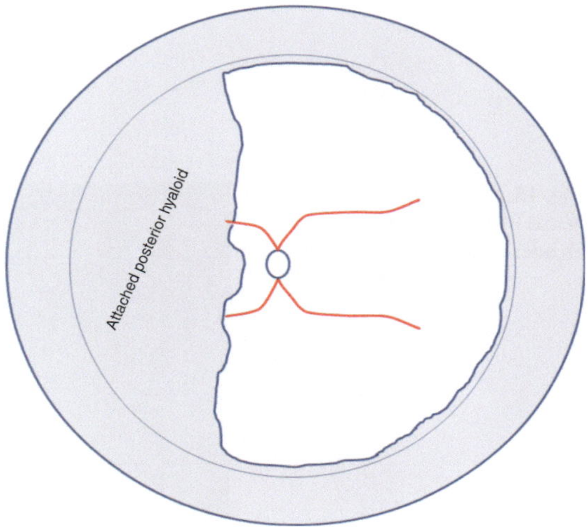

Fig. 15.20 In the initial steps, a vitreous rhexis was performed, and the vitreous was removed to the arcades. Then the fibrovascular membranes together with the central posterior were removed. The final step is the removal of the attached posterior hyaloid in the periphery—often on the nasal side

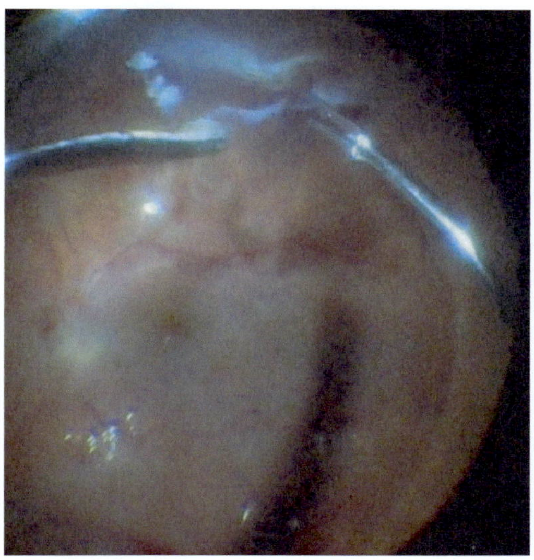

Fig. 15.21 Using bimanual technique—with an endgripping forceps and a knob spatula—the residual posterior hyaloid is removed from the disc to the ora serrata

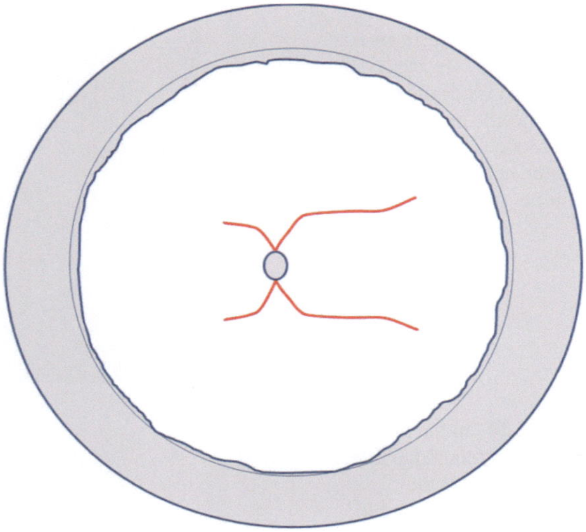

Fig. 15.22 Now a complete PVD has been performed

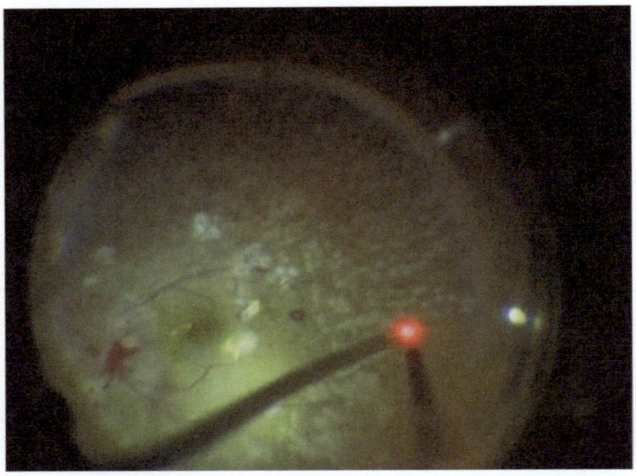

Fig. 15.23 Perform a dense PRP from the arcades to the ora serrata

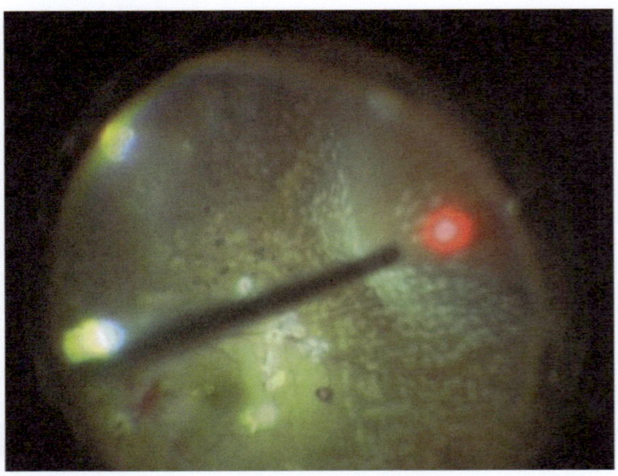

Fig. 15.24 Use preferably a curved laser probe in order to perform a laser treatment up to the ora serrata

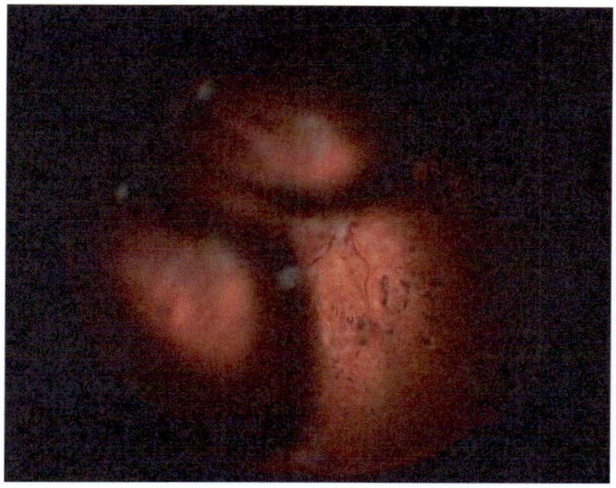

Fig. 15.25 We perform in almost all cases a fluid against air exchange. If the vitreous cavity is filled with PFCL, we perform a PFCL against air exchange and then the tamponade. In this case with a detached retina, we would use 1000 csts silicone oil

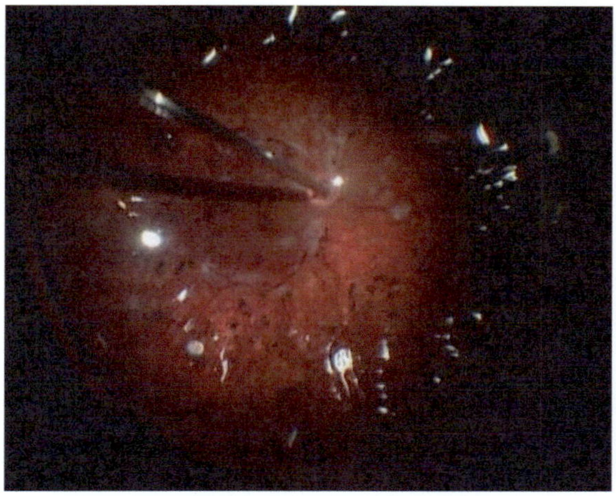

Fig. 15.26 For 23G we use a Charles flute needle with passive aspiration. For 25G and 27G, we use Charles flute needle with active aspiration

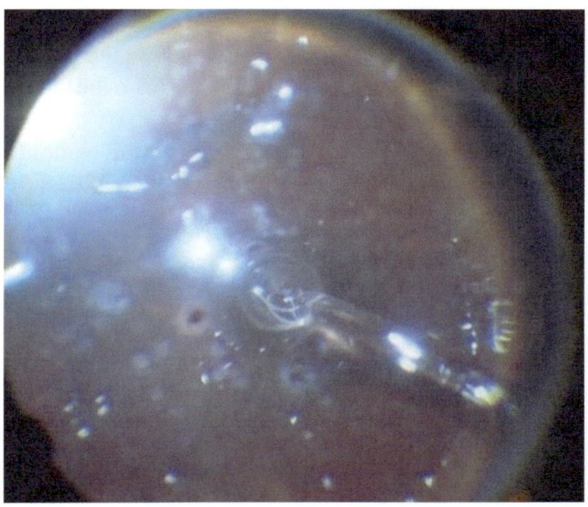

Fig. 15.27 Injection of 1000 csts silicone oil into an air-filled vitreous cavity. If possible, try to perform an air against silicone oil exchange. It is technically much easier than a PFCL against silicone oil exchange

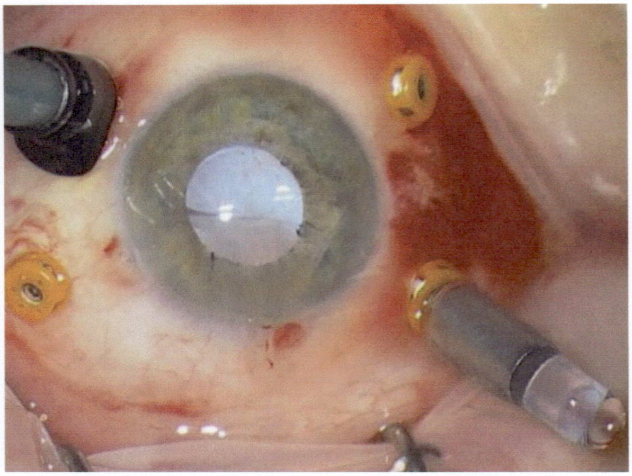

Fig. 15.28 The excessive silicone oil can escape, and overfill is avoided. Then 0.2 mL Avastin is injected into the silicone oil bubble

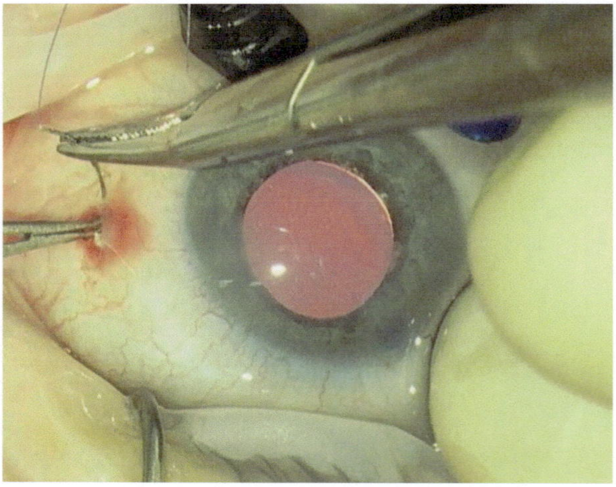

Fig. 15.29 The sclerotomies are sutured with Vicryl 8-0

constant level in a circular fashion (posterior hyaloid rhexis). Do not perform a posterior hyaloid rhexis in the area where the posterior hyaloid is attached.

Then carefully vitrectomize further from the periphery toward the beginning of the tractional membranes. Be careful that you do not exert any strain on the membranes. If the surgeon succeeds with the posterior hyaloid rhexis, he or she can continue removing the tractional membranes bimanually.

3. **Removal of tractional membranes**

The fibrovascular membranes are usually located along the vascular arcades. The membranes are removed together with the posterior hyaloid. The way to success is bimanual delamination (Fig. 15.4).

4. **Instruments for removal of proliferations**

For lifting the membranes, both the 27G endgripping forceps and the backflush instrument are suitable. The forceps grasp the membrane, and the flute needle elevates the membrane through aspiration force. For manipulation of the membrane, use the vacuum cleaner, the 27G retrobulbar cannula (Atkinson, Beaver Visitec), the curved scissors, and the vitreous cutter.

- **Delamination of membranes with 27G Atkinson cannula and 27G vacuum cleaner or 25G knob spatula**

This instrument is suitable for opening of the posterior hyaloid or delamination of flat membranes. The membrane can be lifted up with the blunt cannula and then removed with the micro forceps (Figs. 15.5, 15.6, and 15.7).

Grasp the peripheral portion of the membrane with the Eckardt forceps or a backflush instrument in one hand, and delaminate the membrane with the knob spatula (Figs. 15.8, 15.9, and 15.10) or the vacuum cleaner in the other hand (Figs.15.11, 15.12, and 15.13).

- **Dissection of membranes with 27G curved or 25G straight scissors**

The membranes are partially attached by “tissue bridges” to the retina. These bridges have to be identified by careful delamination and then be cut with the straight or curved scissors (Fig. 15.14 and 15.15). The vertical scissors can be used for horizontal tissue bridges. The tractional membranes are dissected and removed through a constant change of instruments between delamination and cauterization. If a bleeding occurs during this step, then perform a hemostasis.

- **Removal of dissected membranes with vitreous cutter**

Grasp the membrane with intravitreal forceps and hold it in the middle of the vitreous cavity. Then cut it with the vitreous cutter (1000–2000 cuts/min) (Figs. 15.16 and 15.17).

Surgical Pearls No. 103

Peeling and choroidal hemorrhage: Do not pull a membrane forward to the lens—you may cause a choroidal hemorrhage. Pull the membrane parallel to the retina.

5. **Hemostasis**

There are different methods to stop intraoperative bleeding, depending on its severity:

- **Slight bleeding:**
- Increase the intraocular pressure to approximately 40 mmHg,
- aspirate the blood with the left hand, and cauterize the bleeding source with endodiathermy or the laser probe in the right hand. Inside the arcades, we cauterize the bleeding sites with laser. Outside the arcades, we cauterize retinal bleeding sites with endodiathermy (Figs. 15.18 and 15.19). Start with relatively low energy, as too vigorous endodiathermy may create breaks in ischemic retinal tissue. Avoid diathermy on the disc; this may cause destruction of nerve fiber bundles. If the bleeding occurs within the temporal vascular arcades, then use a laser probe to cauterize the bleeding instead. Often you have to work bimanually.

- **Moderate bleeding and bleeding at the optic disc:**
- In the case of a strong bleeding source, hold the knob spatula or the vitreous cutter for about 1 min onto the bleeding source (1 min is longer than most people think).
- **Severe bleeding:**
- If the bleeding is so severe that there is no view of the fundus, and despite aspiration with the flute needle it does not clear up, then you should perform a fluid x air exchange. The bleeding will stop. Now try to cauterize the bleeding source with endodiathermy or compress it mechanically with the knob spatula. The vitrectomy can also be continued in an air-filled vitreous cavity. Another alternative is silicone oil. One can either work under silicone oil or end surgery with a silicone oil tamponade with Avastin.

Surgical Pearls No. 104
Intraoperative hemorrhage and adrenaline: If there is constant bleeding from several vessels under surgery, then add adrenaline to the BSS bottle. Adrenaline will constrict the vessels and reduce the bleeding.

6. **Removal of attached posterior hyaloid in the periphery** (Figs. 15.20, 15.21, and 15.22)

Trim the peripheral vitreous and the vitreous base with a bimanual technique. Indent the sclera with the sclera depressor and cut the vitreous with the vitreous cutter.

After removal of the posterior hyaloid from the posterior pole, remove the residual attached posterior hyaloid in the periphery. Remember: the posterior hyaloid in the periphery is in the most cases only partially detached. The detached part with a posterior hyaloid rhexis was opened in the beginning. Now the attached part must be removed. This part is firmly attached to the retina (Fig. 15.20). Simply inducing a PVD with the vitreous cutter does not work because this creates retinal tears. The surgeon must delaminate the posterior hyaloid with a bimanual technique (Fig. 15.21). The posterior hyaloid has to be removed up to the vitreous base (Fig. 15.22).

The most difficult part of the surgery has been completed.

7. **Panretinal photocoagulation (PRP) under BSS** (Figs. 15.23 and 15.24)

The next step is a PRP. Perform a dense PRP from the arcades up to the ora serrata. By using the scleral depressor, the surgeon can laser treat up to the ora serrata.

After endolaser photocoagulation check if a new hemorrhage has occurred at the central pole, and treat it before moving on to the tamponade.

Surgical Pearls No. 105
Postoperative vitreous hemorrhages are the number one problem following vitrectomy for proliferative diabetic retinopathy. In order to lower the rate of this complication, be meticulous with hemostasis. Watch out for small oozing bleeding sites after PRP has been performed. Even small collections of blood point at continuous bleeding sites that should be treated before closing up.

9. **Fluid against air exchange** (Figs. 15.25 and 15.26)

Perform a fluid against air exchange. In case of 25G or 27G, use active aspiration with backflush instrument or use the vitreous cutter.

Air bubbles behind IOL: During a fluid-air exchange, the water condenses at the posterior surface of the IOL in the area of the capsulotomy, thereby greatly impairing the view of the fundus. It can either be removed with a flute instrument or injection of viscoelastics onto the posterior surface of the IOL.

10. **Intravitreal Avastin**

We always inject 0.2 mL Avastin intravitreally at the end of a diabetic case. We use 0.2 mL and not 0.1 mL because the vitreous is removed.

10. **Internal postoperative tamponade**

In young type 1 diabetics, we prefer 15% C2F6 as postoperative tamponade because it causes less postoperative secondary glaucoma compared to silicone oil. Silicone oil may result in secondary glaucoma after silicone oil removal. We use silicone oil in difficult cases, extensive retinal bleeding and in functionally only eyes. In old type 2 diabetics, we use in the most cases only an air tamponade.

- **Silicone Oil Tamponade** (Figs. 15.27 and 15.28)

In case of a silicone oil, we use in most cases 1000/1300csts silicone oil. Inject the silicone oil under BIOM view. In case of overfill, cut the infusion line, and excessive silicone oil will escape. Inject a 0.1–0. 2 mL Avastin bubble into the silicone oil bubble.

Surgical Pearls No. 106
Lens sparing vitrectomy: In young diabetic patients, we experienced good results with a lens-sparing vitrectomy and then a C_2F_6 gas or 1000 csts silicone oil tamponade. Even after 10–20 years, the lens hardly opacifies.

11. **Removal of trocars** (Fig. 15.29)

If silicone oil is used, one should suture the sclerotomies; otherwise oil might flow under the conjunctiva. Suture 25G sclerotomies with Vicryl 8-0. 27G sclerotomies require usually no suture.

15.3 Complications

1. Injury of a retinal artery during peeling. Fibrovascular membranes may hide the temporal arcade. Be careful with delamination here. Begin with blunt instruments such as a knob spatula or a vacuum cleaner. Prefer a curved scissors (27G curved scissors, DORC).
2. Extensive bleeding: (1) Try to cauterize the bleeding vessel. (2) Place the tip of the vitreous cutter or the knob spatula onto the bleeding vessel for 1 min. (3)

Perform a BSS against air exchange and try to cauterize the vessel. (4) Inject silicone oil and anti-VEGF, and close the case; reoperate when the bleeding has subsided.

15.4 FAQ

Which type of silicone oil you use?

We use routinely 1000/1300 csts silicone oil. We remove the oil after 3 months. We see no advantage of using 5000 csts oil in diabetic cases, even with tractional detachment.

What procedure do you recommend in case of an eye with iris rubeosis, cataract, and vitreous hemorrhage?

Do not operate this eye before the iris rubeosis is treated and has disappeared. We would inject immediately 0.1 mL Avastin. After 1 month, we would perform a combined phacoemulsification + IOL implantation + intravitreal 0.1 mL Avastin. Again 1 month later, we would perform a vitrectomy.

What procedure do you recommend in case of a young type 1 diabetic with PDR and poor compliance?

I would perform an immediate Avastin injection in both eyes. One month later I would schedule a laser coagulation (LIO) in general anesthesia (Figs. 15.30 and 15.31). And again 1 month later, I would perform a lens-sparing vitrectomy if necessary.

What procedure do you recommend in case of an old type 2 diabetic with vitreous hemorrhage secondary to diabetes?

I would schedule a phaco + Avastin. One month later I would perform a vitrectomy with laser, Avastin, and air tamponade.

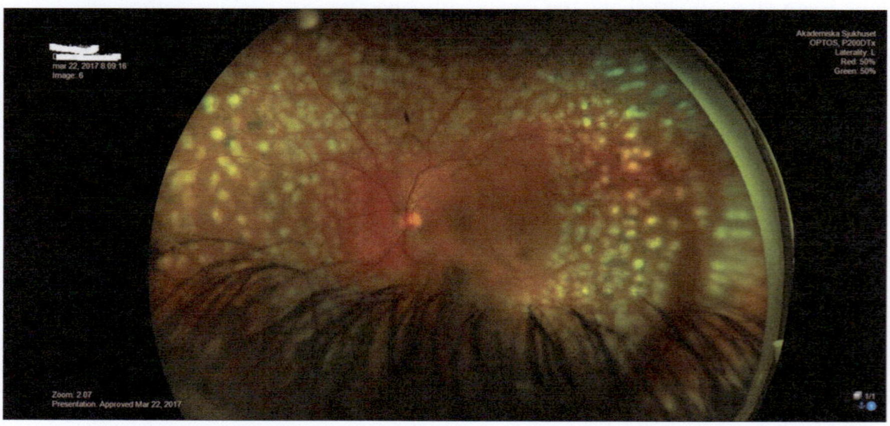

Fig. 15.30 The retina was treated from the temporal arcades to the ora serrata with 1879 laser effects

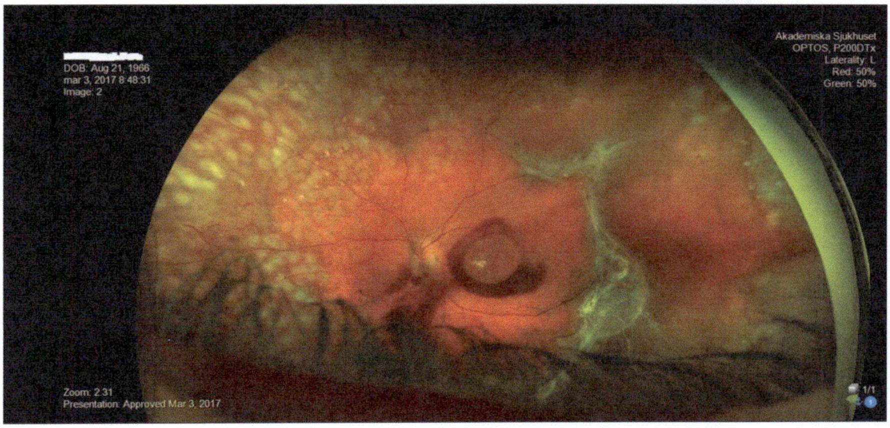

Fig. 15.31 This eye was treated with 1500 laser effects

Anti-VEGF may cause a retinal detachment in diabetic eyes. Why do you wait 4 weeks before you perform a vitrectomy?

Anti-VEGF and laser photocoagulation close the proliferative vessels resulting in a shortening of the membranes and increased traction. This effect is, however, limited. In those eyes, which are pretreated with anti-VEGF, there is a reduced risk of intraoperative bleeding facilitating the removal of fibrovascular membranes. The increased visibility reduces the risk for creating an iatrogenic break. In addition, the risk for a postoperative rebleeding is reduced. The advantages of an anti-VEGF and laser treatment before vitrectomy outweigh the disadvantages. Arevalo et al. conclude that a pretreatment with anti-VEGF results in improved anatomical and functional outcome regardless of increased traction on some severe PDR cases [1]. Da R Lucena and colleagues demonstrate that a pretreatment with anti-VEGF prior to vitrectomy results in a reduced intraoperative bleeding compared to eyes which received no anti-VEGF treatment [2].

References

1. Arevalo JF, Maia M, Flynn HW, et al. Tractional retinal detachment following intravitreal bevacizumab (Avastin) in patients with severe proliferative diabetic retinopathy. Br J Ophthalmol. 2008;92:213–6.
2. da R Lucena D, Ribeiro JAS, Costa RA, et al. Intraoperative bleeding during vitrectomy for diabetic tractional retinal detachment with versus without preoperative intravitreal bevacizumab (IBeTra study). Br J Ophthalmol. 2009;93:688–91.

Part X
Submacular Hemorrhage

Chapter 16
Submacular Hemorrhage Secondary to CNV

Extras: Videos 16.1, 16.2, 16.3, and 16.4.

16.1 Introduction

Timing and procedure are important for this pathology. Try to treat a submacular hemorrhage within 1–2 weeks. The medication is called recombinant (tissue) plasminogen activator (rPA = rtPA, Actilyse®) and acts as a fibrinolytic agent.

There are two possible methods: (1) pneumatic displacement, which comprises the intravitreal injection of rtPA, anti-VEGF, and gas, and (2) vitrectomy, which comprises a vitrectomy, subretinal injection of rtPA, intravitreal injection of anti-VEGF, and gas.

There is an ongoing debate which method (intravitreal or subretinal rtPA) for which size of hemorrhage (small, large, massive) is superior. The actual data indicates that pneumatic displacement is superior for small hemorrhages, but it is unclear which method is the best for a large and a massive hemorrhage.

Regarding small and large hemorrhages, both methods are effective in removing the subretinal hemorrhage but only partially effective in removing the sub-RPE hemorrhage. The consequence is that an anti-VEGF therapy has to be continued after surgery. Eylea® is especially effective for a sub-RPE hemorrhage.

Regarding a massive hemorrhage, two surgical methods are used: (1) peripheral 180° retinotomy and removal of the subretinal hemorrhage. If you remove the blood clot with surgical extraction, you will at the same time remove the underlying pigment epithelium resulting in a geographic atrophy. The next problem is that for removal of a large blood clot, a peripheral retinectomy is required, which may result in a PVR detachment. (2) Injection of intravitreal rtPA prior surgery. A few days

---

Electronic Supplementary Material The online version of this chapter (https://doi.org/10.1007/978-3-319-89677-9_16) contains supplementary material, which is available to authorized users.

U. Spandau, H. Heimann, *Practical Handbook for Small-Gauge Vitrectomy*,
https://doi.org/10.1007/978-3-319-89677-9_16

later, vitrectomy with removal of the subretinal liquefied blood through an iatrogenic hole.

The definition of the size of a submacular hemorrhage varies. Our definition is as follows:

Small hemorrhage: Hemorrhage inside macular region

Large hemorrhage: Hemorrhage including temporal arcades

Massive hemorrhage: Hemorrhage outside temporal arcades and hemorrhagic retinal detachment

There are several different surgical approaches available. Our procedure is as follows:

Small hemorrhage: Pneumatic displacement with rtPA and anti-VEGF; head-down posture for 1 week. See Table 16.1.

Exception: Patients which cannot perform a head-down posture. Procedure: rtPA and anti-VEGF without gas.

Large hemorrhage: Vitrectomy with subretinal injection of rtPA and gas tamponade and anti-VEGF; head-down posture for 1 week. See Table 16.2.

Massive hemorrhage: (1) 1–7 days preoperatively: rtPA. (2) Vitrectomy + iatrogenic hole + drainage of subretinal blood + laser + anti-VEGF + silicone oil. (3) Add rtPA in case of residual thick blood and repeat surgery 1 week later. See Table 16.3.

Other surgical options

Small and large bleedings; submacular rtPA (25micogramm in 0.2 mL) + and aspiration of blood

Massive hemorrhage: 180–360° retinectomy + removal of hemorrhage + reattachment of retina with PFCL + laser + silicone oil; the latter surgery may cause large RPE defects because the hemorrhage is attached to the RPE.

Table 16.1 Our treatment algorithm for treatment of small hemorrhages

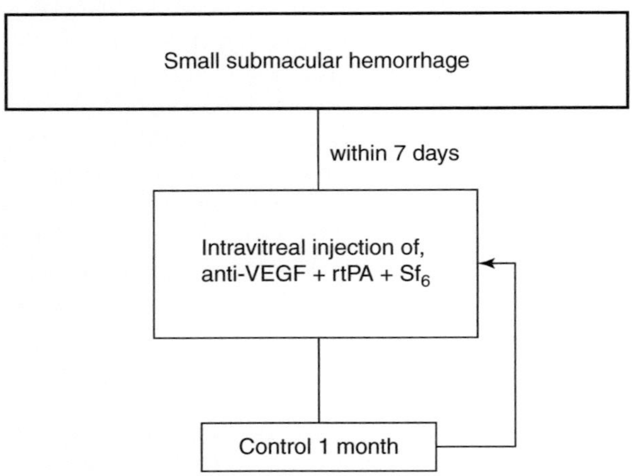

Table 16.2 Our treatment algorithm for large submacular hemorrhages

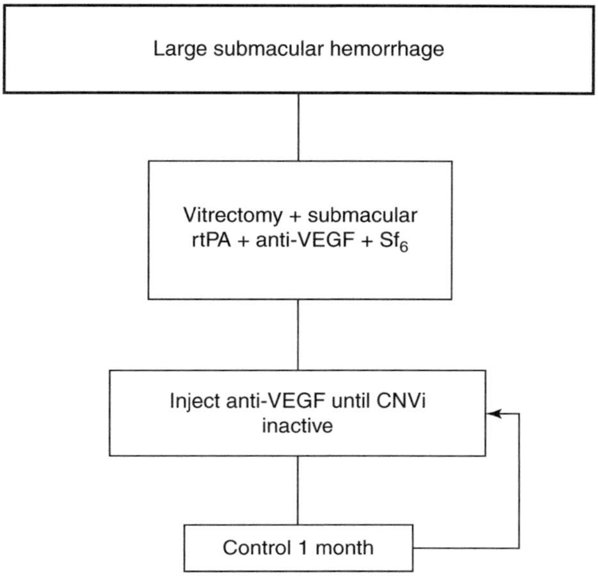

Table 16.3 Our treatment algorithm for massive submacular hemorrhages

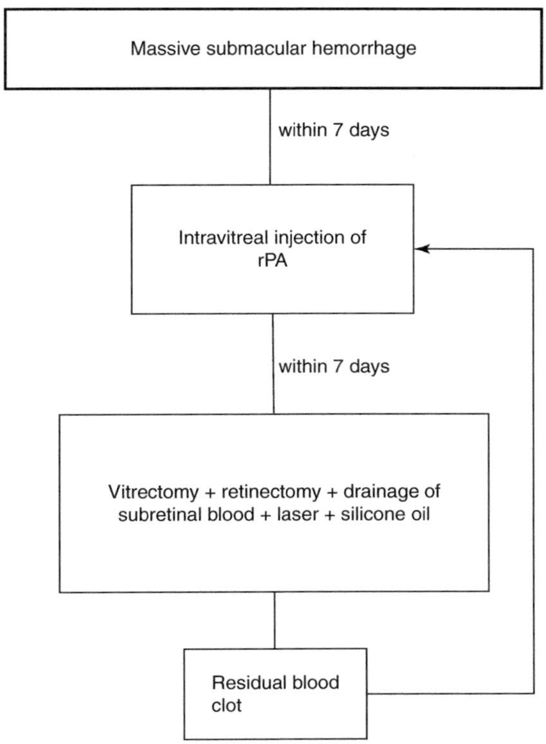

16.2 Surgery of a Small Submacular Hemorrhage

Medication

1. rtPA (Actilyse®) dose: 50 microgram/0.1 mL
2. anti-VEGF: 0.1 mL Avastin, Lucentis, Eylea
3. Gas: 100% Sf_6, use alternatively air

Surgical procedure

Inject anti-VEGF (regular dose) into the vitreous cavity. Perform a paracentesis. Inject 0.1 mL rtPA into the vitreous cavity. Then inject 0.4 mL 100% SF_6 into the vitreous cavity.

Postoperative therapy: 2 tablets Acetazelomid 250 mg.

Head-down posture for 1 week.

Follow-ups

Continue with anti-VEGF treatment until the hemorrhage is resorbed.

16.3 Surgery of a Large Submacular Hemorrhage

16.3.1 Instruments

1. Hybrid 27G and 23G three-port trocar system
2. 120D lens
3. Laser probe
4. 41G subretinal injection needle (23G), DORC 1270.EXT

16.3.2 Usage of the 41G Subretinal Injection Needle (Figs. 16.1 and 16.2)

Attach the syringe with rtPA to the end of the handpiece of the 41G needle (Fig. 16.2). The surgeon holds the handpiece of the needle, and the assistant or scrub nurse holds the syringe and injects slowly the rtPA.

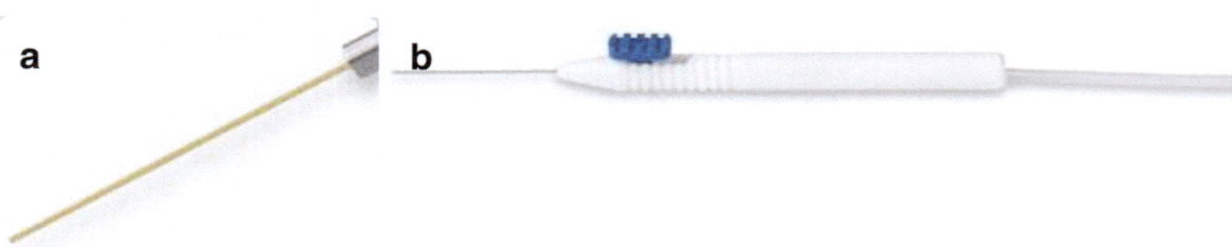

Fig. 16.1 (**a**) 41G cannula (DORC, 1290 BTD23). (**b**) The metal cannula is 23G. The 41G cannula is retractable. Also, available from Medilens

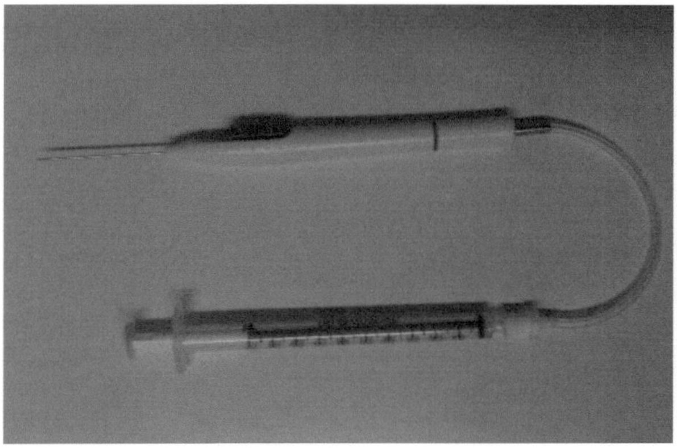

Fig. 16.2 The syringe with rtPA is connected to the 41G cannula

16.3.3 Medication

rtPA (Actilyse®) dose: 25 microgram/0.1 mL
anti-VEGF: 0.1 mL Avastin, Lucentis, Eylea

16.3.4 Tamponade

Gas: 20% SF_6

16.3.5 Surgical Procedure

1. **Vitrectomy with PVD**
2. **Subretinal injection of 0.2 mL rtPA**
3. **Fluid × air exchange**
4. **Tamponade with 20% SF_6**
5. **Intravitreal injection of anti-VEGF**

The surgery step-by-step: Figs. 16.3 and 16.4

1. **Vitrectomy with PVD**
2. **Subretinal injection of 0.2 mL rtPA**

Insert one 27G infusion trocar, one 27G instrument trocar, and one 23G instrument trocar for the dominant hand. Continue with a vitrectomy. Insert then the 41G cannula into the 23G trocar. Test that the cannula is free from air. Then pierce the hemorrhage close to the inferior arcade. Be careful not to injure the pigment epithelium. Inject slowly 0.2 mL rtPA. The subretinal bubble grows slowly. Do not inject too fast because you may create a macular hole.

3. **Fluid × air exchange**
4. **Tamponade with 20% SF_6**
5. **Intravitreal injection of anti-VEGF**

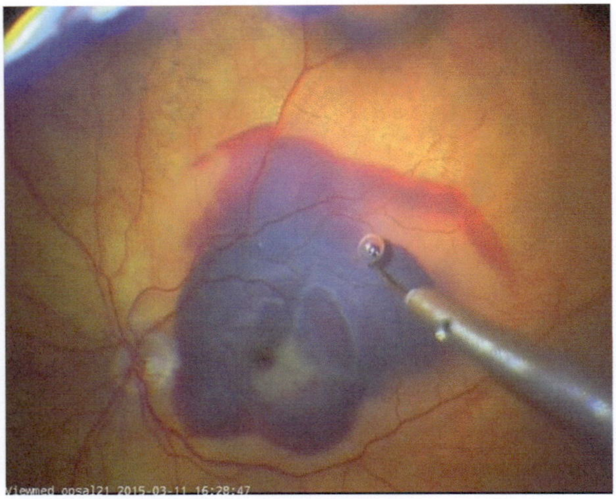

Fig. 16.3 Eject first air bubbles from the cannula, pierce the retina, and inject slowly 0.2 mL rtPA

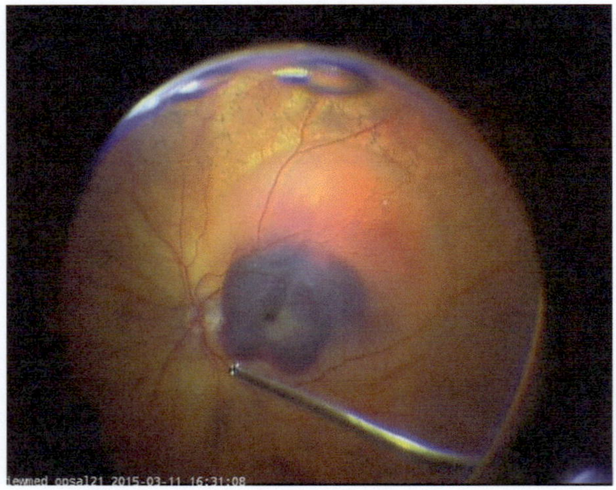

Fig. 16.4 Note the subretinal rtPA bubble

Perform a fluid × air exchange. Leave 25–33% residual fluid. Then add 0.1–0.2 mL Avastin and flush the vitreous cavity with 20% SF_6. Remove finally the trocars.

16.3.6 Postoperative Posture

First 2 h on the back, so that the blood can liquefy and then head-down posture for 1 week so that the blood can drain downwards.

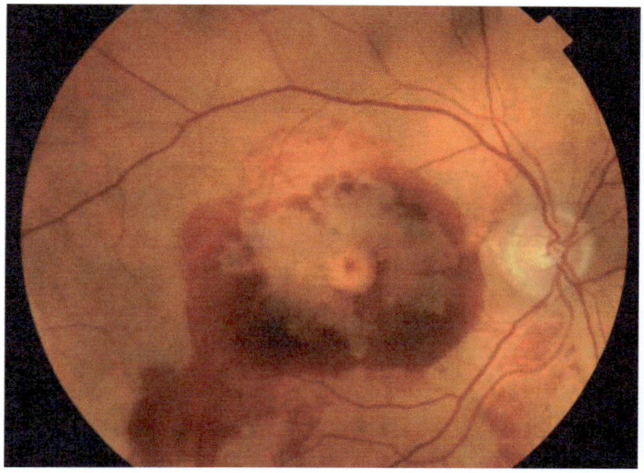

Fig. 16.5 Four-week follow-up. The subretinal hemorrhage is displaced. VA=0,02. The patient is satisfied about the VA improvement

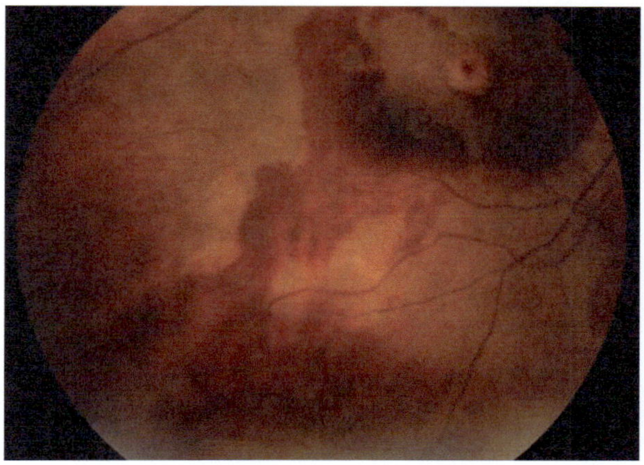

Fig. 16.6 The hemorrhage is displaced to the inferior periphery. Further anti-VEGF injections were scheduled

16.3.7 One-Month follow-up: Figs. 16.5 and 16.6

Continue with anti-VEGF injections until CNV is inactive.

16.3.8 FAQ

Do you aspirate the submacular blood through an iatrogenic hole?
No. The only induced hole is a 41G hole for subretinal injection.
Do you recommend to aspirate the subretinal blood?

No. For a central located hemorrhage you need a central hole. If the blood is not completely liquefied, then the extraction may become difficult. The tear will enlarge intraoperatively and even more postoperatively. The gas bubble and the rtPA will do its job and displace the blood into the periphery.

16.4 Surgery of a Massive Submacular Hemorrhage

16.4.1 Introduction

Inject rtPA 1–7 days before vitrectomy. Then drain the liquefied blood through a small retinotomy. The drainage is very time-consuming; if a (not liquefied) blood clot remains at the end of the surgery, you can inject again rtPA and repeat a drainage surgery a few days later. The advantage of this approach is that you avoid a large retinotomy and do not damage the underlying RPE when removing the blood clot.

16.4.2 Instruments

1. 27G three-port trocar system with chandelier light
2. 120D lens
3. Laser probe

16.4.3 Medication

50 μg/0.1 mL rtPA and anti-VEGF

16.4.4 Tamponade

1000csts silicone oil

16.4.5 Surgical Procedure

1. **Vitrectomy with PVD**
2. **Injection of PFCL**
3. **Iatrogenic hole**
4. **Aspiration of subretinal blood**
5. **Laser treatment**
6. **PFCL × air exchange**
7. **1000 csts silicone oil tamponade**
8. **Inject anti-VEGF and if necessary rtPA**

The surgery step-by-step: Figs. 16.7–16.17

1. **Vitrectomy with PVD**
2. **Injection of PFCL**

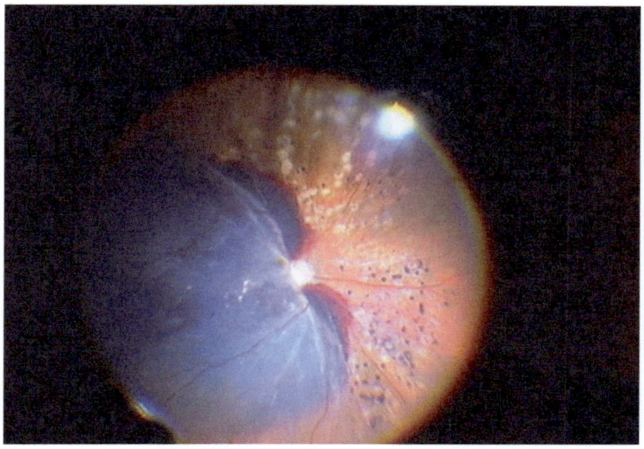

Fig. 16.7 A massive subretinal hemorrhage secondary to CNV. The retina was treated earlier on with a scatter laser due to a diabetic retinopathy

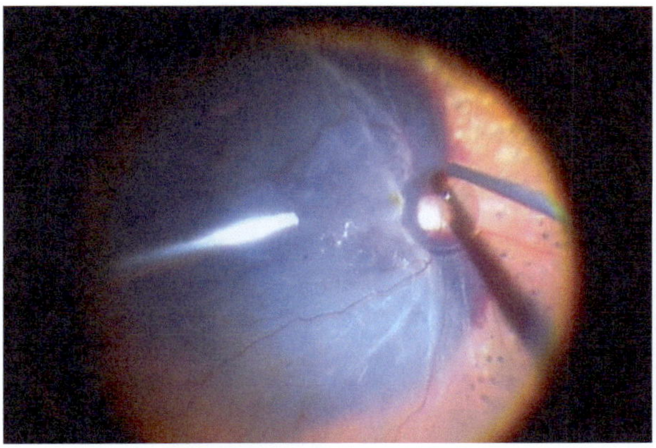

Fig. 16.8 One day before the first vitrectomy, a rtPA injection was performed. Now PFCL is injected to displace the blood from the posterior pole

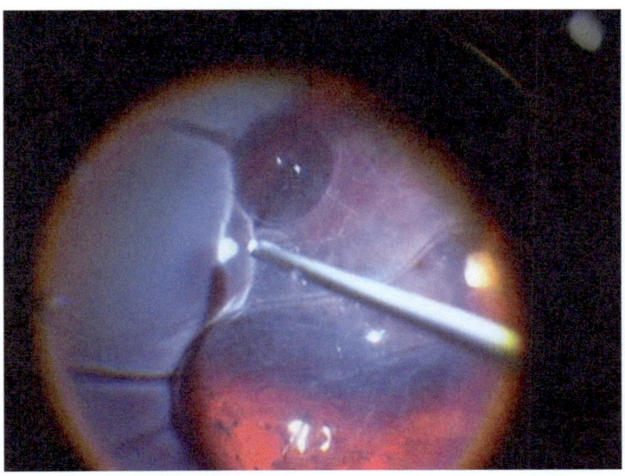

Fig. 16.9 The blood is displaced into the periphery. In the area of the bullous detachment, choose a site for retinotomy, cauterize it, and create a small hole with the vitreous cutter (approx. 200 cuts/min)

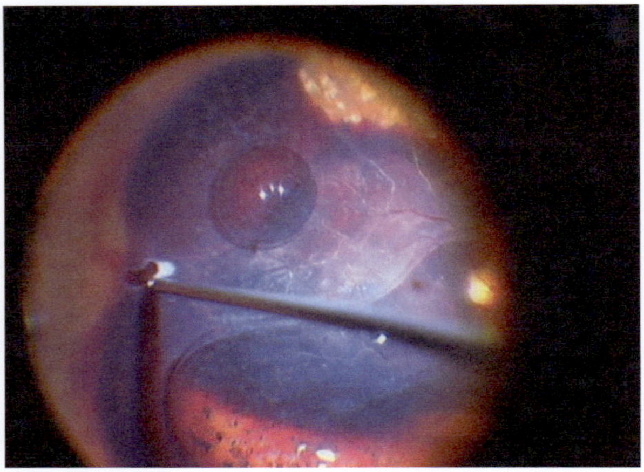

Fig. 16.10 The subretinal blood is aspirated with the vitreous cutter. This maneuver can take approximately 30–60 min

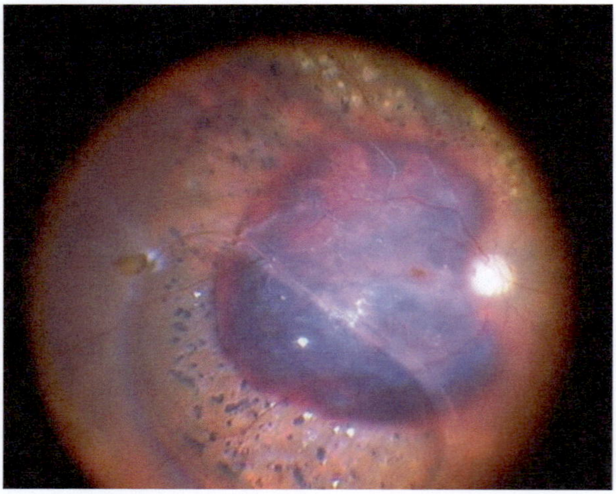

Fig. 16.11 The liquefied blood is removed. It remains a clotted hemorrhage at the posterior pole

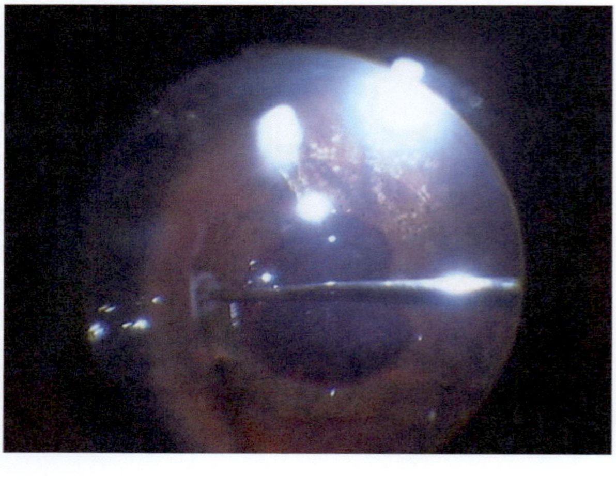

Fig. 16.12 A fluid × air exchange is performed, and the break is laser treated

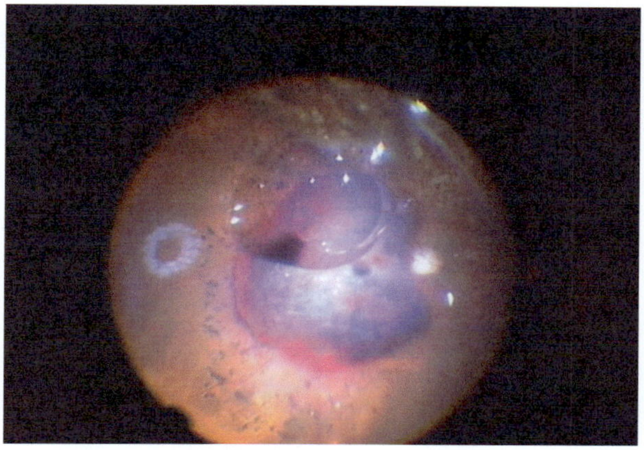

Fig. 16.13 1000 csts silicone oil is injected and then a 0.1 mL rtPA bubble to liquefy the residual hemorrhage

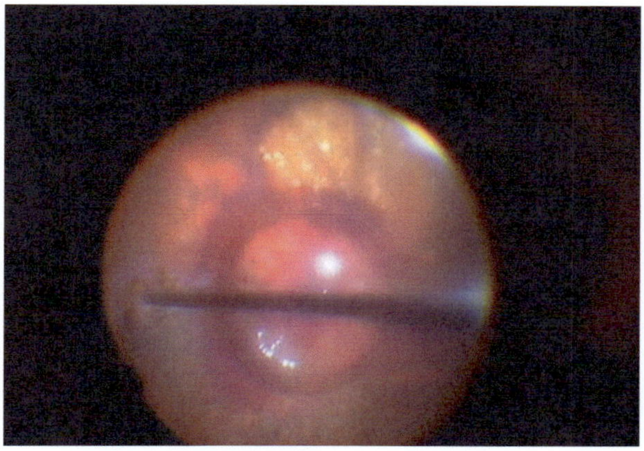

Fig. 16.14 Five days later: Second vitrectomy. The silicone oil is removed

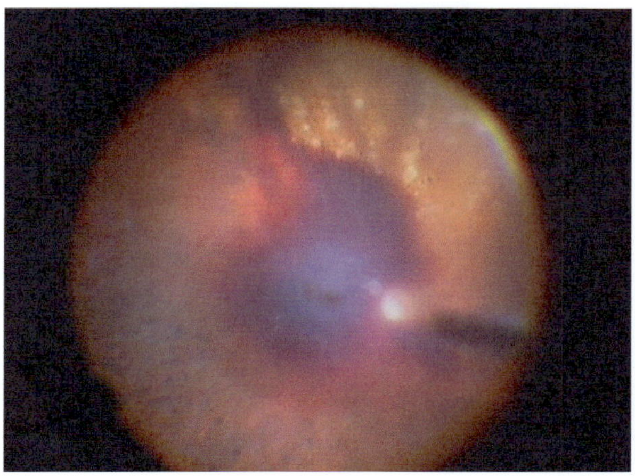

Fig. 16.15 PFCL is injected to displace the liquefied blood, the break is reopened, and the blood aspirated

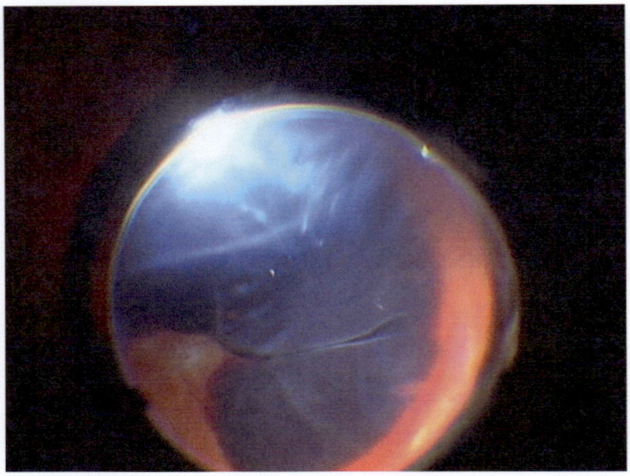

Fig. 16.16 Case report 1: A massive submacular hemorrhage secondary to CNV. The eye is first treated with rtPA

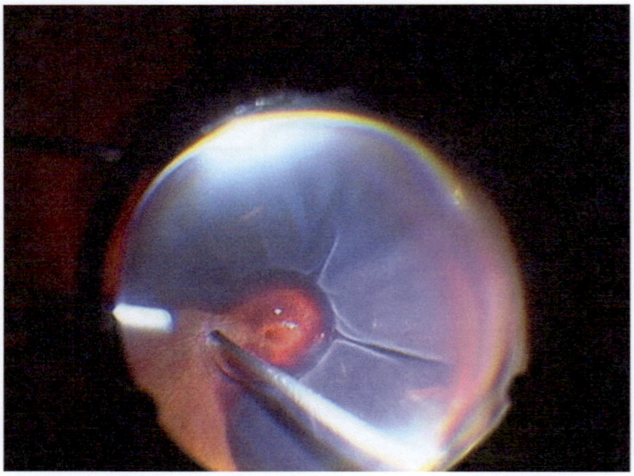

Fig. 16.17 Case report 1: A PFCL bubble is injected onto the posterior pole

Insert three 27G trocars and then a chandelier light. Begin with a core vitrectomy and continue with a PVD and then trimming of the vitreous base (Fig. 16.7). Inject PFCL onto the posterior pole in order to press the submacular blood toward the periphery (Fig. 16.8).

3. **Iatrogenic hole**

Search for a good place for the iatrogenic hole. It should be outside the temporal arcades and ideally inside the bullous detachment. Cut then an iatrogenic hole with the following settings: 400 mmHg vacuum and 100–200 cuts/min (Fig. 16.9).

4. **Aspiration of subretinal blood**

Aspirate then the subretinal blood. This procedure is time-consuming; it may take 15–30 min (Fig. 16.10). Do not enlarge the hole or create a retinectomy because these procedures will increase the PVR risk. In some cases, there is residual thick blood which cannot be aspirated. This blood clot can be removed in a second surgery 1 week later (Fig. 16.11).

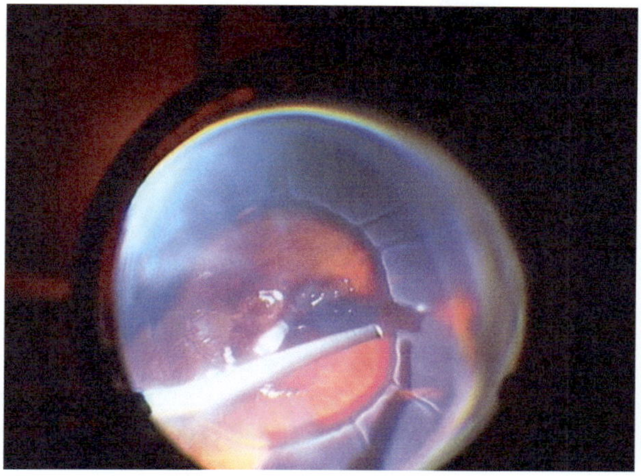

Fig. 16.18 Case report 1: An iatrogenic break is created, and the liquefied hemorrhage is aspirated

5. **Laser treatment** (Fig. 16.12)
6. **PFCL × air exchange** (Fig. 16.12)
7. **1000 csts silicone oil tamponade** (Fig. 16.18)
8. **Inject anti-VEGF and if necessary rtPA** (Fig. 16.13)

Inject PFCL anterior to the tear and continue with laser treating the iatrogenic tear. The next step is a PFCL against air exchange and injection of 1000 csts silicone oil. Inject anti-VEGF medication into the silicone oil bubble to stop the bleeding source. If a residual blood clot is present, then inject also 0.1 mL rtPA. Then remove the trocars.

Postoperative posture

We recommend a head-down posture for 1 week.

Residual submacular hemorrhage

Schedule the next surgery within 7 days.

Individual steps

1. **Removal of silicone oil**
2. **Reopen the iatrogenic hole**
3. **Injection of PFCL**
4. **Aspiration of subretinal blood**
5. **Laser treatment**
6. **1000 csts silicone oil tamponade**
7. **Inject anti-VEGF**

The surgery step-by-step: Figs. 16.14 and 16.15

Remove the silicone oil and reopen the iatrogenic hole. Then inject PFCL to push the blood toward the iatrogenic hole. Then aspirate the residual blood. Continue with a fluid × air exchange and remove the PFCL. Laser treat the break and inject 1000 csts silicone oil. Do not forget to add 0.2 mL Avastin because the CNV is still active.

We recommend again head-down posture for 1 week and removal of the silicone oil after 3 months. If the CNV remains active, continue with anti-VEGF injections every month.

16.5 Brief Case Reports

Case Report No. 1: Massive Submacular Hemorrhage 1

Figs. 16.16–16.21

A 77 y/o female patient lost her left eye due to a wet AMD. The right eye was treated eight times with Lucentis due to wet AMD, and the eye was stable since March 2011 (Fig. 16.18). She visited in April 2014 our outpatient department because of an acute vision loss. Visual acuity was 0.02, and a massive submacular hemorrhage secondary to a CNV was diagnosed (Fig. 16.16). She was treated the same day with rtPA and gas. Two days later a combined vitrectomy with aspiration of subretinal blood + Avastin + heavy silicone oil (Densiron 68) was performed (Figs. 16.16–16.18). I chose heavy silicone oil because she was unable to lie with face down posture. Two months later a Lucentis injection was repeated because the

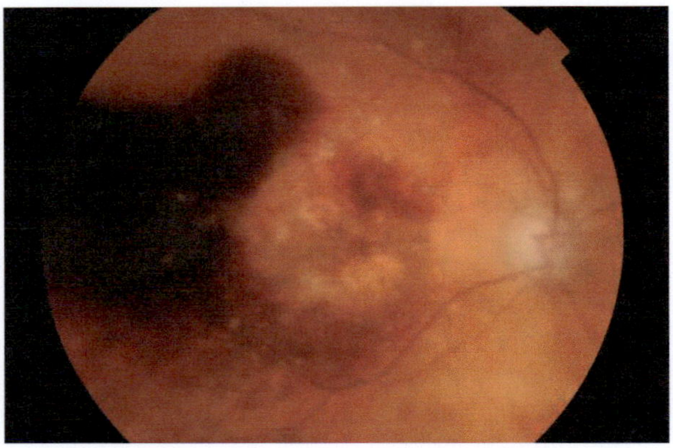

Fig. 16.19 Case report 1: 1-month follow-up. The subretinal blood could be completely removed. Note the residual blood temporal to the macula

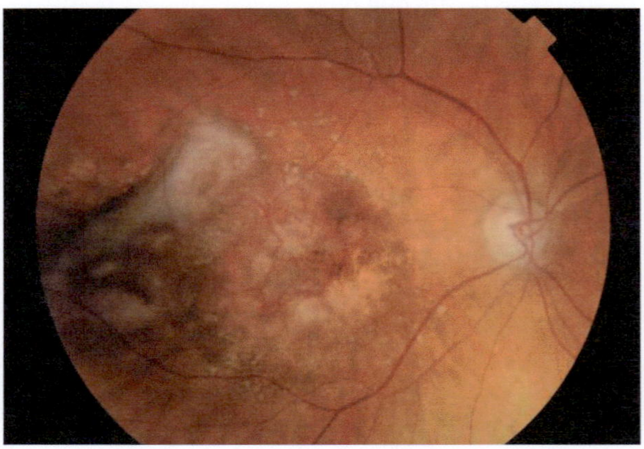

Fig. 16.20 Case report 1: 6-month follow-up. The membrane has formed to a scar

Fig. 16.21 Case report 1: 2-year follow-up. A new hemorrhagic CNV has formed next to the old scar. It was treated successfully with bevacizumab

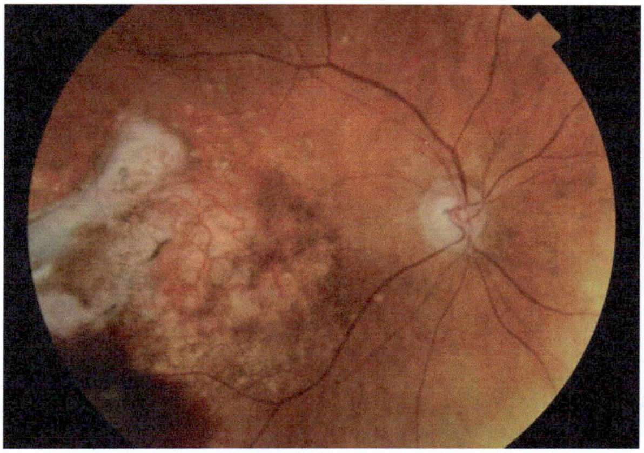

CNV membrane was still bleeding (Fig. 16.24). Six weeks later the silicone oil was removed. The visual acuity was for 2 years stable with 0.4–0.5 (Fig. 16.19). Recently she complained about a slight visual acuity decrease. A visual acuity of 0.3–0.4 was measured, and a recurrent subretinal hemorrhage was diagnosed (Figs. 16.20 and 16.21). An intravitreal injection of Avastin was immediately performed. One month later the bleeding had resorbed significantly, and a CNV could be visualized.

Case Report No. 2: Traumatic Choroidal Hemorrhage (Figs. 16.22–16.24)

A 39 y/o male patient presented to our outpatient department with a closed globe trauma secondary to a fist punch. Visual acuity was measured with 0.2 without correction and 0.4 with + 1.5D sph. A slit-lamp examination revealed a subretinal bleeding at the lower temporal vascular arcade that thinned out toward the macula. There was no sign of a globe rupture.

At the 2-week follow-up, the visual acuity decreased to 0.02 due to a vitreous hemorrhage in the visual axis. At the 3-week follow-up, the VA was stable with 0.02, and the decision was made to perform a vitrectomy + rtPA + gas. I chose vitrectomy because the patient is young, and I feared a retinal detachment from a gas injection without vitrectomy.

Two days later, 3½ weeks after trauma, a lens-sparing vitrectomy with rtPA and gas was performed. No subretinal blood was removed (Fig. 16.22).

The 1-month follow-up showed a visual acuity increase to 0.4–0.5 and a significant decrease of the subretinal blood clot. We decided to repeat the treatment (Fig. 16.23).

Ten days later a rtPA + gas injection was repeated. At the 1-month follow-up, the visual acuity was 0.6 uncorrected and +1.0D sph = 0.8 (Fig. 16.24). The patient was not satisfied; he claimed that the visual acuity hardly improved after the last gas injection and that he had severe 3-D problems and difficulties to coordinate the eyes. His latent diplopia disappeared with a +1.5D glass.

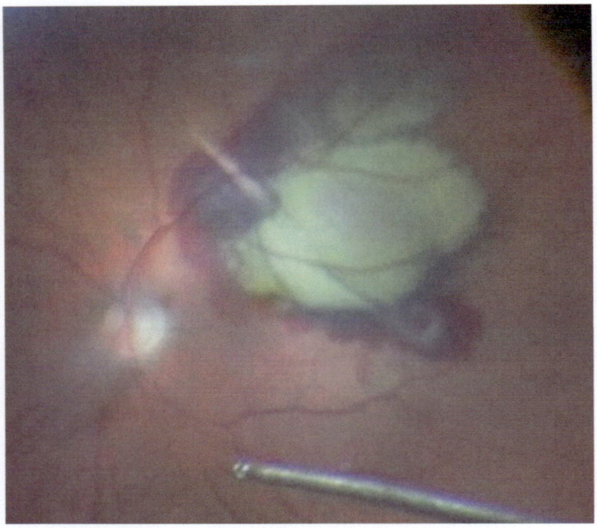

Fig. 16.22 Case report 2: A 4-week-old traumatic subretinal hemorrhage: old and fresh blood is located under the inferior arcade. VA = 0.02. A vitrectomy was performed, rtPA and 20% SF_6 injected

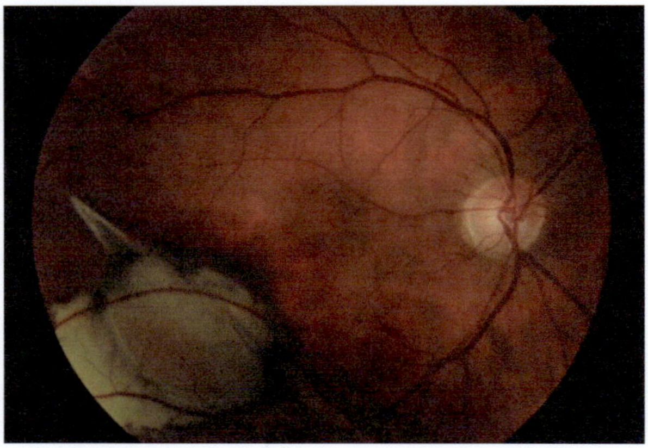

Fig. 16.23 Case report 2: 1-month follow-up: the subretinal hemorrhage is significantly reduced. Note the choroidal defect. A rtPA and gas injection is repeated

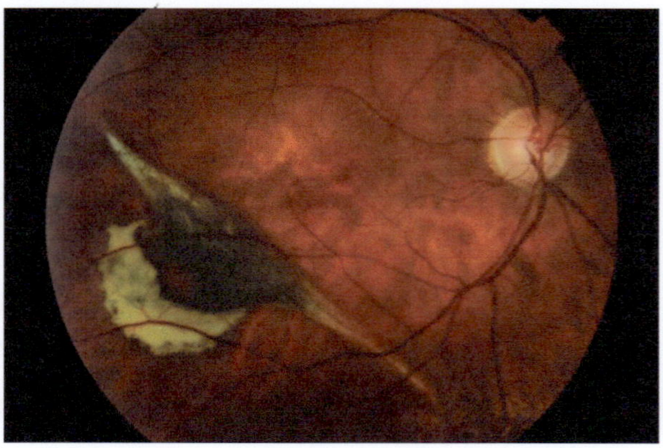

Fig. 16.24 Case report 2: 3-month follow-up: the large amount of subretinal blood is removed and resorbed. The VA increased to 0.8

16.6 Complications

1. Avoid extraction of thick clotted blood within the temporal arcades. You will induce RPE defects with subsequent visual field defects. To prevent this complication, inject rtPA and aspirate the unclotted blood.
2. The surgery is simple but time-consuming. The above described method has a low complication profile. There is a PVR risk due to the iatrogenic hole. The PVR risk is low if you only aspirate the liquefied blood.
3. Do not attempt to cut a central hole and extract subretinal clotted blood with active aspiration or forceps. The hole will enlarge intra- and postoperatively.

16.7 FAQ

Which procedure is better, intravitreal or subretinal Actilyse (rtPA)?

The actual data suggests that a minimal invasive method such as pneumatic displacement is superior to an invasive method such as vitrectomy and subretinal rtPA for small hemorrhages. A minimal invasive surgery is likely superior to a maximal invasive surgery because the macula is severely damaged and has a poor prognosis.

What about the follow-up?

The CNV is not inactive after the primary surgery. It is important to continue with anti-VEGF injections until the membrane is completely dry.

Chapter 17
Submacular Hemorrhage Secondary to Arterial Macroaneurysm

Extras: Video 17.1.

17.1 Introduction

A retinal macroaneurysm has a better prognosis than a subretinal CNV and is usually caused by high blood pressure. It results into a subretinal, sub-ILM, subhyaloidal, and preretinal hemorrhage. The latter may break into the vitreous body. It is tempting to perform a vitrectomy, inject rtPA into the subretinal space, and aspirate the blood. It is however difficult to treat the macroaneurysm because it may easily bleed, destroying all the surgical progress you made.

We perform only a treatment with rtPA and gas. Our treatment algorithm is depicted in Table 17.1. First the preretinal and intravitreal hemorrhage subsides. Then a subhyaloidal hemorrhage persists because the retinal macroaneurysm is still open. You can treat now with gas and Avastin. If the subhyaloidal and the sub-ILM hemorrhage do not resorb, you can remove it with a vitrectomy. Remark: The use of anti-VEGF (Avastin) is questionable in macroaneurysms because the effect of anti-VEGF agents on physiologic vessels is limited.

Conclusion: Be reluctant with a vitrectomy and be generous with intravitreal treatments.

17.2 Brief Case Reports

Case Report No. 1: Retinal Macroaneurysm 1 (Figs. 17.1–17.6)

This 93-year-old female patient presented with an acute vision loss of light perception. A fundus examination showed a large pre- and subretinal hemorrhage with

---

Electronic Supplementary Material The online version of this chapter (https://doi.org/10.1007/978-3-319-89677-9_17) contains supplementary material, which is available to authorized users.

U. Spandau, H. Heimann, *Practical Handbook for Small-Gauge Vitrectomy*,
https://doi.org/10.1007/978-3-319-89677-9_17

Table 17.1 Our treatment algorithm treatment for retinal macroaneurysm

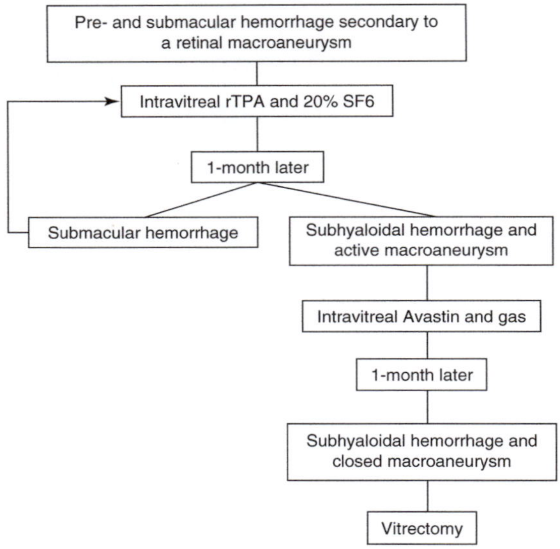

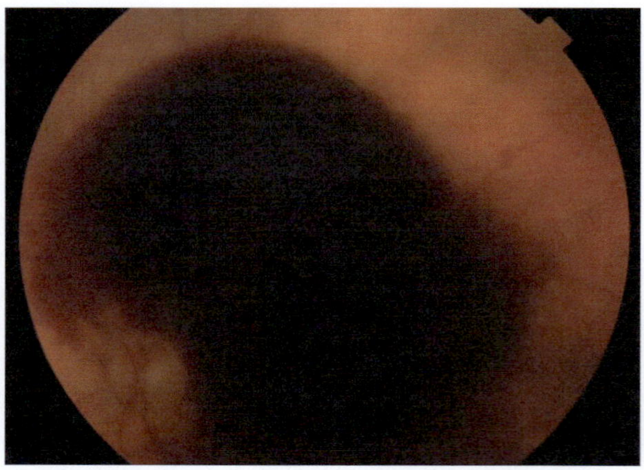

Fig. 17.1 Case report 1: A small preretinal and large subretinal hemorrhage secondary to a retinal macroaneurysm. rtPA and gas are injected

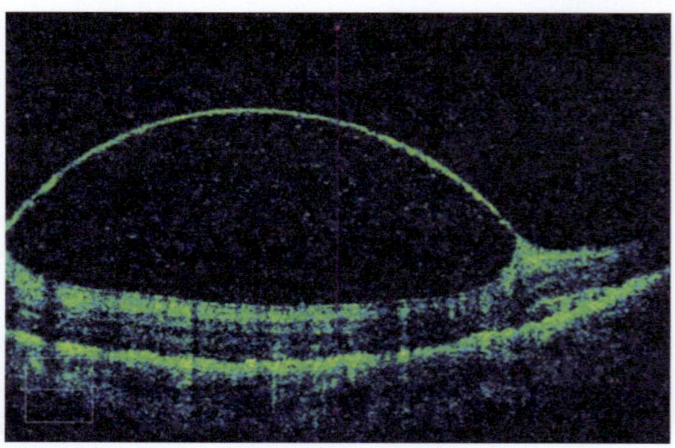

Fig. 17.2 Case report 1: 1-month follow-up. A subhyaloidal hemorrhage. A gas injection is repeated

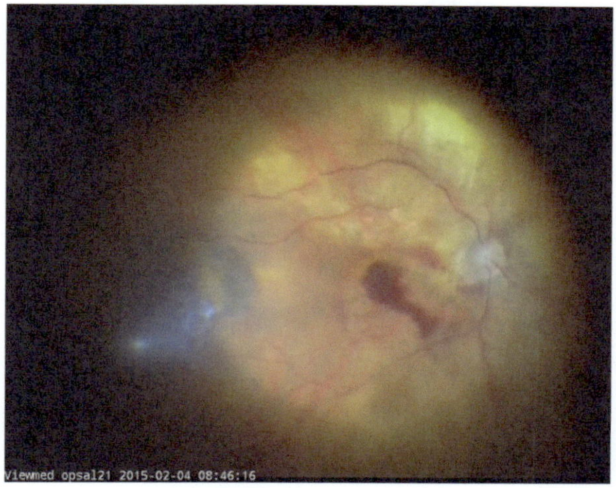

Fig. 17.3 Case report 1: 1-month follow-up after the second gas injection. No difference. A vitrectomy is scheduled

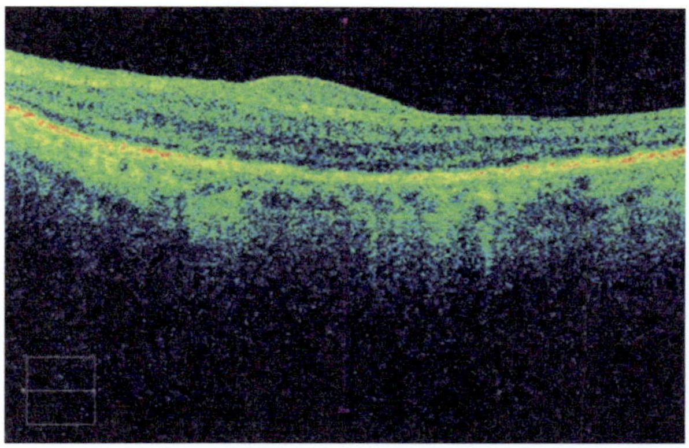

Fig. 17.4 Case report 1: Intraoperative OCT. The subretinal hemorrhage is displaced. Note the preretinal hemorrhage

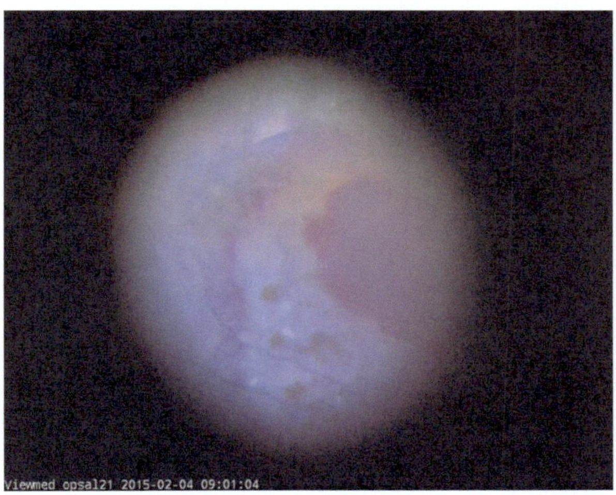

Fig. 17.5 Case report 1: Intraoperative photograph: A preretinal hemorrhage. Note the ILM defect at 11 o'clock which was created with a 27G Atkinson needle

Fig. 17.6 Case report 1: After ILM peeling and aspiration of blood the macula is free

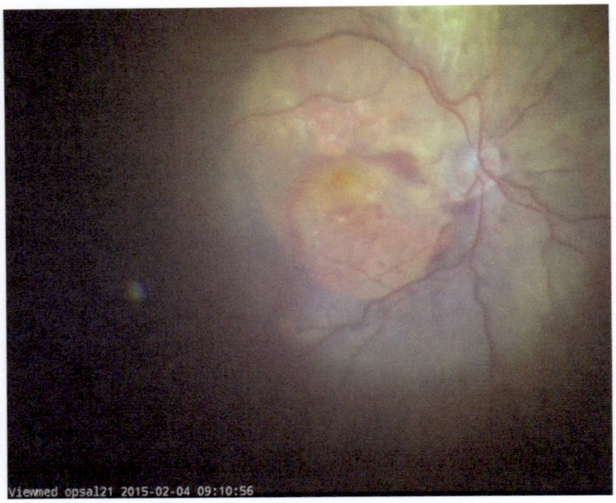

suspicion of a retinal macroaneurysm (Fig. 17.1). Six days later an intravitreal rtPA + 0.5 mL 20% Sf_6 injection was performed. The 1-month follow-up showed a visual acuity of hand movement. The fundus examination showed a reduction of the preretinal hemorrhage and persisting subhyaloidal blood (Fig. 17.2). One day later a second injection with rtPA + Avastin + gas was performed. The 1-month follow-up showed a visual acuity of counting fingers and an unchanged fundus (Fig. 17.3). Six weeks later a vitrectomy with peeling was performed. The residual blood was located between ILM and the retina (Figs. 17.4 and 17.5). After an ILM peeling, this residual blood could be aspirated (Fig. 17.6). At the 1-month follow-up, the visual acuity was measured with 0.2. The hemorrhage was resorbed, and macular function was limited due to a focal pigment epithelium atrophy.

Case Report No. 2: Retinal Macroaneurysm 2 (Figs. 17.7–17.10)

An 83-year-old male patient visited the outpatient department because of a sudden vision loss on the right eye. The visual acuity was measured with 0.02, and a sub- and preretinal hemorrhage in the macula and a retinal macroaneurysm at the inferior arcade was detected. The systemic blood pressure was elevated.

The next day an intravitreal injection with rtPA and 0.4 mL 20% SF_6 was performed.

The 1-month follow-up showed a visual acuity of counting fingers and a bullous subhyaloidal hemorrhage. The retinal macroaneurysm was still bleeding (Figs. 17.7 and 17.8).

Four days later an intravitreal injection of 0.2 mL Avastin and 0.4 mL 20% SF_6 was performed.

The 1-month follow-up showed a VA of 0.1, and a residual subhyaloidal hemorrhage temporal to the macula was detected. This hemorrhage was in contact with the retinal macroaneurysm. The fovea showed a thin bleeding (Figs. 17.9 and 17.10). No further treatment was performed because the macula was free of blood.

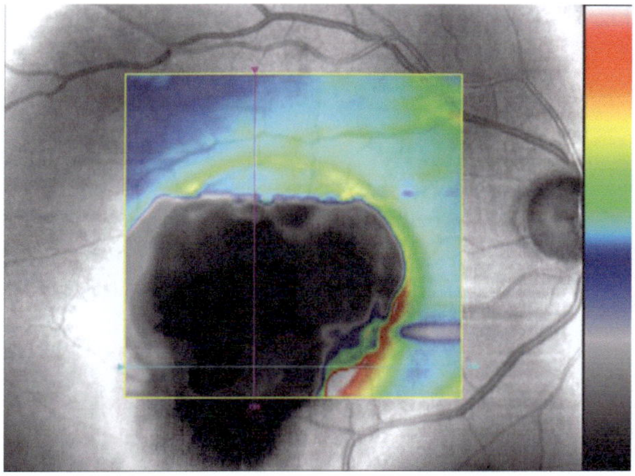

Fig. 17.7 Case report 2: 1-month follow-up after rtPA and gas. OCT: bullous subhyaloidal hemorrhage

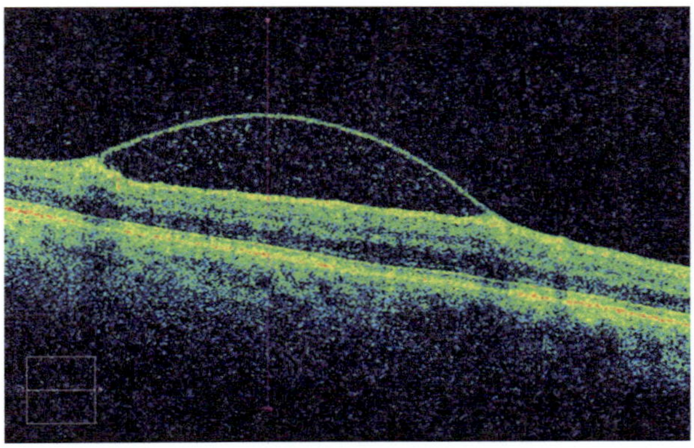

Fig. 17.8 Case report 2: 1-month follow-up. OCT: bullous subhyaloidal hemorrhage

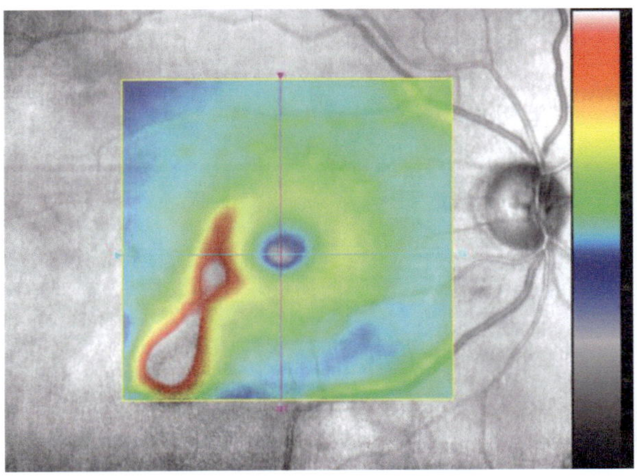

Fig. 17.9 Case report 2: 2-month follow-up. OCT: residual hemorrhage. Free macula

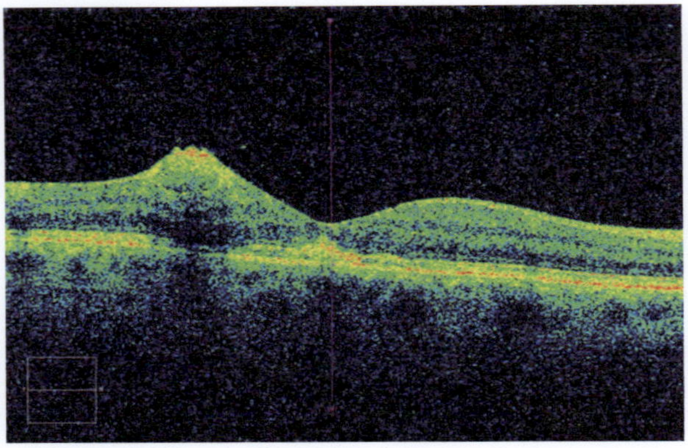

Fig. 17.10 Case report 2: 2-month follow-up. OCT: residual subhyaloidal hemorrhage close to the macula

Part XI
Endophthalmitis and Intraocular Tumor Biopsy

Chapter 18
Endophthalmitis

Extras: Videos 18.1 and 18.2.

18.1 Introduction

The Endophthalmitis Vitrectomy Study recommends intravitreal antibiotics if the visual acuity is > hand motion and PPV if visual acuity = light perception. In practice, most colleagues tend to perform a vitrectomy at earlier stages with a better visual acuity. Due to the increasing number of intravitreal injections, the incidence of endophthalmitis is rising. In every tertiary vitreoretinal center, clear treatment guidelines should be established; all necessary antibiotics and an examination of the microbiological specimens should be available at all times.

In recent years, there is a significant increase of endophthalmitis in patients following intravitreal injections of anti-VEGF agents. In contrast to the previously more common endophthalmitis following cataract surgery, the majority of these patients are still phakic, and the lens or opacified vitreous adjacent to the lens might impair the view of the posterior segment for vitrectomy. If you perform a phaco, then open the posterior capsule, and do not insert an IOL in order to improve the outflow of aqueous and reduce bacterial growth in the capsular bag.

The aim of a vitrectomy for endophthalmitis is the complete removal of the vitreous because the bacteria grow in the vitreous. Therefore, a PVD is necessary. The main obstacle of a vitrectomy for endophthalmitis is the poor view. The poor view is caused by corneal edema, pus, and fibrin in the anterior chamber and often a miotic pupil.

If you are contacted from a peripheral institution regarding a patient with presumed endophthalmitis and a delay of several hours before the patient can be seen in your institution is to be expected, it is advisable to ask the referring ophthalmologist to perform an intravitreal injection of antibiotics before sending the patient.

Electronic Supplementary Material The online version of this chapter (https://doi.org/10.1007/978-3-319-89677-9_18) contains supplementary material, which is available to authorized users.

U. Spandau, H. Heimann, *Practical Handbook for Small-Gauge Vitrectomy*,
https://doi.org/10.1007/978-3-319-89677-9_18

Time is of paramount importance in treating endophthalmitis, and the benefit of earlier antibiotic injection overrides the disadvantages of a short delay in the referral and possibly the failure to obtain a specimen for microbiology.

18.2 Antibiosis [1]:

1 mg/0.1 cc vancomycin
2.25 mg/0.1 cc Ceftazidime (Fortum)

18.2.1 Preparation of Antibiotic Therapy

18.2.1.1 Vancomycin

You need: 1× vancomycin 500 mg and 2× plastic ampoules 10 mL NaCl 9 mg/mL (9%)

1. Dissolve 500 mg of vancomycin in 10 cc NaCl 9 mg/mL (first ampoule).
2. Aspirate 2 cc of the second NaCl 9 mg/mL ampoule and discard it.
3. Add 2 cc of the dissolved vancomycin (first ampoule) into 8 cc of NaCl 9 mg/mL (second ampoule). The ampoule contains now 10 cc of vancomycin 10 mg/mL
4. Inject 0.1 cc (=1 mg) vancomycin into the vitreous cavity.

(Remark: cc = mL)

18.2.1.2 Ceftazidime

You need: 1× Fortum 500 mg and 2× plastic ampoules 10 mL NaCl 9 mg/mL (9%)

1. Dissolve 500 mg of Fortum in 10 cc NaCl 9 mg/mL (first ampoule).
2. Aspirate 8.8 cc of the second NaCl 9 mg/mL ampoule and discard it. The second ampoule contains now 1.2 cc NaCl 9 mg/mL.
3. Draw 1 cc of the dissolved Fortum and inject it into the second ampoule. The second ampoule contains now 2.2 cc Fortum 22.7 mg/mL.
4. Inject 0.1 cc (=2.27 mg) Fortum into the vitreous cavity.

18.3 Surgery

Instruments:

1. Three-port or four-port trocar system
2. Insulin syringe for sampling

Potential Tamponade:

Silicone oil

Individual Steps:

1. 23G–27G three ports with chandelier light
2a. Pseudophakic eye: Flushing of the anterior chamber and the capsular bag
2b. Phakic eye: Phacoemulsification without IOL
3. Specimen from the vitreous cavity
4. Vitrectomy
5. Induction of posterior vitreous detachment
6. Intravitreal antibiotics
7. Tamponade with silicone oil

18.3.1 *The Surgery Step-by-Step* (Figs. 18.1, 18.2, 18.3, 18.4, 18.5, and 18.6)

1. **23G–27G three ports with chandelier light**

If you use a silicone oil tamponade, a chandelier light is advisable.

2a. Pseudophakic eye: Flushing of the anterior chamber and the capsular bag

After performing a paracentesis, rinse the anterior chamber and the capsular bag thoroughly with BSS and irrigation/aspiration (I/A). With foudroyant endophthalmitis, it is appropriate to explant the IOL with the capsular bag.

2b. Phakic eye: Phacoemulsification without IOL

Perform a phaco and cut a round hole in the posterior capsule with the vitreous cutter from pars plana.

Surgical Pearls No. 107
Bad view to fundus: The main surgical difficulty of an endophthalmitis surgery is the poor view. Assess if the vitreous cutter is clearly visible behind the IOL. If not, then a corneal edema, fibrin, and pus in the anterior chamber are most likely responsible. Perform a corneal abrasion with a cotton wool swab or a crescent knife. Then remove pus or fibrin from the anterior chamber. A fibrin membrane may be present in the pupil plane. Remove it with an endgripping forceps.

3. **Specimen from the vitreous cavity**

Take a sample from the central vitreous with a 3 cc syringe (Figs 18.1 and 18.2). Connect the syringe to the vitreous cutter and aspirate manually while performing vitrectomy. Alternatively, you can send the vitrectomy cassette to microbiology.

4. **Vitrectomy**

Start with an anterior vitrectomy. Hold the vitreous cutter directly behind the IOL and remove the retrolental vitreous. In cases of severe endophthalmitis, it is

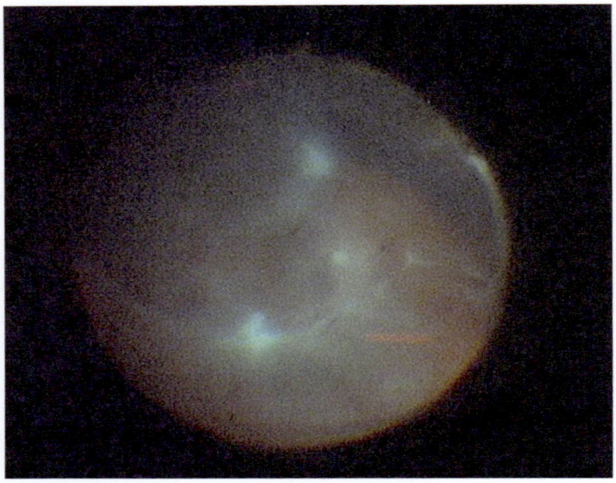

Fig. 18.1 Bad view to fundus is typical in eyes with endophthalmitis

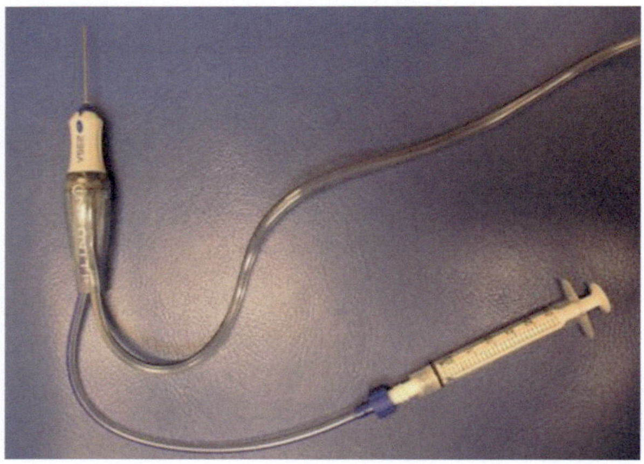

Fig. 18.2 Attach a 3 cc syringe to the vitreous cutter and take a sample. Send the syringe to the microbiology lab

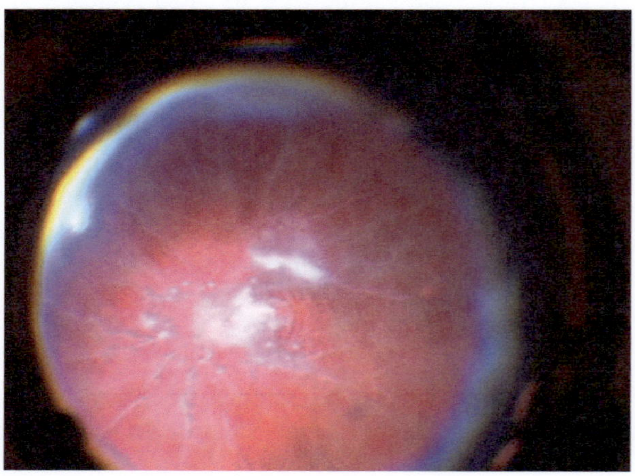

Fig. 18.3 The posterior hyaloid is attached. A PVD is required

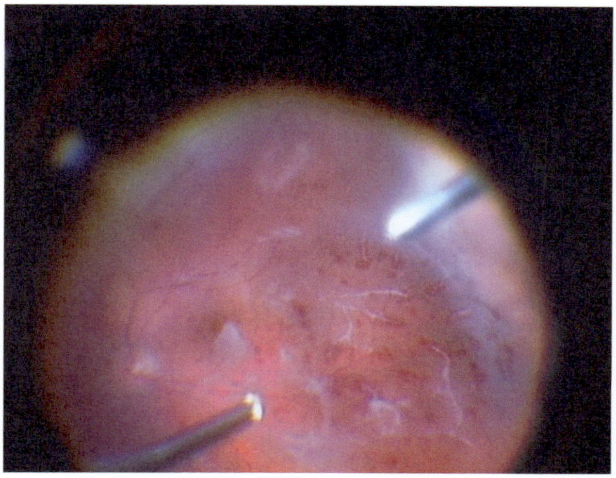

Fig. 18.4 After successful PVD

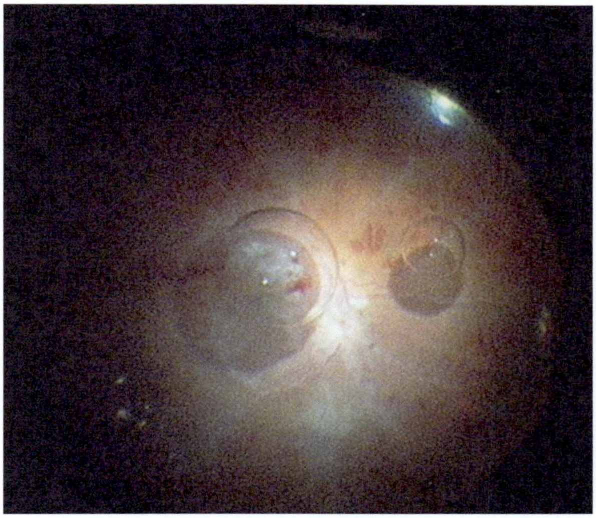

Fig. 18.5 A silicone oil-filled eye. The two bubbles are 0.1 mL vancomycin and 0.1 mL Fortum within the silicone oil bubble. Soon they will reach the space between retina and silicone oil and disappear

sometimes impossible to identify all structures correctly. Focus on identifying retinal vessels as your guideline as early as possible.

Surgical Pearls No. 108
Do not open the pars plana infusion without visualizing it first. If you are unable to see the internal opening of the infusions port, then try to visualize it with a light pipe or the vitreous cutter.

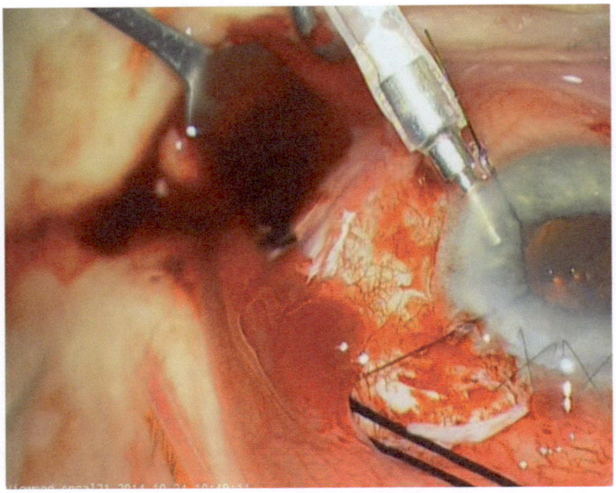

Fig. 18.6 Case report 1: Anterior chamber maintainer, holding sutures and then drainage of subchoroidal blood

5. **Induction of posterior vitreous detachment**

This is the most difficult step in endophthalmitis surgery because you can injure the retina. An induction of the posterior vitreous detachment is an important step in endophthalmitis surgery in order to remove the basis of bacterial growth (Figs. 18.3 and 18.4). This step is difficult because epiretinal pus reduces the visualization of the posterior vitreous. **Caution**: The retina in endophthalmitis is very fragile. It is easy to induce breaks. Be very careful not to induce iatrogenic retinal breaks, as these will necessitate a silicone oil tamponade in endophthalmitis cases. It is not necessary to perform a thorough trimming of the vitreous base. The possible harm is greater than the possible benefit.

6. **Intravitreal antibiotics**

Now 0.1 mL vancomycin and 0.1 mL ceftazidime are injected into the eye (Fig. 18.5).

7. **Potential tamponade: silicone oil**

Some surgeons suggest silicone oil as tamponade, because it is attributed with bacteriostatic properties. Others use no tamponade. In the latter, one has no or only a reduced view of the fundus during the first postoperative days; after about 3 days, the eye will clear up. If you have identified or created a retinal break, we recommend silicone oil tamponade. The antibiotics can be injected into the anterior chamber or into the silicone oil. There is no place for a gas tamponade in endophthalmitis cases because it causes ocular irritation.

Conclusion: The main problem in endophthalmitis is poor visualization. In many cases a corneal abrasion improves visualization. The most important surgical step is a PVD. The PVD, however, is difficult due to poor visualization and an inflamed retina, which is easily injured.

18.4 Brief Case Reports

Case Report 1: Endophthalmitis and Choroidal Hemorrhage
Figs. 18.6–18.9

A 72-year-old male patient was admitted to us due to suspicion of an endophthalmitis. He was operated 2 weeks ago, for phaco + IOL. A posterior capsular defect occurred; an anterior vitrectomy was performed when a subchoroidal hemorrhage developed. An IOL was implanted and then the case was closed. The patient experienced first a visual acuity increase but after 10 days the vision got worse. He visited the outpatient clinic and an endophthalmitis was diagnosed. Visual acuity was light perception, no hypopyon was present, and the view to fundus was bad due to

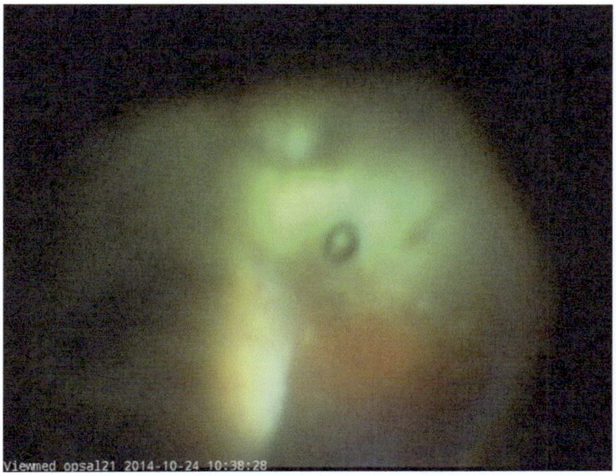

Fig. 18.7 Case report 1: On the left side, a choroidal detachment is visible and a superior vitritis/endophthalmitis is present

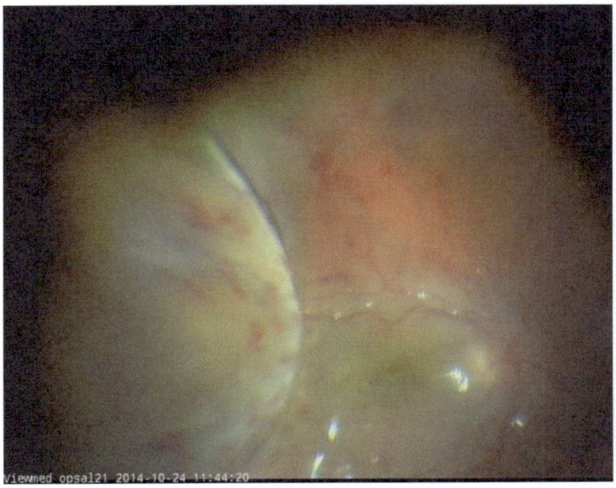

Fig. 18.8 Case report 1: A silicone oil-filled eye. There is residual subchoroidal hemorrhage present

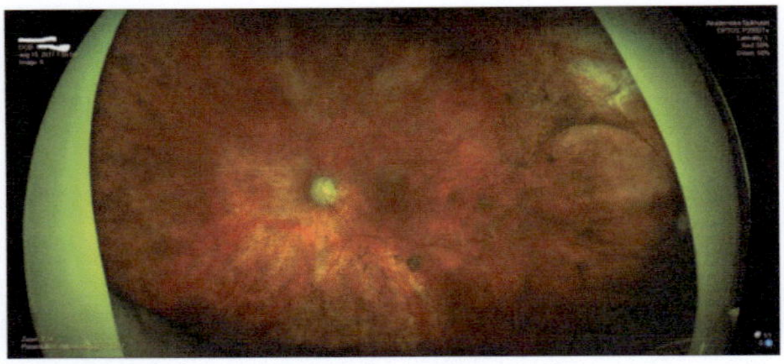

Fig. 18.9 Case report 1: A 15-month follow-up. The silicone oil is removed, VA is 0.3, but the patient is unhappy about his visual function

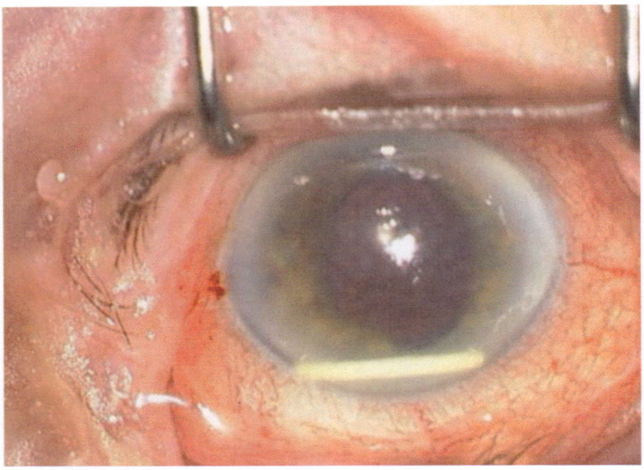

Fig. 18.10 Case report 2: This patient was submitted for an endophthalmitis. A hypopyon is present, the cornea was inflamed, and the view to fundus was poor

the choroidal hemorrhage. The patient complained of ocular discomfort. It was not really clear that an endophthalmitis was present. There are several options now: If only a subchoroidal hemorrhage was present, we could simply wait. If we suspected an endophthalmitis, we could inject antibiotics. This option was tricky due to the large choroidal detachment. And of course, we had the option of vitrectomy which was a difficult option due to the subchoroidal detachment. I decided for the last option. Unfortunately, there was no anesthesia available on this day so that the surgery had to be performed in general anesthesia. A removal of subchoroidal blood + vitrectomy + injection of antibiotics + 1000 csts silicone oil was performed. An endophthalmitis was present.

Case Report No. 2: A Pseudo-endophthalmitis

Figs. 18.10–18.12

A 76-year-old female patient was admitted to our surgical ward with the suspicion of an endophthalmitis with hypopyon. The examination revealed that the eye was painful, the visual acuity was decreased to HM, the cornea was edematous, and a “hypopyon” was present. The hypopyon was, however, an Ozurdex pellet which was lying horizontal in the inferior cornea mimicking a hypopyon.

The patient underwent a complicated phaco 2 months prior. An iris-claw IOL (Artisan®, Verisyse®) was implanted, and then, 6 weeks later, an Irvine-Gass macular

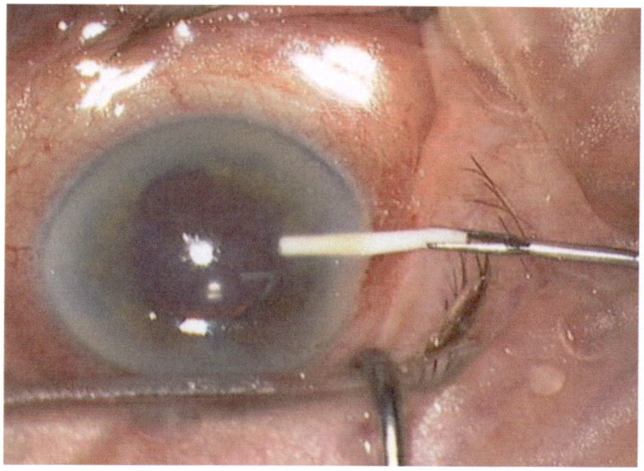

Fig. 18.11 Case report 2: The Ozurdex can be easily removed with an intravitreal forceps. A vitritis was not present

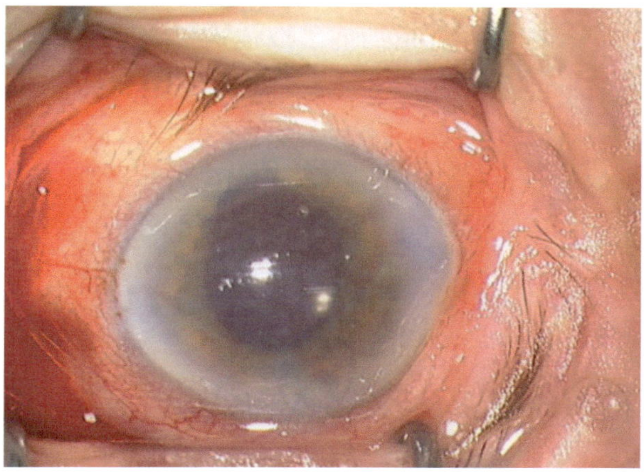

Fig. 18.12 Case report 2: The cornea took months to clear up partially but never became completely clear. Note that a retropupillary Artisan IOL is present

edema occurred. The macular edema was treated with Ozurdex. Ten days after injection, the patient presented with the abovementioned symptoms. The Ozurdex pellet was immediately removed, but the recovery of the cornea was very slow, and the last visual acuity was measured with 0.3. Remark: Do not inject an Ozurdex pellet in an eye with posterior capsular defect or aphakia.

18.5 Complications

Retinal detachment: The retina is very fragile when inflamed. It is easy to create a hole during PVD (central hole!). Do not perform a thorough trimming of the vitreous base. The vitreous cutter causes much dragging to the peripheral retina which may result later into a retinal detachment. *Conclusion*: It is important to perform a PVD, but do not insist to remove every leukocyte in the vitreous base.

18.6 FAQ

Can You Comment Intravitreal Antibiotics vs Vitrectomy Regarding Endophthalmitis?

If you are a retina clinic, then pursue the complete way and perform a vitrectomy. If you are an anterior segment clinic or do not have immediate access to vitrectomy, then inject intravitreal antibiotics. *Important*: Treat the patient immediately after arrival at the ward with intravenous antibiotics (e.g., 1,5 g Zinacef® ×3/d). There is always a considerable delay between the time point of arrival of the patient and the time point of injection. Add also subconjunctival cortisone (e.g., 1 ampoule Betapred®) to reduce the inflammation.

Reference

1. Endophthalmitis Vitrectomy Study Group. Results of the endophthalmitis vitrectomy study. A randomized trial of immediate vitrectomy and of intravenous antibiotics for the treatment of postoperative bacterial endophthalmitis. Arch Ophthalmol. 1995;113(12):1479–96.

Chapter 19
Intraocular Tumor Biopsies

Extras: Videos 19.1, 19.2, 19.3, 19.4, 19.5, and 19.6.

- Transretinal tumor biopsy
- Transscleral tumor biopsy
- Anterior chamber tumor biopsy
- Vitreous biopsy
- Chorioretinal biopsy
- Intraocular biopsy in suspected lymphoproliferative disease

19.1 Introduction

Intraocular tumor biopsies are mainly performed for lesions affecting the uvea (choroid, ciliary body, and iris). The other major indication is suspected intraocular lymphoma, which can affect vitreous, retina, and choroid.

Choroidal tumor biopsies can be performed for diagnostic or prognostic purposes. A diagnostic tumor biopsy is indicated if an intraocular malignancy is suspected, but the diagnosis cannot be established based on the clinical examination alone. A prognostic tumor biopsy is performed in cases in which the clinical diagnosis of a uveal melanoma has been established, and additional testing of a biopsy specimen enables a prognostication regarding the risk for extraocular metastatic disease by examining the gene expression profile or chromosome status.

Electronic Supplementary Material The online version of this chapter (https://doi.org/10.1007/978-3-319-89677-9_19) contains supplementary material, which is available to authorized users.

U. Spandau, H. Heimann, *Practical Handbook for Small-Gauge Vitrectomy*,
https://doi.org/10.1007/978-3-319-89677-9_19

Biopsy techniques have evolved significantly over the past years but vary greatly between centers. Some surgeons recommend a full standard vitrectomy with photocoagulation of the biopsy site and internal gas or oil tamponade in every choroidal biopsy. Others prefer fine-needle aspiration biopsies for posterior as well as anterior segment tumors. For posterior segment tumors, we have minimized the surgical intervention to a transretinal approach without vitrectomy, photocoagulation, and tamponade, which has proven to be effective and safe over the past years. In choroidal tumors at or anterior to the equator, we prefer a transscleral biopsy approach. For tumors in the anterior chamber, our current technique involves an anterior chamber maintainer with a vitrectomy cutter or forceps approach.

Pearls

Prognostic tumor biopsies are usually performed following active treatment of the tumors, i.e., radiotherapy, in order to minimize the risk of local tumor dissemination. In contrast, diagnostic biopsies are performed before any treatment. In such cases, it is mandatory to fast-track the biopsy work-up and possible treatment of the patient in order to minimize the time period until treatment and the risk for a local tumor dissemination of untreated tumor cells.

Pearls

Intraocular biopsies commonly obtain only paucicellular samples, which are difficult to stain and analyze. Cooperation with a pathology lab and a pathologist experienced in the work-up and interpretation of such samples is essential to avoid a high rate of nondiagnostic biopsies. It is mandatory to coordinate the timing of the biopsy, the fixation of the specimen if required, the transport to the pathology lab, and the work-up of the specimen before the biopsy. If a local work-up is not available, the specimen can be send to specialized laboratories using cytology fixation fluid. Contact our lab for more information (www.loorg.org).

Pearls

Patients are extremely disappointed when the biopsy doesn't reveal a diagnostic result, and there is a significant learning curve for surgeons and pathologists dealing with such specimen before a "positive" biopsy can be obtained in the majority of cases. Further, there is a risk of local tumor spread with inadequate surgical techniques. We, therefore, recommend to perform such biopsies only in centers with the adequate experience, backup, and patient numbers to perform biopsies on a regular basis.

Pearls

Waiting for the biopsy result can be an extremely distressing for the patient. The patient should be informed about the usual turnaround times until a biopsy result becomes available. A system for checking on the biopsy result and communication with the patient needs to be established before the biopsy. We recommend to discuss the mode of communication beforehand. Some patients prefer to receive the result over the phone in order not to lose any time; others would like to be informed during a personal conversation with the treating ophthalmologist. Support by a professional psychologist is extremely helpful, as ophthalmologists are usually not trained to provide the adequate support in cases of malignant disease.

Pearls

Tumor biopsies in children have to be approached with extreme caution and should only be performed in centers with experience in pediatric ocular oncology. This is because retinoblastoma may occur with a broad variety of sometimes unusual clinical presentations; a tumor biopsy of an intraocular retinoblastoma carries a high risk for extraocular seeding along the surgical wounds that may lead to systemic dissemination of the disease. In a worst-case scenario, the intraocular tumor biopsy can lead to the death of the patient.

19.2 Transretinal Tumor Biopsy

This is our most commonly used biopsy technique for choroidal tumors affecting the posterior pole up to the equator. In the majority of cases, the diagnosis has previously been established based on the clinical examination, and the biopsy is performed for prognostication. We then perform a biopsy immediately following the radiotherapy. In diagnostic biopsies, the specimen is fast-tracked, and the therapy must be initiated soon after the diagnosis has been confirmed.

Instruments:

1. Standard 25G–27G system
2. Three-way tap inserted into the suction line
3. CryoProbe (optional)

Individual steps:

1. Introduction of three-way tap into suction line
2. 25G–27G three-port system
3. Transretinal penetration into choroid
4. Tumor biopsy with vitreous cutter
5. Hemostasis
6. Backflush of biopsy specimen
7. Review of biopsy site
8. Port removal and cryotherapy (optional)

1. **Introduction of 3-Way Tap into Suction Line**

Transretinal tumor biopsies are performed with a standard 3-port vitrectomy system. The only addition is the insertion of a standard 3-way tap between the tubing of the cutter and the suction line leading to the vitrectomy machine (Fig. 19.1). The 3-way tap is used to backflush the specimen through the cutter.

Pearls

Transretinal tumor biopsy specimens are paucicellular. The best bits of the biopsy specimen usually get stuck in the cutter or in the tubing near the cutter. It is much more effective to backflush the specimen through the cutter opening than trying to suck the specimen all the way up through the cutter and the tubing.

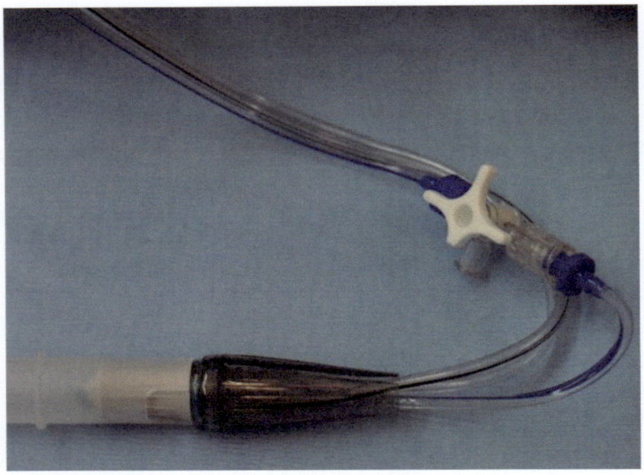

Fig. 19.1 Three-way tap inserted into the suction line of the vitreous cutter

2. **25G–27G Three-Port System**

We recommend the use of 25G–27G systems. They are effective in obtaining adequate biopsy specimen in the majority of cases. In addition, they create smaller retinal breaks and better sealing sclerotomies compared to 23G.

It is important to plan the trocar placement according to the tumor size and location. This is either done by reviewing a wide-angle photograph or indirect ophthalmoscopy and then adjusting the port placement, i.e., moving to a temporal approach or place the infusion nasally. It is mandatory to avoid penetration of the tumor during trocar insertion or a trocar tumor touch in large tumors. In addition, the leading instrument (vitreous cutter) should have a straight path into the tumor tissue without the need of bending the instrument or the risk of lens touch in phakic patients.

The biopsy is performed with a standard three-port setup (infusion line, handheld light source, vitreous cutter) and viewing system (wide-angle for tumors at the vascular arcades or anterior, higher magnification for posterior pole tumors).

Following trocar placement, the infusion line is connected and opened after standard verification of the correct position of the trocar opening in the vitreous cavity. The light pipe is inserted and the viewing system is moved in.

Pearls

Don't start your biopsy in autopilot three-port trocar insertion mode. Plan your trocar placement carefully, in particular in large tumors, tumors extending into the ciliary body, or tumors between 10 and 2 o'clock. Avoid penetrating tumor tissue or touching the tumor surface with the trocars. Aim to achieve a straight path into the tumor with your cutter and avoid a lens touch in phakic patients.

3. **Transretinal Penetration into the Choroid**

The biopsy is performed without a core vitrectomy or shaving of the vitreous base. As little vitreous as possible should be removed. Following insertion of the light pipe and an adequate viewing of the tumor, the vitreous cutter is inserted and pushed through the vitreous toward the tumor (Figs. 19.2 and 19.3). A retinal penetration site is chosen, and the cutter is pushed through the retina into the tumor and through the tumor tissue, until a resistance is felt when the tip of the cutter reaches the sclera.

Pearls

When choosing the penetration point, stay away from larger retinal blood vessels (which might also get caught in the cutter when you withdraw the cutter from the tumor). Aim to penetrate into the thickest part of the tumor to increase your chances for obtaining sufficient biopsy material. In tumors close to the fovea, think about your worst-case scenario of a subretinal hemorrhage – i.e., if you have a choice of penetration above or temporal to the fovea, go temporal, so a potential subretinal hemorrhage does not run into the fovea.

Pearls

Check if cutter and suction are working correctly before you enter the trocar. The next time you will activate it, the cutter will be deep inside the tumor tissue. Then it will be difficult to correct any malfunction.

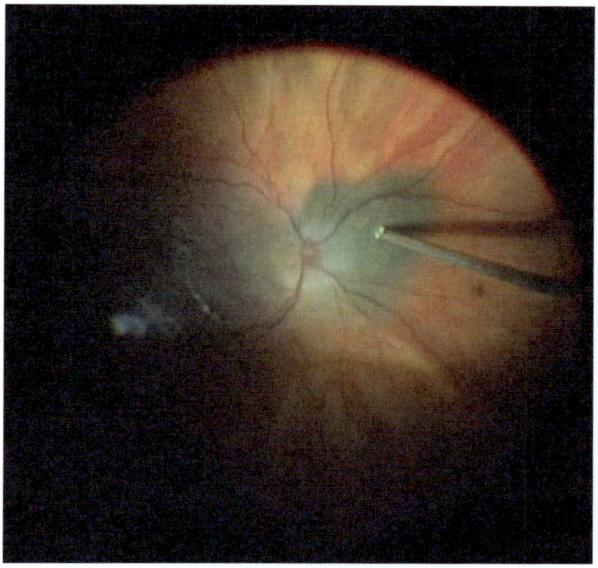

Fig. 19.2 Approach of the vitreous cutter to the tumor. No vitrectomy is performed and the cutter is pushed through the vitreous

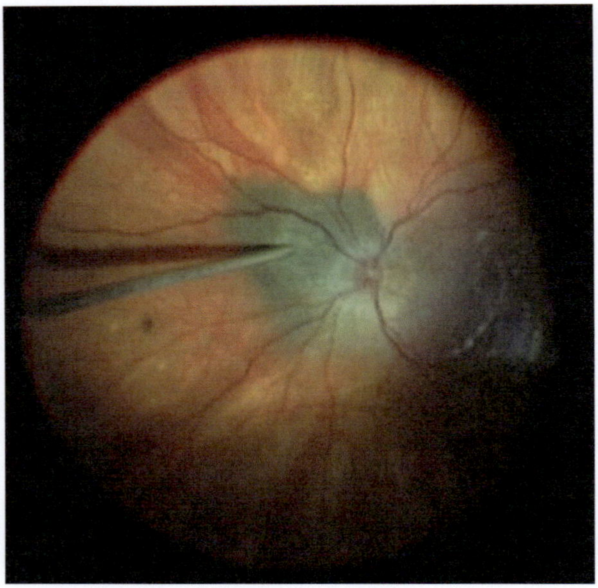

Fig. 19.3 Penetration of the cutter through the retina

Pearls

Know the orientation of your cutter opening before you enter the eye. You cannot see it once inside the tumor. Most vitrectomy cutters have a little mark on the grip of the cutter to indicate its orientation.

Pearls

Choroidal tumors vary greatly in their consistency. They can be fluid, jelly-like, mushy, solid, or leathery. The more solid the tumor, the easier the retinal penetration, but the more difficult the biopsy. In very soft tumors, the retina can be difficult to penetrate, and it is sometimes just pushed away and not penetrated by the tip of the cutter. Try to enter it with greater speed (think of an arrow penetrating the retina, it won't penetrate at a snail's pace). If you cannot purely penetrate the retina by pushing the tip through, cut a small hole into it with the cutter. Start with suction only, lift a bit of the retina, and activate cutting at very low cutting speeds to reduce the number of cuts to a minimum.

4. **Tumor Biopsy with the Vitreous Cutter**

The opening of the cutter should now sit deep inside the tumor as close to the sclera as possible. Activate the vitrectomy with your standard infusion and vitrectomy settings and minimal suction on the foot pedal. Most of the time, you will not see much happening. If no major problem is seen, increase the suction with your foot pedal to your usual maximum suction. Just cut away for about a minute to two. As you are focusing on the tumor, ask the assistant or scrub nurse to monitor the suction line. After some time, blood and tumor material will appear in the suction line. You should stop the cutter once the visible material in the suction line is about to reach the three-way tap.

Surgical Pearls No. 109
How long should you stay inside the tumor if you cannot see any changes at all? A positive sign to stop is when tumor material and/or blood is moving up the suction line and reaches the three-way tap. However, this can take several minutes in solid/leathery tumors. If absolutely nothing can be seen in the suction line or in the tumor, we usually cut away for about 2 min before we stop the cutter.

Surgical Pearls No. 110
Stay as close to the sclera as possible. This is the part of the tumor where you have the best chance of getting a biopsy out of the tumor itself (and not blood or exudates). It is the best place for a hemorrhage to stay localized, as the choroid and anterior tumor can tamponade the hemorrhage and keep it away from the subretinal space. There also is a natural tendency for most surgeons to subconsciously withdraw the cutter toward the retina, which can in the worst of cases result in sucking the retina into the cutter opening and creating a large retinal hole. Try to avoid this by keeping the tip as close to the sclera as you can.

Surgical Pearls No. 111
Once you cut away for about 30–40 s without any major changes, try to rotate the cutter opening by rotating the cutter handpiece like a pencil. This enables you to biopsy different parts of the tumor. In larger tumors, you can also slightly withdraw the tip of the tumor during the biopsy to reach different layers of the tumor.

Pearls

In very thin tumors (2 mm or less), it is sometimes not possible to perform a biopsy without sucking the retina into the cutter opening. In such cases, try to grab and lift the retina with your cutter to create a localized retinal detachment. This will give you more space to cut tumor tissue without creating a large retinal hole.

Pearls

The most common change you will see inside the tumor during the biopsy will be a localized choroidal and retinal hemorrhage. Minor hemorrhages should not cause any concern. In cases of a more pronounced hemorrhage or even a very forceful hemorrhage during the biopsy, stop cutting, leave the cutter in place (do not withdraw it from the tumor), and increase the infusion to about 80 mmHg or more. Wait for about a minute or until the hemorrhage does not expand anymore before proceeding. Then slowly lower the infusion to normal levels and continue.

5. **Hemostasis**

A choroidal biopsy almost always leads to a localized choroidal hemorrhage, and subretinal and vitreous hemorrhages are the most common clinically meaningful complications following such biopsies. A meticulous hemostasis is mandatory to lower the incidence of such vision threatening side effects of the surgery.

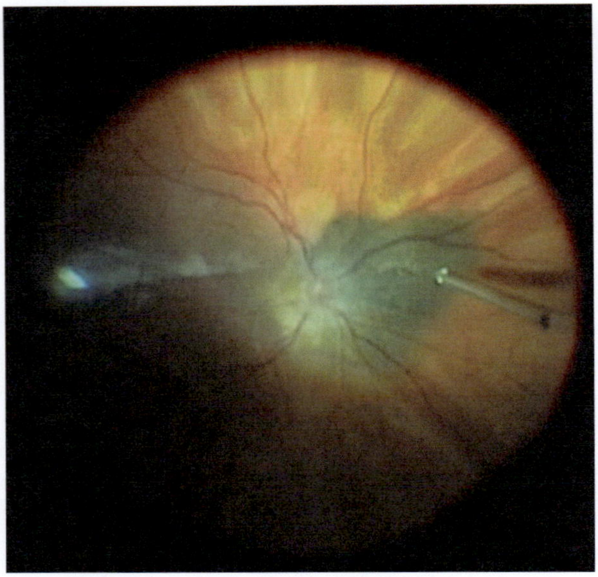

Fig. 19.4 Withdrawing the cutter tip from the choroid and retina

Once the cutting has stopped, leave the cutter within the tumor and increase the infusion to 80 mmHg. Slowly withdraw the cutter until the opening of the cutter reaches the retinal hole, but the tip of the cutter is still within the tumor (Fig. 19.4, Video 19.2). Watch for any hemorrhage appearing in the retinal hole. Then lower the infusion to 60 mmHg and then 40 mmHg, watching for a hemorrhage to appear. If no hemorrhage can be detected, slowly withdraw the cutter through the retinal hole, but stop once the cutter is just in front of the retina. Watch for any hemorrhage to appear in the retinal hole. If so, insert the cutter back into the retinal hole to tamponade the hemorrhage. Increase the infusion again and wait for the hemorrhage to stop.

Once you are able to withdraw the cutter without any active hemorrhage, wait with the cutter in front of the retinal hole; lower the infusion to about 25 mmHg. If no active hemorrhage appears, you can withdraw the cutter. We do not recommend to perform a standard vitrectomy, retinopexy of the retinal break, or endotamponade before or following the biopsy.

Pearls

Mastering hemostasis following the tumor biopsy is the key to lower the rate of postoperative vitreous hemorrhages. Withdraw the cutter from the retinal hole as slowly as possible. Use the cutter like a finger to plug the hole and stop the hemorrhage if it appears. Be patient, use the infusion pressure to stop a hemorrhage, and withdraw the cutter from the eye only when you are sure that the hemorrhage has stopped.

Pearls

The higher the infusion pressure, the more likely retina will get caught in the cutter opening while removing it from the retinal hole. Use active reflux to

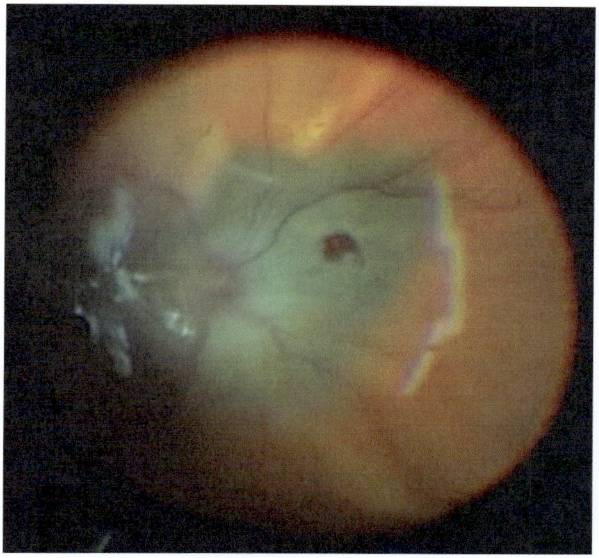

Fig. 19.5 Small preretinal hemorrhage after the biopsy, no vitrectomy required

remove the retina from the cutter. Try to find a balance between hemostasis, infusion pressure, and retinal incarceration into the cutter opening. If you cannot free the retina from the cutter, cut the retina to free the cutter with a very low cutting rate.

Pearls

Minor vitreous hemorrhages in front of the retinal hole do not require any active intervention (Fig. 19.5). In more pronounced hemorrhages, a limited vitrectomy to remove the hemorrhage should be performed straight away before withdrawing the cutter from the eye.

Pearls

It is unusual for tumor material to spread into the vitreous during and after the biopsy. Even if tumor cells can be seen in the vitreous, we usually do not actively chase and remove them, as they almost never cause a local recurrence. It is, however, mandatory to avoid translocation of tumor cells onto the conjunctiva through the sclerotomies. The conjunctiva is an ideal breeding environment for choroidal tumors and local recurrences are common.

6. **Backflush of Biopsy Specimen**

Once the cutter has been removed from the eye, a 5 mL syringe filled with BSS is connected to the open port of the three-way tap. The three-way tap is then rotated to block the suction to the vitrectomy machine and connect the BSS syringe to the cutter line. The BSS is then injected into the cutter line to backflush the biopsy material through the opening of the cutter into the biopsy pot (Fig. 19.6). This can be repeated

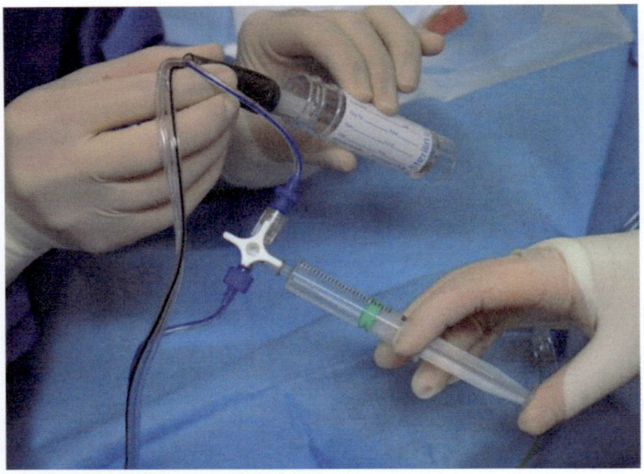

Fig. 19.6 Changing the three-way tap to backflush biopsy specimen through the cutter with a BSS injection through the three-way tap

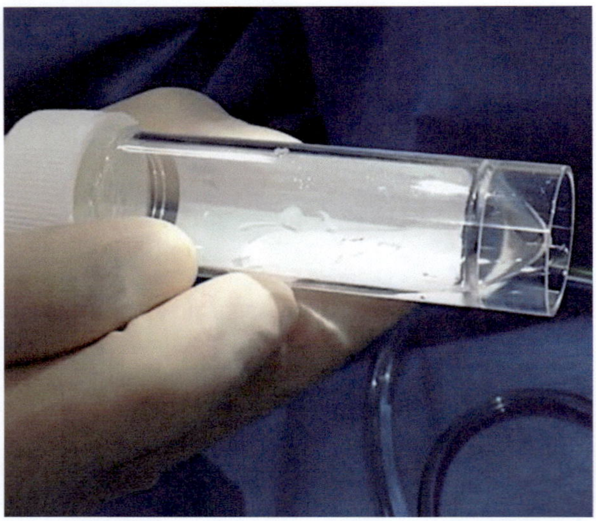

Fig. 19.7 Checking the specimen pot for visible tumor bits and pieces

multiple times until all biopsy material has been removed from the cutter. The biopsy pot is then checked under the microscope for visible tumor parts (Fig. 19.7).

Pearls

In positive biopsies, one can usually spot tumor bits in the biopsy vial without the microscope. This can sometimes be challenging in very hemorrhagic specimen. If no tumor material can be identified, we recommend to go back inside the tumor, using the same penetration site, and repeat the biopsy until tumor material can be identified.

7. **Review of Biopsy Site**

Following the backflush of the biopsy specimen, we routinely review the biopsy site though the operating microscope using the viewing system with endoillumination probe. Minor hemorrhages that may have occurred after the port and the endoillumination have been withdrawn are left alone (Fig. 19.5). In cases of more significant hemorrhages, these can now be removed with the cutter (Video 19.3).

Pearls

When removing the light pipe and the cutter following the biopsy, the intraocular pressure will go down a bit, even when using valved trocars. This may trigger a hemorrhage from the biopsy site. We, therefore, recommend to review the biopsy site with endoillumination in every case at the end of the surgery.

Pearls

There is no need to perform a vitrectomy, retinopexy of the biopsy site, or endotamponade. The vitreous forms a plug in front of the retinal hole, and most tumors are treated with radiotherapy, which ensures a chorioretinal scar formation to prevent access of fluid into the subretinal space. Choroidal tumors usually also act like a buckle to prevent a rhegmatogenous retinal detachment. In addition, the remaining vitreous keeps potentially seeding tumor cells localized in front of the tumor compared to a free-floating intraocular dissemination in vitrectomized eyes.

8. **Port Removal and Optional Cryotherapy**

Because no vitrectomy has been performed despite the three-port vitrectomy setup, there is a higher risk for vitreous prolapse through the wounds and vitreous wick formation. This increases the risk for postoperative endophthalmitis and tumor dissemination to the ocular surface. Great care has to be taken that the ports are sealed appropriately and no vitreous is protruding. Prolapsing vitreous may be removed with the cutter. In cases of potential or suspected dissemination of tumor cells, cryotherapy should be applied to the sclerotomy sites. Some surgeons perform this routinely to all ports in all cases of intraocular biopsies.

19.3 Transscleral Tumor Biopsy

This is our preferred technique for tumors affecting the ciliary body and/or the choroid between the ora serrata and the equator. For prognostic purposes, we perform the biopsy immediately before insertion of a ruthenium plaque or immediately after proton beam radiotherapy. We try to avoid this technique for diagnostic biopsies if an uveal melanoma is suspected, as this technique potentially disseminates cells to the ocular surface or leaves an open channel to the ocular surface, which may result in local tumor seeding.

Instruments:

1. Biopsy forceps (Fig. 19.8)
2. Feather and hockey blade (Fig. 19.9)
3. Tissue glue

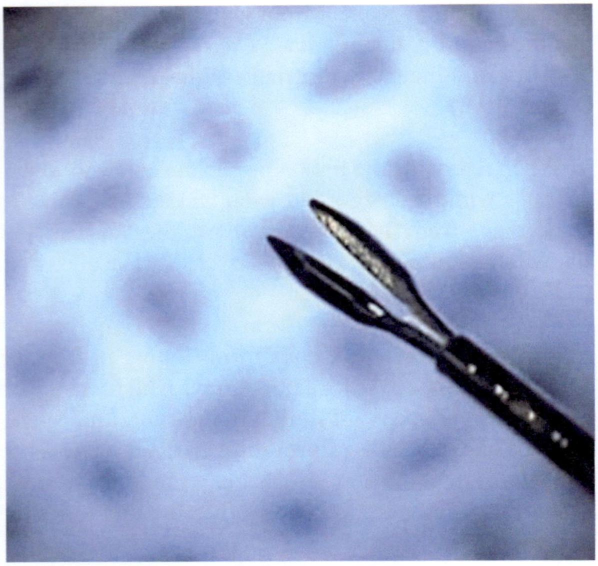

Fig. 19.8 Akgül biopsy forceps (DORC, NL; 1286. ABF)

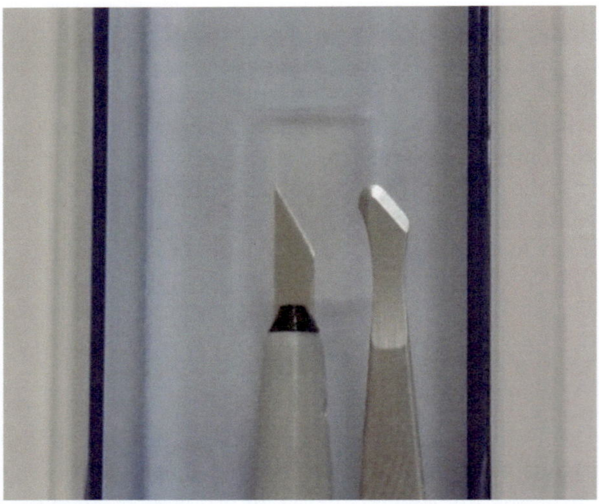

Fig. 19.9 Feather and hockey blades used for transscleral tumor biopsies

Individual steps:

1. **Identification of biopsy site**
2. **Scleral flap**
3. **Cutdown to choroid**
4. **Biopsy with forceps**
5. **Flap closure**

Pearls
We perform transscleral tumor biopsies routinely for tumors of the ciliary body and choroid between the limbus and the equator. Transscleral biopsies posterior to the equator are also possible in selected cases but depend on the individual anatomical situation and safe access to the biopsy site with the biopsy forceps. We recommend to perform these biopsies under the operating microscope for routine anterior segment surgery.

Pearls
Some tumors may be "invisible" in theatre, for example, nonpigmented lesions of the ciliary body. It is mandatory that the exact location for the planned biopsy is clearly identified and can be reproduced in theater before the patient is prepared for the surgery.

Pearls
We strongly advise against transscleral fine-needle aspiration biopsies. This can leave an open channel connecting the tumor to the ocular surface, which may lead to local seeding.

1. **Identification of biopsy site**

The location of the tumor should be confirmed either with ophthalmoscopy or based on the previous examination (ultrasound, photography, drawings). A peritomy is performed in the area of the biopsy. In tumors located between the insertion of the recut muscles and the equator, we recommend to sling the two neighboring rectus muscles with 2–0 silk in order to expose the biopsy site. In lesions between the limbus and the rectus muscles, this is usually not required.

In pigmented lesions, a transillumination with a light source (diaphanoscopy or vitrectomy light source) is performed to identify the shadow of the tumor. Usually the center of the tumor is marked with a marker pen as the location for the biopsy. In more posterior tumors, the biopsy is commonly performed in the anterior third of the lesion. In nonpigmented tumors, the identification of the biopsy site is usually based on the preoperative anterior segment ultrasound examination in combination with the location of the lesion in relation to the limbus, for example, lesion at the 8 o'clock meridian 3–6 mm posterior to the limbus based on the ultrasound examination.

2. **Scleral flap**

A scleral flap is prepared similar to trabeculectomy flaps with the flap opening pointing toward the limbus (Fig. 19.10). The biopsy site should be located at the base of the flap. We usually aim to create a scleral flap with a thickness of about 50–80% of the sclera and a width of about 3 mm. The flap margins are created with a slightly beveled cutdown with the feather or hockey blade. We then prepare the flap with a hockey blade.

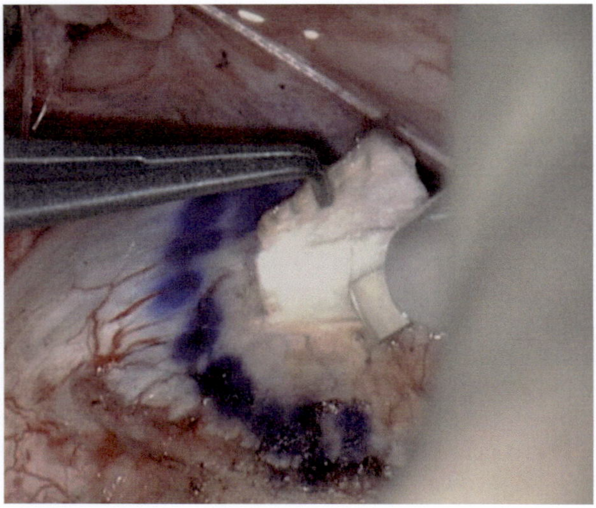

Fig. 19.10 Scleral flap and choroidal cutdown for transscleral tumor biopsy

Surgical Pearls No. 112
Don't be too aggressive with the scleral cutdown toward the choroid. In thin scleras you can cut into or expose the tumor tissue with the risk of seeding to the ocular surface.

Surgical Pearls No. 113
At the same time, try to avoid a very thin scleral flap. A good flap is needed to cover the biopsy channel in order to avoid a seeding of the tumor onto the ocular surface.

Surgical Pearls No. 114
Avoid the scleral areas immediately posterior to the insertions of the rectus muscles. Here the sclera is significantly thinned and it is easy to perforate.

3. **Cutdown to choroid**

Once the flap is prepared, a slit-like cutdown to the choroid is performed with the feather blade (Fig. 19.10). It is important that the choroid/ciliary body is exposed and all scleral lamellae are separated. One can "push" the sclera to the side with the hockey blade once the choroid is exposed. The choroid has to be exposed before you can biopsy it.

Pearls

Make sure that all scleral lamellae have been separated in the slit that exposes the choroid. If scleral trabeculae are left, they form a resistance to the forceps entering the wound. The forceps are then pushed with greater force, which may result in a sudden jolt of the forceps into the eye with the risk of retinal penetration. Don't try to force the forceps through the sclera.

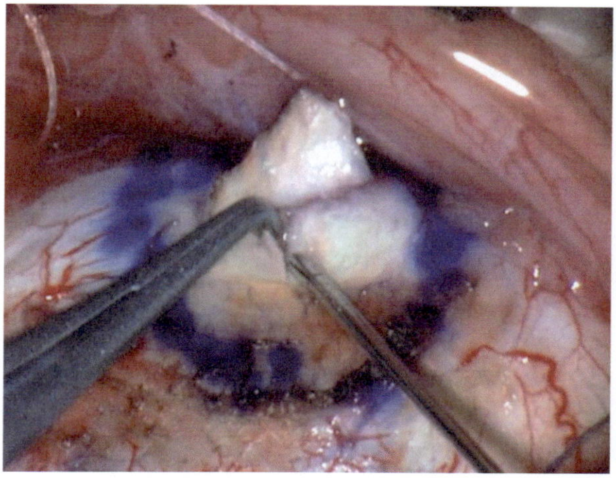

Fig. 19.11 Transscleral tumor biopsy using Akgül forceps

4. **Biopsy with Forceps**

The forceps are pushed into the tumor tissue and tumor material is removed (Fig. 19.11). An assistant should hold a cotton bud or similar very close to the wound in order to immediately swab up any hemorrhage or protruding tumor tissue that may appear once the forceps are withdrawn through the sclera. The biopsy is flushed off the forceps into the biopsy pot with a syringe and BSS. The biopsy spot is inspected for visible tumor material, and the biopsy is repeated until two or three pieces of tumor tissue are identified.

Pearls

We perform our biopsies using the 23G Akgül intraocular biopsy forceps (Fig. 19.8, DORC, www.dorc.eu). Alternatively, we recommend using strong serrated "crocodile" style forceps used for intraocular foreign body removals or peeling of thick epiretinal membranes in order to retrieve sufficient material.

Pearls

More often than not, the biopsy material is stuck to the forceps. Make sure to flush it off with a jet stream of BSS and a blunt cannula before reentering the eye. Check the forceps for remaining tumor tissue under the microscope before reentering the biopsy site. The worst thing that could happen is that you inadvertently touch conjunctiva or sclera with the tumor material on the forceps, thereby risking dissemination of the tumor onto the ocular surface.

5. **Flap closure**

Once enough biopsy material has been returned, the flap is closed with tissue glue (histoacrylic or fibrin glue, Fig. 19.12). The idea behind using the glue is to seal the biopsy wound in order to prevent a seeding of the tumor onto the ocular surface (Courtesy of Prof Bertil Damato, San Francisco, USA). Suturing of the flap is not required.

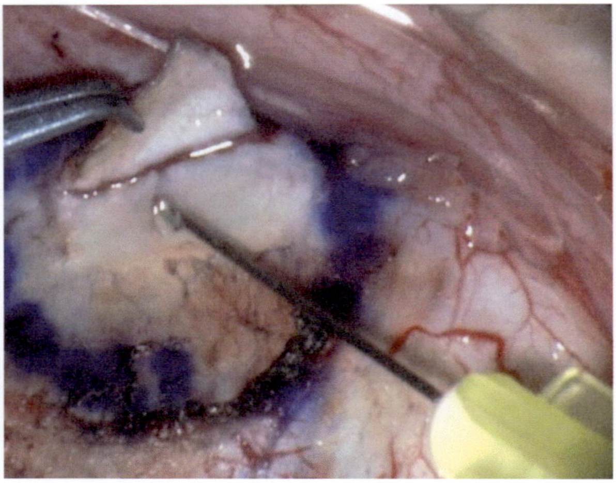

Fig. 19.12 Tissue glue to seal flap after transscleral tumor biopsy

Pearls

When using histoacrylic glue, use only one drop placed in the biopsy wound. This is sufficient to seal the wound and close the flap. Excess histoacrylic glue can form rock-hard granular foreign bodies that easily irritate and perforate the conjunctiva and are extremely difficult to remove surgically at a later stage.

19.4 Anterior Chamber Tumor Biopsy

Iris and ciliary body tumors with infiltration of the chamber angle can be biopsied through the anterior chamber. The setup includes an anterior chamber maintainer. The biopsy is performed with a 25G cutter or the biopsy forceps. Relatively bully lesions can be performed with a viscoelastic substance and forceps only.

Anterior chamber biopsies should be performed in selected cases only. This is because tumor seeding is a much more common event in the anterior chamber, more biopsy material is required for diagnosis, and the histopathological distinction between benign and malignant iris tumors can be extremely challenging with a lot higher rate of nondiagnostic biopsies. In addition, the vast majority of iris melanomas are associated with a low risk of metastatic spread – a prognostic tumor biopsy is less informative and consequential compared to choroidal or ciliary body melanoma.

Instruments:

1. MVR blade
2. Standard 25G vitrectomy pack
3. Anterior chamber maintainer
4. Three-way tap
5. Biopsy forceps (optional)

Individual Steps:

1. **Corneal incisions**
2. **Insertion of anterior chamber maintainer**
3. **Biopsy with cutter or forceps**
4. **Backflush of biopsy specimen**
5. **Removal of anterior chamber maintainer**

Pearls

We now prepare a routine 25G vitrectomy pack with vitrectomy setup in all cases of anterior chamber biopsies in order to remove any significant hemorrhages.

1. **Corneal Incision**

Two corneal incisions are placed for the anterior chamber maintainer and the cutter using a standard MVR blade. The position of the anterior chamber maintainer should be away from the tumor. The incision for the cutter or forceps should enable a straight access to the tumor without crossing the lens in phakic patients.

2. **Insertion of Anterior Chamber Maintainer**

The anterior chamber maintainer is inserted into the anterior chamber (Fig. 19.13). We routinely use 25mmHG infusion pressure. This can be adjusted according to the anterior chamber depth, iris prolapse, hemorrhages, etc.

Pearls

Iris tumors have a tendency to bleed profusely, and, in contrast to posterior segment tumors, there is no retinal cover to contain the hemorrhage. Although we performed some biopsies in bulky tumors with injection of a viscoelastic substance and forceps only, we now recommend using an anterior chamber infusion and a vitrectomy setup in the case of more advanced anterior chamber hemorrhages.

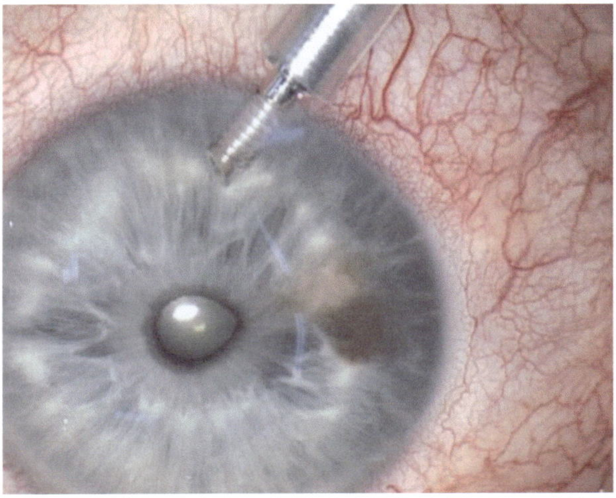

Fig. 19.13 Positioning of the anterior chamber maintainer for iris biopsy

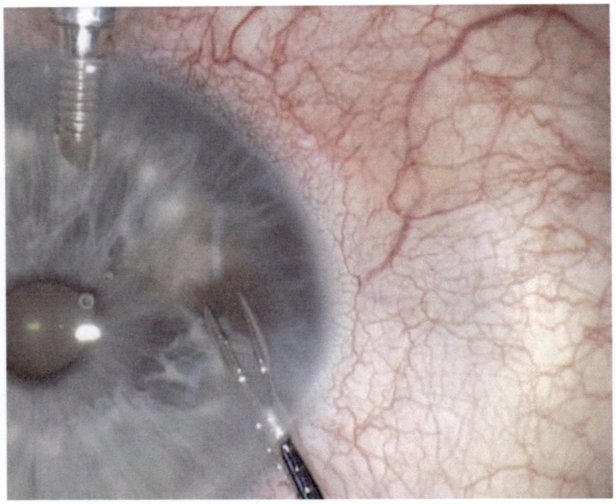

Fig. 19.14 Iris biopsy using Akgül forceps

Increasing the infusion pressure allows hemostasis, and the cutter can be used to remove any hemorrhage and blood clots.

3. **Biopsy with Cutter or Forceps**

The three-way tap is inserted into the infusion line (see transretinal tumor biopsy above), and the cutter is inserted into the tumor. The biopsy is performed using standard setting until sufficient tumor material is obtained.

When using forceps, the forceps are advanced deep into the tumor tissue and then withdrawn after grabbing the tissue (Video 19.5, Fig. 19.14).

Pearls

Iris tumors are often of leathery consistency and the iris itself can be very brittle. Act with caution when pulling the biopsy forceps from the tumor in order to avoid an iridodialysis at the iris base. In the case of doubt, use a vitreous cutter for the biopsy.

Pearls

From a pathologist's point of view, the diagnostic work-up of iris tumors is more challenging compared to choroidal tumors. Therefore, more biopsy material is usually required.

4. **Backflush of Biopsy Specimen**

When using a cutter, the specimen is back flushed via the three-way tap (see transretinal tumor biopsies). When using the biopsy forceps, the specimen is sprayed of the forceps with a jet of BSS (see transscleral biopsies). Again, make sure all tissue has been cleared from the tip of the forceps before reentering the eye.

5. **Removal of Anterior Chamber Maintainer**

The anterior chamber maintainer is removed and the anterior chamber is left with BSS. An appropriate closure of the corneal wounds is reassured. We do not inject intracameral antibiotics routinely.

19.5 Vitreous Biopsy

A vitreous biopsy without a retinal or choroidal biopsy is performed in suspected vitreoretinal lymphoma with a significant cellular component in the vitreous, or cases of acute or chronic endophthalmitis. The advantages of this technique are that it has a relatively low complication rate and avoids a more invasive biopsy of affected retinal or choroidal tissue. The disadvantage is that it has a higher rate of nondiagnostic specimen.

Instruments:

1. Standard 25G–27G vitrectomy pack
2. Three-way tap

Individual Steps:

1. **Insertion of trocars**
2. **"Dry" biopsy of vitreous specimen**
3. **Vitrectomy**
4. **Intraocular tamponade**

1. **Insertion of trocars**

A standard three-port setup with 25G or 27G instruments with the addition of a three-way into the suction line (see above transretinal biopsy) is used. The infusion remains closed for the first part of the "dry" biopsy.

2. **"Dry" Biopsy of Vitreous Specimen**

In cases of associated retinal infiltration, the area of interest is the vitreous immediately in front of the infiltrated retina and choroid. The cutter is placed as close to the retina as it is deemed safe, and the vitrectomy with suction but without infusion is started. As the infusion line remains closed initially, the intraocular pressure can be maintained by manual pressure with globe indentation using a squint hook or cotton bud (assistant or scrub nurse, or bimanual technique with chandelier endoillumination). Once sufficient vitreous has been removed, the infusion line is opened, and the manual pressure on the globe is slowly withdrawn. The biopsy specimen is back flushed through the three-way tap as described in transretinal biopsies above.

Pearls

Try to perform the vitreous biopsy immediately over the affected retina and choroid. There is a kind of "spill over" of cells from the retina/choroid into the vitreous. This is why the best chance of harvesting affected cells in the vitreous is in this area.

3. **Vitrectomy**

Following the "dry" biopsy of the vitreous, we perform a standard vitrectomy including induction of a posterior vitreous detachment and trimming of vitreous base. The vitrectomy cassette is also send for histopathological and/or microbiological analysis.

Pearls

Do not forget to send in the vitrectomy cassette for analysis following the initial vitreous biopsy. The vitrectomy fluid can be prepared by the pathology lab like a cytology specimen. A lot of cells are caught in the cassette which may be able to establish the diagnosis even if the "dry" biopsy specimen fails.

4. **Intraocular Tamponade**

The choice of intraocular tamponade depends on the vitreoretinal morphology. If retinal breaks are not present, we only use air to seal the vitrectomy ports. In cases with retinal breaks, a gas or silicone tamponade is used.

19.6 Chorioretinal Biopsy

This technique is reserved for advanced cases of suspected retino-choroidal diseases, for example, vitreoretinal lymphoma or advanced inflammatory chorioretinal diseases in which the treatment would depend on a specified diagnosis that could not be established with other measures. The aim of the biopsy is to retrieve a relatively large "en bloc" piece of retinal and choroidal tissue or bigger chunks of tissue with the cutter.

Pearls

Chorioretinal biopsies are usually performed in advanced disease, often following previously failed vitreous or choroidal biopsies. The aim is to establish the diagnosis by harvesting relatively large samples with a more aggressive approach compared to other biopsies. Potential anatomical complications or a poor visual outcome has to be accepted in some cases in order to establish the diagnosis.

Instruments:

1. Standard 25G–23G vitrectomy pack with chandelier illumination and three-way tap
2. Scissors (optional)
3. Endolaser and endodiathermy probes
4. Silicone oil tamponade

Individual Steps:

1. **Vitrectomy**
2. **Chorioretinal biopsy**
3. **Endolaser and silicone oil tamponade**

1. **Vitrectomy**

A standard three-port vitrectomy with induction of a posterior vitreous detachment and trimming of vitreous base is performed. If an "en bloc" biopsy of the retina and choroid is planned, a chandelier illumination is inserted with a fourth port, and a peritomy is performed over the port used to retrieve the specimen. If a cutter biopsy is planned, a three-way tap is inserted into the suction line (see transretinal biopsy).

2. **Chorioretinal Biopsy**

An "en bloc" biopsy is performed similar to the preparation of an RPE transplant patch, just with the retina still attached to the specimen. The biopsy site is surrounded by heavy, continuous laser in order to lower the choroidal perfusion and the risk for hemorrhage. Any major retinal vessels running over or through the biopsy site are coagulated with endodiathermy. The retina and choroidal tissue is grasped with a forceps and cut out with horizontal or vertical scissors. Any significant retinal and choroidal bleeding is coagulated with endodiathermy. Once the specimen has been freed from the surrounding tissue, one trocar is removed, and the specimen is retrieved through the sclerotomy. The sclerotomy may have to be enlarged with an MVR blade depending on the size of the biopsy.

In a cutter biopsy, the chorioretinal biopsy material is removed with the cutter. The biopsy specimen is flushed back using a three-way tap as described for transretinal biopsies.

Pearls

In the case of doubt, make a larger sclerotomy in order to retrieve the specimen smoothly through the scleral opening for "en bloc" biopsies. If you lose the biopsy tissue at the sclerotomy site, it can be difficult to retrieve it, as it may get stuck to the remaining vitreous at the vitreous base or disintegrate floating around in the vitreous cavity. Use larger forceps with a good grip of the tissue for this step.

Pearls

We now routinely perform our chorioretinal biopsy with a cutter. In cooperation with out pathologists, we achieve a high rate of "positive" results with this technique, which is much easier to perform than an "en bloc" biopsy.

19.7 Endolaser and Silicone Oil Tamponade

The edges of the chorioretinal biopsy are treated with endolaser. If the retina has detached, we recommend to reattach it with heavy liquid rather than fluid air exchange. We routinely use silicone oil tamponade in such cases. The choice of silicone oil (heavy oil, 1000cts vs. 2000cts or 5000cts) depends on the location of the biopsy, the individual case, and the surgeon's preferences.

Pearls

Be aware of the dangers of air embolism via the vortex veins in cases with open choroidectomies ("PAVE syndrome"). If the chorioretinal biopsy site is near a vortex vein, we urgently recommend never to perform a fluid air exchange or a gas tamponade. A direct heavy liquid-silicone oil exchange is recommended in such cases.

Pearls

At the end of the surgery, don't forget to send the vitrectomy cassette for cytology in addition to the chorioretinal biopsy material. Diagnostic cells may be contained in the bag of fluid and may aid in the diagnosis.

19.8 Intraocular Biopsy in Suspected Lymphoproliferative Disease

Intraocular lymphomas are sometimes difficult to diagnose. In addition, hemato-oncologists are often reluctant to initiate any active treatment without a biopsy-proven diagnosis. In broad terms, two different presentations of intraocular lymphoma can be distinguished:

- Vitreoretinal lymphoma is an extremely aggressive malignant disease. It can affect one or both eyes and the central nervous system. It usually infiltrates the retina and vitreous and is often difficult to diagnose. Typical clinical signs are multifocal vitreoretinal infiltrates and cells. Commonly, patients are seen in uveitis clinics for prolonged periods of time before the correct diagnosis can be established.
- Choroidal lymphomas are even less frequently seen than vitreoretinal lymphoma but usually have a more benign clinical course. The typical presentation is that of a painless diffuse swelling of the choroid.

The mode of biopsy depends on the stage of the disease and the anatomical location of the planned biopsy:

- If the clinical presentation includes mainly vitreous cells, we recommend a "dry" vitreous biopsy of the cellular vitreous infiltration, followed by a vitrectomy as described in the vitreous biopsy section above.
- If a significant choroidal swelling can be detected on ultrasound examination, we recommend a transscleral choroidal biopsy for choroidal but also for suspected vitreoretinal lymphoma.
- In advanced cases and urgent cases or if one of the above techniques have previously failed, we usually proceed to a chorioretinal biopsy with silicone oil tamponade.

Pearls

Always perform an anterior segment UBM ultrasound examination in cases of suspected intraocular lymphoma. You may be surprised by the amount of choroidal thickening present in such cases. If the choroidal swelling is present within 10 mm posterior to the limbus, we recommend a transscleral choroidal biopsy for diagnosis. This is much safer than entering the vitreous cavity and a lot more material can be retrieved.

Part XII
Macular Translocation and Choroidal Detachment

Chapter 20
Macular Translocation

Extras: Videos 20.1 and 20.2.

20.1 Introduction

A macular translocation surgery is recommended in an only eye with submacular CNV. The second eye is typically lost due to a large AMD scar. Surgery in general anesthesia is recommended. The second surgery is scheduled in 2 months with silicone oil removal and muscle surgery.

20.2 Instruments and Materials

1. Four-port trocar system (2 × 20G sclerotomies)
2. 41G injection cannula (DORC, Medilens)
3. PFCL

20.3 Tamponade

Silicone oil

Electronic Supplementary Material The online version of this chapter (https://doi.org/10.1007/978-3-319-89677-9_20) contains supplementary material, which is available to authorized users.

U. Spandau, H. Heimann, *Practical Handbook for Small-Gauge Vitrectomy*,
https://doi.org/10.1007/978-3-319-89677-9_20

20.4 The Surgery

1. **Four-port trocar system**
2. **PVD up to the ora serrata**
3. **Meticulous vitrectomy**
4. **Induction of retinal detachment with 41G cannula**
5. **Fluid × air exchange**
6. **Circular diathermy posterior to ora serrata**
7. **Circular retinectomy**
8. **Anterior vitrectomy and removal of residual anterior retina**
9. **Unfolding of retina**
10. **Removal of CNV membrane**
11. **PFCL instillation**
12. **Rotation of retina and macula**
13. **Circular laser photocoagulation**
14. **PFCL × silicone oil exchange**
15. **Muscle surgery**

The Surgery Step-by-Step

1. **Four-port trocar system**

We recommend a hybrid system with one 25G infusion trocar and two 20G instrument trocars (DORC, NL). A chandelier light is also required.

2. **PVD up to the ora serrata**
3. **Meticulous vitrectomy**

In the most cases of macula translocation surgeries, the posterior vitreous is attached; a PVD is absent. The PVD must be performed meticulously and completely up to the ora serrata. The following step is a meticulous vitrectomy. A test for successful removal of vitreous up to the ora serrata is a diathermy (see also next step). Diathermy does not work on retina with residual vitreous.

4. **Induction of retinal detachment with 41G cannula** (Figs. 20.1 and 20.2)
5. **Fluid × air exchange**

The 41G cannula is pierced through the retina, BSS is injected, and a retinal detachment is induced. Where to pierce the retina? At the superior and inferior temporal arcade. Before piercing the retina, assess that no air is left inside the cannula. Eject BSS while piercing the retina, and when a bleb occurs, keep your hand stable and create a large bullous detachment. Create two or three large bullous detachments. Then continue with a fluid × air exchange. This maneuver presses the subretinal fluid toward the posterior pole and detaches the posterior pole. Optimally a “Mercedes star” is visible in the middle of all blebs signifying a complete detachment. The fluid against air maneuver may be repeated several times until a complete attachment is achieved.

6. **Circular diathermy posterior to ora serrata**

The diathermy marks the retina before the retinotomy. In addition, the cautery prevents bleeding of the retinal edges. Important: Retina with residual vit-

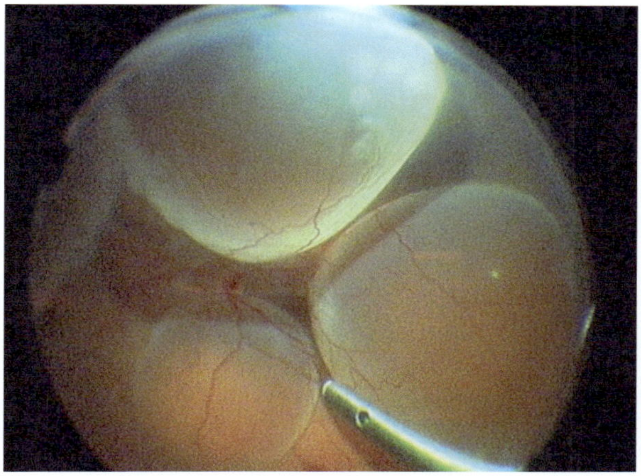

Fig. 20.1 Inject BSS with a 41G cannula under the retina until a bullous detachment has developed

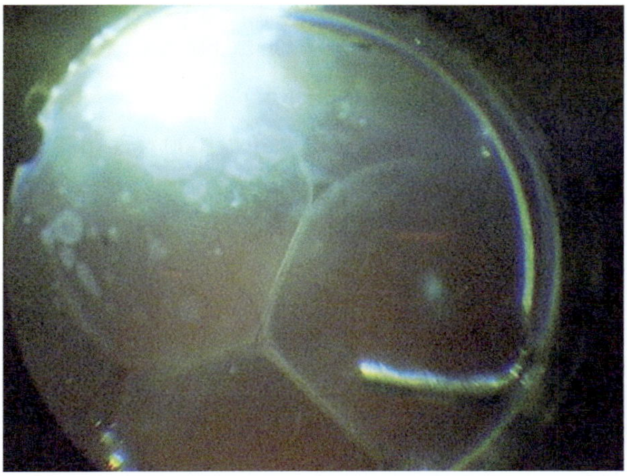

Fig. 20.2 Continue with a fluid × air exchange. The subretinal fluid is pressed toward the macula until the posterior pole is detached. Note the central Mercedes star sign

reous cannot be cauterized. In this case remove the residual vitreous and repeat diathermy.

7. **Circular retinectomy**

This maneuver can be performed with the vertical microscissors (20G Dorc). Alternatively, you can use a 25G or even better a 27G vitreous cutter. Be cautious not to injure the choroid. If a bleeding occurs, then cauterize it at once.

8. **Anterior vitrectomy und removal of residual anterior retina**

The anterior retina may overlap with the rotated retina and cause a PVR. Remove therefore the anterior retina with the vitreous cutter.

9. **Unfolding of retina**

Fold the retina up with a vitreoretinal forceps with circular tips (Geuder (Germany), 36242). At the end, the retina is 360° folded up exposing the subretinal CNV.

10. **Removal of CNV membrane**

Remove the subretinal blood with a backflush instrument and aspirate the membrane. Fixate the membrane in the middle of the eye and remove it with the vitreous cutter. If a feeder vessel is present, then cauterize it.

11. **PFCL instillation**
12. **Rotation of retina and macula (macular translocation)**

Instill PFCL up to the equator. Then rotate the retina and macula with a knob spatula (Eye Tech, UK) or with a vacuum cleaner (extrusion cannula with silicone tip). Rotate the retina clockwise and approximately 30°. Observe that the macula is located on healthy RPE.

13. **Circular laser photocoagulation**

Instill PFCL up to the ora serrata and confirm that the retinotomy edges are completely attached. The best instrument for this maneuver is the knob spatula (Eye Tech, UK). If not, then a membrane is present which must be removed before laser photocoagulation. Then perform a 360° laser cerclage. Apply three rows of laser.

14. **PFCL x silicone oil exchange**

The final step is a PFCL against 1000 csts silicone oil exchange. When the silicone oil reaches the retinotomy edges, aspirate the edges thoroughly from BSS. Then continue with final complete PFCL removal.

15. **Muscle Surgery**

Two months later a silicone oil removal and a muscle surgery of all six eye muscles are performed. To find the right angle for the globe rotation, the vitreoretinal surgeon marks the sclera or cornea along the line optic disc and macula (Fig. 20.3). Then the strabismus surgeon can assess the angle between the marking and the lateral rectus (Fig. 20.4).

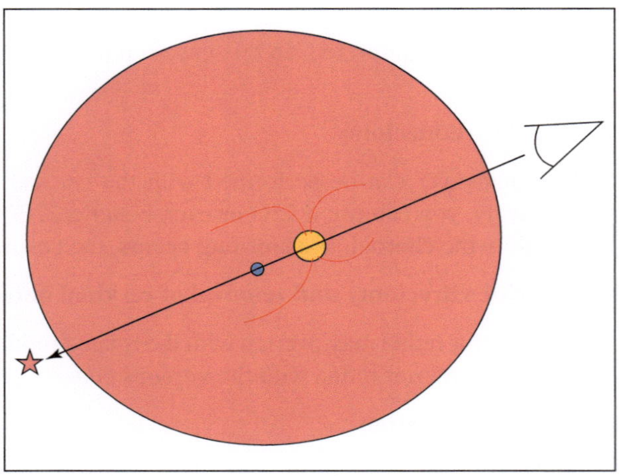

Fig. 20.3 The vitreoretinal surgeon marks the sclera or cornea with a marking pen on the line of optic disc and macula. He can do this step using a binocular indirect ophthalmoscope

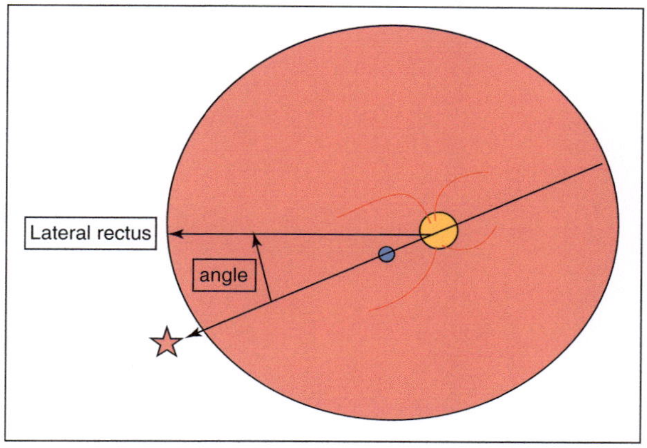

Fig. 20.4 Then the strabismus surgeon can assess the angle between the marking and the lateral rectus and performs a muscle surgery of all six muscles

Chapter 21
Choroidal Detachment: Surgical Management of a Serous Choroidal Detachment

Extras: Video 21.1.

21.1 Introduction

The choroidal detachment may be caused by hypotony, for example, after a trabeculectomy. The IOP is lower than 6 mmHg. Clear fluid is present between sclera and choroid. A so-called choroidal effusion or serous choroidal detachment has developed (Table 21.1). As a basic rule, the subchoroidal fluid is removed from the scleral side, and not transretinal. The surgery of a choroidal effusion has a low complication profile because the serous fluid can be removed easily and complete.

Table 21.1 Diagram of the anatomy of a choroidal detachment

Sclera
Serous fluid in the subchoroidal space
Choroid
Retina
Vitreous

Electronic Supplementary Material The online version of this chapter (https://doi.org/10.1007/978-3-319-89677-9_21) contains supplementary material, which is available to authorized users.

U. Spandau, H. Heimann, *Practical Handbook for Small-Gauge Vitrectomy*,
https://doi.org/10.1007/978-3-319-89677-9_21

21.2 Surgery

A surgery is recommended when kissing choroids are present. If kissing choroids occur after a trabeculectomy, then the first surgical approach is to close the scleral flap with extra sutures. If the IOP improves and increases over 8 mmHg, then the choroidal detachment will disappear.

21.2.1 Instruments

1. 23- or 25-gauge four-port trocar system
2. Anterior chamber maintainer
3. Extra-long 6 mm trocars (23G and 23G from Alcon)

An anterior chamber maintainer is an infusion, which is inserted in the limbus and injects BSS into the anterior chamber.

21.2.2 Tamponade

PFCL, 1000csts silicone oil

21.2.3 The Surgery Step-by-Step

1. **Limbal peritomy**
2. **Place traction sutures beneath all four rectus muscles**
3. **Insert an anterior chamber maintainer**
4. **Sclerotomies between insertion of the muscle and the equator**
5. **Drainage of serous fluid**
6. **Insertion of trocars**
7. **Core vitrectomy**
8. **Injection of PFCL**
9. **Trimming of vitreous base**
10. **Exchange of PFCL against silicone oil**

1. **Limbal peritomy**
2. **Place traction sutures beneath all four rectus muscles**

Perform a 360° peritomy and place traction sutures underneath all horizontal muscles.

3. **Insert an anterior chamber maintainer.**

An inferotemporal paracentesis is performed, the anterior chamber maintainer is inserted, and the infusion line is opened (Fig. 21.1). Now the eyeball becomes

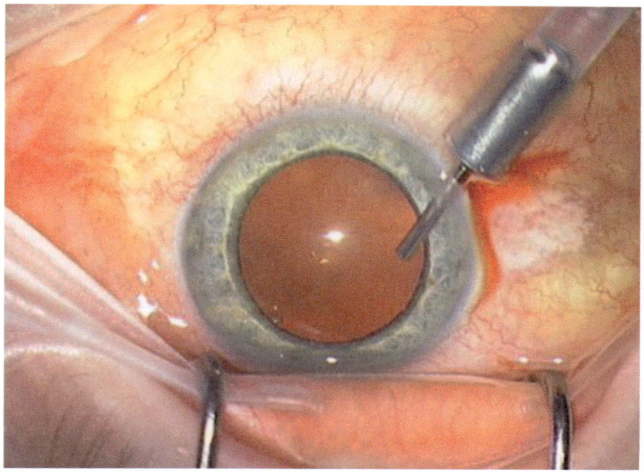

Fig. 21.1 Insert an anterior chamber maintainer to increase IOP

normotensive. An infusion of the anterior chamber works particularly well when there is a pseudophakia.

4. **Sclerotomies between insertion of the muscle and the equator**
5. **Drainage of serous fluid**

Before performing a sclerotomy you should ascertain the location of the choroidal bullae in the eye (Fig. 21.2). It is in the most times temporally and nasally.

A small sclerotomy of 2–3 mm in length is sufficient (Fig. 21.3). Place the sclerotomies between the insertion of the muscle and the equator. For example, if a temporal and nasal choroidal detachment is present, you should perform a temporal and nasal sclerotomy. The sclerotomy is located in the middle between the muscle insertion and equator. The sclerotomies should be 1–2 mm in length and extend in a radial direction. Once the sclerotomy is performed, clear fluid will flow out the sclerotomy. Repeat the maneuver on the nasal side if necessary.

The sclerotomies do not need to be sutured at the end of the surgery.

6. **Insertion of trocars**

When no more blood flows out of the sclerotomy, you can try to insert the trocars at the pars plana if you have not done this before (Fig. 21.4). Due to the detachment of the pars plana epithelium, this is a difficult procedure. Choose an area with little choroidal detachment and select a sutureable, longer infusion cannula (see above). Use preferably 6-mm-long trauma trocars from Alcon. Check if the trocar is located in the vitreous cavity. If the trocar cannula is not in the vitreous cavity, it can be freed from the surrounding tissue with a membrane pic from the opposite trocar cannula. The same procedure can now be performed with the second trocar cannula. Remove the anterior chamber maintainer and insert a pars plana infusion line. Then insert a second trocar opposite to the infusion cannula.

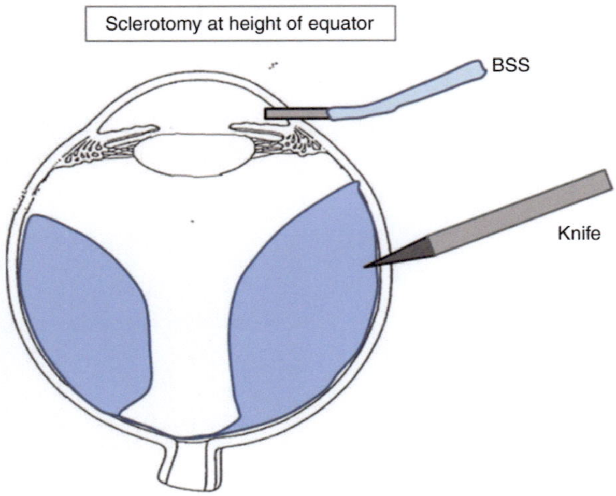

Fig. 21.2 Perform a 1–2 mm sclerotomy on height of the equator

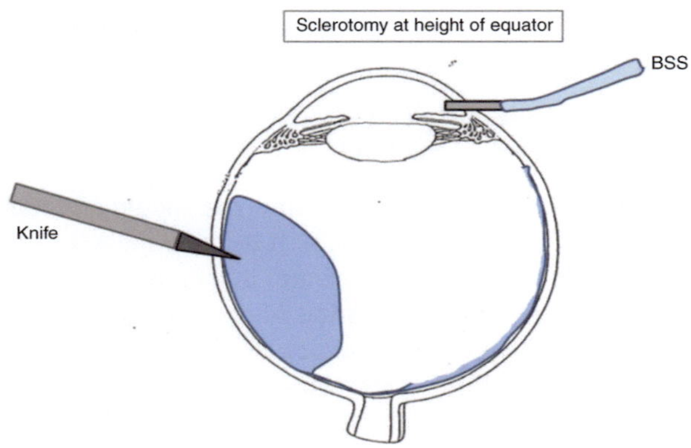

Fig. 21.3 The same maneuver on the other side

7. **Core vitrectomy**
8. **Injection of PFCL**

If the choroidal detachment has regressed, a vitrectomy can be performed (Fig. 21.5). You may need to insert a chandelier light. Then PFCL is injected, which pushes the residual suprachoroidal blood through the sclerotomies outside. You should now check the sclerotomies (flick the BIOM out and rotate the globe with the traction sutures).

9. **Trimming of vitreous base**

Perform a thorough trimming of the vitreous base because a long-lasting or even permanent silicone oil tamponade is required.

10. **Exchange of PFCL for silicone oil**

If there is only a minor residual choroidal detachment, perform a PFCL/silicone oil exchange. The silicone oil is injected through the infusion cannula. Suture the sclerotomies with a Vicryl 8-0 stitch.

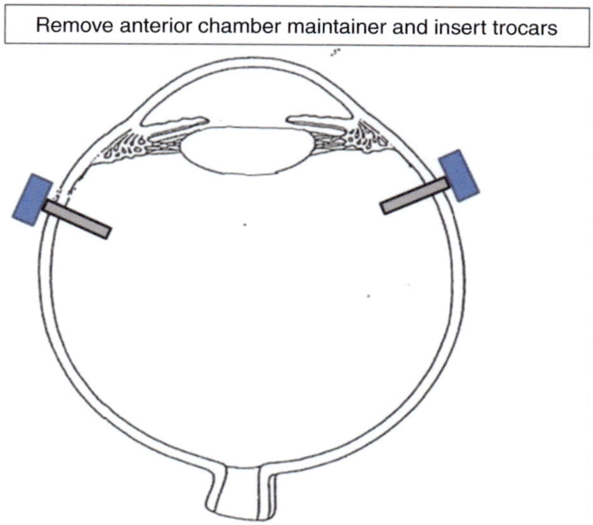

Fig. 21.4 Insert trocars and remove the anterior chamber maintainer

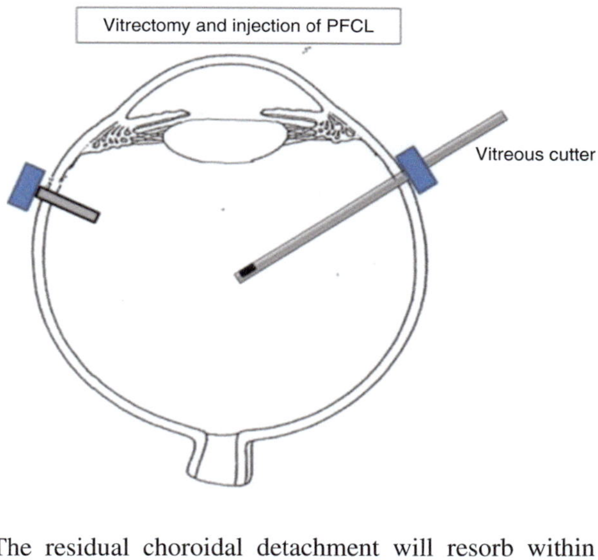

Fig. 21.5 Continue with a vitrectomy

Postoperative course: The residual choroidal detachment will resorb within 3 months. We recommend a silicone removal after 3–6 months.

Surgical Pearls No. 115

Hypotony: A hypotony is defined with an IOP < 6 mmHg. A choroidal detachment develops. A possible treatment is a drainage of the subchoroidal fluid and a permanent silicone oil tamponade.

Part XIII
Trauma

Chapter 22
Open Globe Injury

Extras: Videos 22.1, 22.2, 22.3, 22.4, 22.5, and 22.6.

22.1 Introduction

Trauma presents with a huge variety. Not one traumatic case can be compared with the other. This makes trauma surgery exciting and demanding but makes also recommendations for surgical procedure rather difficult. Generally, a globe injury is divided up in an open globe injury and a closed globe injury. Here we will only talk about open globe injuries. For open globe injury, two major traumas are possible: (1) a small ocular injury secondary to an intraocular foreign body (IOFB) and (2) a large globe injury affecting the sclera (=scleral injury) or the cornea (=corneal injury). Remark: A corneal injury is often called a perforation and a scleral rupture is also named a globe rupture. See Fig. 22.1.

The IOFB causes in the most cases only a small defect in the cornea or sclera which is good for the prognosis of the globe. But if the IOFB is of organic material such as wood then the risk for endophthalmitis is high and the prognosis is poor. If the IOFB is of metal, then the prognosis is better. An endophthalmitis is seldom (Fig. 22.1). The surgery for a small perforation with an IOFB is described in detail in the following chapter.

In the following the surgery for an open globe rupture is described. In case of a globe injury affecting only the cornea, the prognosis is good because the endophthalmitis risk is low and the posterior segment is not affected. In case of a scleral injury, the prognosis is poor because the retina may be incarcerated and a subchoroidal, subretinal, or intravitreal hemorrhage may be present. Many eyes get lost in a hypotony.

Electronic Supplementary Material The online version of this chapter (https://doi.org/10.1007/978-3-319-89677-9_22) contains supplementary material, which is available to authorized users.

U. Spandau, H. Heimann, *Practical Handbook for Small-Gauge Vitrectomy*,
https://doi.org/10.1007/978-3-319-89677-9_22

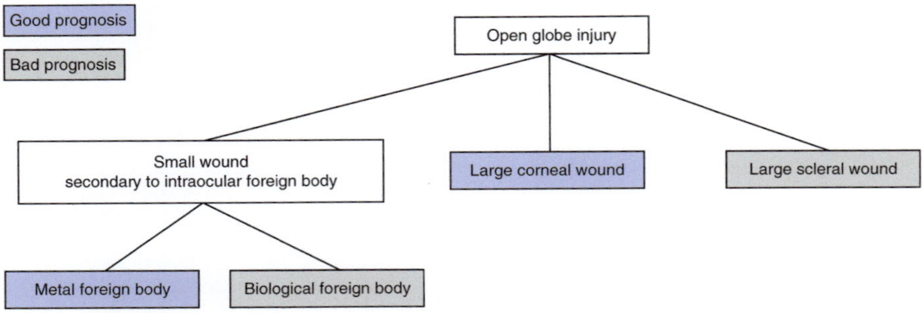

Fig. 22.1 Open globe injury and different prognosis

22.1.1 Indication to Vitrectomy

The indication for surgery is a retinal detachment. Not every eye with open globe has a retinal detachment. If the scleral defect is located at the height of the limbus, then the retina is not involved. If you are insecure, then measure the distance between limbus and scleral rupture with the caliper. If the distance is shorter than 4 mm (pars plana), then a retinal engagement is unlikely. If the distance is larger than 4 mm (adult), then a retinal defect is likely. It is helpful to perform a preoperative ultrasound. In addition, control if light perception in all directions exists.

Why not perform a prophylactic vitrectomy? An eye which suffered a trauma is very inflamed. A vitrectomy in an inflamed tissue (vitreous and retina) increases the risk of a retinal detachment. Example: Vitreous hemorrhage after open globe injury. A clinical example: <ZA corneal wound from 11 to 1 o'clock is sutured successfully. Two days later you perform an ultrasound and suspect a retinal detachment. You perform a vitrectomy and find an attached retina. One week later the eye has a PVR retinal detachment.

22.1.2 Timing of Surgery

In an initial surgery, we close the globe and 2 weeks later we perform vitrectomy. See our treatment algorithm in Fig. 22.2. Other authors recommend to operate after 5–7 days [1]. Even eyes with minimal or no light perception can be operated because visual acuity often increases after surgery. Perform an ultrasound: Is a subchoroidal hemorrhage (SCH) present? Is a vitreous hemorrhage present? Is a retinal detachment present? This information will help you to find your way during vitrectomy.

But the prognosis is often poor. The main reason for failure in the long run is hypotony and corneal decompensation. But the spectrum of trauma is very large which makes it very difficult to generalize. We use to inform the patient that the prognosis is very poor but that in the majority of cases the outcome is better than without surgery. In our experience patients with open globe rupture are postoperatively much more satisfied than patients with chronic and total retinal detachment.

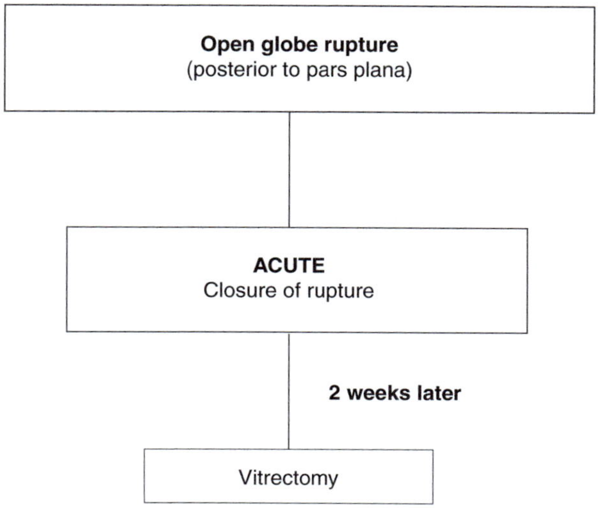

Fig. 22.2 Our treatment algorithm for open globe injuries without IOFB

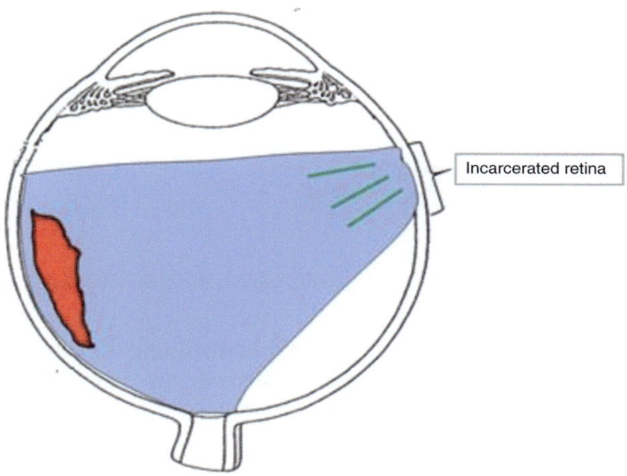

Fig. 22.3 The retina is incarcerated in the scleral wound on the right side and a large break is present on the left side

Anatomical characteristics of the posterior segment in open globe injuries are an attached posterior hyaloid, an incarcerated retina, and a napkin ring (subretinal annular ring around the optic disc) (Figs. 22.3, 22.4, and 22.5).

22.1.3 Planning of Surgery

The main indication for surgery is a retinal detachment. Silicone oil is the most common tamponade. The situation of the anterior chamber, therefore, is very important for surgery. Assess whether a cataract surgery has been performed or not.

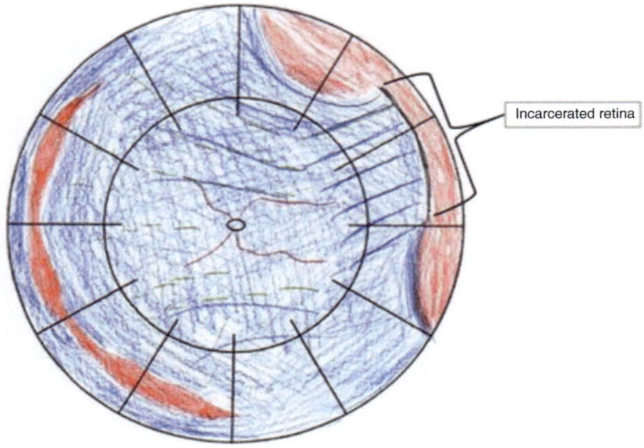

Fig. 22.4 A large retinal break on the left side and a retinal incarceration on the right side

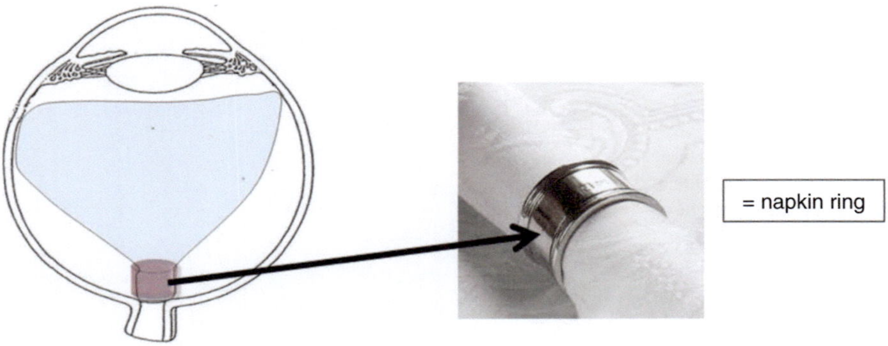

Fig. 22.5 A subretinal fibrotic ring around the retina located at the optic disc = napkin ring

In many cases aphakia due to a luxated lens/IOL and sometimes even aniridia are present. Aniridia and aphakia, however, are a big hinder for silicone oil tamponade. In case of aphakia an Artisan IOL can prevent a silicone, oil prolapse. In case of aphakia and aniridia, an iris-IOL prosthesis (Opthec, NL) or a suture net is a good option.

22.1.4 Characteristics of Surgery

The surgery is difficult due to poor visualization secondary to a cloudy media and blood. Due to the extensive intravitreal, subretinal, and subchoroidal hemorrhage, it is very difficult to see the difference between blood, vitreous, retina, and choroid. The retina may be incarcerated in the wound and has to be relieved from the wound through a retinotomy. A PVD is usually not present.

A napkin ring may form subretinally at the optic disc. It has the shape of a ring and constricts the retina (Fig. 22.5). The annular membrane occurs after a chronic detachment. In order to remove the napkin, ring a 360° circumferential retinotomy is required.

Another important part of surgery is the anterior segment. In case of an iris defect, repair the iris defect so that a round pupil is present. Then insert a retropupillar IOL in order to prevent a silicone oil prolapse into the anterior chamber.

The surgery should be performed in general anesthesia and the surgical time is 2–4 h.

The Surgical Management of an Open Globe with Scleral Injury
Material and Instruments

1. **23G or 25G trauma trocars (Alcon)**
2. **Chandelier light**
3. **Maybe: Artisan IOL**
4. **PFCL**
5. **Silicone oil**

The Surgery

1. **Insertion of anterior chamber maintainer**
2. **Removal of hyphema**
3. **Inspection of posterior segment**
4. **Core vitrectomy**
5. **Insertion of trauma trocars**
6. **Peripheral vitrectomy and PVD**
7. **Endodiathermy of traumatic retinal edges**
8. **Retinotomy of incarcerated retina**
9. **Removal of subretinal membranes**
10. **Removal of napkin ring**
11. **Instillation of PFCL**
12. **Attachment test and rotation test**
13. **Laser treatment**
14. **Preparation of anterior chamber before silicone oil tamponade**
15. **PFCL against air and exchange**
16. **1000 csts silicone oil tamponade**

Every Step in Detail

1. **Insertion of anterior chamber maintainer**
2. **Removal of hyphema**

In many trauma cases, a hyphema is present. Remove the hyphema with irrigation and aspiration. If the cornea is cloudy perform a corneal abrasion. If the view does not improve, then a hemorrhagic cornea is likely. The only solution is now a corneal transplantation. Examine the iris and the lens status. If the iris is hemorrhagic do not insist to remove the blood but cut only a central pupil with the vitreous cutter.

3. **Inspection of posterior segment**
4. **Core vitrectomy**

Insert the light fiber through a side incision and examine the retina, i.e., try to examine the retina. If you do not see anything, then work carefully because the retina may be totally detached. Start to cut centrally on height of the pars plana. Try to identify the retina, choroid, and hemorrhagic vitreous from each other. If you cannot identify any structures in the center behind pars plane, then continue to work in the periphery. Even if you cut retina in the periphery, this is not a problem because a large retinotomy is required in the end.

5. **Insertion of trauma trocars**
6. **Peripheral vitrectomy and PVD**
7. **Endodiathermy of traumatic retinal edges**

Assess the periphery for a suitable area to insert the trocars. Try to insert at least two instrument trocars so that you can work easier in the posterior segment. As trocars, we use 23G or 25G trauma trocars from Alcon. Then continue with a vitrectomy. In many cases a PVD is absent. Induce a PVD and then instill PFCL to flatten the central retina. Perform a thorough peripheral vitrectomy as possible. If you leave peripheral vitreous and use silicone oil as tamponade, then the silicone oil will press the peripheral vitreous against the ciliary body causing ciliary body insufficiency and hypotony. Perform a meticulous diathermy of bleeding retinotomy edges in order to prevent recurrent PVR.

8. **Retinotomy of incarcerated retina** (Figs. 22.6 and 22.7)
9. **Removal of subretinal membranes**
10. **Removal of napkin ring** (Fig. 22.8)
11. **Instillation of PFCL**

If the retina is incarcerated into the scleral wound, then perform a retinotomy at the scleral wound in order to mobilize the incarcerated retina (Figs. 22.6 and 22.7). Continue with removal of subretinal membranes. Finally remove the fibrous ring around the optic disc. Then reattach the retina through instillation of PFCL over the

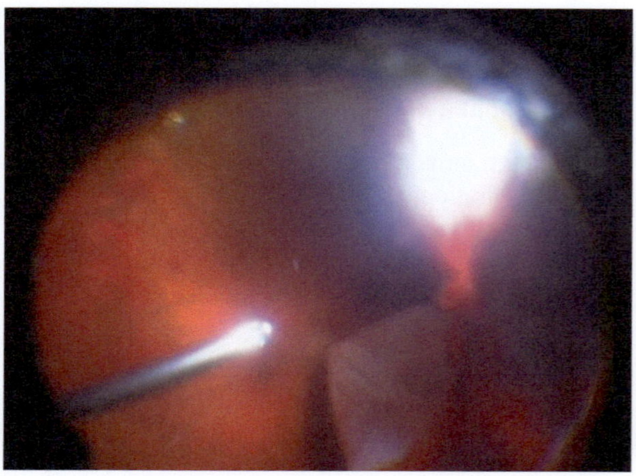

Fig. 22.6 The retina is incarcerated on the right side into the scleral wound

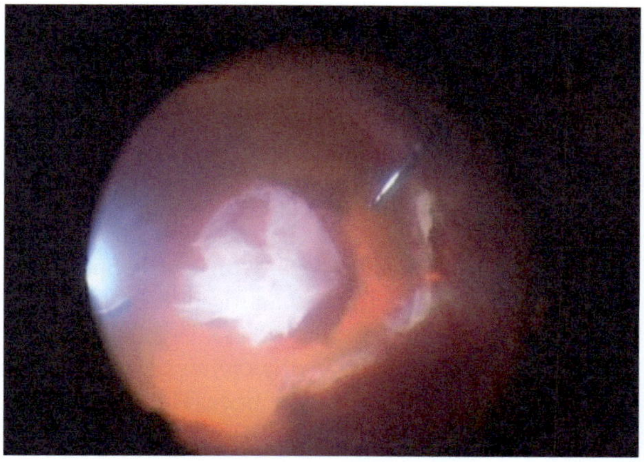

Fig. 22.7 After retinotomy: Note the residual retina in the scleral wound on the right side

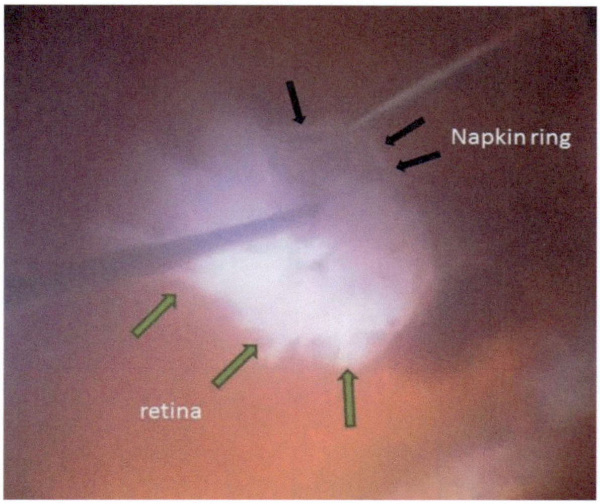

Fig. 22.8 Note the napkin ring which is located subretinally around the optic disc

retinotomy edges. Check if the retina is completely attached at the optic disc. If not, then you did not remove the complete napkin ring (Fig. 22.8). This procedure is difficult because the retina is mobile. Check also the retinal edges. Are they attached or enrolled? Flatten the distorted retina with a Charles flute needle with silicone tip or a knob spatula. If a membrane causes a radial retinal distortion, then remove the membrane.

12. **Attachment test and rotation test**
13. **Laser treatment**

Check now if the macula is correctly located or if a rotation is present. If you observe a rotation, then rotate the retina with the vacuum cleaner or a knob spatula. Continue with three rows of laser along the retinotomy edges. For retinal edges a laser duration of 300 ms is required. Remark: The usual laser duration for retinal breaks is 200 ms.

14. **Preparation of anterior chamber before silicone oil tamponade** (Figs. 22.9, 22.10, and 22.11)
15. **PFCL against air and exchange**
16. **1000 csts silicone oil tamponade** (Fig. 22.12)

Before continuing with a tamponade, the anterior chamber must be prepared for the tamponade. Is an aphakia present? If aphakia is present and you plan to use silicone oil, then an iridectomy is required to prevent a pupillary block. If possible, insert an Artisan iris-claw IOL with a retropupillary implantation (Fig. 22.9). If aniridia is present then implant an iris-IOL prosthesis (Opthec, NL) (Fig. 22.10). An alternative is a suture net (Fig. 22.11). If you plan a silicone oil tamponade, then fill the anterior chamber with methylcellulose to prevent an intraoperative prolapse of silicone oil into the anterior chamber. The next step is a PFCL against silicone oil exchange. If you prefer first a PFCL against air exchange, then perform a meticulous fluid aspiration at the retinotomy edges. Close the case with a 1300 St or 5000 csts silicone oil tamponade (Fig. 22.12).

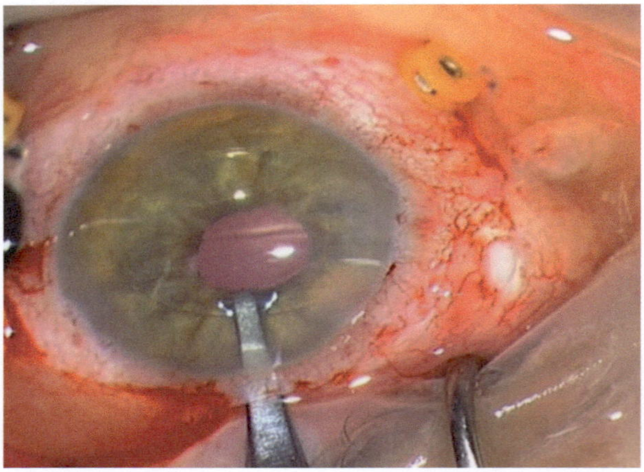

Fig. 22.9 In case of aphakia insert an IOL, in this case an Artisan IOL with retropupilar fixation. It will prevent a silicone oil prolapse

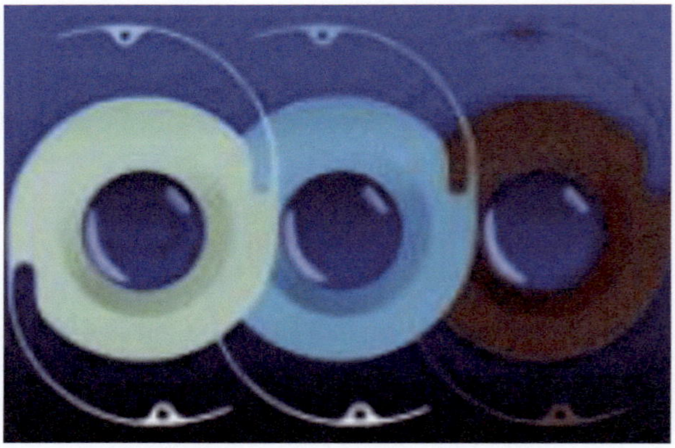

Fig. 22.10 An IOL-iris prosthesis from Opthec, Netherlands. The diameter is 9 mm. A large incision is therefore required. The color of the prosthesis turns out brighter when inserted in the eye. We use only the brown iris. The prize is approximately 400 Euros

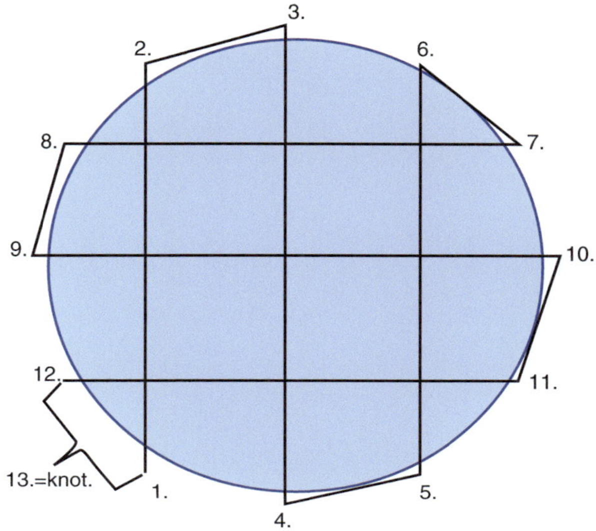

Fig. 22.11 A drawing of the suture. Start with 1 and end with 12. Number 13 is the knot. One continuous suture

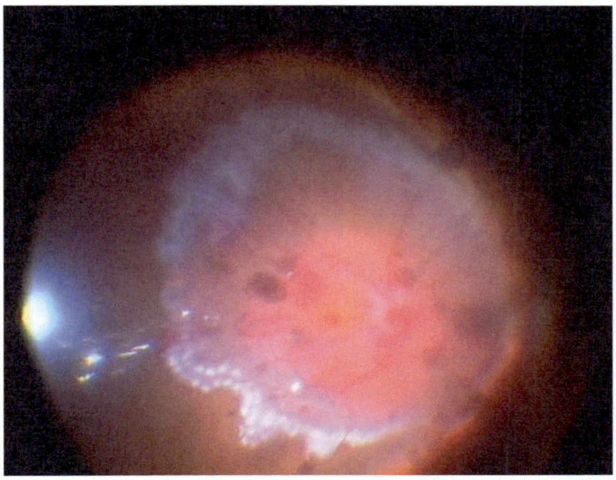

Fig. 22.12 The final view to retina. Visual acuity is 0.1, the globe is normotensive and the patient is satisfied. The minority of these cases have such a good outcome

Reference

1. Kuhn F. The timing of reconstruction in severe mechanical trauma. Ophthalmic Res. 2014;51(2):67–72.

Chapter 23
Surgical Management of a Suprachoroidal Hemorrhage (SCH)

Extras: Video 23.1.

23.1 Introduction

The choroidal detachment may also be caused by an expulsive hemorrhage. This is a hemorrhage in the suprachoroidal space (Table 23.1) which is located between the sclera and the detached choroid. Sometimes the term "suprachoroidal" is used synonymously to "subchoroidal" and the abbreviation is SCH. As a basic rule, these hemorrhages are removed from the scleral side, and not transretinal. The removal of the blood in a hemorrhagic detachment is difficult and incomplete.

23.1.1 Indication for Surgery

We would not operate a quadrant detachment or a 50% detachment. But if both sides have a bullous detachment with kissing choroids then we would operate. The main surgical problem is the complete removal of the hemorrhage and that the pars plana epithelium is detached which makes the insertion of trocars very difficult. Therefore, an anterior chamber maintainer is used and trocars are inserted later when the choroidal detachment is reduced.

Table 23.1 Diagram of the anatomy of a suprachoroidal hemorrhage

Sclera
Hemorrhage in the subchoroidal space
Choroid
Retina
Vitreous

Electronic Supplementary Material The online version of this chapter (https://doi.org/10.1007/978-3-319-89677-9_23) contains supplementary material, which is available to authorized users.

U. Spandau, H. Heimann, *Practical Handbook for Small-Gauge Vitrectomy*,
https://doi.org/10.1007/978-3-319-89677-9_23

23.1.2 Instruments

1. 23- or 25-gauge four-port trocar system
2. Anterior chamber maintainer
3. Extra-long 6 mm trocars (23G and 23G from Alcon)

An anterior chamber maintainer is an infusion, which is inserted in the limbus and injects BSS into the anterior chamber.

23.1.3 Tamponade

PFCL, 1000csts silicone oil

23.2 The Surgery Step-by-Step

1. **Limbal peritomy**
2. **Place traction sutures beneath all four rectus muscles**
3. **Insert an anterior chamber maintainer**
4. **Sclerotomies between insertion of the muscle and the equator**
5. **Drainage and expression of subchoroidal blood**
6. **Insertion of trocars**
7. **Core vitrectomy**
8. **Injection of PFCL**
9. **Trimming of vitreous base**
10. **Exchange of PFCL against silicone oil**

1. **Limbal peritomy**
2. **Place traction sutures beneath all four rectus muscles**

Perform a 360° peritomy and place traction sutures underneath all horizontal muscles.

3. **Insert an anterior chamber maintainer**

An inferotemporal paracentesis is performed, the anterior chamber maintainer is inserted, and the infusion line is opened (Fig. 23.1). Now the eyeball becomes normotensive. An infusion of the anterior chamber works particularly well when there is a pseudophakia.

4. **Sclerotomies between insertion of the muscle and the equator**
5. **Drainage and expression of subchoroidal blood**

Before performing a sclerotomy, you should ascertain the location of the SCH in the eye. You can confirm your ultrasound examination by inspecting the vitreous cavity with a light pipe (Fig. 23.2). Search for the quadrant with the highest bullous choroidal detachment.

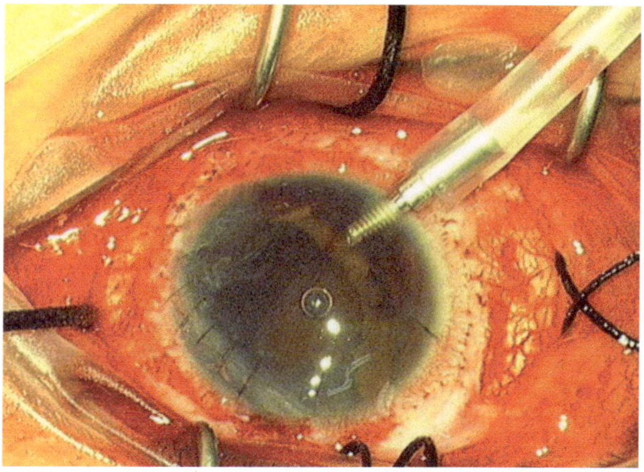

Fig. 23.1 Eye with a perforating trauma from a stick. In a first operation the temporal limbus was sutured with Ethilon 10-0 and the sclera at 5 o'clock from the limbus to the insertion of the inferior rectus muscle was sutured with Vicryl 8-0. Prior to the second operation, a 360-degree suprachoroidal hemorrhage was detected. Now four traction sutures were placed beneath the four horizontal muscles. An anterior chamber maintainer was inserted to maintain normal IOP

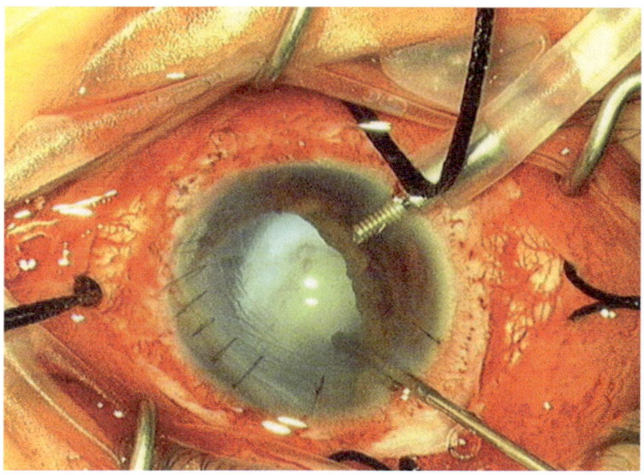

Fig. 23.2 With help of a light pipe, which is inserted through a paracentesis, the situation in the posterior segment is explored

The sclerotomy should be 3–4 mm in length and extend in a radial direction (Fig. 23.3). Concerning the location of these sclerotomies, there are different preferences. Some surgeons perform the sclerotomies 4 mm posterior the limbus, other place the sclerotomies equatorial, since there is more suprachoroidal blood. We place the sclerotomies between the insertion of the muscle and the equator. For example, if a temporal and nasal choroidal detachment is present, you should perform a temporal and nasal sclerotomy at 3:30 and 8:30. Once the sclerotomy is performed, liquefied blood (Fig. 23.4) and blood clots (Fig. 23.5) will flow out the sclerotomy.

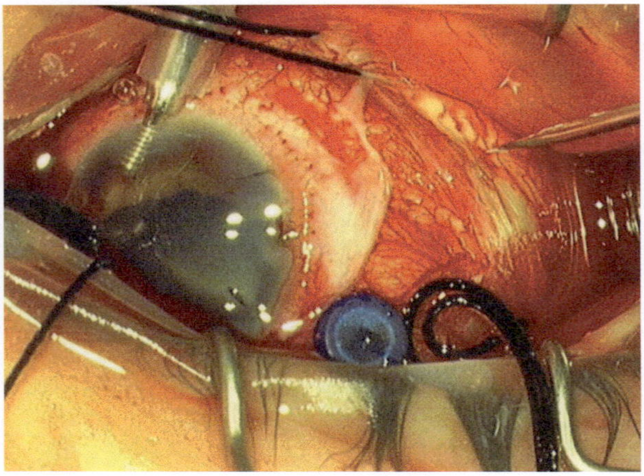

Fig. 23.3 A 3 mm sclerotomy is performed between the insertion of a straight eye muscle and the equator

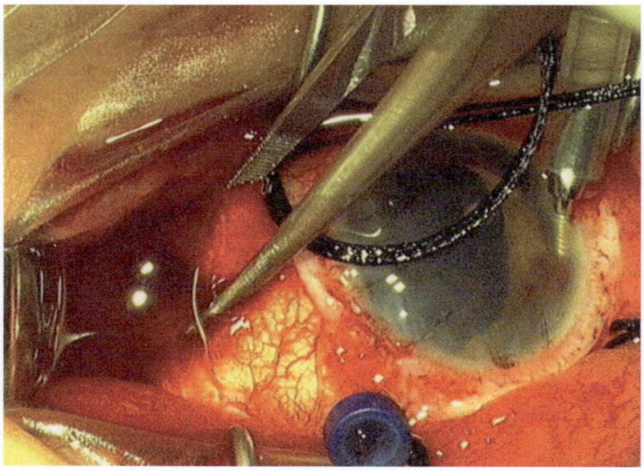

Fig. 23.4 Liquefied blood flows out of the second sclerotomy on the other side of the globe. Extract the blood by compressing the globe with a forceps or cotton swabs

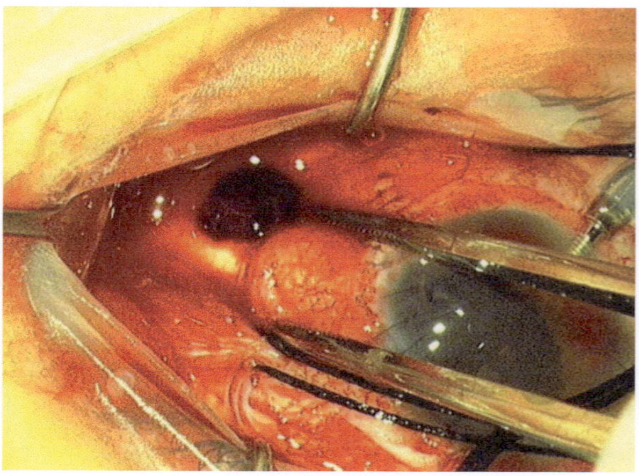

Fig. 23.5 Thick blood clots can be pressed through a larger 4 mm incision. If the sclerotomy is too small you cannot extract thicker blood clots. This sclerotomy needs to be sutured with 1–2 Vicryl 8-0 cross sutures

If only liquefied blood flows out and no clots, you should enlarge the sclerotomy to 4–5 mm and then massage the eyeball firmly with two cotton swabs in the direction of the sclerotomies. With this technique, you can extract the large blood clots.

These large sclerotomies should be sutured at the end of the surgery.

Surgical Pearls no 116

The most common mistake in case of a SCH are too small sclerotomies. Large blood clots cannot be removed through small 3 mm sclerotomies; they require 4–5 mm sclerotomies. So, if the choroidal detachment is not reduced after drainage of liquefied blood, then large blood clots are present. Enlarge the sclerotomies to 4–5 mm.

6. **Insertion of trocars**

When no more blood flows out of the sclerotomy, you can try to insert the trocars at the pars plana if you have not done this before. Due to the detachment of the pars plana epithelium, this is a difficult procedure. Choose an area with little choroidal detachment and select a sutureable, longer infusion cannula (see above). Use preferably 6-mm-long trauma trocars from Alcon. Check if the trocar is located in the vitreous cavity. If the trocar cannula is not in the vitreous cavity, it can be freed from the surrounding tissue with a membrane pic from the opposite trocar cannula. The same procedure can now be performed with the second trocar cannula. Remove the anterior chamber maintainer and insert a pars plana infusion line. Then insert a second trocar opposite to the infusion cannula.

Surgical Pearls No. 117

Subepithelial location of trocars: Especially in eyes with choroidal detachment an initially correctly placed trocar cannula may move subepithelially during a later stage of the operation. Double-check the trocars several times during surgery.

7. **Core vitrectomy**
8. **Injection of PFCL**

If the choroidal detachment has regressed, a vitrectomy can be performed. You may need to insert a chandelier light. Then PFCL is injected, which pushes the residual suprachoroidal blood through the sclerotomies outside. You should now check the sclerotomies (flick the BIOM out and rotate the globe with the traction sutures). If little or no blood flows out in an area with a high choroidal detachment, try to expel blood clots with a forceps or cotton swabs.

9. **Trimming of vitreous base**

Perform a thorough trimming of the vitreous base in trauma patients, in particular the anterior part of the vitreous base which extends over the ciliary body. Otherwise the eye will develop cyclitic membranes which grow on the ciliary body and result in hypotony. Cyclitic membranes are very difficult to remove. The development of cyclitic membranes will increase if you use silicone oil as a tamponade.

10. **Exchange of PFCL for silicone oil**

If there is only a minor residual choroidal detachment, perform a PFCL/silicone oil exchange. The silicone oil is injected through the infusion cannula. Suture the sclerotomies with a Vicryl 8-0 stitch.

Postoperative course: The residual choroidal detachment will resorb within 3 months. We recommend a silicone removal after 3–6 months.

Chapter 24
Penetrating Eye Injury by Metal Intraocular Foreign Bodies (IOFB): Delayed and Stepwise Surgery

Extras: Videos 24.1, 24.2, 24.3, 24.4, 24.5, 24.6, and 24.7.

24.1 Introduction

Penetrating eye injuries should be treated by experienced surgeons. These cases are associated with a high complication rate, and a guarded prognosis and the initial surgical intervention are of vital importance. There has been a long debate about the timing and the extent of the initial surgical intervention.

24.2 Delayed Vitrectomy ↔ Immediate Vitrectomy

We prefer a delayed vitrectomy. A traumatized eye is very inflamed. Inflammation increases the risk for PVR. Delaying surgery results in reducing the risk for PVR. When performing a vitrectomy in an eye with IOFB, a posterior vitreous detachment (PVD) is required. The most patients with IOFB, however, are young and have an attached posterior vitreous. But if you wait 4 weeks, then the metallic IOFB will induce a posterior vitreous detachment. So, the surgical delay results in less PVR and a PVD. We wait maximal 4 weeks. In addition, an air tamponade is sufficient. This procedure applies to metallic IOFB only. Organic IOFB should be operated immediately, as the endophthalmitis risk is high.

We do not prefer the immediate surgery because (1) the experienced retinal team is often not present when the trauma case arrives at the clinic, (2) a PVD is not

---

Electronic Supplementary Material The online version of this chapter (https://doi.org/10.1007/978-3-319-89677-9_24) contains supplementary material, which is available to authorized users.

U. Spandau, H. Heimann, *Practical Handbook for Small-Gauge Vitrectomy*,
https://doi.org/10.1007/978-3-319-89677-9_24

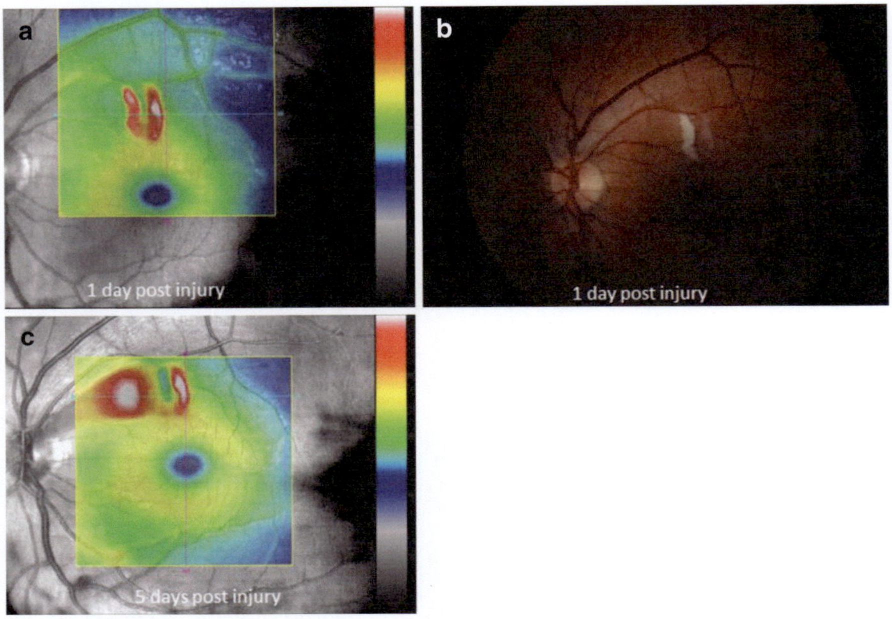

Fig. 24.1 OCT examinations of a retinal wound after trauma with a metal IOFB. The OCT after 1 day shows moderate wound swelling (**a**, **b**). After 5 days the wound swelling is much more pronounced (**c**)

present, and (3) if retinal wounds are present and if the foreign body sticks in the retina, then immediate extraction will cause bleeding from the exit wound and result in PVR from the wound edges. (4) A silicone oil tamponade is required.

Four weeks of waiting will quieten the retinal wound, and the foreign body can be extracted without bleeding or PVR from the wound edges. This notion is confirmed by OCT examinations showing the reduction of retinal wound swelling within 1 month (Figs. 24.1 and 24.2).

24.3 Our Treatment Algorithm at the University of Uppsala (Fig. 24.3)

The first step is the primary closure of the wound (cornea or sclera). We do not remove a traumatic cataract in the same session. If there is suspicion of a non-sterile penetration, we inject intravitreal antibiotics. We treat the patient then for 10 days with intravenous antibiotics (1.5 g Zinacef® three times daily). In the most cases, there is view to fundus. In case of vitreous hemorrhage an ultrasound, examination is necessary. If

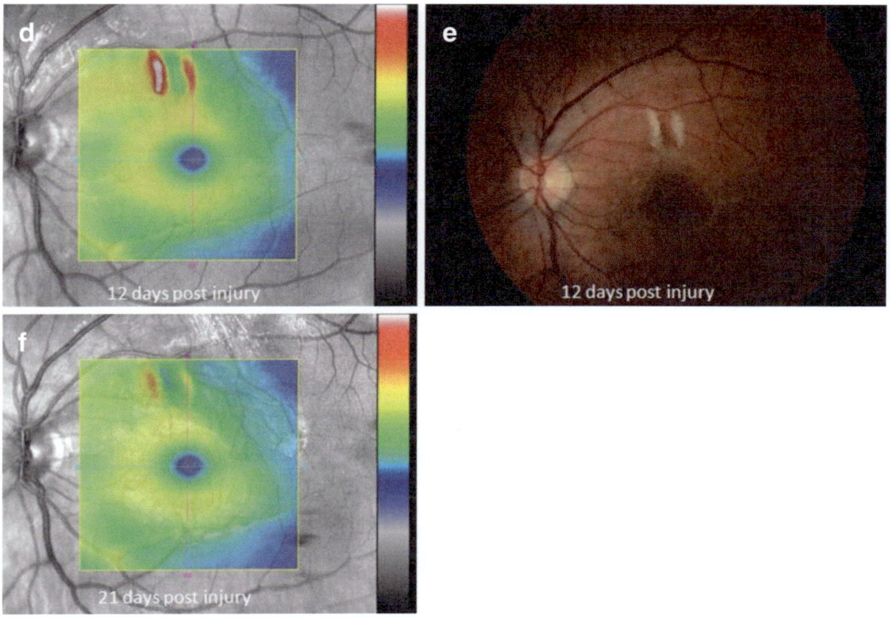

Fig. 24.2 After 12 days the retinal swelling is markedly reduced (**d**, **e**) and almost disappeared after 21 days (**f**)

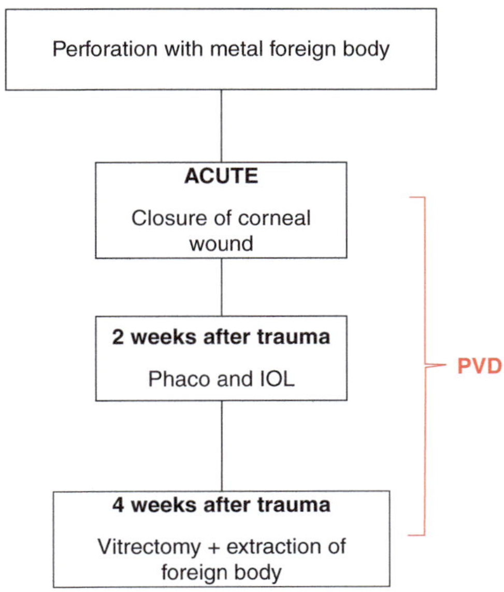

Fig. 24.3 Our treatment algorithm for stepwise IOFB surgery. After 4 weeks, a PVD is present, the eye is quiet, and the PVR risk is low when extracting the IOFB. If the retina is detached, we operate at once

the retina is attached, we continue to wait; if the retina is detached, we operate immediately. But retinal detachments during the natural course of IOFB are seldom.

After approximately 2 weeks, we perform a cataract surgery and implant an IOL. In many cases the lens capsule is partially injured. We try to implant the IOL into the bag or into a stable sulcus position. A scleral fixated IOL is rarely necessary. Then approximately 2 weeks after phacoemulsification, we perform a vitrectomy with foreign body extraction. The vitrectomy is easy because a PVD is present and the retinal wound has healed. The risk of bleeding from the retinal/choroidal wound is much less and the risk of PVR from the wound edges is highly reduced.

We prefer to perform phacoemulsification and vitrectomy at different time points because the posterior capsule is often damaged. Vitrectomy worsens therefore the result of the phacoemulsification if both are performed at the same time points. If phacoemulsification and vitrectomy are performed at the same time, then the extensive vitrectomy with gas tamponade will tamper with the IOL. The gas may luxate the IOL into the anterior chamber, the vitrectomy may cause posterior synechiae, and so on.

Surgical Pearls No. 118
Avoid operating an inflamed or vascularly active eye. If the retina is attached, wait and treat the inflammation and vascularization; use steroids and anti-VEGF. If the retina is detached, you have to operate.

24.4 IOFB Extraction, Delayed Surgery

In the following the surgical procedure for a stepwise and delayed surgery is demonstrated.

It is advisable to perform the vitrectomy in general anesthesia.

24.4.1 Instruments

1. 25G or 27G trocars with chandelier illumination
2. Endo magnet (Synergetics, USA) **OR**
3. Diamond dust coated foreign body forceps (Fig. 24.4)
4. Laser probe

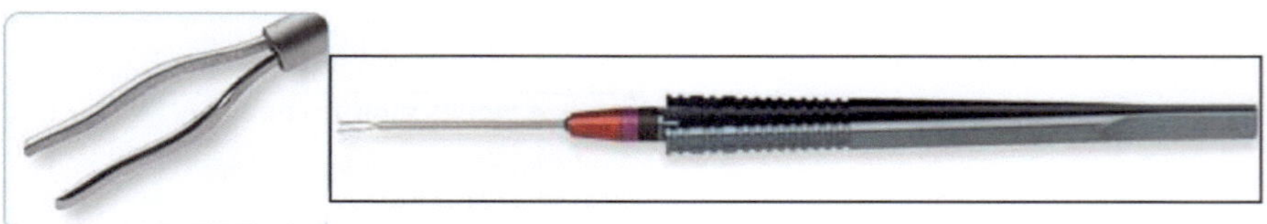

Fig. 24.4 A IOFB forceps with a diamond dusted grip. The foreign body is extracted through a 20G sclerotomy (without trocar). Available are 17G, 19G, and 20G foreign body forceps (DORC, Geuder, Synergetics). The sclerotomy must be enlarged according to the size of the IOFB

24.4.2 *Tamponade*

Intraoperative: maybe PFCL

Postoperatively: Air

Individual Steps

1. **25G or 27G three-port system with chandelier light**
2. **Vitrectomy, PVD**
3. **Exposure of IOFB**
4. **Prepare the exit sclerotomy**
5. **Extraction of IOFB through sclerotomy**
6. **Apply laser at the impact site**
7. **Air tamponade**

24.4.3 *The Surgery Step-by-Step* (Figs. 24.5, 24.6, 24.7, 24.8, 24.9, and 24.10)

1. **Three-port system with chandelier light**

   We use the three-port trocar system with chandelier light.

2. **Vitrectomy, PVD**

   The advantage of a delayed surgery is that a PVD is almost always present. It is very important to induce a posterior vitreous detachment, otherwise there is an increased risk of PVR.

3. **Exposure of IOFB** (Figs. 24.5 and 24.6)

   One has to resist the urge to remove the IOFB as soon as you can see it. An extensive vitrectomy should be performed first and in particular around the IOFB. Only

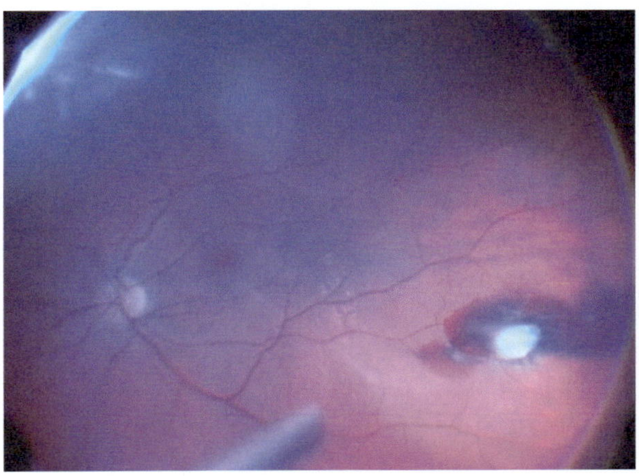

Fig. 24.5 After 4 weeks there is still a retinal hemorrhage at the perforation site

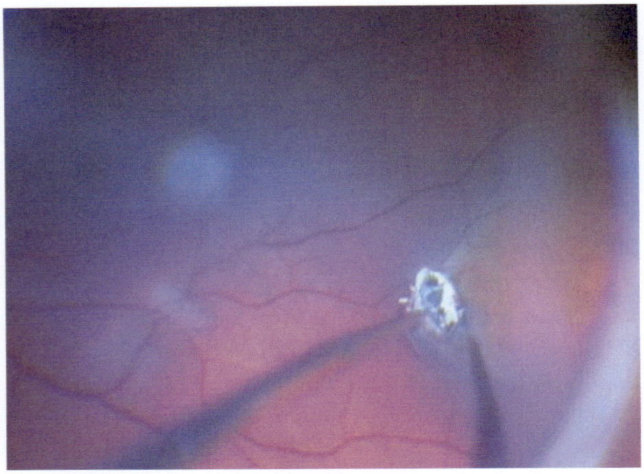

Fig. 24.6 Note that the IOFB is inside a retinal pocket

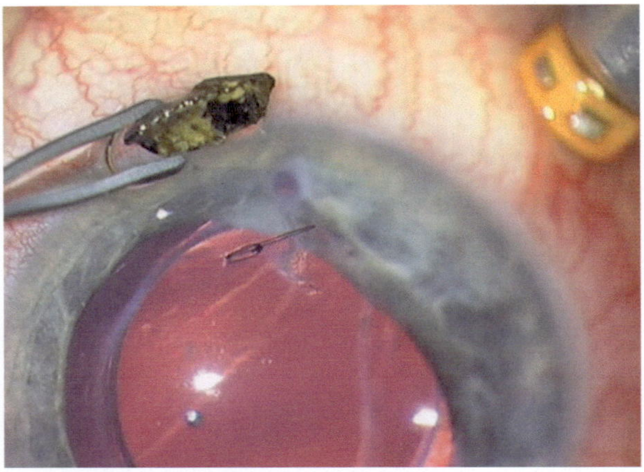

Fig. 24.7 The IOFB which was inside the eye for 4 weeks: no PVR, no endophthalmitis

remove the IOFB when no more vitreous is attached or surrounding it and around the sclerotomy through which it will be removed.

4. **Prepare the exit sclerotomy**

Before grasping and extracting the IOFB, decide where the exit sclerotomy is placed. Open here the conjunctiva and perform a limbus-parallel sclerotomy. The sclerotomy is as wide as the IOFB.

5. **Extraction of IOFB through sclerotomy** (Fig.24.7)

The foreign body can be extracted with the forceps (serrated or diamond dusted) or the endomagnet. Before extraction of the foreign body, it is advisable to inject a PFCL bubble to protect the macula. Then enlarge the sclerotomy sufficiently parallel to the limbus. Insert the forceps through this sclerotomy, grasp the IOFB, and extract it through the sclerotomy. In many cases a bimanual extraction is necessary. One forceps (e.g., 27G endgripping forceps, DORC) is inserted through a trocar and extracts the IOFB from the retina. The IOFB forceps is inserted through the large

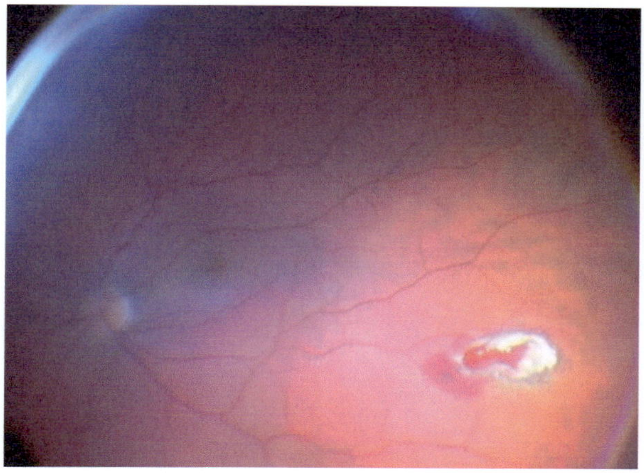

Fig. 24.8 The perforation site after removal of the IOFB

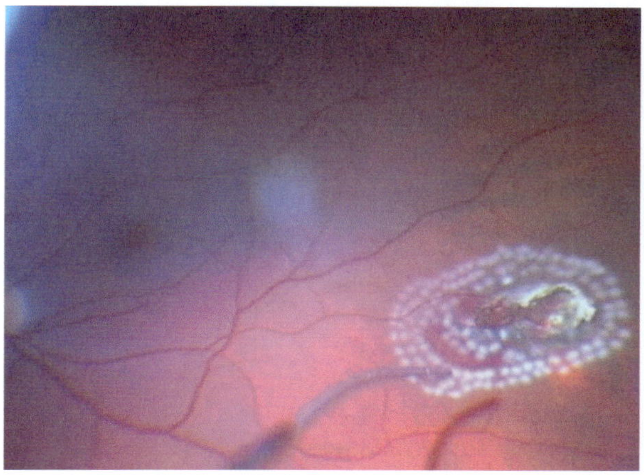

Fig. 24.9 Three rows of laser photocoagulation. After 4 weeks the retinal edges cause no PVR

sclerotomy, takes over the IOFB from the endgripping forceps, and extracts it through the sclerotomy.

Congratulations! The worst part is done. Take a deep breath and continue with closing the exit sclerotomy with Vicryl 8-0 cross sutures.

6. **Apply laser at the impact site** (Figs. 24.8 and 24.9)

Then you have to photocoagulate the retina around the impact site. If the retina is detached in the area of laser treatment, you must first inject PFCL in order to flatten the retina.

7. **Air tamponade** (Fig. 24.10)

We use in most cases an air tamponade.

Fig. 24.10 An air tamponade is sufficient

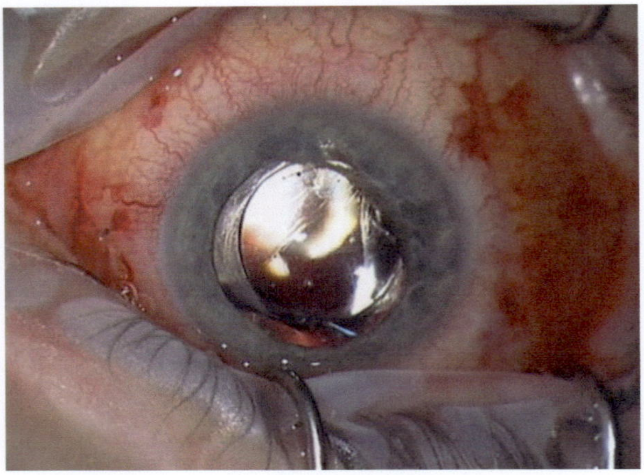

24.5 IOFB Extraction, Immediate Surgery

In the following the surgical procedure is presented if you choose to perform an immediate surgery. See Fig. 24.11:

24.5.1 The Surgery

24.5.1.1 Instruments

1. 25 g or 27G trocars with chandelier illumination
2. Endomagnet **OR**
3. Diamond dust coated foreign body forceps
4. Diathermy
5. Laser probe

24.5.1.2 Tamponade

Intraoperative: maybe PFCL

Postoperatively: 1000 or 5000 csts silicone oil

24.5.1.3 Individual Steps

1. **23G–27G three-port system with chandelier light.**
2. **Vitrectomy.**
3. **Induction of PVD.**

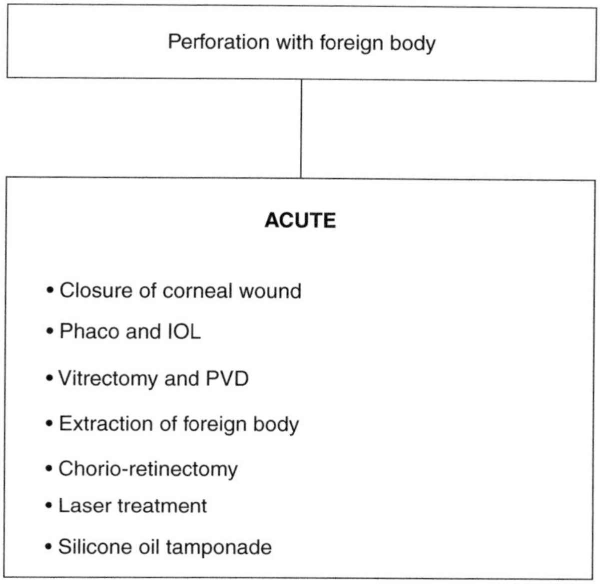

Fig. 24.11 Our treatment algorithm in case of immediate surgery. The main difference is that a 1 mm retinectomy around the wound edges followed of diathermy of the choroid has to be performed (Ferenc Kuhn technique)

4. **Exposure of IOFB.**
5. **Extraction of IOFB through sclerotomy or cornea.**
6. **1 mm retinectomy around the impact site and diathermy of the exposed choroid.**
7. **Apply laser at the impact site.**
8. **Silicone oil tamponade.**

<u>**The Surgery Step-by-Step:**</u> Figs. 24.12 and 24.13

1. **Three-port system with chandelier light.**

We use the three-port trocar system and insert a chandelier light.

2. **Vitrectomy.**
3. **Induction of PVD.**

It is very important to induce a posterior vitreous detachment; otherwise there is an increased risk of PVR. As it can be difficult to determine a posterior vitreous detachment in young eyes, it is advisable to use dyes such as triamcinolone or trypan blue.

4. **Exposure of IOFB.**

One has to resist the urge to remove the IOFB as soon as you can see it. An extensive vitrectomy should be performed first and in particular around the IOFB. Only remove the IOFB when no more vitreous is attached or surrounding it and no vitreous is in the way at the sclerotomy through which the IOFB will be removed. If the IOFB is stuck in the choroid and sclera, you may apply laser around it in order to lower the intraocular hemorrhage that will occur when you pull the IOFB out of the sclera.

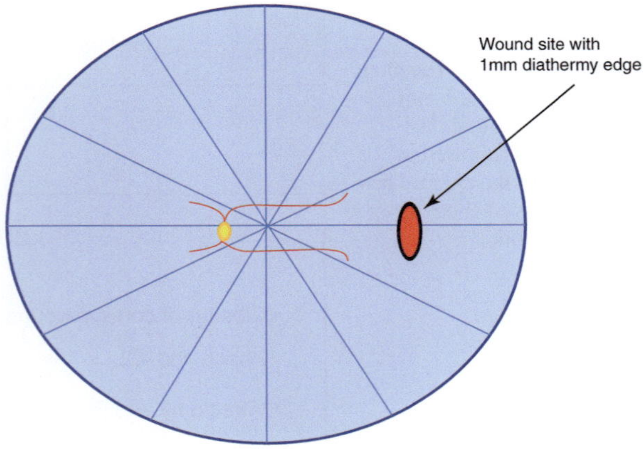

Fig. 24.12 In immediate surgery, a 1 mm diathermy around the wound edges are recommended (Ferenc Kuhn technique)

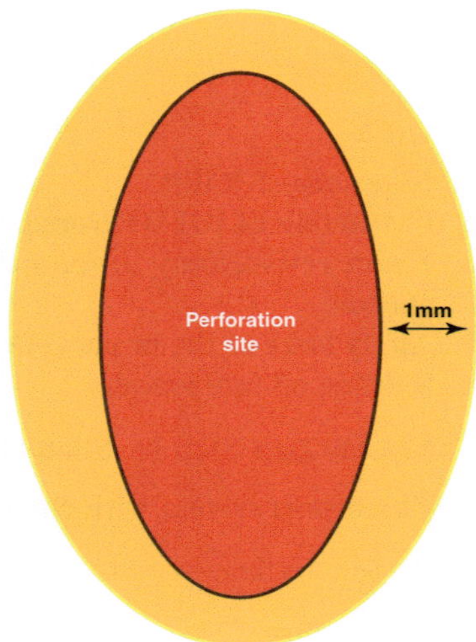

Fig. 24.13 The retina and choroidea is cauterized 1 mm around the perforation site

5. **Extraction of IOFB through sclerotomy or cornea.**

Before extraction of the IOFB, decide whether to extract the IOFB through the sclera or a corneal main incision. The latter is possible if a posterior capsular defect is present. Extract then the IOFB through the main incision. In this case the IOL is implanted after extraction of the IOFB.

6. **1 mm retinectomy around the impact site and diathermy of the exposed choroid** (Figs. 24.12 and 24.13).

After successful extraction of the IOFB, a 1 mm retinectomy is performed around the impact site. You should also cauterize the underlying choroid. This is thought to reduce the rate of postoperative PVR. First, cauterize the retina 1 mm distant from the edge of the impact, then cut the retina with the 25G/27G vitreous cutter at a low cutting rate (about 200 cuts/min). Finally, the underlying choroid is cauterized with diathermy or laser.

7. **Apply laser at the impact site.**

After successful retinectomy and cauterization of the choroid you must photocoagulate the retina around the impact site. If the retina is detached in the area of laser treatment, inject first PFCL in order to flatten the retina.

8. **Silicone oil tamponade.**

If you perform a vitrectomy immediately after surgery, we recommend a 1000 or 5000 csts silicone oil as tamponade. This is due to the high postoperatively risk of developing PVR from the wound edges.

24.5.2 Complications

The possible complications of immediate vitrectomy are:

Perioperative choroidal bleeding from exit wound

Postoperative PVR from wound edges

Postoperative anterior segment inflammation with posterior synechiae and dislocation of IOL

FAQ:

What about the risk of retinal detachment?

In our experience the retina is often injured but detaches very seldom. If the retina is attached, there is no reason for an immediate surgery. And the retina is attached in most cases. If the retina is detached immediate surgery is necessary. Assess the retina once a week with slit lamp or ultrasound.

Is the risk of endophthalmitis not increased if you wait 4 weeks for vitrectomy?

The highest risk of endophthalmitis is within the first week after injury. We had four cases of endophthalmitis in 10 years and two foreign bodies were wood and two were metal. In all four cases, an endophthalmitis was present at the initial examination. The endophthalmitis was present within 1 day in case of a wooden foreign body and within 3 days in case of a metal foreign body.

What about the timing of surgery (Fig. 24.14)?

The penetrating wound has to be sutured acute. When to extract the foreign body? Two schools: At once. Our treatment algorithm: As long as the retina is attached, we wait. And the retina is usually attached after a penetration with a foreign body. Usually we extract the foreign body after 1 month. Advantages: The eye is quiet, the posterior hyaloid is usually detached, and the impact site is usually very quiet resulting in a lower risk of PVR from the wound edges. An air tamponade is

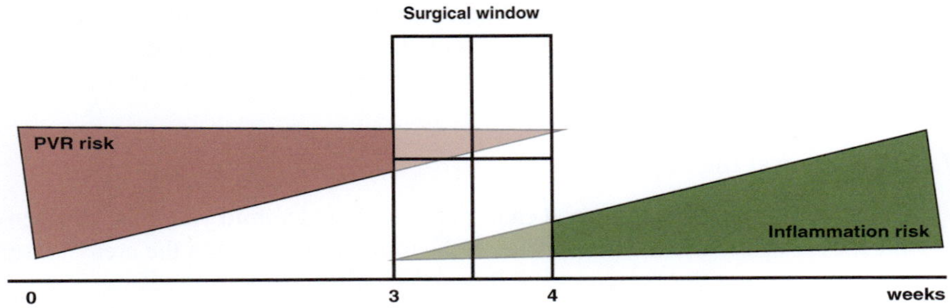

Fig. 24.14 The timing of vitrectomy for penetrating injuries with IOFB is important. Do not operate too early and do not wait too long. A surgical window between 3 and 4 weeks is an optimal time point for IOFB extraction

sufficient. What happens if you wait longer than 4 weeks for surgery? The IOFB causes a sterile inflammation which increases the risk for a PVR detachment.

24.5.3 A retrospective study from the University of Uppsala, Sweden, in the time period from 2008 to 2016 showed:

Number of penetrating injuries with IOFB: 21

Type of IOFB: 2 wooden IOFB, 19 metal IOFB.

Localization: Central and peripheral

Our treatment algorithm is as follows: Acute: Suturing of the corneal and scleral injury. Then 1 week iv antibiotics. Then weekly follow-ups. There is view to the retina under the complete follow-up. After 2 weeks: Phaco + IOL, after 4 weeks ppV + removal of foreign body.

Endophthalmitis: Two patients with wooden IOFB and two patients with metal IOFB. The patients with wooden IOFB came directly after injury to the hospital and an endophthalmitis was present. In case of metal IOFB, the endophthalmitis was present after 3 days. All other patients had no endophthalmitis.

Retinal detachment: One patient with endophthalmitis developed a retinal detachment after vitrectomy. The eyes of the two patients with wooden foreign body were enucleated. All other 18 patients had no retinal detachment.

PVR: The PVR arises from the perforation site. The retinal swelling at the perforation site disappears within 4 weeks and then you can operate with minimal PVR risk. In addition, after 4 weeks a PVD is present, which is an advantage in case of young patients.

Surgical technique: The first patient was operated immediately according to Ferenc Kuhns technique with retinochoroidectomy. Three weeks later the eye developed a PVR reaction at the perforation site. All other patients were operated after 4 weeks with delayed vitrectomy. There were no postoperative complications such as PVR. Only one patient developed a postoperative retinal detachment which could be reattached with a second vitrectomy.

Surgical Pearls No. 119

Anterior chamber hemorrhage. A fresh ACH is not easy to remove, because the fibrin is difficult to aspirate. Inject rtPA at the beginning, wait a few minutes, and then the blood can be removed easier.

Surgical Pearls No. 120

Timing of surgery (Fig. 24.14). An endophthalmitis risk is high in the first week. The patient should receive oral and local antibiotics. Then perform a weekly follow-up. If the retina detaches then operate at once. If the retina remains attached, which is the regular course of this pathology, then plan surgery after 3–4 weeks. Now the PVR risk from the perforation site is minimal. It is not recommended to wait longer because the metal IOFB causes a focal sterile inflammation with engagement of the retina.

24.5.4 Case Report

A 5-year-old boy presented in OPD with visual acuity decrease and a total retinal detachment was diagnosed. A combined phaco/vitrectomy with inferior segmental buckle was performed. A metallic intraocular foreign body was detected and extracted (Fig. 24.15). Two weeks later a recurrent detachment was observed. A membrane peeling and an additional radial buckle was performed. The silicone oil was removed 2 months later, and the final follow-up, 4 months later, showed a completely attached retina with a visual function of 0.3.

Remark: The father reported that 2 months earlier he and his son worked in the garage and something hit his son's eye but after 1 day he complained of no pain.

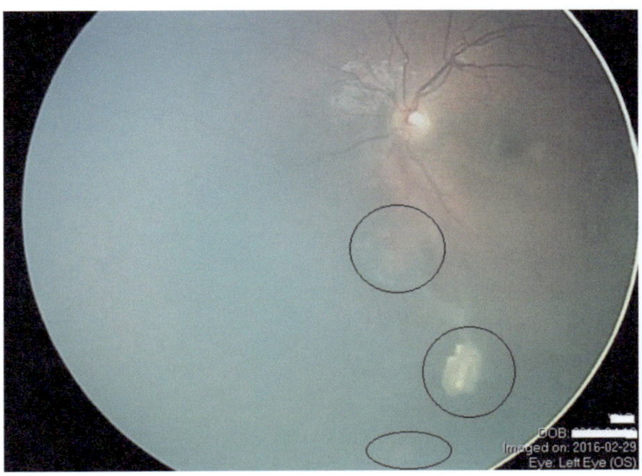

Fig. 24.15 Note the IOFB at the inferior pole. The other round markings indicate a retinal tear caused by the IOFB

Chapter 25
FAQ

Gas tamponade in aphakia: how do you keep it out of the AC? Face Down posture? Any other recommendations?

You cannot prevent gas in the AC. I have no other suggestions.

Phakic patient with sutured 20G pars plana infusion (inferotemporal quadrant) that is blocked with ciliary epithelium: how do you clear the tissue covering the tip? Would you use the cutter or the MVR blade entering from the same side sclerotomy, i.e., the superotemporal one, in order to avoid the lens?

I use the spatula from the other side. If you work in a phakic eye it is difficult. Question: Why is the trocar covered by epithelium? Choroidal detachment? Did the infusion trocar go out under the operation and you got a choroidal detachment? If the latter is the case, I recommend following trick: Remove the infusion trocar, replace the infusion to an instrument trocar, increase the infusion, take a trauma trocar from Alcon (23G, 6 mm long) and use this as a new infusion trocar, and set the infusion back. You will have no problems with the epithelium.

During removal of the last trocar in a gas filled eye, the eye becomes extremely decompressed and soft. A sutured is placed to the sclerotomy and the eye is filled again with gas through a 30G needle. Any useful tips?

You will not have this problem with 25G. You have this problem with 23G. And the reason is the bigger sclerotomy. It is therefore important to insert the trocar in a 15° angle before operation. After operation compress the sclerotomy with an anatomic forceps or scleral depressor, if it leaks make a suture. Remove first both instrument trocars. If the eye is soft, add more gas and remove as last maneuver the infusion trocar, but remove first the infusion and then the trocar.

If the eye is still soft, your idea with the postoperative injection is perfect.

Could the 23G cutter be used during fluid-air exchange to aspirate the SRF (active aspiration mode) instead of a 23G backflush cannula (passive aspiration)?

Yes of course. Even better (easier to maneuver) is a flute needle with active aspiration.

U. Spandau, H. Heimann, *Practical Handbook for Small-Gauge Vitrectomy*,
https://doi.org/10.1007/978-3-319-89677-9_25

When injecting PFCL, do you reduce the infusion pressure or not?

No. I work bimanual. One hand injects PFCL and the other hand aspirates BSS with the flute needle. This works only, if you use a chandelier light. If you do not have/use a chandelier light, I recommend a double-barreled infusion cannula (see material section in my book).

Any tips on avoiding slippage during PFCL × silicone oil exchange?

The danger of slippage from PFO to silicone oil is low. The danger of slippage is high from PFO to air to gas and especially if it is a giant tear. Look in the book: Retinectomy. The main point is to aspirate the PFCL until it is just posterior to the edge of the giant tear (posterior edge of the tear). Now aspirate thoroughly the residual subretinal fluid from the tear. Only when the tear is completely dry you can continue with aspiration of PFCL.

In addition, strict head posture for 3–5 days.

How would you deal with a retinal incarceration?

This is difficult. Best is to avoid it in the first place when you suture a trauma case. The only solution is retinectomy. In detail: Oraparallel diathermy posterior to the incarceration. Retinectomy along the diathermised retina. I would then cut/remove the retina from the anterior part of the incarcerated retina. Then PFCL, then laser, and then PFCL against silicone oil exchange.

In the case of a very dense vitreous hemorrhage <u>in a phakic eye</u>, when infusion cannot be visualized and thus opened, would you start the vitrectomy using an AC maintainer? Will the BSS in the AC keep sufficient tone of globe?

You can do a short vitrectomy. BSS flows through the zonules to the posterior segment but only slowly. Therefore, no, you cannot do a long vitrectomy. An alternative is to check the tension of the globe constantly with your index finger and wait if the globe is soft.

If you are sure that the retina is attached (ultrasound), then I would definitely set the infusion in the pars plana. I would double check the infusion trocar with a light pipe or even use the long trauma trocar from Alcon.

Remark: In my personal experience the location of the trocars (in vitreous cavity or subepithelial) is difficult in eyes with choroidal detachment (hypotensive eyes, trauma eyes). I always check if the trocar is located in the vitreous cavity, but this was never necessary except of eyes with choroidals. And in these eyes, I use now only these long trauma trocars from Alcon.

So coming to your question: If the eye has choroidals, I would insert an anterior chamber maintainer, and if the eye has no choroidals, I would insert a pars plana infusion.

What do you do in case of subretinal PFCL?

<u>Remark:</u> The most common reason that PFCL gets under the retina is continuing traction with open standing rupture.

<u>Solution 1:</u> Aspirate PFCL with 41G cannula (Figs. 25.1 and 25.2). Attach a 41G cannula (DORC, Synergetics) on active aspiration, insert the cannula transretinally into the PFCL bubble, and aspirate it. The retinal hole requires no laser.

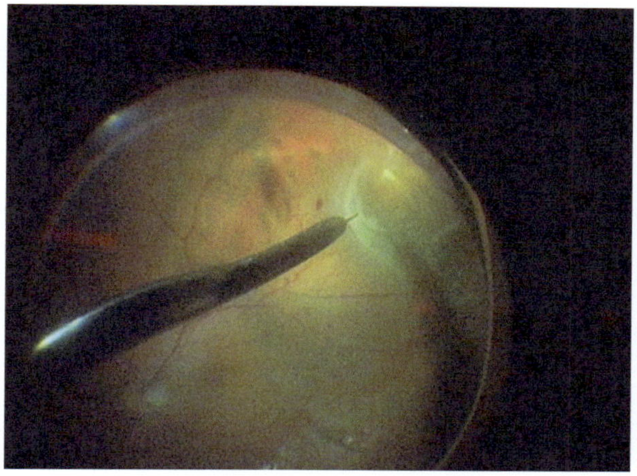

Fig. 25.1 The cannula is inserted into the vitreous cavity and is located just above the subretinal PFCL bubble

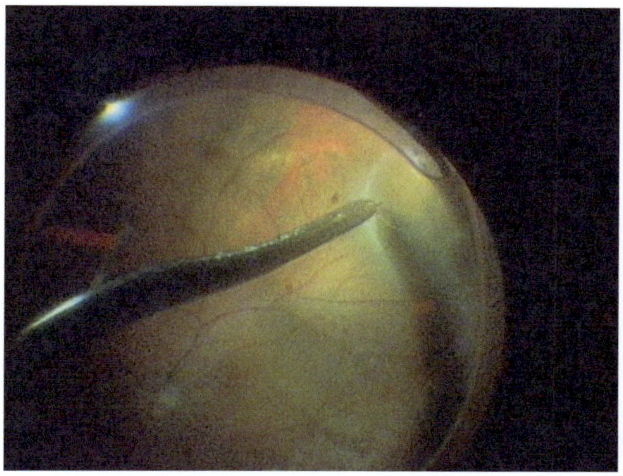

Fig. 25.2 The cannula is placed transretinal into the PFCL bubble and the PFCL aspirated

Solution 2: Make a tiny hole with a CRVO knife or an intravitreal scissors. Then aspirate the subretinal PFCL with the backflush instrument and laser treat the tear afterwards.

How do you deal with subretinal silicone oil (behind a retinal tear)?

Inject BSS between the big silicone oil bubble in the vitreous cavity and the small silicone oil bubble under the retina. The BSS will separate the big bubble from the small bubble. Then squeeze the small oil bubble out through the retinal tear with the spatula. If the silicone oil bubble is not located under the tear, then move it there with the knob spatula.

Is there a prophylactic treatment of PCO?

If you perform a combined phaco/PPV, you may intraoperatively cut a hole in the posterior capsule (Figs. 25.3–25.5). Cut a round hole in the center of the posterior

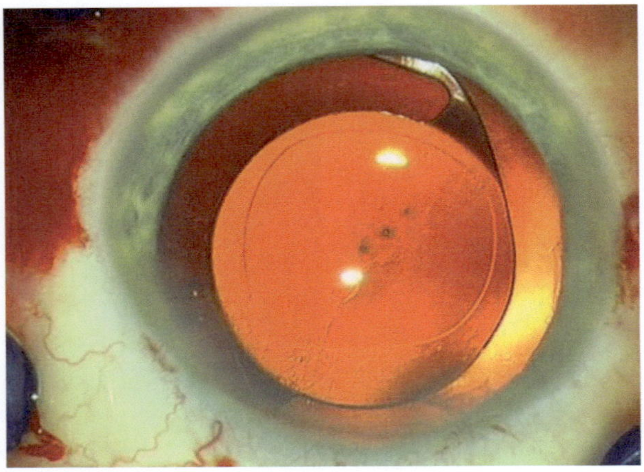

Fig. 25.3 A combined phaco + PPV due to a macular hole

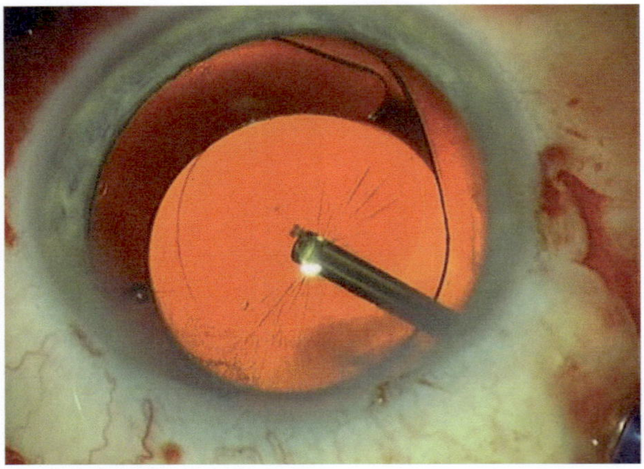

Fig. 25.4 The posterior capsule is aspirated by the vitreous cutter

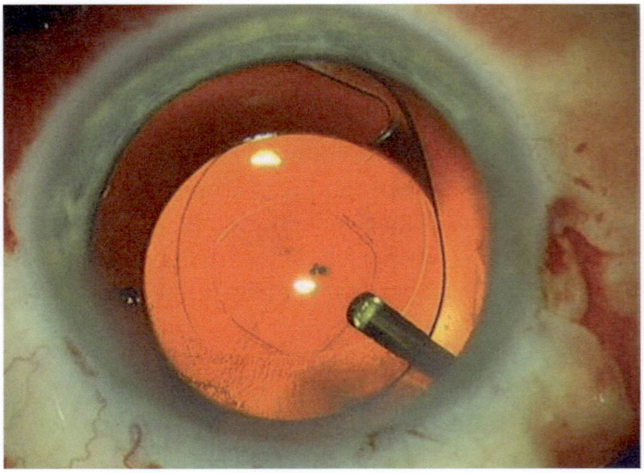

Fig. 25.5 A round hole is cut in the posterior capsule

capsule with the vitreous cutter (cut: 400/min). The IOL will not luxate and the posterior opening because circular will not tear.

Iris capture after combined phaco/PPV.

Attach a 27G cannula (gray cannula) onto a 2 mL syringe. Place patient behind the slit lamp. Drop topical anesthesia + povidone iodine. Perform a paracentesis and press the optic with the cannula behind the iris.

Retinal fold after PPV for retinal detachment. Postoperative slippage of the retina may occur in PPVs for retinal detachment secondary to a giant tear (Figs. 25.6–25.8 and Video 20.2).

Induce a retinal detachment with a 41G active injection cannula (DORC). Perform a fluid-air exchange in order to increase the detachment at the posterior pole. Inject PFCL and massage the retina with a knob spatula or Tano diamond dusted membrane scraper. Perform a gas or silicone oil tamponade.

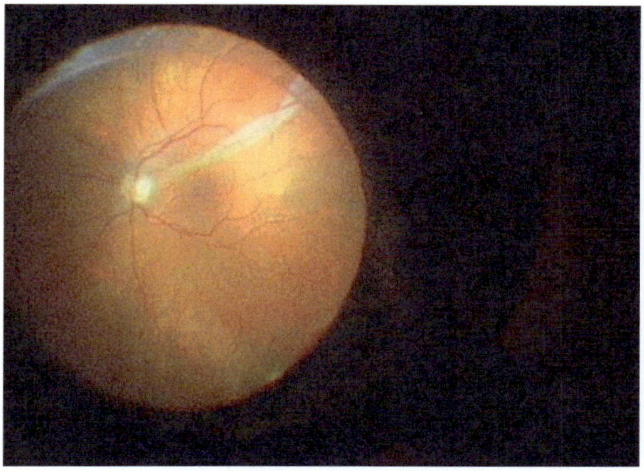

Fig. 25.6 Retinal fold after vitrectomy for a retinal detachment secondary to a giant tear

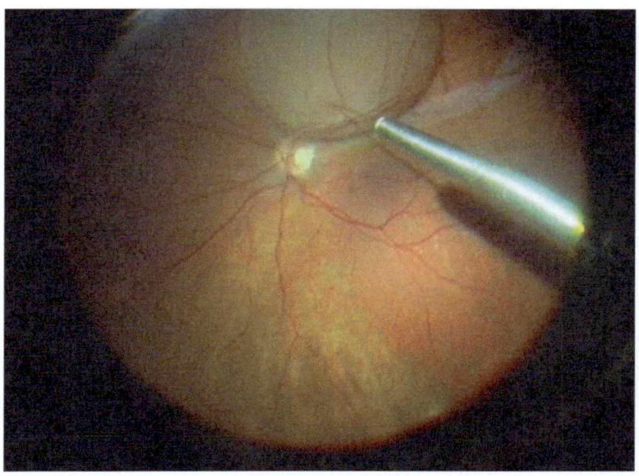

Fig. 25.7 Injection of subretinal fluid with a 41G active injection cannula (DORC) to induce an artificial retinal detachment

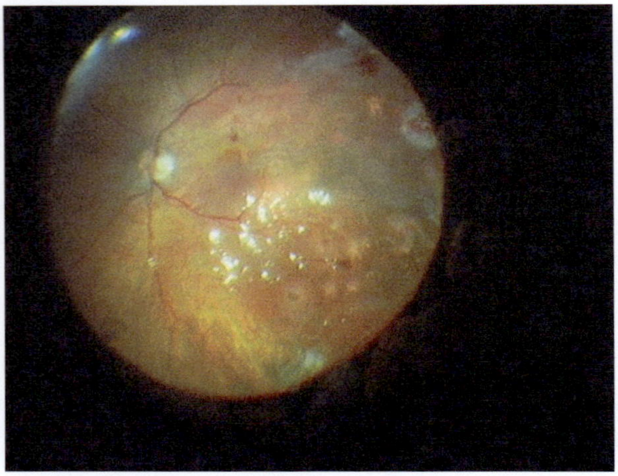

Fig. 25.8 Fundus picture at the end of the operation. No visible retinal fold at the posterior pole

Dear Ulrich,
Modern retina surgery is=
A: Anti-VEGF
B: Biom
C: Chandelier light
D: Dye (Dual!)
E: Eckardt-23G-trocars
F: Fantastic: Your-book!
Greetings
Yaser (from Abu Dhabi)

I would like to ask the following question regarding your technique for peeling in PVR detachment cases: Following vitrectomy, you perform a fluid x air exchange: do you drain the SRF through the retinal break and try to make the retina completely flat? Then, under air, you inject Trypan Blue on the PVR area; then you perform an air x fluid exchange; then you peel the PVR. Is the sequence correct?

The procedure for PVR is:

1. Vitrectomy.
2. Staining. In order to perform a good peeling, we like to stain the membranes. Because the membranes are spread all over the retina, the usual method does not work well. We therefore make a fluid × air exchange and then drop the dye on the PVR areas (Fig. 25.9). The dye is very concentrated on these areas and you always get a good staining of the membranes. Wait 30 s and then aspirate the excessive dye at the posterior pole and then return to fluid filled eye. And then perform the peeling. There are different “ideologies” between peeling and retinectomy. But, in any case, you have to remove the membranes posterior to the retinectomized retina.
3. Peeling. Start in the center and continue to the periphery.

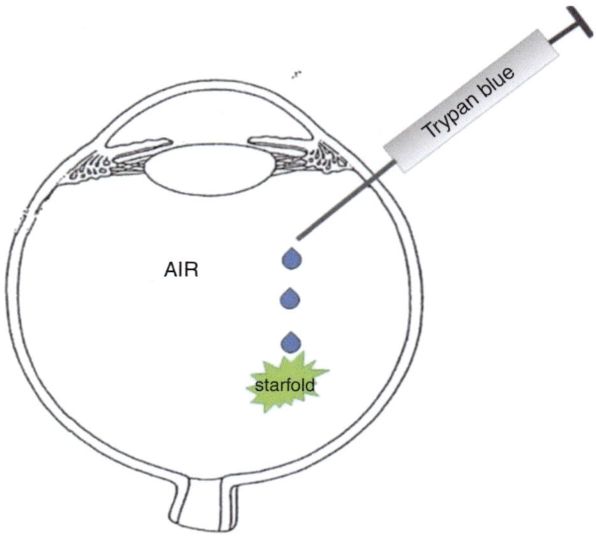

Fig. 25.9 The vitreous cavity is filled with air. Then the dye is dropped on peripheral located membranes. This method increases the concentration of the dye

No, the retina does not become more bullous. This is only a temporary effect from air × fluid to fluid x air exchange because you press the subretinal fluid to the posterior pole under air.

Appendices

Materials (in Alphabetical Order)

41G aspiration and injection cannula. DORC: Disposable Dual bore BSS injection needle (41G). 1270.01

42G injection cannula. Synergetics REF: 12.03

Brilliant Peel®: (Brilliant Blue G) Geuder, Heidelberg

BSS Plus®: Alcon

C_2F_6: many providers, for example Alcon

C_3F_8: many providers, for example Alcon

Caliper of CASTROVIEJO Geuder No: 19135

Cannula, silicone oil 23-Gauge: Med One: 3241st PolyTip Cannula 23-Gauge 10 mm (Sanisoglu) or DORC: 1272.VFI06. 23-Gauge 7 mm

Cannula, Silicone oil 16-Gauge: "High viscosity injector cannula (Peyman)". Ref- No. 585002. Beaver-Visitec International Ltd. Bidford on Avon, UK

Cannula, 23G for injection of dye: DORC 1281.A5D06

Cannula, 25G for injection of dye: MedOne. Ref. 3225 or DORC 1272.SD25

Cannula, double-barrel injection Dual bore 23-Gauge cannula for injection of PFCL. DORC: EFD.06

Capsular tension ring: DORC, Corneal

Celoftal® (for cornea): Alcon

Chandelier light in trocar: ALCON: Chandelier Accurus 8065751574 or Chandelier Constellation 8065751577; DORC: 23-gauge Chandelier light 3269. EB06 and Synergetics 25G Awh Chandelier. 56.51.23P or 56.51.25P

Chandelier light in sclera: 27-gauge twinlight from Eckhardt 3269.MBD27; Synergetics: 25-Gauge Awh Chandelier 56.20.25

Contact Lens, Plano: DORC: Disposable vitrectomy lens: Flat. 1284.DD

Densiron 68®: Fluoron

U. Spandau, H. Heimann, *Practical Handbook for Small-Gauge Vitrectomy*,
https://doi.org/10.1007/978-3-319-89677-9

Foreign body forceps: (1) 17G Microforceps: Avci Foreign Body. DORC. 2286.H; (2) 20G intravitreal foreign body forceps: Geuder 36264; (3) 19G Foreign body forceps. Synergetics REF 11.20PIN (Single use instrument)

Fragmatome: Alcon (Accurus Fragmentation Handpiece), DORC

ILM-Blue®: (Brilliant Blue G) DORC

Knives:

2.4 mm wide main incision knife. Indication: Main incision. Slit knife. Alcon. 8065992445

Crescent bevel up knife. Indication: Preparation of a frown-incision. Crescent angled bevel up. Alcon. 8065990002

V-lance. Knife for 1.3 mm wide scleral and corneal incisions. Indication: Paracentesis and 20G sclerotomy. 20G V-lance. Alcon. 8065912001

15° knife: Indication: paracentesis. Alcon. 8065921501

Membrane Blue®: (Trypan blue) DORC

Membrane BlueDual®: (Trypan blue + Brilliant Blue G) DORC

Monoblue®: (Trypan blue) Arcadophta, Toulouse, France

Ocucoat® (for cornea): Bausch&Lomb

Oxane Hd®: Bausch & Lomb

Silicone oil 1000csts: Fluoron. G-80 710, DORC or Bausch & Lomb

Silicone oil 5000csts: Fluoron. G-80 810

SF_6: many providers, for example Alcon

Suture for sclerafixated IOL: Alcon. Polypropylene, blue monofilament, double armed. 8065307601

Triamcinolone acetonide (Volon A®): Pfizer

Trocar forceps for the removal of trocars. DORC. 1278

Valved Trocar System by Alcon: 23G, 8065751657

Valved Trocar System by Alcon for trauma: 23 G trocar 6 mm 3-pack: 8065751445

Valved Trocar System by DORC: 23G, 1272.ED206

Valved Trocar System by Geuder: 23G, G 33 445

Valved Trocar System by Oertli: 23G, Autoseal PMS®

Company Addresses (in Alphabetical Order)

Alcon

Alcon Laboratories (U.K.) Ltd.
Pentagon Park
Boundary Way
Hemel Hempstead
Herts HP2 7UD, England
Phone: 44+1442.341.234
www.alcon.com

Arcadophta
293, route de Seysses
F-31100 Toulouse
Phone: 0033/561/405235
Fax: 0033/5617 408 466
info@arcadophta.com
www.arcadophta.com

Bausch & Lomb
United Kingdom
Europe, Middle East & Africa Division European Headquarters
Bausch & Lomb House
106-114 London Road
Kingston-Upon-Thames
Surrey KT2 6QJ, England
Phone: 44-20-8781-5500
Fax: 44-20-8781-2989
www.bausch.com

DORC
Dutch Ophthalmic Research
Center International BV
Scheijdelveweg 2
3214 VN Zuidland
The Netherlands
Phone: +31 181 458080
Fax: +31 181 458090
www.dorc.nl

Eye Technology Ltd.
19 Totman Crescent
Brook Road Industrial Estate
Rayleigh
Essex SS6 7UY
United Kingdom
sales@eye-tech.co.uk

Fluoron GmbH
Magirus-Deutz-Strasse 10
89077 Ulm
Phone: 0731/20,559,970
Fax: 0731/205 599 728
info@fluoron.de
www.fluoron.de

Geuder AG
Hertzstr. 4

69126 Heidelberg
Phone: 06221/3066
Fax: 06221/303 122
info@geuder.de
www.geuder.de

IRIDEX Corporation
1212 Terra Bella Avenue
Mountain View, CA 94043, USA
www.iridex.com

MedOne Surgical Inc.
Sarasota, FL USA 34 243
www.MedOne.com

Oculus, Inc. GmbH
Münchholzhäuser 29 st
D-35582 Wetzlar
Phone: 0641/20 050
Fax: 0641/2005255
sales@oculus.de
www.oculus.de

Oertli Instrumente AG
Hafnerwisenstr. 4
CH-9442 Berneck
Tel: 0041/71/74742 2000
Fax 0041/71/74742 90
E-mail: info@oertli-instruments.com
www.oertli-instruments.com

Ophtec BV
Schweitzerlaan 15
9728 NR Groningen
The Netherlands
www.ophtec.com

Synergetics France GmbH
Synergetics France SARL
6 Place de la Madeleine
75008 Paris
France
Phone: 825 825 250
Fax: 1 64 11 16 99
E-mail: plecharpentier@synergeticsusa.com
www.synergeticsusa.com

List of Important Surgical Pearls (S & P)

S & P 43: Sclerotomy
S & P 44: Leaking sclerotomies
S & P 45: Choroidal injury from the infusion fluid
S & P 46: SCH (suprachoroidal hemorrhage)
S & P 47: Removal time
S & P 48: Postoperative hypotony
S & P 49: Removing Densiron 68®
S & P 50: Passive removal of light silicone oil
S & P 51: Residual oil bubbles
S & P 52: Posterior capsulotomy with the vitreous cutter
S & P 53: "Sticky silicone oil"
S & P 54: Silicone IOL
S & P 55: PVD
S & P 56: Membrane & dye
S & P 57: Peeling of ERM and ILM
S & P 58: PVD
S & P 59: Staining in air filled eye
S & P 60: ILM peeling and dot-hemorrhages
S & P 61: Peeling with chandelier light
S & P 62: Backflush instrument
S & P 63: Tamponade for macular hole
S & P 64: Difficult IOLin-the-bag extraction from posterior pole
S & P 65: Chandelier light
S & P 66: Complicated cataract surgery
S & P 67: Dropped nucleus
S & P 68: Residual nuclear fragment
S & P 69: 1-piece IOL vs 3-piece IOL
S & P 70: Retinal tear under a muscle
S & P 71: Phaco or no phaco
S & P 72: Corneal suture
S & P 73: Corneal lubrication
S & P 74: PVD in RRD
S & P 75: Triamcinolone and RRD
S & P 76: Unseen breaks and Schlieren phenomenon
S & P 77: PFCL
S & P 78: Iatrogenic break
S & P 79: Laser
S & P 80: Lasercerclage
S & P 81: Laser necrosis
S & P 82: Trimming of vitreous base
S & P 83: Air test for detachment
S & P 84: Active aspiration
S & P 85: Removal of PFCL
S & P 86: 27G and air tamponade
S & P 87: Gas vs silicone oil

S & P 88: Management of miotic pupil
S & P 89: Laser cerclage ≠ encircling band
S & P 90: Cryopexy versus laser photocoagulation
S & P 91: Shake gas syringe
S & P 92: Silicone oil overfill
S & P 93: Too tight encircling band
S & P 94: Laser photocoagulation for retinotomy
S & P 95: Bilateral PDR
S & P 96: B-scan
S & P 97: Blocked infusion
S & P 98: Removal of anterior hyaloid
S & P 99: How should epiretinal blood be removed
S & P 100: Small pupil
S & P 101: BSS damages the phakic lens
S & P 102: Corneal lubrication
S & P 103: Peeling and choroidal hemorrhage
S & P 104: Intraoperative hemorrhage and adrenaline
S & P 105: Postoperative vitreous hemorrhages
S & P 106: Lens sparing vitrectomy
S & P 107: Bad view to fundus
S & P 108: pars plana infusion
S & P 109: Tumour biopsy with vitreous cutter
S & P 110: Tumour biopsy with vitreous cutter
S & P 111: Tumour biopsy with vitreous cutter
S & P 112: Transscleral tumour biopsy
S & P 113: Transscleral tumour biopsy
S & P 114: Transscleral tumour biopsy
S & P 115: Hypotony
S & P 116: SCH too small sclerotomies
S & P 117: Subepithelial location of trocars
S & P 118: Inflamed or vascularly active eye
S & P 119: Anterior chamber hemorrhage
S & P 120: Timing of surgery

Index

U. Spandau, H. Heimann, *Practical Handbook for Small-Gauge Vitrectomy*,
https://doi.org/10.1007/978-3-319-89677-9

R

S

MIX
Papier aus verantwortungsvollen Quellen
Paper from responsible sources
FSC® C105338

If you have any concerns about our products,
you can contact us on
ProductSafety@springernature.com

In case Publisher is established outside the EU,
the EU authorized representative is:
Springer Nature Customer Service Center GmbH
Europaplatz 3, 69115 Heidelberg, Germany

Printed by Libri Plureos GmbH
in Hamburg, Germany